Caring for the Hospitalized Child

A Handbook of Inpatient Pediatrics

Author
American Academy of Pediatrics
Section on Hospital Medicine

Editors
Daniel A. Rauch, MD, FAAP
Jeffrey C. Gershel, MD, FAAP

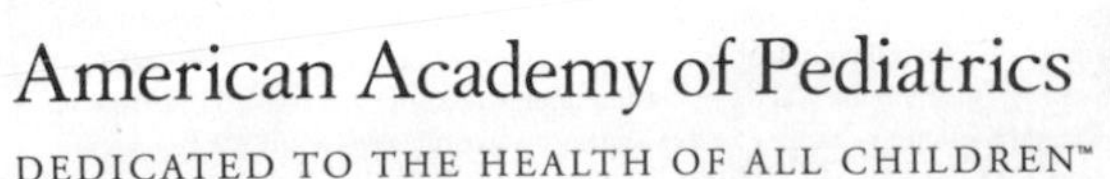

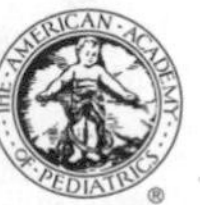

American Academy of Pediatrics Department of Marketing and Publications Staff

Library of Congress Control Number: 2012941475
ISBN: 978-1-58110-754-8
MA0652

The recommendations in this publication do not indicate an exclusive course of treatment or serve as a standard of medical care. Variations, taking into account individual circumstances, may be appropriate. The mention of product names in this publication is for informational purposes only and does not imply endorsement by the American Academy of Pediatrics.

Every effort has been made to ensure that the drug selection an dosage set forth in this text are in accordance with the current recommendations and practice at the time of publication. It is the responsibility of the health care provider to check the package insert of each drug for any change in indications and dosage and for added warnings and precautions.

9-332/1212 2 3 4 5 6 7 8 9 10

Reviewers/Contributors

Editors

Daniel A. Rauch, MD, FAAP, FHM
Associate Professor of Pediatrics
Mount Sinai School of Medicine
Associate Director of Pediatrics
Elmhurst Hospital Center
Elmhurst, NY

Jeffrey C. Gershel, MD, FAAP
Vice Chairman, Department of Pediatrics
Jacobi Medical Center
Professor of Clinical Pediatrics
Albert Einstein College of Medicine
Bronx, NY

American Academy of Pediatrics Board of Directors Reviewer

Michael V. Severson, MD, FAAP

American Academy of Pediatrics

Errol R. Alden, MD, FAAP
Executive Director/CEO

Roger F. Suchyta, MD, FAAP
Associate Executive Director

Maureen DeRosa, MPA
Director, Department of Marketing and Publications

Mark Grimes
Director, Division of Product Development

Jeff Mahony
Manager, Digital Strategy and Product Development

S. Niccole Alexander, MPP
Manager, Section on Hospital Medicine

AAP Reviewers

Committee on Adolescence

Committee on Coding and Nomenclature

Committee on Drugs

Committee on Hospital Care

Committee on Infectious Diseases

Committee on Medical Liability and Risk Management

Council on Children With Disabilities

Council on Communications and Media

Council on Injury, Violence, and Poison Prevention

Disaster Preparedness Advisory Council

National Center for Medical Home Implementation

Section on Adolescent Health

Section on Allergy & Immunology

Section on Anesthesiology & Pain Medicine

Section on Bioethics

Section on Clinical Pharmacology & Therapeutics

Section on Dermatology

Section on Endocrinology

Section on Gastroenterology, Hepatology & Nutrition

Section on Hematology/Oncology

Section on Hospice and Palliative Medicine

Section on Infectious Diseases

Section on Nephrology

Section on Nutrition

Section on Pediatric Pulmonology

Section on Rheumatology

Section on Transport Medicine

Section on Young Physicians

Copy Editor

Kate Larson

Cover Design and Book Design

Peg Mulcahy

Chapter Authors

Jamilet Alegria, MD
Assistant Professor of Clinical Pediatrics
University of California, Irvine, School of Medicine
Pediatric Hospitalist
Division of Hospital Medicine and Division of Neonatology
CHOC Children's – Children's Hospital of Orange County
Pomona Valley Hospital Medical Center
Pomona, CA
Chapter 43: Immunodeficiency

Brian Alverson, MD, FAAP
Associate Professor of Pediatrics
Brown University
Director, Division of Pediatric Hospital Medicine
Hasbro Children's Hospital
Providence, RI
Chapter 64: Urinary Tract Infection

David Amrol, MD, FAAAAI, FACAAI
Associate Professor of Internal Medicine and Adjunct Assistant Professor of Pediatrics
Director, Allergy and Clinical Immunology Division
University of South Carolina School of Medicine
Columbia, SC
Chapter 43: Immunodeficiency

Moises Auron, MD, FAAP, FACP
Assistant Professor of Medicine and Pediatrics
Cleveland Clinic Lerner College of Medicine
Cleveland Clinic Children's Hospital
Cleveland, OH
Chapter 63: Nephrotic Syndrome

Gabriella C. Azzarone, MD, FAAP
Assistant Professor of Pediatrics
Albert Einstein College of Medicine
Pediatric Hospitalist
Children's Hospital at Montefiore
Bronx, NY
Chapter 60: Hemolytic Uremic Syndrome

Ara Balkian, MD, MBA
Chief Medical Director, Inpatient Operations
Associate Chair, Inpatient Pediatrics
Children's Hospital Los Angeles
Assistant Professor of Pediatrics
Keck School of Medicine at the University of Southern California
Los Angeles, CA
Chapter 34: Gastrointestinal Bleeding

Sheldon Berkowitz, MD, FAAP
Medical Director, Minneapolis Children's Clinic
Children's Hospitals and Clinics of Minnesota
Assistant Professor of Pediatrics
University of Minnesota
Minneapolis, MN
Chapter 30: Do Not Resuscitate/Do Not Intubate
Chapter 31: Informed Consent: Permission, Assent, and Confidentiality

Shimona Bhatia, DO, MPH
Pediatric Hospitalist Attending
Children's National Medical Center
Clinical Instructor of Pediatrics
The George Washington University School of Medicine
Washington, DC
Chapter 81: Fractures

Genevieve L. Buser, MD, MSHP
Fellow, Pediatric Infectious Diseases
Children's Hospital of Philadelphia
Philadelphia, PA
Chapter 82: Osteomyelitis
Chapter 83: Septic Arthritis

Douglas W. Carlson, MD, FAAP, SFHM
Professor of Pediatrics
Director, Division of Hospital Medicine
Washington University
St Louis Children's Hospital
St Louis, MO
Chapter 26: Noninvasive Monitoring
Chapter 97: Sedation

Scott Carney, MD, FAAP
Assistant Professor of Pediatrics
University of South Carolina School of Medicine
Assistant Program Director
Palmetto Health Richland Pediatric Residency
Columbia, SC
Chapter 45: Fever of Unknown Origin

Julie Cernanec, MD, FAAP
Associate Staff
Center for Pediatric Hospital Medicine
Children's Hospital, Cleveland Clinic
Cleveland, OH
Chapter 62: Nephrolithiasis

Lindsay Chase, MD, FAAP
Assistant Professor of Pediatrics
Director of Pediatric Hospital Medicine Fellowship
Baylor College of Medicine
Texas Children's Hospital
Houston, TX
Chapter 12: Skin and Soft Tissue Infections
Chapter 17: Neck Masses
Chapter 19: Parotitis
Chapter 20: Peritonsillar Abscess
Chapter 21: Retropharyngeal Abscess

Vincent W. Chiang, MD, FAAP, FHM
Associate Professor of Pediatrics
Harvard Medical School
Chief, Inpatient Services, Department of Medicine
Boston Children's Hospital
Boston, MA
Chapter 71: Seizures

Daniel T. Coghlin, MD, FAAP
Assistant Professor of Pediatrics
The Warren Alpert Medical School of Brown University
Pediatric Hospitalist
Hasbro Children's Hospital
Providence, RI
Chapter 64: Urinary Tract Infection

Eyal Cohen MD, MSc, FRCP(C)
Associate Professor of Pediatrics and Health Policy, Management & Evaluation
University of Toronto
The Hospital for Sick Children
Toronto, ON, Canada
Chapter 73: Feeding Tubes and Enteral Nutrition

Laurie S. Conklin, MD
Assistant Professor of Pediatrics
George Washington University School of Medicine
Pediatric Gastroenterologist
Children's National Medical Center
Washington, DC
Chapter 35: Inflammatory Bowel Disease

Edward E. Conway Jr, MD, MS, FAAP, FCCM, FCCP, FHM
Chairman, Milton and Bernice Stern Department of Pediatrics
Professor of Clinical Pediatrics at the Albert Einstein College of Medicine
Chief Pediatric Critical Care Medicine
Beth Israel Medical Center
New York, NY
Chapter 68: Altered Mental Status

Matthew A. Cunningham, MD
Fellow in Vitreoretinal Surgery and Diseases
University of Iowa Hospitals and Clinics
Iowa City, IA
Chapter 77: Acute Vision Loss in the Hospitalized Child

Shani Cunningham, DO
Iowa City, IA
Chapter 73: Feeding Tubes and Enteral Nutrition
Chapter 75: Obesity
Chapter 76: Parenteral Nutrition

Sharon Dabrow, MD
Professor of Pediatrics
Director, Residency Program
Department of Pediatrics
University of South Florida
Tampa, FL
Chapter 49: Acute Liver Failure
Chapter 99: Pyloric Stenosis

Jennifer Daru, MD, FAAP
Assistant Clinical
Professor of Pediatrics
University of California San Francisco
Chief, Division of Pediatric Hospital Medicine
California Pacific Medical Center
San Francisco, CA
Chapter 54: Leading a Team

Paola Dees, MD
Pediatric Hospitalist
All Children's Hospital Johns Hopkins Medicine
St Petersburg, FL
Chapter 99: Pyloric Stenosis

Carla N. DeJohn, MD, FAAP
Assistant Professor of Pediatrics
Baylor College of Medicine
Texas Children's Hospital
Houston, TX
Chapter 52: Family-Centered Rounds
Chapter 86: Child Abuse: Physical Abuse and Neglect
Chapter 87: Sexual Abuse

Kelly DeScioli, MD
Houston, TX
Chapter 13: Acute Bacterial Sinusitis

Marcella M. Donaruma-Kwoh, MD, FAAP
Assistant Professor, Pediatrics
Baylor College of Medicine
Texas Children's Hospital
Houston, TX
Chapter 86: Child Abuse: Physical Abuse and Neglect
Chapter 87: Sexual Abuse

Lindsey C. Douglas, MD, FAAP
Attending Physician, Pediatric Hospital Medicine
Assistant Professor of Pediatrics
The Children's Hospital at Montefiore
The Pediatric Hospital for Albert Einstein College of Medicine
Bronx, NY
Chapter 6: Endocarditis

Nora Esteban-Cruciani, MD, MS, FAAP
Associate Professor of Clinical Pediatrics
Albert Einstein College of Medicine
Assistant Director, Pediatric Hospital Medicine
Children's Hospital at Montefiore
Bronx, NY
Chapter 74: Fluids and Electrolytes

Bryan R. Fine, MD, MPH, FAAP, FHM
Associate Professor of Clinical Pediatrics
Adjunct Assistant Professor in Public Health
Eastern Virginia Medical School
Director, Division of Pediatric Hospital Medicine
Children's Hospital of The King's Daughters
Norfolk, VA
Chapter 51: The Economics of Pediatric Hospitalist Medicine
Chapter 56: Pediatric Hospitalists in Transport
Chapter 73: Feeding Tubes and Enteral Nutrition

Brock C. Fisher, MD
Pediatric Critical Care and Pediatric Anesthesia
Anesthesia Services Medical Group
Divisions of Pediatric Critical Care and Anesthesia
Rady Children's Hospital San Diego
Associate Clinical Professor, Department of Anesthesia
University of California San Diego
San Diego, CA
Chapter 95: Ventilation and Intubation

Erin Stucky Fisher, MD, FAAP, MHM
Professor of Clinical Pediatrics and Vice Chair for Clinical Affairs
Associate Pediatric Residency Program Director
Pediatric Hospital Medicine Fellowship Director
Department of Pediatrics
University of California San Diego,
Medical Director for Quality Improvement
Rady Children's Hospital San Diego
San Diego, CA
Chapter 55: Patient Safety
Chapter 95: Ventilation and Intubation

Jason L. Freedman, MD
Fellow, Pediatric Hematology & Oncology
Children's Hospital of Philadelphia
University of Pennsylvania
Philadelphia, PA
Chapter 40: Acute Complications of Cancer Therapy

Jason A. French, MD, FAAP
Clinical Instructor, Pediatrics
Children's Hospital Colorado
Section of Pediatric Hospital Medicine
Department of Pediatrics
University of Colorado School of Medicine
Denver, CO
Chapter 70: Headache

Blake A. Froberg, MD
Assistant Professor of Pediatrics
Assistant Professor of Emergency Medicine
Associate Director of the Indiana Poison Center
Indiana University School of Medicine
Indianapolis, IN
Chapter 48: Toxic Exposures

Sarah Gaethke, MD, FAAP
Attending Physician
ProHealth Care
Mukega, WI
Chapter 65: Acute Ataxia

Sandra Gage, MD, PhD, FAAP
Assistant Professor of Pediatrics
Section of Hospital Medicine
Medical College of Wisconsin
Milwaukee, WI
Chapter 65: Acute Ataxia
Chapter 67: Acute Weakness

Rachel Gallagher, MD, RDMS
Instructor of Pediatrics
Harvard Medical School
Staff Physician
Division of Emergency Medicine
Boston Children's Hospital
Boston, MA
Chapter 71: Seizures

Matthew Garber, MD, FAAP, FHM
Associate Professor of Pediatrics
University of South Carolina School of Medicine
Director, Pediatric Hospitalists
Children's Hospital, Palmetto Health Richland
Columbia, SC
Chapter 45: Fever of Unknown Origin

Laurie Gordon, MD, MA, FAAP
Assistant Professor of Pediatrics
Weill Cornell Medical School
New York, NY
Director, Pediatric Inpatient Unit
New York Hospital Queens
Site Director, Weill Cornell Pediatric Residency Program
New York Hospital Queens
Flushing, NY
Chapter 11: Rashes Associated With Serious Underlying Disease

Elizabeth Hart, MD, FAAP
Assistant Clinical Professor of Pediatrics
George Washington University Children's National Medical Center
Washington, DC
Chapter 35: Inflammatory Bowel Disease

Daniel Hershey, MD
Assistant Professor
University of California, San Diego
Rady Children's Hospital and Health Center
San Diego, CA
Chapter 98: Acute Abdomen

Vanessa L. Hill, MD, FAAP
Assistant Professor of Pediatrics
UT Health Science Center—San Antonio
Medical Director of Inpatient Services
CHRISTOS Santa Rosa Children's Hospital
San Antonio, TX
Chapter 92: Bronchiolitis

Margaret E. Hood, MD, FAAP
Clinical Professor
Department of Pediatrics
University of Washington
Seattle, WA
Chapter 57: Pediatric Palliative Care

Jonathan T. Johnson, MD
Assistant Professor of Pediatrics
Baylor College of Medicine
Pediatric Hospital Medicine
Texas Children's Hospital
Houston, TX
Chapter 79: Red Eye
Chapter 80: White Eye

Quan Johnson, MD
Hospitalist Division
Children's National Medical Center
Instructor of Pediatrics
George Washington University Medical Center
Washington, DC
Chapter 81: Fractures

Vanitha I. Johnson, MD
Resident–PGY-4
Department of Ophthalmology
Baylor College of Medicine & Cullen Eye Institute
Houston, TX
Chapter 78: Ocular Trauma

Valerie Jurgens, MD
Pediatric Hospital Medicine Fellow
Clinical Instructor of Pediatrics
George Washington University School of Medicine and Health Sciences
Childrens National Medical Center
Washington, DC
Chapter 33: Gastroenteritis

Daran Kaufman, MD
Instructor of Clinical Pediatrics
Jacobi Medical Center
Albert Einstein College of Medicine
Bronx, NY
Chapter 96: Pain Management

Erica C. Kaye, MD
Resident in Pediatrics
Department of Medicine
Boston Children's Hospital
Harvard Medical School
Boston, MA
Chapter 57: Pediatric Palliative Care

Caryn A. Kerman, MD, FAAP
Pediatric Hospitalist
The Children's Hospital of Philadelphia
Philadelphia, PA
Chapter 40: Acute Complications of Cancer Therapy

Jacquelyn C. Kuzminski, MD, FAAP
Associate Professor of Pediatrics
Medical College of Wisconsin
Milwaukee, WI
Chapter 41: Anemia

Kyle Lamphier, MD
Clinical Instructor of Pediatrics
University of Southern California Keck School of Medicine
Children's Hospital of Los Angeles
Los Angeles, CA
Chapter 34: Gastrointestinal Bleeding

Vivian Lee, MD
Assistant Professor of Clinical Pediatrics
University of Southern California Keck School of Medicine
Pediatric Hospitalist
Children's Hospital Los Angeles
Los Angeles, CA
Chapter 59: Acute Glomerulonephritis

Carly Levy, MD, FAAP
Clinical Assistant Professor of Pediatrics
Division of General Pediatrics
Palliative and Supportive Care
Thomas Jefferson University
A.I. duPont Hospital for Children
Wilmington, DE
Chapter 44: Fever in Infants Younger Than 60 Days

Stephanie R. Lichten, MD, FAAP
Associate Program Director
Advocate Children's Hospital
Oak Lawn, IL
Chapter 1: Anaphylaxis
Chapter 14: Cervical Lymphadenopathy
Chapter 16: Mastoiditis
Chapter 18: Orbital Cellulitis

Sheila K. Liewehr, MD, FAAP
Assistant Professor of Pediatrics
Albert Einstein College of Medicine
Pediatric Hospitalist
Children's Hospital at Montefiore
Bronx, NY
Chapter 60: Hemolytic Uremic Syndrome

Julie Lin, MD, FAAP
Pediatrician
Dallas, TX
Chapter 50: Neonatal Hyperbilirubinemia

Michelle A. Lopez, MD
Assistant Professor of Pediatrics
Baylor College of Medicine
Texas Children's Hospital
Houston, TX
Chapter 12: Skin and Soft Tissue Infections

Cara Lye, MD
Assistant Professor of Pediatrics
Baylor College of Medicine
Texas Children's Hospital
Houston, TX
Chapter 19: Parotitis

Sanjay Mahant, MD, MSc, FRCPC
Division of Paediatric Medicine
Hospital for Sick Children
Associate Professor of Paediatrics
Department of Paediatrics
University of Toronto
Toronto, ON, Canada
Chapter 73: Feeding Tubes and Enteral Nutrition

Jennifer Maniscalco, MD, MPH, FAAP
Assistant Professor of Clinical Pediatrics
University of California Keck School of Medicine
Director, Pediatric Hospital Medicine Fellowship
Children's Hospital Los Angeles
Los Angeles, CA
Chapter 59: Acute Glomerulonephritis

Kristie Manning, MD, FAAP
Pediatric Hospitalist
Associate Transport Director
California Pacific Medical Center
San Francisco, CA
Chapter 56: Pediatric Hospitalists in Transport

Michelle Marks, DO, FAAP, FHM
Head, Center of Pediatric Hospital Medicine
Department of General Pediatrics
Cleveland Clinic Children's Hospital
Cleveland, OH
Chapter 94: Complications of Cystic Fibrosis

Joelle Mast, MD, PhD, FAAP
VP, Chief Medical Officer
Blythedale Children's Hospital
Lecturer
School of Health Sciences
New York Medical College
Valhalla, NY
Assistant Clinical Professor Pediatrics
Weill Cornell Medical Center
New York, NY
Chapter 96: Pain Management

Erich C. Maul, DO, FHM, FAAP
Associate Professor of Pediatrics
University of Kentucky College of Medicine
Medical Director, Pediatric Progressive Care
Kentucky Children's Hospital
Lexington, KY
Chapter 2: Arrhythmias
Chapter 5: Electrocardiogram Interpretation

Sonaly Rao McClymont, MD, FAAP
Pediatric Hospitalist Attending
Children's National Medical Center
Clinical Instructor of Pediatrics
The George Washington University School of Medicine
Washington, DC
Chapter 3: Congestive Heart Failure

Jerry McLaughlin, MD
Department of Pediatric Critical Care
Swedish Medical Center
Seattle, WA
Chapter 89: Acute Respiratory Failure

Oliver F. Medzihradsky, MD, MPH, MSc, FACP
Assistant Clinical Professor
Division of Hospital Medicine
University of California San Francisco
San Francisco, CA
Chapter 84: Acute Agitation

Scott Miller, MD, FAAP
Pediatric Hospitalist
Jacobi Medical Center
Instructor of Clinical Pediatrics
Albert Einstein College of Medicine
Bronx, NY
Chapter 46: Kawasaki Disease
Chapter 85: Depression

Brent A. Mothner, MD, FAAP
Assistant Professor of Pediatrics
Baylor College of Medicine
Texas Children's Hospital
Houston, TX
Chapter 37: Pancreatitis

Meaghan E. Mungekar, MD, FAAP
Assistant Attending in Pediatrics
Beth Israel Medical Center
New York, NY
Chapter 68: Altered Mental Status

Anuj Steve Narang, MD, MHCM, FAAP
Chief Medical Officer
Banner Health System
Cardon Children's Medical Center
Phoenix, AZ
Chapter 58: Quality Improvement

Joanne M. Nazif, MD, FAAP
Assistant Professor of Pediatrics
Albert Einstein College of Medicine
Pediatric Hospitalist
Children's Hospital at Montefiore
Bronx, NY
Chapter 7: Myocarditis
Chapter 8: Pericarditis

Jennifer Nead, MD
Fellow, Pediatric Endocrinology
Washington University School of Medicine
St Louis, MO
Chapter 15: Infectious Croup
Chapter 17: Neck Masses
Chapter 19: Parotitis
Chapter 20: Peritonsillar Abscess
Chapter 21: Retropharyngeal Abscess

Roger Nicome, MD, FAAP
Assistant Professor of Pediatrics
Section of Pediatric Hospital Medicine
Texas Children's Hospital
Houston, TX
Chapter 22: Diabetes Insipidus
Chapter 23: Diabetic Ketoacidosis

Katherine M. O'Connor, MD, FAAP
Assistant Professor of Pediatrics
Albert Einstein College of Medicine
Attending Physician
Pediatric Hospital Medicine
The Children's Hospital at Montefiore
Bronx, NY
Chapter 32: Gallbladder Disease

Jennie G. Ono, MD, FAAP
Instructor in Pediatrics
Weill Cornell Medical College
New York Presbyterian Hospital
New York, NY
Chapter 38: Dysfunctional Uterine Bleeding
Chapter 39: Sexually Transmitted Infections

Snezana Nena Osorio, MD, MS, FAAP
Associate Professor of Clinical Pediatrics
Weill Cornell Medical College
Medical Director, General Inpatient Pediatrics
The New York-Presbyterian Hospital
New York, NY
Chapter 38: Dysfunctional Uterine Bleeding
Chapter 39: Sexually Transmitted Infections

Mary C. Ottolini, MD, MPH, FAAP
Vice Chair for Medical Education
Professor of Pediatrics
George Washington University
School of Medicine and Health Sciences
Childrens National Medical Center
Washington, DC
Chapter 33: Gastroenteritis

Philip Overby, MD
Assistant Professor of Neurology and Pediatrics
Albert Einstein College of Medicine
Bronx, NY
Chapter 66: Acute Hemiparesis

Nancy Palumbo, MD, FAAP
Assistant Professor of Pediatrics
Hofstra North-Shore LIJ School of Medicine
Director of Pediatric Hospitalist Program
Associate Pediatric Residency Program Director
Steven and Alexandra Cohen Children's Medical Center of New York
New Hyde Park, NY
Chapter 27: Suprapubic Bladder Aspiration
Chapter 29: Urinary Bladder Catheterization

Rita M. Pappas, MD, FAAP
Staff, Pediatric Hospital Medicine
Children's Hospital, Cleveland Clinic
Assistant Professor of Pediatrics
Cleveland Clinic Lerner College of Medicine of Case Western Reserve University
Cleveland, OH
Chapter 91: Bacterial Tracheitis

Binita Patel, MD, FAAP
Assistant Professor, Pediatrics
Section of Pediatric Emergency Medicine
Baylor College of Medicine
Houston, TX
Chapter 9: Shock

Jack M. Percelay, MD, MPH, FAAP
Pediatric Hospitalist
E.L.M.O. Pediatrics
New York, NY
Chapter 25: Lumbar Puncture

Andrew M. Perry, MD, FAAP
Assistant Professor of Pediatrics
University of Hawaii John A. Burns School of Medicine
Emergency Physician
Kapiolani Medical Center for Women and Children
Honolulu, HI
Chapter 9: Shock

Sarah Phillips, MS, RD, LD
Instructor of Pediatrics
Baylor College of Medicine
Manager of Nutrition Support
Texas Children's Hospital
Houston, TX
Chapter 76: Parenteral Nutrition

Stacy B. Pierson, MD, FAAP
Assistant Professor of Pediatrics
Baylor College of Medicine
Attending Physician, Section of Pediatric Hospital Medicine
Texas Children's Hospital
Houston, TX
Chapter 61: Henoch-Schönlein Purpura

Gregory Plemmons, MD
Associate Professor of Pediatrics
Vanderbilt University School of Medicine
Nashville, TN
Chapter 75: Obesity

Kevin Powell, MD, PhD, FAAP
Associate Professor of Pediatrics
St Louis University
Pediatric Hospitalist
SSM Cardinal Glennon Children's Medical Center
St Louis, MO
Chapter 30: Do Not Resuscitate/Do Not Intubate
Chapter 31: Informed Consent: Permission, Assent, and Confidentiality

Ricardo Quinonez, MD, FAAP, FHM
Associate Professor of Pediatrics
Section of Pediatric Hospital Medicine
Section Director of Research and Quality
Baylor College of Medicine
Texas Children's Hospital
Houston, TX
Chapter 76: Parenteral Nutrition
Chapter 93: Community-Acquired Pneumonia

Shawn L. Ralston, MD, FAAP
Chief, Section of Pediatric Hospital Medicine
Children's Hospital at Dartmouth
Associate Professor of Pediatrics
Geisel School of Medicine at Dartmouth
Hanover, NH
Chapter 92: Bronchiolitis

David I. Rappaport, MD, FAAP
Associate Professor of Pediatrics
Jefferson Medical College
Hospitalist and Associate Residency Program Director
Nemours/AI duPont Hospital for Children
Wilmington, DE
Chapter 44: Fever in Infants Younger Than 60 Days

Hai Jung H. Rhim, MD, MPH, FAAP
Assistant Professor of Pediatrics
Albert Einstein College of Medicine
Pediatric Hospitalist
Children's Hospital at Montefiore
Bronx, NY
Chapter 47: Esophageal Foreign Body

Jay Riva-Cambrin, MD, FRCSC
Assistant Professor of Neurosurgery
University of Utah
Primary Children's Medical Center
Salt Lake City, UT
Chapter 69: Cerebrospinal Fluid Shunt Complications

W. LeGrande Rives, MD
Assistant Professor of Pediatrics
Washington University School of Medicine
St Louis Children's Hospital
St Louis, MO
Chapter 26: Noninvasive Monitoring

Kenneth Rivlin, MD, PhD, FAAP
Chief, Division of Pediatric Hematology/Oncology
Jacobi Medical Center
Clinical Assistant Professor of Pediatrics
Albert Einstein College of Medicine
Bronx, NY
Chapter 42: Sickle Cell Disease

Mary E. M. Rocha, MD, MPH, FAAP
Assistant Professor of Pediatrics
Baylor College of Medicine
Texas Children's Hospital
Houston, TX
Chapter 28: Tracheostomies

Helen Maliagros Scott, MD, FAAP
Assistant Professor of Pediatrics
North Shore–LIJ School of Medicine at Hofstra University
Pediatric Hospitalist
Steven and Alexandra Cohen Children's Medical Center of New York
New Hyde Park, NY
Chapter 24: Intravenous Lines

Mitzi Scotten, MD, FAAP
Associate Professor of Pediatrics
Director, Medical Student Clerkship
Director, Pediatric Cystic Fibrosis Clinic
University of Kansas Medical Center
Kansas City, KS
Chapter 53: Hospitalist Comanagement

Samir S. Shah, MD, MSCE, FAAP
Professor of Pediatrics
University of Cincinnati College of Medicine
Director, Division of Hospital Medicine
Attending Physician in Infectious Diseases and Hospital Medicine
Cincinnati Children's Hospital Medical Center
Cincinnati, OH
Chapter 82: Osteomyelitis
Chapter 83: Septic Arthritis

Anjali Sharma, MD, FAAP
Assistant Professor in Pediatrics
Medical College of Wisconsin
Milwaukee, WI
Chapter 67: Acute Weakness

Alyssa H. Silver, MD, FAAP
Assistant Professor of Pediatrics
Albert Einstein College of Medicine
Pediatric Hospitalist
Children's Hospital at Montefiore
Bronx, NY
Chapter 7: Myocarditis
Chapter 8: Pericarditis

Tamara D. Simon, MD, MSPH, FAAP
Assistant Professor of Pediatrics
University of Washington School of Medicine and Children's Hospital
Center for Clinical and Translational Research
Seattle Children's Research Institute
Seattle, WA
Chapter 69: Cerebrospinal Fluid Shunt Complications

Geeta Singhal, MD, MEd, FAAP
Associate Professor of Pediatrics
Section Head and Service Chief
Pediatric Hospital Medicine Associate Director
BCM Office of Professional Development
Baylor College of Medicine
Texas Children's Hospital
Houston, TX
Chapter 13: Acute Bacterial Sinusitis
Chapter 52: Family-Centered Rounds

Laurie Bernard Stover, MD
Associate Professor of Pediatrics
UC San Diego School of Medicine
Hospitalist
Rady Children's Hospital
San Diego, CA
Chapter 10: Erythema Multiforme and Stevens-Johnson Syndrome

Anu Subramony, MD, MBA, FAAP
Assistant Professor of Pediatrics
Assistant Director, General Pediatrics Inpatient Service
Columbia University School of Physicians & Surgeons
New York Presbyterian Morgan Stanley Children's Hospital
New York, NY
Chapter 40: Acute Complications of Cancer Therapy

Rana Tabassum, MD
Senior Physician
Pinellas County Health Department
St Petersburg, FL
Chapter 49: Acute Liver Failure

E. Douglas Thompson Jr, MD, MMM, FHM, FAAP
Chief, Section of Hospital Medicine
St Christopher's Hospital for Children
Assistant Professor of Pediatrics
Drexel University College of Medicine
Philadelphia, PA
Chapter 42: Sickle Cell Disease

Joel S. Tieder, MD, MPH
Assistant Professor
Department of Pediatrics
Division of Hospital Medicine
University of Washington and Seattle Children's Hospital
Seattle, WA
Chapter 90: Apparent Life-Threatening Events

Jayne S. Truckenbrod, DO
Pediatric Hospital Medicine Fellow
Children's National Medical Center
Clinical Instructor of Pediatrics
The George Washington University School of Medicine
Washington, DC
Chapter 3: Congestive Heart Failure

Joyee G. Vachani, MD, MEd, FAAP
Assistant Professor of Pediatrics
Baylor College of Medicine
Associate Director of Pediatric Hospital Medicine Fellowship
Texas Children's Hospital
Houston, TX
Chapter 72: Failure to Thrive

Wendy Van Ittersum, MD, FAAP
Assistant Professor of Pediatrics, General Pediatrics
Cleveland Clinic Lerner College of Medicine Case Western Reserve University
Cleveland Clinic
Cleveland, OH
Chapter 36: Meckel Diverticulum

Tamara Vesel, MD, FAAHPM
Director, Pediatric Palliative Fellowship
Dana Farber Cancer Institute and Children's Hospital
Instructor in Pediatrics
Harvard Medical School
Boston, MA
Chapter 57: Pediatric Palliative Care

Yakov Volkin, MD, FAAP
Assistant Professor of Pediatrics
Mount Sinai School of Medicine
Attending Physician
Elmhurst Hospital Center
Elmhurst, NY
Chapter 4: Deep Venous Thrombosis

Colleen M. Wallace, MD, FAAP
Assistant Professor of Pediatrics
Washington University School of Medicine
St Louis, MO
Chapter 97: Sedation

Susan C. Walley, MD, FAAP
Assistant Professor of Pediatrics
University of Alabama at Birmingham
Chair, Continuing Medical Education Program
Children's of Alabama
Birmingham, AL
Chapter 88: Acute Asthma Exacerbation

Susan Wu, MD, FAAP
Assistant Professor of Clinical Pediatrics
University of Southern California Keck School of Medicine
Division of Hospital Medicine
Children's Hospital Los Angeles
Los Angeles, CA
Chapter 43: Immunodeficiency

Derek Zhorne, MD
Fellow, Pediatric Hospital Medicine
Baylor College of Medicine
Texas Children's Hospital
Houston, TX
Chapter 20: Peritonsillar Abscess
Chapter 21: Retropharyngeal Abscess

Table of Contents

Ear, Nose, Throat

Endocrinology

Equipment and Procedures

Ethics

Gastroenterology

Gynecology

Hematology

Immunology

Infectious Diseases

Ingestion

Liver Diseases

Miscellaneous Issues

Nephrology

Neurology

Nutrition

Ophthalmology

Orthopaedics

Psychiatry

Psychosocial

Pulmonary

Preface

Care for the hospitalized child has evolved significantly since the term *hospitalist* was first used more than 15 years ago. Most pediatric teaching services use hospitalists for the care of general pediatric inpatients, but the scope of practice often extends to comanagement of subspecialty and surgical patients, as well as coverage in intensive care units and newborn nurseries. Community hospitals are also employing hospitalists to improve the quality and efficiency of care while expediting admissions from ambulatory physicians who are becoming less eager to care for inpatients.

Today's hospitalized children tend to be sicker and more complicated than before. As a result of pressures from payers, previously well patients must now be more seriously ill to justify admission, while complex care and technology-dependent children represent an ever-increasing percentage of inpatients. Furthermore, decreasing hospital days and lengths of stay have become priorities for both hospitals and insurance companies. At the same time, all parties insist on care that is safe, efficient, timely, cost-effective, patient-centered, and equitable. The net result is that providing care for the hospitalized child has become increasingly challenging.

The care of pediatric inpatients is addressed in many available resources, including textbooks, handbooks, and the Internet. However, very few provide concise, specific, point-of-care recommendations about the most common diagnoses encountered, and none have relied solely on hospitalists as contributors. The book was conceived as a resource that was written and edited by experts in the field of pediatric hospital medicine, whose primary focus is the care of hospitalized children. The authors all have hands-on experience with their topics and represent leaders in the field. Their practice settings vary from children's hospitals to private community hospitals to general pediatric services in public hospitals, so that their recommendations can be used in any of these settings. The clinical chapters are meant to be directive in immediate care and specific about when to either escalate care or begin discharge planning.

Written specifically for the hospitalist, this book includes chapters beyond just clinical care to address the "whole" of a hospitalist's work. We have included discussions about activities, such as leadership, economics, consent, and management of the inpatient service, and have incorporated other facets of patient care beyond laboratory tests and treatments. Comprehensive care for hospitalized children must include attention to systems of care, procedures, and ethics, because no sick child exists in a vacuum, and non-bedside activities can have a profound effect on patient outcomes.

No clinical manual, textbook, or online resource can be all-encompassing, and this one is no different. Every child is unique. Although this book gives specific direction for most cases, no one resource can account for every clinical possibility. We all learn very early in our careers that there are many ways to address a given clinical issue. We present the approaches of our contributors while recognizing there are many equally satisfactory alternatives.

Daniel A. Rauch, MD, FAAP
Jeffrey C. Gershel, MD, FAAP

Allergy

Anaphylaxis

Introduction

The term anaphylaxis applies to both anaphylactic (immunoglobulin [Ig] E mediated) and anaphylactoid (non–IgE mediated) reactions resulting in the release of immune mediators from basophils and mast cells. It is a severe, potentially fatal, multi-organ system allergic reaction. Therefore, it is imperative to recognize the signs and symptoms of anaphylaxis and treat it rapidly and appropriately. The most common causes are peanuts, tree nuts, and shellfish, although anaphylaxis in an inpatient may be triggered by latex, radiocontrast material, medications, or foods (Table 1-1).

As many as 20% to 30% of patients will have a biphasic response, with most responses occurring within 1 to 8 hours after the initial reaction has abated. Protracted anaphylaxis (up to 72 hours) is rare and usually occurs when there is continued exposure to the trigger.

Clinical Presentation

History

The patient usually presents with some combination of flushing, pruritus, urticaria and/or angioedema, tightness of the throat, respiratory distress, vomiting and/or diarrhea, and a sense of impending doom (Table 1-2). Ask about possible triggers and previous episodes, as well as treatment given and whether the patient is receiving any chronic medications, especially a β-blocker.

Table 1-1. Agents That Can Trigger Anaphylaxis in Inpatient Setting

Trigger	Examples
Antibiotics	β-lactams (cephalosporins, penicillins), sulfonamides
Foods	Egg whites, fish and shellfish, milk, peanuts, sesame, soy, tree nuts (pecans, pistachios, walnuts)
Hormones	Estrogen, progesterone
Infusions	Blood transfusion, dextran, infliximab, intravenous immunoglobulin, radiocontrast material
Latex	Balloons, gloves
Medications	Aspirin, muscle relaxants, nonsteroidal anti-inflammatories, opioids
Physiological factors	Cold, exercise, heat, pressure, sunlight

Table 1-2. Presentation of Anaphylaxis	
Organ System	**Presentation**
Cardiovascular	Hypotension, syncope, arrhythmias
Central nervous system	Confusion, dizziness, lightheadedness, behavior changes
Gastrointestinal	Nausea, abdominal pain, vomiting, diarrhea
Other	Sense of impending doom, seizures, headache, rhinitis, metallic taste
Respiratory	Cough, stridor, dyspnea, wheezing
Skin	Urticaria, angioedema, flushing, pruritus without rash, diaphoresis

Physical Examination

Perform a rapid examination, assessing vital signs, airway patency, respiratory sufficiency, cardiac rhythm, and mental status. Otherwise, the most frequently involved organ system is the skin, followed by the respiratory and gastrointestinal tracts (including oral mucosa).

Differential Diagnosis (Table 1-3)

The diagnosis of anaphylaxis is based on specific signs and symptoms of involvement of, by definition, at least 2 organ systems. If any of the following 3 criteria are present, the diagnosis of anaphylaxis is likely:

- Rapid onset of illness involving hives and/or mucosal tissue changes along with any of the following:
  - Respiratory compromise
  - Cardiovascular involvement
  - Evidence of end organ dysfunction
- Two or more organ systems involved following a known exposure
- Hypotension minutes to hours after an allergen exposure

Treatment

Anaphylaxis is a medical emergency and requires immediate care and attention. Address the ABCs, provide oxygen as needed, discontinue all ingoing intravenous (IV) antibiotics or contrast infusions, avoid any latex products, remove any indwelling latex catheters, and begin continuous cardiorespiratory monitoring and pulse oximetry. If the patient has stridor at rest or respiratory compromise despite epinephrine (see page 5), prepare to intubate. Place a hypotensive patient in the supine position with elevation of the lower extremities. Note that treatment may prove especially challenging if the patient is receiving a β-blocker.

Table 1-3. Differential Diagnosis of Anaphylaxis

Diagnosis	Clinical Features
Angioedema	May have had previous similar episodes Swelling of face, neck, and extremities without pruritus No acute respiratory or cardiovascular symptoms
Asthma	May have had previous similar episodes No acute dermatologic, gastrointestinal (GI), or cardiovascular symptoms
Cardiac tamponade	Muffled heart sounds Pericardial friction rub No acute dermatologic or GI symptoms
Cholinergic urticaria	Urticaria and wheezing Occurs within 30 minutes of vigorous exercise
Croup	Barking cough, stridor, fever No acute dermatologic, GI, or cardiovascular symptoms
Food poisoning	Vomiting, diarrhea, may have flushing No acute dermatologic, respiratory, or cardiovascular symptoms
Mastocytosis	Skin involved most often May have bone marrow and solid organ infiltration
Panic attacks	Feeling of impending doom No acute dermatological symptoms
Red man syndrome	Infusion with Vancomycin may mimic anaphylaxis Slowing rate of infusion decreases symptoms
Urticaria	No acute GI, respiratory, or cardiovascular symptoms

Epinephrine

Epinephrine is the first and most important treatment; there are no contraindications. It will reverse peripheral vasodilatation and bronchoconstriction, decrease angioedema and urticaria, shrink upper airway edema, enhance myocardial contractility, and suppress further release of immune mediators from mast cells and basophils.

Normotensive patient: Give 0.01 mL/kg (0.5 mL maximum) of *1:1,000* epinephrine *intramuscularly* into the lateral thigh. Repeat the dose every 5 to 15 minutes, as needed.

Hypotensive patient: Arrange for transfer to an intensive care unit and give 0.01 mg/kg (0.1 mL/kg, 10 mL maximum) of *1:10,000* epinephrine *intravenously*. Repeat every 3 to 5 minutes and increase subsequent doses to 0.1 to 0.2 mg/kg (0.1–0.2 mL/kg of *1:1,000*). In the absence of IV access, give 0.01 mg/kg of *1:1,000* epinephrine *intramuscularly* (0.1 mL/kg, 3 mL maximum). If the patient remains hypotensive, initiate an IV drip, starting with 0.1 mcg/kg/min (1.5 mcg/kg/min maximum).

Vasopressor Infusion

If the patient remains hypotensive despite epinephrine and volume repletion, start a dopamine drip (2–20 mcg/kg/min).

Antihistamines

Histamine 1 (H_1) and H_2 antihistamines block the effect of circulating histamines without affecting further mediator release. Antihistamines are therefore secondary treatment, and epinephrine is still necessary. In addition, antihistamines do not exert an immediate effect. Give diphenhydramine (H_1), 1 to 2 mg/kg (100 mg maximum) intravenously or orally every 6 hours *and* ranitidine (H_2), 2 mg/kg (50 mg maximum) every 6 to 8 hours intravenously or orally.

Albuterol

If the patient continues to have bronchospasm after epinephrine has been given, treat with nebulized albuterol (0.15 mg/kg/dose; 2.5 mg minimum, 10 mg maximum), either hourly or continuously.

Corticosteroids

Give either IV or oral methylprednisolone or oral prednisone (1–2 mg/kg/day divided every 6 hours, 80 mg/day maximum) for 3 days. This will decrease the risk of recurrent or protracted anaphylaxis but has no effect on the immediate reaction.

Glucagon

A patient taking β-blockers will have a limited response to epinephrine, increasing the risk for bronchospasm, hypotension, and paradoxical bradycardia. Give a loading dose of 20 to 30 mcg/kg (1 mg maximum) intravenously over 5 minutes, followed by a continuous infusion of 5 to 15 mcg/min, titrating the dose to the ideal blood pressure.

Indication for Consultation

- **Allergist:** First or severe episode of anaphylaxis, recurrent anaphylaxis, unknown etiology/exposure

Disposition

- **Intensive care unit transfer:** Severe respiratory distress requiring intubation, continuous epinephrine drip, hypotension requiring vasopressor infusion, patient on a β-blocker
- **Discharge criteria:** Normotensive on oral therapy after minimum observation period of 24 hours, without respiratory distress or significant end-organ dysfunction; family has a prescription for an epinephrine autoinjector and are educated about its use (store at room temperature, administer through clothing at the anterolateral aspect of the thigh and avoid holding thumb over the tip), as well as the importance of avoidance of food and environmental triggers; family instructed on ordering a MedicAlert bracelet (888/633-4298 or www.medicalert.org).

Discharge Management

- Continue the diphenhydramine and H_2 antihistamine for 2 to 3 days after discharge.
- Stop glucocorticoids after 3 days without a taper.

Follow-up

- **Allergist:** 2 to 3 weeks
- **Primary care:** 2 to 3 days

Pearls and Pitfalls

- The resuscitation will be challenging if the patient is taking a β-blocker.
- Anaphylaxis can be triggered by foods or medications received while on an inpatient service.
- Response may be seen as late as 72 hours postexposure.
- A biphasic response most occurs within 8 hours following resolution of initial symptoms.

Coding

ICD-9

- Anaphylaxis **995.0**
- Angioedema **995.1**

Bibliography

Ben-Shoshan M, Clarke AE. Anaphylaxis: past, present and future. *Allergy.* 2011; 128:661–614

Liberman DB, Teach SJ. Management of anaphylaxis in children. *Pediatr Emerg Care.* 2008;24:861–866

Simons FER. Anaphylaxis. *J Allergy Clin Immunol.* 2010;125:S161–S181

Simons KJ, Simons FE. Epinephrine and its use in anaphylaxis: current issues. *Curr Opin Allergy Clin Immunol.* 2010;10:354–361

Walker DM. Update on epinephrine (adrenaline) for pediatric emergencies. *Curr Opin Pediatr.* 2009;21:313–319

Cardiology

CHAPTER 2

Arrhythmias

Introduction

Arrhythmias are encountered in 2 types of inpatients. One is the patient with a history of known heart disease or recently diagnosed heart disease who is admitted for medical or surgical management of the heart disease or a complication of either the heart disease or its treatment. The second type of patient may not have a history of heart disease and the arrhythmia is either an incidental finding or related to a noncardiac disease process such as hyperthyroidism, fever, toxic ingestion, or medication side effect.

Clinical Presentation

When a child presents with a suspected arrhythmia (see Table 2-1 on page 12), it is critical to focus on the history and physical examination findings. However, the detail is determined by the stability of the patient. In an unstable patient, a directed history and examination are critical so as not to delay lifesaving treatment.

History

A patient with an arrhythmia can present in a variety of ways, depending on the age and underlying rhythm/heart disease. An infant may have nonspecific signs and symptoms, such as tachypnea, diaphoresis and/or cyanosis with feeds, irritability, and inconsolability. An older patient may complain of chest pain, nausea, palpitations, syncope/near syncope, or shortness of breath. Any age patient can present with cardiovascular collapse.

Have the patient or family describe the episode and whether there were any previous similar episodes. Assess for other symptoms, including chest pain, lightheadedness, dyspnea, palpitations, fatigue, irritability, and altered mental status. Ask about recent illnesses and review any medications or possible ingestions. Determine the medical history, especially if there are any chronic illnesses, as well as a family history of heart disease or sudden or unexplained death.

Physical Examination

Perform a directed physical examination to determine stability, focusing on the vital signs and ABCs. A stable patient has a maintainable airway, minimal to no respiratory distress, and adequate perfusion. Adequate perfusion is defined as appropriate mental status, capillary refill of 2 seconds or less, appropriate minimal blood pressure for age, appropriate heart rate for age, normal oxygen saturation, and adequate urine output. Auscultate for breath sounds as well as heart rate, rhythm, murmur, and additional sounds such as clicks or gallops. Check for hepatosplenomegaly, jugular venous distension, and peripheral edema.

Table 2-1. ECG Findings in Arrhythmias

Rate (bpm)	Rhythm	PR	QRS	Causes
Asystole				
0	None	Absent	Absent	See Box 2-1.
Atrial fibrillation				
Atrial: 350–600 Ventricular: variable	Irregularly irregular	Absent, fibrillation waves present	Normal	Cardiac surgery, valvular or ischemic disease, idiopathic, WPW
Atrial Flutter				
Atrial: 240–360 Ventricular: depends on degree of block (2:1–4:1)	Saw-tooth flutter waves with regular ventricular conduction at fixed ratio (2:1–4:1)	Absent	Normal	Same as atrial fibrillation
1° AV Block				
Normal for age	Regular	Prolonged for age	Normal	Normal variant, ARF, CM, CHD, digitalis toxicity, CTD
2° AV Block Type I				
Normal for age	Progressive lengthening of PR interval until non-conduction of a QRS	Progressively lengthening	Normal	Normal variant, myocarditis, CM, CHD, AMI, SLE, Lyme disease, digitalis or ß-blocker toxicity
2° AV Block Type II				
Normal to bradycardic for age	AV conduction cycles between normal and complete block, resulting in dropped QRS	Normal	Normal	Same as type I
3° AV Block				
Dissociation between atrial and ventricular rates Rate of Ps > QRS	Rate of Ps and QRSs are regular, but independent of each other	Variable	Congenital: normal Acquired: prolonged	Congenital: maternal SLE or CTD, CHD Acquired: ARF, myocarditis, Lyme disease, CM, AMI, digitalis toxicity
Long QT Syndrome				
Normal for age	Regular Prolonged QTc interval >0.45	Normal	Normal	Drug toxicity, ↓K, ↓Ca, JLNS, RWS

Table 2-1. ECG Findings in Arrhythmias, continued				
Rate (bpm)	**Rhythm**	**PR**	**QRS**	**Causes**
Sinus Arrhythmia				
Normal for age	Regularly irregular; rhythm changes with respirations	Normal	Normal	Normal respiration
Sinus Bradycardia				
Infant: <80 Child: <60	Regular	Normal	Normal	Normal in athletes Increased ICP See Box 2-1.
Sinus Tachycardia				
Infant: 140–200 Child: 120–180	Regular	Normal	Normal	Shock, sepsis, pain, fever, anxiety, AMI, drug toxicity
Supraventricular Tachycardia				
Infant: >220 Child: >180	Regular Does not vary	Masked by tachycardia	Normal	Idiopathic, CHD, postoperative
Ventricular Fibrillation				
150–300	Chaotic No organized electrical activity	Absent	Absent	See Box 2-1.
Ventricular Tachycardia				
120–200	Regular	Masked by tachycardia	Widened	Myocarditis, AMI, CM, LQTS, CHD, drug toxicity; see Box 2-1

Abbreviations: AMI, acute myocardial infarction; ARF, acute rheumatic fever; AV, atrioventricular; CHD, congenital heart disease; CM, cardiomyopathy; CTD, connective tissue disease; ICP, intracranial pressure; JLNS, Jervell and Lange-Nielsen; LQTS, long QT syndrome; RWS, Romano-Ward syndrome; SLE, systemic lupus erythematosus; WPW, Wolff-Parkinson-White syndrome

Treatment of Specific Arrhythmias

The priority is determining whether a patient with an arrhythmia is stable, with palpable pulses, adequate perfusion with a normal blood pressure for age, normal urine output, normal oxygen saturation, and normal mental status. In such a case there is time to systematically evaluate the situation. In addition, many arrhythmias have underlying reversible causes for which the American Heart Association has coined the mnemonic of "Hs and Ts" (Box 2-1). It is imperative that these conditions are diagnosed and treated.

Asystole

Confirm that the monitor leads are properly attached to the patient's chest and the monitor, then change the monitor lead setting (change from lead I to lead II or lead II to lead III) and confirm asystole in a second lead. Initiate CPR,

Box 2-1. Hs and Ts of Reversible Causes of Arrhythmias	
Hypoxemia	**T**rauma
Hypovolemia	**T**amponade (pericardial)
Hyper-/**H**ypokalemia	**T**oxic ingestion
Hypoglycemia	**T**hrombosis, pulmonary
Hydrogen (acidosis)	**T**ension pneumothorax
Hypothermia	**T**hrombosis, coronary

secure an airway, obtain intravenous/intraosseous (IV/IO) access, and provide oxygen and adequate ventilation.

Give 0.01 mg/kg (0.1 mL/kg, 1 mg maximum = 10 mL maximum) of *1:10,000* epinephrine intravenously or intraosseously. If there is no IV/IO access, use 0.1 mg/kg (0.1 mL/kg, 3 mg maximum = 3 mL maximum) of *1:1,000* epinephrine followed by 5 to 10 mL of normal saline via the endotracheal tube every 3 to 5 minutes until vascular access is achieved.

Atrial Fibrillation and Atrial Flutter

Investigate for underlying medical conditions. The goals are to convert the atrial rhythm, control the ventricular response, and prevent recurrences. The approach varies, depending on the patient's clinical status.

In an acute, life-threatening situation, attempt direct current cardioversion (0.5–1 J/kg). Consult with a pediatric cardiologist to initiate anticoagulation with heparin and ventricular rate control with digoxin, a β-blocker, or a calcium channel blocker. If the patient is stable, with atrial fibrillation or flutter of unknown duration, consult with a pediatric cardiologist and delay cardioversion until the patient is adequately anticoagulated.

First-Degree Atrioventricular (AV) Block

No treatment is needed except in the setting of structural heart disease and drug toxicity.

Second-Degree AV Block, Type I

Treat the underlying disease causing the arrhythmia.

Second-Degree AV Block, Type II

Treat the underlying disorder. Be aware that this has a high risk for progression to third-degree AV block. Refer the patient to a pediatric cardiologist for potential pacemaker placement.

Third-Degree AV Block

Treat with atropine 0.02 mg/kg intravenously every 5 minutes for 2 to 3 doses (minimum dose 0.1 mg; maximum single dose 0.5 mg in children, 1 mg in adolescents; maximum total dose of 1 mg for children and 2 mg for adolescents). Use this to increase heart rate while arranging for transcutaneous or transvenous pacing until a permanent pacemaker can be placed. Indications for pacemaker therapy include

- Signs and symptoms of congestive heart failure
- Infant with a structurally normal heart and a ventricular rate less than 50 bpm
- Infant with structural heart disease and a ventricular rate less than 70 bpm
- Patient with a wide QRS escape rhythm, ventricular ectopy, or ventricular dysfunction

Long QT Syndrome

If the patient presents with torsades de pointes, obtain serum electrolytes and urine drug screens and treat with magnesium sulfate 25 to 50 mg/kg IV (2 g maximum). Contact pediatric cardiology and monitor the patient closely, as further resuscitation may be necessary.

If the long QT is an incidental finding or discovered during the evaluation for syncope, immediately refer the patient to pediatric cardiology and arrange to screen all first-degree relatives.

Symptomatic Sinus Bradycardia

Initiate basic life support, obtain IV/IO access, provide oxygen, and place the patient on a monitor. Assess for reversible causes (Hs and Ts) and treat the underlying disease. Start transcutaneous pacing, if readily available. Otherwise, treat with epinephrine as described for asystole.

If there is increased vagal tone or the patient has an AV block, give atropine as described above for third-degree AV block. Situations where increased vagal tone is encountered include inferior myocardial disease, hypoglycemia, hypothyroidism, increased intracranial pressure, sick sinus syndrome, and potassium abnormalities. Numerous drugs, such as digoxin and β-blockers, can also cause increased vagal tone.

Supraventricular Tachycardia (SVT)

Initiate basic life support, obtain IV/IO access, provide oxygen, and place the patient on a monitor. Assess for reversible causes (Hs and Ts) and treat the underlying disease. Initial treatment depends on whether or not the patient is well perfused.

If the patient is well perfused, initially attempt vagal maneuvers, such as covering the face with a bag full of slushy ice water, attempting a Valsalva maneuver, or performing unilateral carotid artery massage. If unsuccessful, give adenosine 0.1 mg/kg rapid IV push (6 mg maximum) with the syringe as close to the IV site as possible, followed by a rapid IV push of 5 to 10 mL of normal saline. Using a stopcock can facilitate the rapid infusion of the adenosine and flush. If the first dose is not successful, repeat at a dose of 0.2 mg/kg rapid IV push (12 mg maximum). If the second dose of adenosine does not convert the rhythm, give another 0.2 mg/kg rapid IV push (12 mg maximum). If the patient continues in SVT, consult a pediatric cardiologist to discuss the next step (further antiarrhythmics or synchronized cardioversion).

If the patient is poorly perfused, use synchronized cardioversion at 0.5 to 1 J/kg. If unsuccessful, increase to 2 J/kg. If cardioversion is unsuccessful or the SVT recurs, consult with a cardiologist whenever possible and give either amiodarone 5 mg/kg IV over 20 to 60 minutes or procainamide 15 mg/kg IV over 30 to 60 minutes. Be prepared to treat bradycardia or other dysrhythmias that may result following amiodarone or procainamide administration.

Ventricular Fibrillation (VF)

Initiate basic life support, obtain IV/IO access, provide oxygen, ensure adequate ventilation, and place the patient on a monitor. Once VF is noted, proceed to immediate defibrillation. Give a single shock of 2 J/kg followed by 2 minutes of CPR; second shock of 4 J/kg followed by 2 minutes of CPR; subsequent shocks 4 J/kg or greater to a maximum of 10 J/kg or adult levels of energy. After the second defibrillation attempt, give epinephrine every 3 to 5 minutes as for asystole. After the third defibrillation attempt, start an antiarrhythmic, either amiodarone (5 mg/kg IV/IO bolus; may be repeated twice for refractory VF/pulseless VT) or lidocaine 1 mg/kg IV/IO bolus. Continue cycles of "CPR-shock-drug" until return of spontaneous circulation, rhythm change, or termination of resuscitative efforts.

Ventricular Tachycardia (VT)

Initiate basic life support, obtain IV/IO access, provide oxygen, ensure adequate ventilation, and place the patient on a monitor. If the patient is pulseless, treat identically to VF. If the patient has pulse and good perfusion, give amiodarone (5 mg/kg IV over 20 minutes), or consult a pediatric cardiologist to assist with further management (possible procainamide infusion or synchronized cardioversion).

If the patient has a pulse and poor perfusion, use synchronized cardioversion as for SVT. Consult a pediatric cardiologist or intensivist to assist with further management (possible procainamide infusion or synchronized cardioversion).

Disposition

- **Intensive care unit transfer:** Life-threatening arrhythmias (VF, VT, sustained SVT, symptomatic bradycardia, AV block of second degree type II or higher, atrial flutter or fibrillation, asystole)
- **Discharge criteria:** Hemodynamically stable on a regimen that can be managed at home

Indications for Consultation

- **Pediatric cardiology:** Life-threatening arrhythmias (as above), long QT, SVT, heart block

Pearls and Pitfalls

- The stability of the patient determines how rapidly to treat the arrhythmia.
- Always confirm asystole in 2 different leads.
- Symptomatic bradycardia of less than 60 bpm in any age group requires initiation of CPR.

Coding

ICD-9

- Atrial fibrillation **427.31**
- Atrial flutter **427.32**
- Cardiac arrest **427.5**
- Dysrhythmia NOS **427.9**
- Neonatal bradycardia **779.81**
- Neonatal tachycardia **779.82**
- Newborn cardiac arrest **779.85**
- Sinus bradycardia **427.81**
- Supraventricular tachycardia **427.0**
- Ventricular fibrillation **427.41**
- Ventricular tachycardia **427.1**

CPT

- Cardiopulmonary resuscitation **92950**
- Cardioversion/defibrillation, external **92960**
- Transcutaneous pacing **92953**

Bibliography

Doniger SJ, Sharieff GQ. Pediatric dysrhythmias. *Pediatr Clin North Am.* 2006;53:85–105

Kleinman ME, Chameides L, Schexnayder SM, et al. Part 14: pediatric advanced life support: 2010: American Heart Association guidelines for cardiopulmonary resuscitation and emergency cardiovascular care. *Circulation.* 2010;122 (18 suppl 3):S876–S908

O'Connor M, McDaniel N, Brady WJ. The pediatric electrocardiogram part II: dysrhythmias. *Am J Emerg Med.* 2008;26:348–358

Park M. Cardiac arrhythmias. In: *Pediatric Cardiology for Practitioners.* 5th ed. Philadelphia, PA: Mosby Elsevier; 2008:417–444

Park M. Cardiovascular infections. In: *Pediatric Cardiology for Practitioners.* 5th ed. Philadelphia, PA: Mosby Elsevier; 2008:351–380

Park M. Disturbances of atrioventricular conduction. In: *Pediactric Cardiology for Practitioners.* 5th ed. Philadelphia, PA: Mosby Elsevier; 2008:445–448

CHAPTER 3

Congestive Heart Failure

Introduction

Congestive heart failure (CHF) is the inability of the heart to meet the metabolic demands of the body. Rather than a single disease entity, CHF represents a constellation of signs and symptoms arising from a number of etiologies. The most common causes of CHF in children are congenital heart disease (CHD), cardiomyopathies (including genetic, acquired, inherited metabolic, or muscle disorders; infectious diseases; drugs; toxins; Kawasaki disease; and autoimmune diseases), and myocardial dysfunction after surgical repair of heart defects. Other causes include arrhythmias and cardiac valve disease. Regardless of the etiology of CHF, the resulting pathophysiological syndrome requires immediate attention, supportive care, and prompt cardiology consultation.

Clinical Presentation

History

Infants

Feeding difficulty is the most prominent symptom, which is often associated with tachycardia, tachypnea, and diaphoresis. Poor feeding ultimately leads to failure to thrive.

Children/Adolescents

Toddlers and older children often exhibit fatigue, exercise intolerance, poor appetite, and growth failure. Adolescents may have additional symptoms, similar to those of adults, including shortness of breath, orthopnea, nocturnal dyspnea, abdominal pain, or chronic cough.

Physical Examination

All age groups typically present with tachycardia and tachypnea. Hepatomegaly is an early finding, and if the enlargement is relatively acute, there may be flank pain or tenderness due to stretching of the liver capsule. Mild–moderate disease may present with no distress; however, patients with severe disease may be dyspneic at rest. With an acute onset the patient may appear anxious but well nourished, versus calm yet malnourished with chronic CHF.

An infant with severe disease may have nasal flaring, retractions, grunting, and occasionally wheezing. Rales are rare in an infant unless there is coexisting pneumonia. An infant with low cardiac output may have cool and/

or mottled extremities, weakly palpable pulses, a narrow pulse pressure, and delayed capillary refill.

While uncommon in an infant, an older child may exhibit signs of increased systemic venous pressure, including distention of neck veins (venous pulsations visible above clavicle while patient is sitting) and peripheral edema (particularly in the face and dependent parts of the body). Low cardiac output may cause peripheral vasoconstriction leading to cool extremities, pallor, cyanosis, and delayed capillary refill. With more advanced disease, pulmonary edema and rales are more likely.

The cardiac examination can be quite variable depending on the etiology of disease. In cardiomyopathy there is usually a quiet precordium. Shunt lesions (ventricular septal defect, patent ductus arteriosus) usually cause a hyperdynamic precordium. Obstructive lesions (aortic stenosis, coarctation of the aorta) may have a systolic thrill. A third heart sound in mid-diastole can be a normal finding in children but is more frequently noted in those with heart disease. Regardless of the etiology of failure, a holosystolic murmur of mitral regurgitation is often present with advanced disease.

Laboratory

Standard testing to diagnose CHF includes a chest x-ray, electrocardiogram (ECG), and echocardiogram. The chest x-ray will invariably show cardiac enlargement with or without evidence of pulmonary venous congestion. The presence of pulmonary congestion depends on the etiology of disease. It is less likely in early cardiomyopathy but more common with left to right shunt or advanced disease. An echocardiogram is the primary diagnostic modality for confirming CHF (ie, ventricular dysfunction, anatomical abnormality, etc). In contrast, the ECG, while almost always abnormal, is generally not useful in diagnosing heart failure but may provide clues to the etiology.

If it is difficult to determine whether a patient is exhibiting signs of a primary respiratory process versus cardiac-induced respiratory symptoms, obtain a brain natriuretic peptide (BNP) level. BNP is a hormone secreted by the heart in response to volume and pressure overload and is a sensitive marker of cardiac filling pressure and diastolic dysfunction. It will be elevated in heart failure and normal in a primarily respiratory process.

Once a diagnosis of CHF has been established, the remainder of the laboratory testing depends on the age of the patient, presence or absence of CHD, and coexistent systemic disorders. Obtain a complete blood cell count (CBC), electrolytes, liver function tests, renal function tests, a blood gas, and a lactate. The CBC may reveal a leukocytosis secondary to an infection, anemia as an etiology, thrombocytopenia in disseminated intravascular coagulation, or pancytopenia due to viral suppression. CHF can cause electrolyte abnormalities, including hyponatremia (fluid overload) and metabolic acidosis (poor perfusion). Renal failure may be a consequence or cause of CHF, and elevated liver function tests occur with end-organ damage or a viral illness. The blood gas provides objective evidence of impending respiratory failure, while an abnormal lactate can be a sign of poor tissue perfusion or a clue to a metabolic cause of illness.

Differential Diagnosis

It is important to differentiate CHF from possible respiratory and/or infectious illnesses, in which case the patient is unlikely to have hepatomegaly, cardiomegaly, or failure to thrive (Table 3-1). If a patient has a history of structural heart disease and presents with new signs and symptoms of CHF, it may be due to an aggravating condition such as fever, anemia, or an arrhythmia. In a patient without structural heart disease, there are many possible etiologies of CHF, some of which are listed in Box 3-1.

Table 3-1. Differential Diagnosis of Congestive Heart Failure

Diagnosis	Clinical Features[a]
Asthma	Previous episodes Wheezing, tachypnea, retractions Chest x-ray: hyperinflation without cardiomegaly or pulmonary congestion
Bronchiolitis	Rales +/- wheezing, tachypnea, retractions Chest x-ray: atelectasis and hyperinflation without cardiomegaly
Pneumonia	Fever, rales, tachypnea Chest x-ray: focal consolidation
Sepsis	Fever, ill-appearing, poor perfusion Tachypnea, tachycardia

[a]Note the absence of hepatomegaly, cardiomegaly, failure to thrive, and elevated brain natriuretic peptide in all.

Box 3-1. Etiologies of Heart Failure in a Previously Structurally Normal Heart

- Acquired valvular disease (rheumatic heart disease)
- Anemia
- Chemotherapy (anthracyclines)
- Arrhythmia (bradycardia or tachycardia)
- Atrioventricular fistula
- Cardiomyopathy (acquired or genetic)
- Eating disorders/caloric deficiency
- Hypertension
- Hypoglycemia
- Inborn errors of metabolism (disorders of fatty acid oxidation, mitochondria, glycogen storage)
- Kawasaki disease
- Muscular dystrophies
- Myocardial infarction
- Myocarditis (usually viral: adenovirus, coxsackievirus, parvovirus)
- Renal failure
- Sepsis
- Systemic lupus erythematosus
- Thyroid disease (hypothyroidism, thyrotoxicosis)

Treatment

If CHF is suspected, immediately consult with a cardiologist for recommendations regarding appropriate management. Initial stabilization includes intravenous (IV)/intraosseous access (essential), cardiorespiratory monitoring (with telemetry if available), and judicious fluid administration. Volume overload is almost *always* present, so use smaller 5- to 10-mL/kg boluses in place of the typical 20 mL/kg and a slower administration rate while continuously monitoring for signs of pulmonary and hepatic congestion. The overall goals of medical management are decreasing afterload, increasing contractility, and reducing preload volume. The most commonly used medications are diuretics, typically furosemide (1 mg/kg oral or IV) to decrease preload. Give furosemide early, while waiting for the cardiologist.

The cardiologist may recommend giving vasoactive or inotropic medications (dopamine, milrinone, epinephrine) for acute management instead of further IV fluid administration. Other commonly used medications include digoxin to improve contractility and systolic ventricular function and angiotensin-converting enzyme inhibitors to decrease afterload.

If structural heart disease is suspected, use oxygen cautiously and only in consultation with a cardiologist. This is critical in that oxygen, by lowering pulmonary vascular resistance, shunts blood from the systemic to the pulmonary circulation, potentially causing rapid deterioration in certain ductal-dependent or mixing lesions (hypoplastic left heart syndrome, transposition of the great arteries, large ventricular septal defects). Once these etiologies have been ruled out, it is safe to administer oxygen to supplement tissue oxygenation and alleviate respiratory distress. If further respiratory support is required, use a high FiO_2 bag and mask, followed by noninvasive positive pressure ventilation, as the required sedation and vagal effects of endotracheal intubation can be detrimental to cardiac function.

After initiating cardiovascular stabilization, consider noncardiac causes of heart failure and treat accordingly before further intervention. Once a cardiac etiology is confirmed, treatment options are varied based on etiology and severity, and may include medical management, cardiac catheterization, or surgical intervention. Transfer a patient with severe or unresponsive heart failure to an intensive care unit (ICU), where additional modalities, such as extracorporeal membrane oxygenation or left ventricular assist devices, may be available. Regardless of intervention or severity, continued management must address proper nutrition and growth, along with general health measures, such as vaccinations and exercise parameters.

Indications for Consultation

- **Cardiology:** All patients
- **Infectious disease, rheumatology, metabolics/genetics:** Depending on the suspected etiology and severity

Disposition

- **ICU transfer:** Impending respiratory failure, poor perfusion, hypotension, severe electrolyte abnormalities, metabolic acidosis, lethargy, any other evidence of cardiovascular compromise or end-organ damage
- **Interinstitutional transfer:** Diagnostic and treatment modalities or a pediatric cardiologist and/or intensivist are not immediately available.
- **Discharge criteria:** Breathing easily without respiratory distress, taking adequate fluid and nutrition, normal electrolytes and, usually, no oxygen requirement. Discharge ultimately depends on the specific etiology of disease and cardiology plan of care.

Follow-up

- **Primary care:** 1 week
- **Cardiology:** 2 to 3 days, dependent on etiology and severity

Pearls and Pitfalls

- Family members or caretakers who see a patient on a regular basis may not notice subtle changes in appearance or behavior. For example, edema may be mistaken for normal weight gain and exercise intolerance as lack of interest in activities.
- A patient may present with primarily abdominal symptoms (nausea, vomiting, abdominal pain), without respiratory complaints. These can then be mistaken for acute gastroenteritis or another gastrointestinal process, leading to an excessive fluid resuscitation in a fluid-overloaded patient.

Coding

ICD-9

- Acute myocarditis **422.90**
- CHF **428.0**
- Primary cardiomyopathy **425.4**

Bibliography

Blume ED, Freed MD, Colan SD. Congestive heart failure. In: Keane JF, Lock JE, Fyler C, eds. *Nadas' Pediatric Cardiology.* 2nd ed. Philadelphia, PA: Saunders Elsevier; 2006:83–91

Hsu DT, Pearson GD. Heart failure in children. Part II: diagnosis, treatment, and future directions. *Circ Heart Fail.* 2009;2:490–498

Kantor PF, Mertens LL. Clinical practice: heart failure in children. Part I: clinical evaluation, diagnostic testing, and initial medical management. *Eur J Pediatr.* 2010; 169:269–279

Kay JD, Colan SD, Graham TP Jr. Congestive heart failure in pediatric patients. *Am Heart J.* 2001;142:923–928

Macicek SM, Macias CG, Jefferies JL, Kim JJ, Price JF. Acute heart failure in the pediatric emergency department. *Pediatrics.* 2009;124:e898–e904

Madriago E, Silberbach M. Heart failure in infants and children. *Pediatr Rev.* 2010; 31:4–12

O'Connor MJ, Rosenthal DN, Shaddy RE. Outpatient management of pediatric heart failure. *Heart Failure Clin.* 2010;6:515–529

CHAPTER 4

Deep Venous Thrombosis

Introduction

Deep venous thrombosis (DVT) is very unusual in children, although the incidence has risen over the last 10 to 15 years to about 25 to 30 cases per 10,000 hospital admissions. Prompt diagnosis is critical, as an undiagnosed and untreated DVT may be lead to a fatal pulmonary embolism (PE) or cause serious long-term morbidity. The most important risk factors for a DVT are a venous central line, prolonged immobilization (>3–4 days), local infection (osteomyelitis or skin and soft tissue infections), and a family history of DVT (Box 4-1.)

DVT primarily affects the lower extremities and is subdivided in 2 groups: distal (calf veins) and proximal (thigh veins) thrombosis. Up to 90% of PEs originate from a dislodged thrombus from one of the proximal lower extremity veins. Involvement of the upper extremities is much less common and is almost always associated with a central line, total parenteral nutrition, dialysis, a hypercoagulable state, or cancer chemotherapy. Although a PE can be demonstrated in up to 60% of patients with DVTs, most are clinically silent. Nonetheless, maintain a high clinical suspicion as the mortality from clinically apparent PEs approaches 30%.

Box 4-1. Risk Factors for DVT

Acquired Conditions	
Acute osteomyelitis	Medications (oral and transdermal contraceptives)
Diabetes mellitus	Nephrotic syndrome
Family history of DVT	Obesity
Immobilization (post-surgery, post-trauma)	Pregnancy
Indwelling venous catheter, especially central	Prosthetic cardiac valves
Inflammatory diseases (SLE, IBD, RA)	Serious infections (sepsis)
Malignancy	Sickle cell disease
Inherited Hypercoagulable Conditions	
Anti-thrombin deficiency	Protein S and C deficiency
Factor 5 Leiden mutation	Prothrombin gene mutation

Abbreviations: DVT, deep venous thrombosis; IBD, irritable bowel syndrome; RA, rheumatoid arthritis; SLE, systemic lupus erythematosus.

Clinical Presentation

History

Ask about a personal or family history of the risk factors and predisposing conditions listed in Box 4-1. The patient may complain of some combination of leg pain and swelling, pitting edema, warmth and erythema, dilated superficial veins and, on occasion, a palpable cord in the calf, caused by a thrombosed vein. The pain may result in a limp or limitation of activity and it may be worse when the affected limb is dependent due to swelling or during activity.

The most common symptoms of a pulmonary embolism are dyspnea and pleuritic chest pain. Less frequently, the patient may complain of fever, cough, and hemoptysis.

Physical Examination

Carefully inspect the leg, looking for swelling, erythema, tenderness, and dilated superficial veins. Palpate for a cord, which represents subcutaneous venous clots. Measure the circumference of the mid-portion of the affected limb segment (usually 10 cm below the tibial plateau) and compare to the unaffected side. A difference greater than 3 cm is concerning for a DVT. Attempt to elicit Homans sign, which is popliteal calf pain that occurs upon forceful and abrupt dorsiflexion of the ankle while the knee is held in the flexed position. However, these findings are neither sensitive nor specific for DVT. Therefore, determine the Wells score (Table 4-1) based on signs, symptoms, and risk factors.

Table 4-1. The Wells Score[a]

Clinical Feature	Score
Entire leg swollen	1
Calf swelling >3 cm compared to other calf (measured 10 cm below tibial tuberosity)	1
Localized tenderness along the distribution of the deep venous system	1
Pitting edema, greater in the symptomatic leg	1
Collateral superficial veins, not varicose	1
Active cancer, treatment ongoing or within previous 6 months of palliative treatment	1
Paralysis, paresis, or recent plaster immobilization of the lower extremity	1
Recently bedridden for more than 3 days or major surgery within 4 weeks	1
Alternative diagnosis as likely or greater than deep venous thrombosis	*Subtract 2 points*

[a]Interpretation: high probability: score ≥3; moderate probability: score 1 or 2; low probability: score ≤0.

Complications

As noted previously, signs suggestive of a PE include tachypnea and dyspnea, as well as fever, tachycardia, and hemoptysis. Rales and/or an S3 or S4 gallop rhythm may be appreciated.

Laboratory

Obtain a complete blood cell count (CBC), prothrombin time (PT), activated partial thromboplastin time (aPTT), fibrinogen, and quantitative D-dimer if a DVT is suspected. If an inherited hypercoagulable condition is a concern in a patient with either no evident risk factors or recurrent DVTs, also obtain antithrombin III, protein C, protein S, factor 5 Leiden, antiphospholipid antibodies, lupus anticoagulant, homocysteine, alpha$_2$-antitrypsin, and prothrombin 20210.

Radiology

Order a Doppler and compression ultrasonography (sonogram with compression of the major veins) of the affected limb. This is the noninvasive test of choice and is both highly sensitive (89%–96%) and specific (94%–99%) for symptomatic proximal DVT. If the initial study is negative and the clinical suspicion of DVT remains high, either repeat the study in 5 to 7 days or obtain a computed tomography (CT) angiography of the limb. Order a magnetic resonance angiography when the noninvasive tests are equivocal, large central vessels are the site of concern, or contrast studies are contraindicated. If a PE is suspected, discuss with a radiologist to determine the local preference among a ventilation-perfusion lung, thin-cut chest CT (can be difficult to perform in a young child), or a spiral chest CT.

Differential Diagnosis

A clotting activation marker, such as quantitative D-dimer, has high sensitivity and negative predictive value, but a low specificity. The combination of low pretest probability or clinical decision rule (Wells score) and a negative D-dimer has an extremely high negative predictive value for venous thromboembolism (about 99%). However, a positive D-dimer does not confirm the diagnosis of DVT. False-positive levels occur with malignancies, trauma, recent surgery, infections, pregnancy, and acute bleeding.

The differential diagnosis (Table 4-2) of suspected DVT includes a variety of disorders that present in a similar fashion. It is essential to make the diagnosis because an untreated DVT may have serious sequelae.

Table 4-2. Differential Diagnosis of Deep Venous Thrombosis[a]	
Diagnosis	**Clinical Features**
Muscle strain/sprain	History of trauma Localized tenderness Bruising and/or hematoma
Cellulitis	Local area of skin with redness/warmth Clear demarcation between involved/uninvolved areas Constitutional symptoms (fever, malaise)
Baker's cyst	Prior history of knee swelling and/or pain Palpable fluid filled mass behind the knee
Lymphedema	Insidious onset Cutaneous and subcutaneous thickening
Venous insufficiency	Visible dilated veins Chronic skin changes with possible ulceration Muscle cramping, numbness, tingling, or itching
Superficial thrombophlebitis	Palpable superficial veins

[a]In each case, Homans sign will be negative, except with a calf muscle strain.

Treatment

If a DVT is suspected, consult a hematologist. To decrease the chance of embolization, order strict bed rest until the Doppler is performed. Also discontinue any sequential compression device (SCD). The goals of treating DVT are to prevent local extension of thrombus and embolization (usually PE), reduce the risk or recurrent thrombosis, and minimize long-term complication (chronic venous insufficiency, post-thrombotic syndrome, chronic thromboembolic pulmonary hypertension). There is no consensus on DVT management for children, so that the treatment of choice is individualized to the specific circumstances of the patient and the preference of the consultants. Options include thrombolytic therapy for a massive PE, anticoagulation for at least 3 months, vena cava filter to prevent PE, surgical thrombectomy, and supportive care, including compressive stockings, venous compressing pump, and managing skin ulcers.

Low Molecular Weight Heparin (LMWH)

In contrast to unfractionated heparin (UFH), LMWH has high specific activity against factor Xa and less activity against thrombin. DVT treatment dosing is twice that for prophylaxis (<2 months of age: 1.5 mg/kg subcutaneous [SC] every 12 hours; >2 months of age: 1 mg/kg SC every 12 hours). Monitor LMWH with anti-factor Xa levels obtained 4 hours after the dose. The goal is 0.5 to 1.0 units/mL at 4 hours after the last SC injection. Once this is achieved, follow the anti-factor Xa weekly. For a DVT, treat with LMWH for up to 3 months.

LMWH offers several advantages over UFH, including superior bioavailability, with a longer half-life and dose-independent clearance, which results in a more predictable anticoagulation response. It can be administered subcutaneously with minimal laboratory monitoring and dose adjustment. Prior to institution of LMWH therapy, obtain a CBC, PT, aPTT, and platelet count. Do not give the patient salicylates and avoid intramuscular injections and arterial punctures while receiving LMWN. Hold LMWH for 24 hours prior to an invasive procedure, especially lumbar puncture, then resume the therapeutic dose 24 hours (minor surgery or invasive procedure) or 48 to 72 hours (major surgery) later.

Unfractionated Heparin

Use UFH specifically in a neurosurgical patient and as an option in all other children. The loading dose is 75 units/kg intravenous (IV) over 10 minutes, immediately followed by an infusion of 28 units/kg/hour (<1 year of age) or 20 units/kg/hour (>1 year of age). Use the aPTT to closely monitor therapy and always obtain the sample from a different limb than the infusion site. Alternatively, monitor anti-factor Xa, aiming for a therapeutic range of 0.3 to 0.7 units/mL (laboratory dependent).

Obtain an aPTT 4 hours after administration of the UFH loading dose. When the aPTT is 2 to 3 times the mean control value, repeat a CBC with platelet count. If the platelet count is less than 100,000/mm^3, consider discontinuation of heparin and instituting an alternative therapy. The risk of heparin-induced thrombocytopenia is greatest after 5 to 7 days of treatment, so re-check the CBC after a week of therapy. Since UFH has a very short half-life, excessive levels can usually be controlled by stopping the infusion. Treat a symptomatic overdose with protamine (1 mg for each 100 units of UFH).

The duration of UFH therapy for DVT is 5 to 7 days. Institute warfarin therapy on day 1 or 2 (see below) to facilitate the transition to long-term oral treatment. If the patient has a pulmonary embolism, give the heparin therapy for 7 to 14 days and start the warfarin on day 5.

Warfarin

Use warfarin (oral vitamin K antagonist) to transition from IV heparin to oral treatment for outpatient management. It is significantly cheaper than LMWH, but requires more frequent monitoring. The loading/maintenance dose is 0.1 to 0.2 mg/kg (10 mg maximum), as single daily oral doses, over 3 to 5 days. Base subsequent doses on the international normalized ratio (INR) response, measured every 3 to 5 days. When 2 INRs obtained 24 hours apart are between 2 and 3, discontinue the heparin. Continue to measure the INR frequently (weekly) until stable, as well as after *any medication change*. The diet also must be stable. Prior to any surgery, consult with a hematologist to determine appropriate warfarin management.

DVT Prophylaxis

Consider DVT prophylaxis for a patient with identifiable risk factors. Although there are no consensus pediatric protocols, an adolescent may be a candidate for the local adult practice. Mobilization is preferred, when possible. Mechanical methods to decrease venous stasis include compression stockings and sequential SCDs. Efficacy of an SCD is related to duration of use, but many of these devices are poorly tolerated by children. Anticoagulation is more effective and often easier to administer. With LMWH, use half the DVT treatment does (<2 months of age: 0.75 mg/kg SC every 12 hours; >2 months of age: 0.5 mg/kg SC every 12 hours). For unfractionated heparin titrate the dose to an aPTT of 1.2 to 1.5 times control.

Indications for Consultation

- **Hematologist:** All patients
- **Vascular surgeon:** Extensive thrombosis above the knee/elbow and involving any vessels of the chest or abdomen

Disposition

- **Intensive care unit transfer:** Pulmonary embolism
- **Discharge criteria:** Therapeutic range of INR or anti-Xa achieved, parent/patient education completed (DVT, anticoagulants, pulmonary embolism, diet if taking warfarin), and the patient is stable

Coding

ICD-9

- Acute DVT of upper extremity **453.82**
- Acute DVT of proximal lower extremity **453.41**
- Acute DVT of distal lower extremity **453.42**

Follow-up

- **Primary care:** 1 week
- **Hematologist (depending on the outpatient anticoagulant choice):** Within 3 days for warfarin or 1 week for LMWH
- **Vascular surgeon:** If involved per their request

Bibliography

Bates SM, Jaeschke R, Stevens SM, et al. Diagnosis of DVT: antithrombotic therapy and prevention of thrombosis, 9th ed: American College of Chest Physicians evidence-based clinical practice guidelines. *Chest.* 2012;141(2 suppl):e351S–e418S

Graziano JN, Charpie JR. Thrombosis in the intensive care unit: etiology, diagnosis, management, and prevention in adults and children. *Cardiol Rev.* 2001;9:173–182

Raffini L, Huang YS, Witmer C, Feudtner C. Dramatic increase in venous thromboembolism in children's hospitals in the United States from 2001 to 2007. *Pediatrics.* 2009;124:1001–1008

Raffini L, Trimarchi T, Beliveau J, Davis D. Thromboprophylaxis in a pediatric hospital: a patient-safety and quality-improvement initiative. *Pediatrics.* 2011;127:e1326–e1332

Revel-Vilk S. Central venous line-related thrombosis in children. *Acta Haematol.* 2006;115:201–206

Tormene D, Gavasso S, Rossetto V, Simioni P. Thrombosis and thrombophilia in children: a systematic review. *Semin Thromb Hemost.* 2006;32:724–728

Young G. Diagnosis and treatment of thrombosis in children: general principles. *Pediatr Blood Cancer.* 2006;46:540–546

CHAPTER 5

Electrocardiogram Interpretation

Introduction

An electrocardiogram (ECG) is a graphic representation of the progression of electrical activity through the heart. It is often used as a screening test in situations such as suspected congenital heart disease, chest pain, syncope, acquired heart disease, hypertension, and medication monitoring.

Systematic Reading of ECGs (Table 5-1)

1. **Patient identification:** Always confirm that the ECG was performed on the correct patient.
2. **Standardization:** Check the bottom of the ECG for the paper speed, which is typically 25 mm/sec. This makes the x-axis time 0.04 seconds per small box, or 0.2 seconds for each large box, on the tracing paper. Also note the calibration marker, which is usually 10 mm high by 5 mm wide. This is called full standard, but a common variation is to have a stair-step pattern to the calibration with a 10 mm block followed by a 5 mm step-down. This means that the limb leads (I, II, II, aVR, aVL, aVF) are at full standard while the precordial leads (V1-6) are at half standard. When this is the case, remember to multiply the precordial voltage values by 2 for accurate interpretation.
3. **Rate, rhythm, and axis**
   a. Rate: Read the rate in beats per minute (bpm) directly from the computer interpretation or use one of the following methods:
      i. 60/RR interval = rate (in bpm)
      ii. (# of R waves in 6 large boxes) X 50 = rate (in bpm)
   b. Rhythm
      i. Regular vs irregular
      ii. Sinus or non-sinus: Sinus rhythm *always* has a P wave before every QRS, a normal PR interval for age, and a normal P wave axis.
   c. Axis: This refers to the vector of electrical force. Calculate the axis for P waves, QRS complexes, and T waves by using leads I and aVF. To determine axis of any wave
      i. Look at the wave voltage in lead I and aVF and determine if the wave is positive or negative (ie, most of the wave is above [positive] or below [negative] the isoelectric line. Then, determine the quadrant of the axis .

Lead I	aVF	Axis
+	+	0–90 (normal)
+	–	0–$^{-}$90 (left)
–	+	90–180 (right)
–	–	$^{-}$90–180 (superior)

  ii. P wave axis: Normal is upright P wave in lead I and aVF. All other configurations are abnormal (non-sinus).

  iii. QRS axis: Always interpret the QRS axis relative to the patient's age, as normal will vary. Newborns typically have a right axis, while the normal adult ECG form is present by 3 years of age, with most of the changes occurring in the first 3 to 6 months of life.

  iv. T wave axis: Normal is upright in lead I and aVF, except in the first day of life when lead I may be negative.

4. Waves and intervals

  a. P wave morphology: Check the height and duration; look for notched or biphasic waves or changing morphologies.

  b. QRS morphology: Assess the amplitude, duration, presence of Q waves, R/S progression, and the R/S ratio.

  c. ST-T wave morphology: Look for elevated or depressed ST segments, alternating polarity, and notched T waves and note the amplitude.

  d. PR interval: Determine whether it is prolonged or short for age, or varying over time.

  e. QTc interval: Calculate using Bazett formula QTc = QT/√RR interval. Although the QTc varies with age, consider any QTc 0.45 or greater to be abnormal.

5. Chamber hypertrophy

  a. Right atrial hypertrophy

    i. Tall P waves greater than 3 mm in any lead, most commonly II, V1 and V2

  b. Left atrial hypertrophy

    i. Prolonged P wave duration (>0.1 sec) in any lead

    ii. Notched or biphasic P wave in V1

  c. Biatrial hypertrophy

    i. Combination of P wave prolongation and increased P wave amplitude

  d. Right ventricular hypertrophy (RVH)

    i. Right axis deviation

    ii. R in V1 or S in V6 greater than 98th percentile for age

    iii. Upright T in V1 after day of life 3

    iv. R/S ratio greater than reference in V1 or less than reference in V6

Table 5-1. ECG Reference Values[a]

					V_1			V_6		
Age	HR (bpm)	QRS Axis	PR Interval (sec)	QRS Duration (sec)	R wave Amplitude (mm)	S wave Amplitude (mm)	R/S Ratio	R wave Amplitude (mm)	S wave Amplitude (mm)	R/S Ratio
0–7 d	95–160 (125)	30 to 180 (110)	0.08–0.12 (0.10)	0.05 (0.07)	13.3 (25.5)	7.7 (18.8)	2.5	4.8 (11.8)	3.2 (9.6)	2.2
1–3 wk	105–180 (145)	30 to 180 (110)	0.08–0.12 (0.10)	0.05 (0.07)	10.6 (20.8)	4.2 (10.8)	2.9	7.6 (16.4)	3.4 (9.8)	3.3
1–6 mo	110–180 (145)	10 to 125 (70)	0.08–0.13 (0.11)	0.05 (0.07)	9.7 (19)	5.4 (15)	2.3	12.4 (22)	2.8 (8.3)	5.6
6–12 mo	110–170 (135)	10 to 125 (60)	0.10–0.14 (0.12)	0.05 (0.07)	9.4 (20.3)	6.4 (18.1)	1.6	12.6 (22.7)	2.1 (7.2)	7.6
1–3 y	90–150 (120)	10 to 125 (60)	0.10–0.14 (0.12)	0.06 (0.07)	8.5 (18)	9 (21)	1.2	14 (23.3)	1.7 (6)	10
4–5 y	65–135 (110)	0 to 110 (60)	0.11–0.15 (0.13)	0.07 (0.08)	7.6 (16)	11 (22.5)	0.8	15.6 (25)	1.4 (4.7)	11.2
6–8 y	60–130 (100)	-15 to 110 (60)	0.12–0.16 (0.14)	0.07 (0.08)	6 (13)	12 (24.5)	0.6	16.3 (26)	1.1 (3.9)	13
9–11 y	60–110 (85)	-15 to 110 (60)	0.12–0.17 (0.15)	0.07 (0.09)	5.4 (12.1)	11.9 (25.4)	0.5	16.3 (25.4)	1 (3.9)	14.3
12–16 y	60–110 (85)	-15 to 110 (60)	0.12–0.17 (0.14)	0.07 (0.10)	4.1 (9.9)	10.8 (21.2)	0.5	14.3 (23)	0.8 (3.7)	14.7
>16 y	60–100 (80)	-15 to 110 (60)	0.12–0.20 (0.15)	0.08 (0.10)	3 (9)	10 (20)	0.3	10 (20)	0.8 (3.7)	12
	range (mean)	range (mean)	range (mean)	mean (98th %ile)	mean (98th %ile)	mean (98th %ile)		mean (98th %ile)	mean (98th %ile)	

[a]From Tschudy MM, Arcara KM, eds. *The Harriet Lane Handbook*. 19th ed. Philadelphia,PA: Elsevier Mosby; 2012: 170, with permission from Elsevier.

v. Q in V1 (qR or qRs pattern) also suggests RVH
vi. Voltage criteria for RVH with abnormal T wave axis indicates strain pattern

e. Left ventricular hypertrophy (LVH)
i. Left axis deviation
ii. R in V6 or S in V1 greater than 98th percentile for age
iii. R/S ratio less than reference in V1 or greater than reference in V6
iv. Q in V5 or V6 5 mm or greater with tall T waves in those leads
v. Voltage criteria for LVH with abnormal T wave axis indicates strain pattern

f. Biventricular hypertrophy
i. Voltage criteria for LVH and RVH in the absence of a bundle branch block or preexcitation (see below)
ii. Voltage criteria for RVH or LVH and relatively large voltages for the other ventricle
iii. Large, equiphasic QRS complexes in 2 or more limb leads and in V2-V5

6. **Conduction disturbances**

a. Right bundle branch block (RBBB): This is the most common conduction disturbance seen in children. The differential diagnosis includes S/P open heart surgery, right ventricular volume overload, Ebstein anomaly, coarctation of the aorta, cardiomyopathy, myocarditis, heart failure, muscular dystrophies, Kearn-Sayre syndrome, Brugada syndrome, arrhythmogenic right ventricular dysplasia, and congenital hereditary RBBB. Criteria for RBBB include
i. Right axis deviation
ii. Prolonged QRS for age
iii. Terminal slurring of QRS
1. Wide slurred S in I, V5, V6
2. Terminal slurred R' in aVR, V4R, V1, V2
iv. ST depression and T wave inversion (not common in children)

b. Left bundle branch block (LBBB): This is rare in children now that ventriculotomies are rarely performed, but can be seen after cardiac surgery (especially after procedures on the left side of the heart), and in hypertrophic cardiomyopathy and myocarditis. Criteria for LBBB include
i. Left axis deviation
ii. Prolonged QRS for age
iii. Loss of Q in V5 and V6
iv. QS pattern in V1

v. Slurred QRS
   1. Slurred, wide R in I aVL, V5, V6
   2. Wide S in V1, V2

vi. ST depression and T wave inversion in V4-V6

c. Intraventricular block
   i. Prolongation of entire QRS complex
   ii. This suggests a serious underlying diffuse myocardial disease, metabolic derangements such as hyperkalemia, severe hypoxia/ ischemia, or drug toxicity

d. Preexcitation: This occurs when there is accelerated atrioventricular conduction to one ventricle via an accessory pathway, such as Wolff Parkinson White syndrome. Criteria are
   i. Short PR interval for age
   ii. Delta wave
   iii. Wide QRS for age

Common Patterns in Clinical Diseases

1. **Innocent murmurs:** No abnormal ECG changes
2. **Pathologic murmurs** (associated with structural heart disease): See Table 5-2.
3. **Chest pain/ischemia**
   a. Since 96% of all cases of pediatric cases of chest pain are noncardiac, most ECGs will be normal. Clinical manifestations that should be more concerning for underlying cardiac chest pain include chest pain with exertion; diaphoresis; pallor; anxiety; shortness of breath; nausea/ vomiting; radiation of pain to arm, jaw, neck, or back; and syncope.

Table 5-2. ECG Findings in Structural Heart Disease

Heart Condition	ECG Findings
Aortic regurgitation	Normal to LVH, LAH
Aortic valve stenosis	Normal to LVH; strain pattern
Atrial septal defect	RAD, RVH, RBBB
Coarctation of the aorta	LVH; infants may have RBBB or RVH
Endocardial cushion defect	Superior QRS axis, LVH or BVH
Hypertrophic obstructive cardiomyopathy	LVH, deep Q waves in VS and V6
Patent ductus arteriosus	Normal to LVH or BVH
Pulmonary stenosis	Normal to RAD, RVH, (RAH in severe cases)
Tetralogy of Fallot	RAD, RVH or BVH, possibly RAH
Ventricular septal defect	Normal to LVH or BVH

Abbreviations: BVH, biventricular hypertrophy; ECG, electrocardiogram; LAH, left atrial hypertrophy; LVH, left ventricular hypertrophy; RAH, right atrial hypertrophy; RAD, right axis deviation; RBBB, right bundle branch block; RVH, right ventricular hypertrophy.

b. Ischemia follows a progression from elevated ST segments with deep, wide Q waves in the hyperacute phase, followed by deep, wide Q waves with elevated ST segments and biphasic or inverted T waves in the evolving phase, followed by deep, wide Q waves and almost normal T waves.
c. Serial ECGs become important when ischemia is suspected as 40% to 65% of initial ECGs in the setting of myocardial infarction are normal.

4. **Myocarditis**
   a. ECG findings are variable in myocarditis. Any of the following may be seen:
      i. Low voltage QRS
      ii. Nonspecific ST segment changes, T wave inversion possible
      iii. Long QT interval
      iv. Arrhythmias, especially premature atrial or ventricular contractions
5. **Pericarditis**
   a. Low voltage QRS caused by pericardial effusion
   b. ST-T changes follow a time-dependent progression
      i. Initially have ST segment elevation
      ii. Returns to normal over 2 to 3 days
      iii. T wave inversion 2 to 4 weeks after onset of disease
6. **Long QT syndrome**
   a. QTc varies with age; rule of thumb is that any QTc greater than 0.45 is abnormal and requires evaluation by a cardiologist
   b. In addition to prolonged QTc, can also see abnormal T wave morphology, bradycardia, second-degree atrioventricular block, multifocal premature ventricular contractions, and ventricular tachycardia.
   c. Screen all first-degree relatives of the patient to look for familial long QT syndromes such as
      i. Jervell and Lange-Nielsen syndrome: Congenital deafness, syncope, family history of sudden death
      ii. Romano-Ward syndrome: Same findings as Jervell and Lange-Nielsen syndrome but with normal hearing
      iii. Timothy syndrome: Webbed fingers and toes
      iv. Anderson-Tawil syndrome: Muscle weakness, periodic paralysis, ventricular arrhythmias, developmental delays
7. **Electrolyte disorders**
   a. Hyperkalemia: ECG changes vary with level of hyperkalemia
      i. Greater than 6 mEq/L: Tall, peaked T waves
      ii. Greater than 7.5 mEq/L: Widened QRS, PR prolongation, tall T waves

   iii. Greater than 9 mEq/L: Disappearance of P waves and sinusoidal QRS; ultimately leads to asystole
b. Hypokalemia: Changes not apparent until potassium is less than 2.5 mEq/L
   i. Depressed ST segments, biphasic T waves, prolonged QTc, possible appearance of U waves
c. Hypercalcemia: Serum greater than 11 mg/dL or ionized greater than 5mg/dL
   i. Shortened ST segment without changing T wave morphology
   ii. Shortened QTc interval
d. Hypocalcemia: Infant serum greater than 11 mg/dL or ionized greater than 5 mg/dL; child serum less than 8.5 mg/dL or ionized less than 4.5 mg/dL
   i. Prolonged ST segment without changing T wave morphology
   ii. Prolonged QTc interval

8. **Kawasaki disease**
   a. Up to 60% have prolonged PR interval during the acute presentation
   b. May see arrhythmias, nonspecific ST-T wave changes, or ischemic changes with severe disease
9. **Lyme carditis**
   a. PR interval prolongation

Ambulatory Monitoring

1. **Ambulatory monitors,** which can be initiated either in the inpatient setting or at time of discharge, are indicated in the following situations:
   a. Determine if chest pain, palpitation, or syncope are arrhythmic in origin.
   b. Evaluate efficacy of antiarrhythmic therapy.
   c. Screen high-risk cardiac patients (cardiomyopathies, postoperative).
   d. Evaluate implanted pacemaker dysfunction.
   e. Determine the effects of sleep on arrhythmias.
2. **Holter monitors** are for short duration (24–72 hours).
3. **Event recorders** can monitor longer periods. When symptoms are sensed, the patient is expected to press a button. This records the current ECG, as well as a time-limited amount of the ECG preceding and following the event trigger.

Pearls and Pitfalls

- The only way to interpret an ECG correctly is within the context of the clinical history, medical factors, and age-appropriate reference values.
- Use the same interpretation system and calipers for every ECG.
- Look at many normal ECGs, as it is the only way to recognize an abnormal one.
- Leads may be cut lengthwise to ensure proper placement on an infant's chest. If something doesn't seem right, discuss with a pediatric cardiologist.

Coding

CPT

ECG, routine with at least 12 leads, interpretation and report only **93010**

Bibliography

Davignon A, Rautaharju P, Boisselle E, et al. Normal ECG standards for infants and children. *Ped Cardiol.* 1979/80;1:123–131

Frazier A, Southern-Pruette C. Cardiology. In: Custer J, Rau R, eds. *The Harriet Lane Handbook*. 18th ed. Philadelphia, PA: Mosby; 2009:173–202

Park M. Cardiovascular infections. *Pediatric Cardiology for Practitioners*. 5th ed. Philadelphia, PA: Mosby Elsevier; 2008:351–380

Park M. Electrocardiography. *Pediatric Cardiology for Practitioners*. 5th ed. Philadelphia, PA: Mosby Elsevier; 2008:40–65

Park M, Guntheroth W. *How to Read Pediatric ECGs*. 4th ed. Philadelphia, PA: Mosby Elsevier; 2006

CHAPTER 6

Endocarditis

Introduction

Infective endocarditis (IE) is an infection of the endothelium of the heart initiated by endothelial damage, leading to adherence of bacteria and ultimately the entrapment of organisms that evade host defenses. The incidence is approximately 1:1,500 pediatric admissions a year. However, the incidence is increasing as a result of the survival of children with congenital heart disease (CHD) and the more frequent use of indwelling central venous catheters (CVCs), especially in premature infants. Although IE is rare in children, there is significant morbidity and mortality.

The most common organisms causing IE are *Staphylococcus aureus* (especially for acute IE), *Streptococcus viridans*, coagulase-negative staphylococcus, pneumococcus, HACEK organisms (*Haemophilus* species, *Actinobacillus actinomycetemcomitans*, *Cardiobacterium moninus*, *Eikenella corrodens*, and *Kingella kingae*), enterococcus, and *Candida* (especially in newborns). However, blood cultures are negative in 5% to 7% of cases.

IE can be a subacute or acute process. Subacute IE presents with nonspecific symptoms and is caused by less virulent organisms. Acute IE is a fulminant disease presenting with high fever and a toxic-appearing patient. *S aureus* is more often associated with acute IE.

Clinical Presentation

History

Subacute IE usually presents with nonspecific signs and symptoms, such as prolonged fever, fatigue, weakness, arthralgias, myalgias, and weight loss. Occasionally, the presentation is acute with high fever and shock. There is often a history of CHD (especially cyanotic), cardiac surgery, indwelling catheters, prematurity, or previous history of endocarditis.

Physical Examination

There are rarely physical findings in subacute IE. A new heart murmur is neither necessary nor sufficient for the diagnosis. Extracardiac manifestations (Osler nodes, Roth spots, Janeway lesions, petechiae, hemorrhages, splenomegaly, glomerulonephritis) are rare in children, but can represent septic emboli or immune complexes in the brain, kidney, gastrointestinal tract, extremities, and lungs. In contrast, acute IE can present with the physical findings associated with shock, including hypotension, tachycardia, and tachypnea, along with high fever and signs of congestive heart failure.

Laboratory

If IE is suspected, obtain a complete blood cell count (the patient may be anemic secondary to hemolysis or chronic disease), erythrocyte sedimentation rate or C-reactive protein (usually elevated), rheumatoid factor (often elevated), and a urinalysis (an immune complex glomerulonephritis can lead to red blood cell casts and proteinuria).

Obtain 3 blood cultures from separate venipunctures on the first day, then 2 more if the first ones have no growth at 48 hours. If acute IE is suspected, obtain 4 cultures, with at least 1 hour time span from the first one to the fourth. Ensure that the sample size is sufficient (1–3 mL in an infant, 5–7 mL in a young child), but if there is difficulty obtaining an adequate sample, inoculate the aerobic culture only.

Radiology

Order a transthoracic echocardiogram (TTE) when IE is suspected. Although a TTE is sufficient for most pediatric patients, order a transesophageal echocardiogram for a patient who is obese, particularly muscular, is post–cardiac surgery, or has compromised respiratory function.

Differential Diagnosis

The diagnosis of IE can be challenging; use the modified Duke criteria (Table 6-1 and Box 6-1).

Box 6-1. Identifying Infective Endocarditis (IE) Using Modified Duke Criteria
Definite
Pathologic criteria: Microorganism by culture or histology of vegetation or abscess
2 major criteria
1 major criterion and 3 minor criteria
5 minor criteria
Possible
1 major criterion and 1 minor criterion
3 minor criteria
Rejected
Resolution in ≤4 days antibiotics
Not meeting criteria for possible IE
No pathologic evidence of IE at surgery or autopsy with ≤4 days antibiotics
Alternate diagnosis

Consider the diagnosis of IE for a patient with fever of unknown origin, new murmur, history of cardiac disease (especially after cardiac surgery), or history of CVC (Table 6-2).

Table 6-1. Modified Duke Criteria

Major	
Positive blood culture	2 blood cultures with microorganism consistent with infective endocarditis (*Streptococcus viridans*, *Streptococcus bovis*, *Staphylococcus aureus*, HACEK, enterococci) ≥2 positive blood cultures >12 h apart ≥3 positive blood cultures at least 1 h apart Positive blood culture for *Coxiella burnetii* or antiphase-I IgG Ab titer >1:800
Endocardial involvement	Positive echocardiogram: oscillating mass (vegetation), abscess, new dehiscence of prosthetic valve *or* New valvular regurgitation
Minor	
Vascular phenomena	Arterial emboli, intracranial or conjunctival hemorrhage, septic pulmonary infarct, mycotic aneurysm, Janeway lesion
Immunologic phenomena	Glomerulonephritis, Osler nodes, Roth spots, (+) rheumatoid factor
Microbiological evidence	Positive blood culture not meeting major criteria *or* serologic evidence of infection
Predisposition	Heart condition Intravenous drug use
Fever	

Table 6-2. Differential Diagnosis of Infective Endocarditis (IE)

Sign/Symptom	Diagnoses
Prolonged fever	Bartonellosis Collagen vascular diseases Inflammatory bowel disease Kawasaki disease Malignancy Occult abscess Osteoarticular infections
New murmur	Anemia Fever Innocent murmur Previously undiagnosed cardiac anomaly
Positive blood culture	Bacteremia or sepsis without IE Contaminated specimen

Treatment

Consult both a cardiologist and infectious diseases specialist. While antibiotics are the mainstay of treatment for IE, they can generally be held until cultures are positive in a patient with stable, subacute IE. The antibiotic therapy for IE is complex. Choose a regimen in consultation with an infectious diseases specialist, taking into account the organism, sensitivities, and whether the patient has native or prosthetic cardiac material (Tables 6-3 and 6-4). For specific treatment regimens, refer to the American Heart Association statement, *Unique Features of Infective Endocarditis in Childhood* at http://circ.ahajournals.org/cgi/content/full/105/17/2115.

Indications for surgery for IE include large vegetations (>1 cm), anterior mitral valve leaflet vegetation, growing vegetation after therapy, extension of abscess after therapy, valvular dysfunction, heart failure, heart block, embolic events after therapy, fungal endocarditis, and mycotic aneurysm.

Endocarditis prophylaxis is suggested for a limited number of cardiac diseases during dental procedures and some respiratory, skin, and musculoskeletal procedures. Refer to the American Heart Association statement for

Table 6-3. Treatment of Infective Endocarditis of Native Valve Caused by *Streptococcus viridans* or *Streptococcus bovis*

Susceptibility	Antibiotic	Dose: kg/day	Frequency	Duration
Highly penicillin susceptible	Penicillin G *or*	200,000 units	q 4–6 h	4 weeks
	Ampicillin *or*	300 mg	q 4–6 h	4 weeks
	Ceftriaxone *or*	100 mg	q day	4 weeks
	Vancomycin (if unable to tolerate β-lactams)	40 mg	q 6–12 h	4 weeks

Notes

1. If the organism is relatively resistant to penicillin, use the same regimen as above, but increase the dose of penicillin to 300,000 units/kg/day for 4 weeks with gentamicin (3 mg/kg/day divided q 8 h or q day) for first 2 weeks.
2. If the valve is prosthetic, use same regimen as above, but 6 weeks with gentamicin for first 2 weeks.
3. For enterococcus or high level of resistance to penicillin, use the same regimen as above, increase the dose of penicillin to 300,000 units/kg/day plus gentamicin, both for 4 weeks if <3 months duration symptoms or 6 weeks if >3 months.

Table 6-4. Treatment of Infective Endocarditis of Native Valve Caused by Staphylococci

Susceptibility	Antibiotic	Dose: kg/day	Frequency	Duration
Methicillin susceptible	Nafcillin *or* oxacillin, *with or without* gentamicin	200 mg 3 mg IV/IM	q 4–6 h q 8–24 h	4 weeks 4 weeks

Notes

1. If patient is unable to tolerate penicillins, use vancomycin as for *S viridans*.
2. If methicillin resistant, use vancomycin for 6 weeks plus gentamicin for the first 3–5 days.
3. If the valve is prosthetic, add rifampin (20 mg/kg/day PO or IV, divided q 8 h for 6 weeks) to above regimens, with gentamicin for the first 2 weeks.
4. For HACEK organisms, use ceftriaxone (100 mg/kg/day IV q 24 h; 4 weeks native valves, 6 weeks for prosthetic material).
5. For fungal IE, use Amphotericin B, but the patient will often require surgery and long-term imidazole suppressive therapy.

indications and prophylaxis doses at http://circ.ahajournals.org/cgi/content/full/116/15/1736.

Indications for Consultation

- **Cardiology:** All patients (echocardiography interpretation)
- **Cardiothoracic surgery:** If surgery is indicated
- **Infectious disease:** All patients, especially for resistant or unusual organisms

Disposition

- **Intensive care unit transfer:** Shock, embolic events (especially with organ dysfunction), unstable vegetation, cardiothoracic surgery required
- **Interinstitutional transfer:** For cardiology consult, if not available locally
- **Discharge criteria:** Afebrile, blood cultures negative, completed intravenous antibiotic course or the patient is a good candidate for outpatient antibiotics (condition is stable, afebrile, low risk for embolism, peripherally inserted central catheter is placed, home nursing arranged, family is willing)

Follow-up

- **Primary care:** 1–2 weeks
- **Cardiology:** 1 week
- **Repeat echocardiogram:** Clinical deterioration during treatment in a patient with an abnormal echocardiogram and at completion of treatment
- **Repeat blood culture:** 8 weeks after completion of antibiotics to document cure

Pearls and Pitfalls

- Include IE in a fever of unknown origin workup.
- Antibiotic therapy can be delayed until cultures positive in stable, subacute IE.
- IE can be diagnosed in setting of negative blood culture and/or negative echocardiogram.

Coding

ICD-9

- Acute and subacute bacterial endocarditis **421.0**
- Acute endocarditis, unspecified **421.9**
- Endocarditis valve unspecified **424.9**

Bibliography

Day MD, Gauvreau K, Shulman S, Newburger JW. Characteristics of children hospitalized with infective endocarditis. *Circulation.* 2009;119:865–870

Ferrieri P, Gewitz MH, Gerber MA, et al. Unique features of infective endocarditis in childhood. *Pediatrics.* 2002;109:931–943

Li JS, Sexton DJ, Mick N, et al. Proposed modifications to the Duke criteria for the diagnosis of infective endocarditis. *Clin Infect Dis.* 2000;30:633–638

Rosenthal LB, Feja KN, Levasseur SM, et al. The changing epidemiology of pediatric endocarditis at a children's hospital over seven decades. *Pediatr Cardiol.* 2010;31:813–820

Tissières P, Gervaix A, Beghetti M, Jaeggi ET. Value and limitations of the von Reyn, Duke, and modified Duke criteria for the diagnosis of infective endocarditis in children. *Pediatrics*. 2003;112:e467

Wilson W, Taubert KA, Gewitz M, et al. Prevention of infective endocarditis: guidelines from the American Heart Association: a guideline from the American Heart Association Rheumatic Fever, Endocarditis, and Kawasaki Disease Committee, Council on Cardiovascular Disease in the Young, Council on Clinical Cardiology, Council on Cardiovascular Surgery and Anesthesia, and the Quality of Care and Outcomes Research Interdisciplinary Working Group. *Circulation*. 2007;116:1736–1754

Myocarditis

Introduction

Acute myocarditis is inflammation of the muscular wall of the heart, which may also potentially extend to involve the endocardium and pericardium. Most cases in the United States are caused by viruses, historically coxsackievirus and adenovirus. However, more recently, parvovirus B-19, human herpesvirus-6, cytomegalovirus (CMV), Epstein-Barr virus (EBV), and novel H1N1 influenza have become more frequent. Other less common infectious causes include bacteria (meningococcus, *Streptococcus, Staphylococcus, Listeria,* and *Mycobacterium* species), spirochetes (*Borrelia burgdorferi*), *Rickettsia* species (especially scrub typhus), and protozoa (*Trypanosoma cruzi*). In addition, drugs can cause myocardial inflammation either by direct toxic effect (chemotherapeutic agents) or by inducing hypersensitivity reactions (anticonvulsants, antipsychotics, antibiotics). Often, however, the specific agent causing the myocarditis is not identified.

The presentation of myocarditis ranges from subclinical or mild disease with spontaneous resolution to fulminant disease with cardiogenic shock. Mortality can be high (up to 33%). About one-third of patients will have a full cardiac recovery and another one-third will have cardiac sequelae, including dilated cardiomyopathy ultimately necessitating cardiac transplantation. Interestingly, a patient who presents with fulminant myocarditis but survives the initial acute phase of illness is more likely to have a complete cardiac recovery than someone with a less severe acute presentation.

Clinical Presentation

History

The clinical presentation varies according to age and severity of disease. An infant often presents with nonspecific symptoms, including poor feeding, fever, tachypnea, irritability, listlessness, pallor, diaphoresis, vomiting without diarrhea, and episodic cyanosis. In addition, an infant is more likely to have a fulminant presentation requiring advanced cardiorespiratory support early in the course. An older child can present with a nonspecific flu-like illness or gastroenteritis. In more severe cases, there may be symptoms of congestive heart failure (CHF), including malaise, decreased appetite, shortness of breath, and exercise intolerance.

An adolescent may complain of chest pain similar to ischemia, with anterior chest pressure radiating to the neck and arms, in addition to the other symptoms noted previously. An older patient can also present with palpitations, syncope and, rarely, sudden death. A patient with pancarditis (myocarditis and pericarditis) will present with precordial pain that varies with respiration and position.

Physical Examination

Look for signs of heart failure or cardiogenic shock, including hypotension, tachypnea, hepatomegaly, abnormal heart sounds (including an S3 or S4 gallop), a murmur associated with mitral or tricuspid insufficiency, abnormal lung examination with evidence of pulmonary venous congestion (rales), and poor perfusion (weak pulses and prolonged capillary refill time). Tachycardia out of proportion to the fever or hydration status is a frequent, but not universal, finding.

Laboratory

Obtain a complete blood cell count and either a C-reactive protein or erythrocyte sedimentation rate. While inflammatory markers are often elevated, they rarely provide insight into the etiology. To identify a possible pathogen, send a blood culture, polymerase chain reaction of nasal or tracheal aspirates for viruses, viral titers (CMV, EBV, and parvovirus), nasal and rectal viral cultures, and a Lyme titer if epidemiology dictates. Send cardiac troponins (troponin I and T) and cardiac enzymes, including a creatine kinase-MB. Elevated troponins help to confirm the diagnosis, although normal results do not exclude the diagnosis of myocarditis.

Obtain a chest radiograph, which will frequently document cardiomegaly. Other findings include pulmonary venous congestion, interstitial infiltrates, or pleural effusions. Also obtain a 12-lead electrocardiogram (ECG). The most common ECG findings are sinus tachycardia, low voltage QRS complexes, and nonspecific T wave changes. Other ECG changes can mimic those of myocardial infarction or pericarditis, including ST segment changes and pathologic Q waves. Arrhythmias, such as supraventricular or ventricular tachycardia, or varying degrees of atrioventricular block, can also be present.

Order a transthoracic echocardiogram, which can help rule out other causes of cardiac dysfunction, including vegetation (endocarditis) and pericardial effusion (pericarditis). The findings in myocarditis are variable and can include left ventricular or biventricular dysfunction, dilatation, wall motion abnormalities, and mitral and tricuspid valve regurgitation. The loss of right ventricular function is the best predictor of death or need for cardiac transplant. A pericardial effusion, if present, is typically small.

The gold standard for the diagnosis of myocarditis has been endomyocardial biopsy. However, it has fallen out of favor as a result of the low sensitivity for diagnosis and the risk associated with the procedure in a patient with myocardial inflammation. Cardiac magnetic resonance imaging with gadolinium, when available, is becoming a more useful diagnostic tool, since it allows visualization of the entire myocardium and is noninvasive.

Differential Diagnosis

The presentation of myocarditis is variable, depending on disease severity. Since it can be subtle, a high index of suspicion is needed to diagnose a nonfulminant case. Consider myocarditis in any patient with vomiting without diarrhea, respiratory distress, tachycardia out of proportion to the fever or hydration status, new-onset CHF or arrhythmia, or ischemic chest pain. Myocarditis can often be initially mistaken for an acute viral illness or respiratory disorder. Other entities to consider include myocardial ischemia or infarction, pericarditis with or without myocarditis, endocarditis, other causes of CHF (see page 19), dilated cardiomyopathy, and pulmonary embolism. Inflammatory processes such as systemic lupus erythematosus, rheumatic fever, and Kawasaki disease can also present with myocarditis.

Treatment

If myocarditis is suspected, immediately consult a cardiologist who can direct further workup and management. However, the treatment for myocarditis remains largely supportive. If a treatable infectious pathogen is identified, give the appropriate therapy. Closely monitor hemodynamic status for signs of worsening cardiac function or shock. Observe a patient who presents with mild disease for developing signs of heart failure. Depending on the disease severity, recommend bed rest to reduce metabolic needs.

With the guidance of a pediatric cardiologist, treat a patient presenting with heart failure with traditional heart failure therapy, such as diuretics, angiotensin converting enzyme inhibitors, angiotensin receptor antagonists, and β-blockers (see Congestive Heart Failure, page 19). Manage an arrhythmia with the appropriate medications (see Arrhythmias, page 11), although a persistent arrhythmia may require temporary or permanent pacing, and possibly an implantable cardioverter defibrillator.

The consulting cardiologist may suggest steroids and intravenous immunoglobulins, although their use is controversial.

A patient presenting with profound shock may require mechanical ventilation (to reduce metabolic demand), cardiac afterload reduction, and/or inotropic support. Other potential treatment modalities include circulatory support via extracorporeal membrane oxygenation (ECMO) and, if the clinical picture deteriorates despite medical management, a ventricular assist device (VAD). If the patient is refractory to both medical and mechanical circulatory efforts, consider a transfer to a center that performs cardiac transplantation.

Indications for Consultation

- **Cardiology:** Suspected myocarditis
- **Infectious disease:** Myocarditis secondary to sepsis, spirochetes, or protozoa

Disposition

- **Intensive care unit transfer:** Symptomatic myocarditis
- **Interinstitutional transfer:** Patient requires technology or management options not available locally (echocardiogram, pediatric intensive care unit, ECMO, VAD, transplantation), or a pediatric cardiologist is not immediately available
- **Discharge criteria:** Stable or improving cardiac function, managed with oral medication. Advise the patient to refrain from competitive sports and vigorous exercise until cleared by a pediatric cardiologist.

Follow-up

- **Cardiology:** 2 days to 2 weeks, depending on the severity of the illness
- **Primary care:** 3 to 5 days

Pearls and Pitfalls

- Given the often subtle, nonspecific, and variable presentations of a patient with myocarditis, prompt diagnosis requires a high index of suspicion.
- Suspect myocarditis when a patient with presumed gastroenteritis/dehydration worsens after fluid boluses.
- Suspect myocarditis in any patient with unexplained CHF or arrhythmia, especially following an acute viral illness.

Coding

ICD-9

- Acute myocarditis in diseases classified elsewhere **422.0**
- Acute myocarditis, unspecified **422.90**
- Coxsackie myocarditis **074.23**
- Idiopathic myocarditis **422.91**
- Influenza myocarditis **487.8**
- Septic myocarditis **422.92**
- Tuberculous myocarditis **017.9** and **422.0**

Bibliography

Blauwet LA, Cooper LT. Myocarditis: *Prog Cardiovasc Dis.* 2010;52:274–288

Durani Y, Giordano K, Goudie BW. Myocarditis and pericarditis in children. *Pediatr Clin North Am.* 2010;57:1281–1303

Levine MC, Klugman D, Teach SJ. Update on myocarditis in children. *Curr Opin Pediatr.* 2010;22:278–283

Towbin JA. Myocarditis. In: Allen HD, Driscoll DJ, Shaddy RE, Feltes TF, eds. *Moss and Adam's Heart Disease in Infants, Children and Adolescents.* 7th ed. Philadelphia, PA: Lippincott, Williams & Wilkins; 2008:1207–1225

Vashist S, Gautam KS. Acute myocarditis in children: current concepts and management. *Curr Treat Options Cardiovasc Med.* 2009;11:383–391

CHAPTER 8

Pericarditis

Introduction

Acute pericarditis is an inflammatory condition of the fibrous pericardium surrounding the heart, often accompanied by an effusion in the pericardial cavity. It may occur in isolation or as part of a systemic disease. Most cases of pericarditis are considered idiopathic because no source can be identified. However, specific etiologies include viral infection (most often enteroviruses), bacterial infection (purulent pericarditis), tuberculosis, connective tissue or collagen vascular diseases, metabolic diseases, uremia, neoplasms, drug reactions, trauma, and postpericardiotomy syndrome.

Purulent pericarditis is most often associated with infection at another site with hematogenous or direct spread. The most common causative organisms are *Staphylococcus aureus*, group A β-hemolytic streptococcus, pneumococcus, and meningococcus. Complications of pericarditis include pericardial constriction and cardiac tamponade, which is acute compression of the heart from increased intrapericardial pressure due to pericardial effusion.

Clinical Presentation

History

The classic presentation of acute pericarditis is the sudden onset of chest pain that is pleuritic in nature (exacerbated by inspiration), worse when recumbent, and alleviated by sitting upright and leaning forward. The pain can radiate to the neck, arms, back, or shoulders. In a younger child, however, chest pain may be absent. Instead, the patient is more likely to present with tachycardia, tachypnea, and fever. A child with viral pericarditis may have a history of a recent upper respiratory infection or gastroenteritis, while bacterial pericarditis is generally more acute in onset with symptoms developing over a few days.

Physical Examination

A pericardial friction rub is diagnostic, but not always present. Auscultate while the patient is leaning forward. With large effusions the heart sounds may be muffled.

A patient with cardiac tamponade will be ill-appearing with signs of right heart failure (lower extremity edema, hepatomegaly) and poor systemic perfusion (weak pulses, cool extremities, delayed capillary refill) due to decreased cardiac output. Other findings suggestive of tamponade include pulsus paradoxus (a decrease in systolic blood pressure of more than 10 mm Hg with inspiration) and Beck triad (systemic hypotension, elevated jugular venous pressure, and muffled heart sounds).

Laboratory

Obtain a complete blood cell count and either a C-reactive protein or erythrocyte sedimentation rate. While these are often elevated, they rarely provide insight into the etiology, although a markedly elevated white blood cell count can suggest bacterial pericarditis. Obtain a blood culture when sepsis is suspected (fever, tachycardia, toxic appearance). Obtain serologic testing, including antinuclear antibody and rheumatoid factor, in cases with suggestive signs and symptoms, such as arthritis, rash, or weight loss. Obtain cardiac enzymes when the diagnosis is unclear. Troponin I may be mildly elevated in pericarditis, while creatine kinase-MB elevation occurs in myopericarditis.

Obtain a chest radiograph, which may be normal or show an enlarged cardiac silhouette with a characteristic globular ("water bottle") appearance if a large effusion is present.

Obtain a 12-lead electrocardiogram (ECG). The ECG may progress through 4 stages, from diffuse ST elevation and PR depression (the classic finding), to normalization of ST and PR segments, to diffuse T wave inversion, to normalization of T waves (Figure 8-1).

Figure 8-1. 12-Lead Electrocardiogram From a Patient With Acute Pericarditis Demonstrating Diffuse ST Elevation and PR Depression

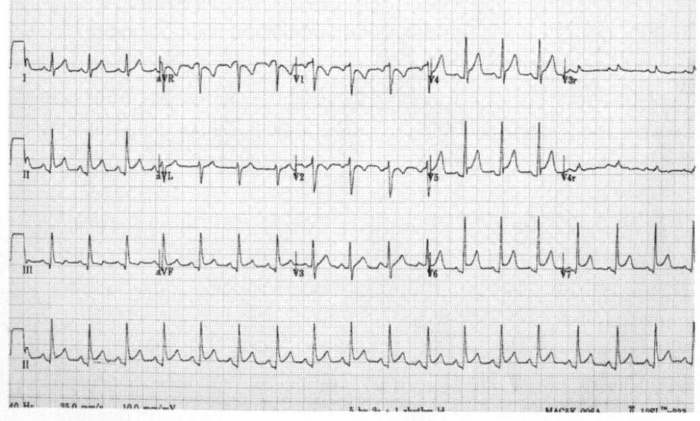

Obtain a transthoracic echocardiogram, which must be performed urgently if pericardial tamponade is suspected. The presence of a pericardial effusion on echocardiogram can support the diagnosis, although absence of an effusion does not exclude pericarditis.

Differential Diagnosis

The cause of chest pain in pediatrics is usually benign, with the most common etiologies being either idiopathic or musculoskeletal. See Table 8-1 for the differential diagnosis.

Table 8-1. Differential Diagnosis of Pericarditis

Diagnosis	Clinical Features
Costochondritis	Chest pain reproducible by palpation at costochondral junction Chest x-ray and electrocardiogram (ECG) normal
Endocarditis	Chest pain rare Echocardiogram may be positive Osler nodes, Janeway lesions, Roth spots, splinter hemorrhages
Myocardial ischemia or infarction	Non-pleuritic chest pain Friction rub absent PR depression rare T wave inversion accompanies localized ST elevation
Myocarditis	Chest pain rare Friction rub absent Signs of congestive heart failure Low QRS voltages and occasional dysrhythmias Enlarged chambers, impaired left ventricular function on echocardiogram
Pneumonia	Decreased breath sounds or other focal findings (rales) ECG normal Chest x-ray usually diagnostic
Pneumothorax	Decreased breath sounds on affected side Decreased QRS voltages, possible right shift of QRS axis Chest x-ray usually diagnostic
Pulmonary embolism	Non-pleuritic chest pain Friction rub rare No PR depression ST elevation with T wave inversion only in leads III, aVF, V1

Treatment

Closely monitor the patient's hemodynamic status. If tamponade is suspected, administer volume resuscitation (20 mL/kg of normal saline infused over 15 min) until the diagnosis is confirmed by echocardiogram and an urgent pericardiocentesis can be performed. If the clinical findings are consistent with tamponade but echocardiogram is not immediately available, do not delay pericardiocentesis. Other indications for pericardiocentesis include suspected purulent, tuberculous, or neoplastic pericarditis, or large pericardial effusions. Send the fluid for cell count, glucose, protein, Gram stain and cultures, acid-fast bacilli stain, viral polymerase chain reaction (most commonly for enterovirus) if available, triglycerides (to evaluate for chylous effusion in a patient with a history of cardiac surgery) and, if indicated, cytology.

If the clinical picture suggests a purulent pericarditis, give empiric parenteral antibiotic therapy and arrange drainage via pericardiocentesis, a pericardial catheter, or an open procedure. Start with vancomycin (60 mg/kg/day divided every 8 hours, 4 g/day maximum) combined with a third-generation cephalosporin (ceftriaxone 100 mg/kg/day divided every 12 hours, 4g/day maximum) until an organism is identified. Consult with an infectious diseases specialist to tailor the duration of antibiotic therapy, which averages about 3 to 4 weeks. At a minimum, continue the antibiotics until there is clinical resolution (no effusion, afebrile, normalization of white blood cell count).

If the patient is well-appearing, with an idiopathic or presumed viral pericarditis and a small or midsize effusion, treat with rest and a nonsteroidal anti-inflammatory agent for relief of the chest pain and inflammation. Give ibuprofen (5–10 mg/kg/dose every 6–8 hours) until symptoms resolve, typically within 1 to 2 weeks. Add ranitidine (2–4 mg/kg/day divided every 12 hours, 300 mg/day maximum) for gastroprotection while ibuprofen is administered. Routine steroid use is controversial. Use prednisone (1 mg/kg/day for 4 weeks with subsequent taper) for a patient with collagen vascular disease, an immune-mediated process, or an idiopathic effusion that is refractory to treatment with ibuprofen.

Indications for Consultation

- **Cardiology:** Suspected pericarditis
- **Infectious disease:** Purulent or tuberculous pericarditis
- **Rheumatology:** Known or suspected collagen vascular disease

Disposition

- **Intensive care unit transfer:** Suspected or confirmed cardiac tamponade
- **Interinstitutional transfer:** For cardiac consultation or drainage, if either is not available onsite

Discharge Criteria

- **Pericarditis:** Asymptomatic (no fever or chest pain)
- **Pericardial effusion:** Effusion resolved or stable
- **Patient has had a drainage procedure:** No fluid reaccumulation during 1 week of observation

Follow-up

- **Primary care:** 1 week
- **Patient with effusion:** Follow-up echocardiogram within 1 week to document resolution
- **Patient with purulent pericarditis:** Cardiology follow-up within 1 to 2 weeks

Pearls and Pitfalls

- The patient may not have the "classic" signs and symptoms of pericarditis, such as a friction rub and pleuritic chest pain that change with position.
- A chest x-ray and echocardiogram may only be useful if an effusion accompanies pericardial inflammation.
- The most reliable study for making the diagnosis of pericarditis is an ECG with characteristic ST and PR segment changes.

Coding

ICD-9

- Acute idiopathic pericarditis (includes benign, nonspecific, or viral) **420.91**
- Acute pericarditis in diseases classified elsewhere (list underlying condition first) **420.0**
- Acute pericarditis, purulent/suppurative **420.99**
- Acute pericarditis, unspecified **420.90**
- Acute rheumatic pericarditis **391.0**
- Cardiac tamponade **423.3**
- Coxsackie pericarditis **074.21**
- Pericardial effusion **423.9**

Bibliography

Demmler G. Infectious pericarditis in children. *Pediatr Infect Dis J.* 2006;25:165–166

Khandaker MH, Espinosa RE, Nishimura RA, et al. Symposium on cardiovascular diseases. Pericardial disease: diagnosis and management. *Mayo Clin Proc.* 2010;85:572–593

Lange RA, Hillis LD. Clinical practice. Acute pericarditis. *N Engl J Med.* 2004;351: 2195–2202

Rheuban KS. Pericardial diseases. In: Allen HD, Driscoll DJ, Shaddy RE, Feltes TF, eds. *Moss and Adam's Heart Disease in Infants Children, and Adolescents.* 7th ed. Philadelphia, PA: Lippincott, Williams & Wilkins; 2008:1290–1298

Shock

Introduction

Shock is a state of systemic tissue hypoperfusion and injury. It represents a final common pathway for several frequently mixed derangements in volume status, vascular tone, venous return to the heart, and cardiac pump physiology. Septic shock, which is the most common type in children, often has a progression through signs and symptoms of compensation until overt hypotension and irreversible cardiovascular collapse ensue (*decompensated shock*). Other types of shock are classified by etiology (anaphylactic, spinal or neurogenic, cardiogenic) or physiology (distributive, low cardiac output, obstructive, hypovolemic) with considerable overlap in clinical presentation. The key to successful shock therapy is the recognization of shock in its *compensated* stages.

Management of shock (along with respiratory failure and cardiac dysrhythmia and arrest) is a core portion of the American Heart Association's Pediatric Advanced Life Support (PALS) program. The American College of Critical Care Medicine's (ACCM) frequently updated pediatric septic shock guidelines have become the standard evidence-based information about shock management. The ACCM septic shock algorithm has become a part of PALS and is featured on the PALS pocket-reference card.

Clinical Presentation

History

Ask about fever, difficulty breathing, skin color (from caregiver's knowledge of baseline), changes in mental status and behavior, and urine output, as well as a history of trauma and potential sources of infection and fluid loss (cough, congestion, vomiting, diarrhea, abdominal pain, bleeding). In addition, confirm that the patient has normal immune status and no history of hemodynamically significant heart disease. If the patient has been in the hospital, review the prior 6 to 12 hours of vital signs; intake-output flow sheets; and observations by bedside nurses, respiratory therapists, and parents.

Physical Examination

The patient typically presents in compensated shock with fever (or hypothermia), tachycardia (persistent and out of proportion to fever, see below), widened pulse pressure (indicating low systemic vascular resistance), difficulty breathing, and signs of altered perfusion (pallor, mottled skin, delayed capillary refill, weak pulses, altered mental status, oliguria), but with a *normal age-approriate blood pressure*. There are a number of trendable, validated measures of ongoing decompensation. One is the pediatric early warning scoring system using 3 domains: behavior, respiratory, and cardiovascular (Table 9-1). An ongoing score 5 or higher indicates the need for intervention, rapid-response team notification and, if not readily improving, intensive care unit (ICU) transfer.

Table 9-1. Pediatric Early Warning Score (PEWS)

	0	1	2	3
Behavior	Playing Appropriate	Sleeping	Irritable	Lethargic/confused *or* ↓response to pain
Cardiovascular	Pink *or* Capillary refill 1–2 s	Pale/dusky *or* Capillary refill 3 s	Grey/cyanotic *or* Capillary refill 4 s *or* Pulse >20 above normal	Grey/cyanotic/mottled *or* Capillary refill ≥5 s *or* Pulse >30 above normal *or* Bradycardia
Respiratory	Within normal parameters No retractions	>10 above normal *or* Accessory muscle use *or* >30% FiO_2 or >3 L/min	>20 above normal *or* Retractions *or* >40% FiO_2 or >6 L/min	≥5 below normal parameters with retractions/grunting *or* >50% FiO_2 or >8 L/min
Score 2 extra for ¼ hourly nebulizers or persistent vomiting following surgery.				
From Monaghan A. Detecting and managing deterioration in children. *Paediatr Nurs.* 2005;17(1):32–35.				

Laboratory

Order a bedside glucose, complete blood cell count with differential, comprehensive chemistries (end-organ hypoperfusion leads to acute renal and hepatic injury as well as electrolyte abnormalities), and a blood culture if sepsis is a possibility. In addition, if sepsis is a concern, send a disseminated intravascular coagulation panel and type and screen. Obtain additional cultures (eg, urine, spinal fluid, cutaneous abscess, joint) depending on the history and physical examination. Obtain blood gas analysis with measurement of serum lactate (variably elevated with tissue hypoperfusion) and ionized calcium (decreased in some cases of sepsis and leading to refractory shock). In general, venous specimens are adequate for the assessment of shock. Order a chest x-ray, which may reveal infiltrates, cardiomegaly, or findings of acute respiratory distress syndrome.

Differential Diagnosis

The priority is recognizing shock early, while it is in the *compensated* stage. Viral, bacterial, and other infectious agents may cause fever and tachycardia in the absence of actual shock. In general, the pulse rises by approximately 9 beats per degree Celsius of temperature elevation. The differential diagnosis is summarized in Table 9-2.

Volume Loss

Vomiting and diarrhea, along with inadequate intake, are common symptoms of hypovolemic shock (hypovolemia is a component of other forms as well). Hemorrhage, including from accidental or inflicted trauma, is another important etiology. Typical signs and symptoms include decreased pulses, dry mucosal surfaces, delayed capillary refill, decreased skin turgor, and late tachycardia and hypotension.

Sepsis

The patient will present with fever (or hypothermia) and signs and symptoms of infection (cough, congestion, vomiting, diarrhea, skin rash, etc). As sepsis may manifest hypovolemic and distributive components (low vascular tone), as well as myocardial depression, a complex mix of phenotypes is seen. These are described as *cold shock (vasoconstricted)* and *warm shock (vasodilated)*, with considerable overlap often best discerned with invasive and/or sonographic monitoring modalities in an ICU. In general, the patient with warm shock presents with bounding pulses and flash capillary refill with wide pulse pressure reflecting low systemic vascular resistance. Cold shock presents with capillary refill delayed more than 2 seconds, cool extremities, and diminished peripheral pulses.

Cardiogenic

The typical findings are tachypnea, dyspnea, tachycardia, rales, hepatomegaly, jugular venous distention, and cardiac murmurs and gallops. Cardiomegaly and poor or delayed pulses may also be seen. Causes include congenital heart lesions, myocarditis, persistent dysrhythmias, and high-outflow conditions (anemia, vascular malformations).

Anaphylactic

The patient presents with difficulty breathing, poor aeration, and an exposure to a known or suspected allergen (food, drug, arthropod, other), with or without urticarial eruption.

Neurogenic

This involves a spinal cord injury, which leads to sympathetic denervation of the vascular bed. Warm extremities from vasodilation and relative or absolute bradycardia accompanies hypotension refractory to fluid boluses, necessitating early vasopressor support.

Obstructive

The pathophysiology is impeded venous return secondary to pneumothorax, hemothorax, pericardial tamponade, and left ventricular outflow obstructive lesions. Heart and/or lung sounds may be diminished, low voltages may be seen on electrocardiogram, and pulsus paradoxus may be noted. Distended neck veins and tracheal deviation away from the side of tension pneumothorax may also be seen.

Table 9-2. Differential Diagnosis of Shock

Diagnosis	Clinical Features
Anaphylaxis	Exposure history Skin rash, urticarial, angioedema Stridor, wheezing, dyspnea Vomiting and diarrhea
Congestive heart failure	Rales Hepatomegaly Cardiomegaly
Hypovolemia	History of fluid loss, poor intake, bleeding (including internal intravascular loss) Delayed capillary refill Dry mucosal surfaces Vital signs respond to fluid bolus(es)
Neurogenic	History of trauma Accompanying paralysis Poor response to fluid bolus(es)
Obstructive	History of trauma or cardiothoracic surgery Prominent dyspnea Muffled heart sounds Distended neck veins, especially in older patients
Sepsis	Fever Widened pulse pressure (warm shock) Poor response to fluids

Treatment

Early in the care process, consult with a critical care specialist or initiate transfer to a tertiary care center. For all forms of shock, initial management is the ABCs, including establishing and maintaining an airway, providing oxygen and ventilatory support, and securing vascular access (peripheral venous, intraosseous, central venous). If there is any concern for sepsis, administer broad-spectrum intravenous (IV) antibiotics. For a normal host give vancomycin (15 mg/kg every 8 hours, or every 6 hours if meningitis is suspected, 2 g/day maximum) and cefotaxime (50 mg/kg, or 75 mg/kg if meningitis is suspected every 8 hours, 12 g/day maximum). If the patient is immunocompromised or has an indwelling vascular access, use vancomycin (as above), pipercillin/tazobactam (80 mg/kg every 8 hours ≤9 months of age; 100 mg/kg every 8 hours ≥9 months or ≤40 kg; or 3 g every 8 hours for ≥40 kg), and gentamicin (2.5 mg/kg every 8 hours, 4 g/day maximum).

Hypovolemic, Septic, and Other Etiologies With Component of Hypovolemia

Give prompt, rapid volume resuscitation with crystalloid fluids (normal saline, lactated Ringer), up to 60 to 80 mL/kg, or more. Use boluses of 20 mL/kg over 5 to 10 minutes, using push-pull technique or rapid infuser systems, as *IV infusion pumps cannot achieve the needed rate for patients in shock.* Try to achieve resuscitation using a "golden hour" approach, minimizing delays between fluid boluses and reassessments. This is associated with decreased mortality and involves rapid volume boluses followed by rapid reassessment. Attempt to normalize capillary refill, pulses, skin temperature, mental status, and blood pressure, but maintain ongoing monitoring for signs of volume overload (rales, jugular venous distension, hepatomegaly). Control temperature with antipyretics when possible.

If hypotension persists or develops despite 60 mL/kg of crystalloid fluid infusion in the golden hour, or if the patient has ongoing signs of shock, administer dopamine (a peripheral vein is satisfactory). Begin dopamine at 5 mcg/kg/min and titrate by 2.5 mcg/kg/min every 5 to 10 minutes to a maximum of 10 mcg/kg/min via peripheral infusion.

Manage dopamine-resistant shock with vasoactive medications administered via central line, ideally in an ICU. For warm shock, give norepinephrine, starting at 0.02 mcg/kg/min and titrate up to 2 mcg/kg/min. For cold shock, use an epinephrine infusion starting at 0.02 mcg/kg/min and titrate up to 1 mcg/kg/min as needed. Until central access is achieved, start the epinephrine infusion through a peripheral line, up to a maximum rate of 0.05 mcg/kg/min. See Figure 9-1 for further vasoactive support, ideally directed with invasive monitoring with mixed venous oxygen saturations in an ICU.

If the hemoglobin is lower than 10 g/dL, consider blood product transfusion support to increase oxygen-carrying capacity. Indications for intubation and mechanical ventilation include respiratory failure, poor airway protection in an obtunded patient, and unreversed shock despite fluid boluses and peripheral dopamine infusion. Correct hypoglycemia, hypocalcemia, and temperature disturbances. Consider the possibility of adrenal insufficiency and the need for hydrocortisone support.

Cardiogenic

See Congestive Heart Failure (page 19), Myocarditis (page 47), and Pericarditis (page 53) for specific therapies. Consult with a cardiologist or intensivist, who may recommend afterload-reducing inotropic support such as milrinone (50–75 mcg/kg infusion over 10–60 minutes, followed by 0.5–0.75 mcg/kg/min). For a neonate with ductal-dependent congenital heart lesions or undifferentiated shock, give a prostaglandin-E infusion (alprostadil 0.05–0.1 mcg/kg/min initially, then 0.01–0.05 mcg/kg/min). Watch for apnea and provide ventilatory support as needed.

Anaphylactic

See Anaphylaxis on page 3 for specific therapies.

Obstructive

Do not delay therapy while awaiting chest radiography. Perform life-saving needle thoracentesis, evacuation of pericardial tamponade, or prostaglandin-E infusion. Treat a pneumothorax with placement of an 18- or 20-gauge angiocatheter in the midclavicular line, second intercostal space (over the top of the third rib), followed by tube thoracostomy. Treat pericardial tamponade with volume support to increase preload, and if unresponsive to fluids, pericardiocentesis by a qualified physician.

Indications for Consultation

- **Cardiology:** Cardiogenic shock or obstructive shock due to cardiac tamponade and need for urgent pericardiocentesis
- **Critical care specialist:** Fluid refractory shock
- **Infectious diseases:** Resistant or complex infections
- **Surgeon, intensivist, other qualified physician:** Need for central venous access or if unable to obtain reliable IV access promptly

Figure 9-1. Management of shock.

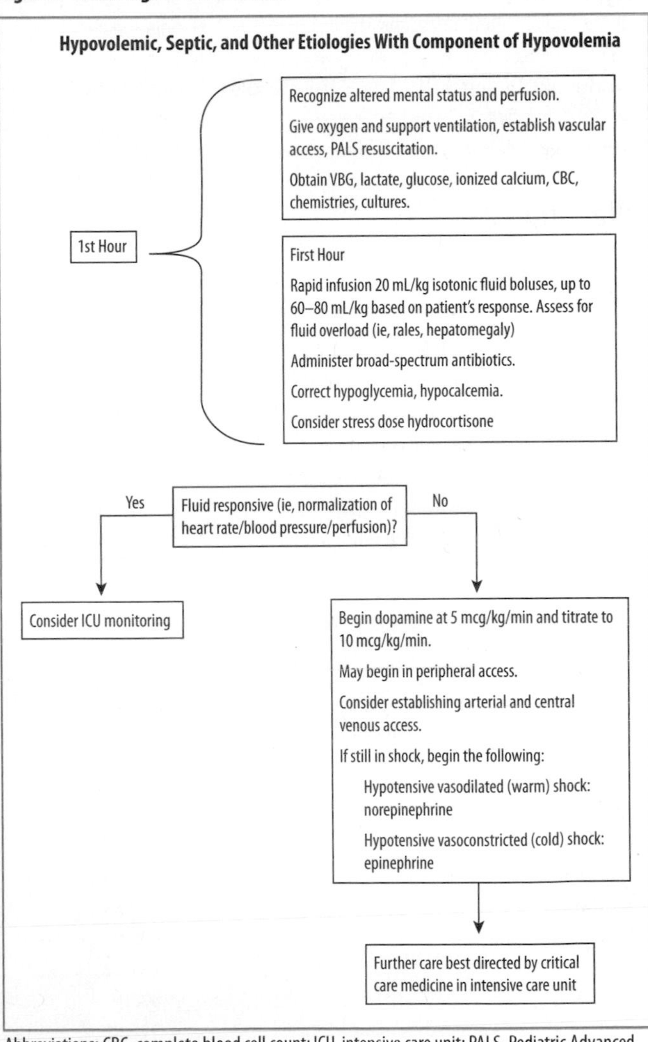

Hypovolemic, Septic, and Other Etiologies With Component of Hypovolemia
1st Hour
Recognize altered mental status and perfusion.
Give oxygen and support ventilation, establish vascular access, PALS resuscitation.
Obtain VBG, lactate, glucose, ionized calcium, CBC, chemistries, cultures.
First Hour
Rapid infusion 20 mL/kg isotonic fluid boluses, up to 60–80 mL/kg based on patient's response. Assess for fluid overload (ie, rales, hepatomegaly)
Administer broad-spectrum antibiotics.
Correct hypoglycemia, hypocalcemia.
Consider stress dose hydrocortisone
Fluid responsive (ie, normalization of heart rate/blood pressure/perfusion)?
Yes
No
Consider ICU monitoring
Begin dopamine at 5 mcg/kg/min and titrate to 10 mcg/kg/min.
May begin in peripheral access.
Consider establishing arterial and central venous access.
If still in shock, begin the following:
Hypotensive vasodilated (warm) shock: norepinephrine
Hypotensive vasoconstricted (cold) shock: epinephrine
Further care best directed by critical care medicine in intensive care unit

Abbreviations: CBC, complete blood cell count; ICU, intensive care unit; PALS, Pediatric Advanced Life Support; VBG, venous blood gas.

Adapted from Carcillo JA, Fields AI, et al. Clinical practice parameters for hemodynamic support of pediatric and neonatal patients in septic shock. *Crit Care Med.* 2002;30(6):1365–1378; Brierley J, Carcillo JA, Choong K, Cornell T, et al. Clinical practice parameters for hemodynamic support of pediatric and neonatal septic shock: 2007 update from the American College of Critical Care Medicine. *Crit Care Med.* 2009;37(2):666–688, with permission from Lippincott, Williams & Wilkins.

Disposition

- **ICU transfer:** Fluid refractory shock (see Figure 9-1), ongoing elevated early warning score
- **Institutional transfer:** Need for ICU or specialist consultation not available locally
- **Discharge criteria:** Normal vital signs and adequate oral intake

Follow-up

- **Primary care:** 2 to 3 days
- **Infectious diseases:** 1 week if long-term antibiotic therapy initiated

Pearls and Pitfalls

- Inadequate recognition of compensated forms of shock (persistent tachycardia being a prime example) is associated with time-dependent mortality. *Early goal-directed therapy saves lives.*
- A patient with persistently abnormal vital signs (tachycardia, wide pulse pressure) or impaired perfusion, even in the absence of hypotension or vasoactive infusion requirement, may require ICU transfer for close monitoring.
- Promptly attempt intraosseous line placement if securing IV access is a problem.

Coding

ICD-9

- Hypotension (do not use with a diagnosis of shock) **458.9**
- Anaphylactic shock NOS **995.0**
- Cardiogenic shock **785.51**
- Hypovolemic shock **785.59**
- Newborn shock **779.89**
- Postoperative shock **998.0**
- Septic shock **785.52**
- Septicemia, unspecified **038.9**
- Sepsis with acute organ dysfunction **995.92**
- Spinal shock, unspecified **953.9**
- Traumatic shock **958.4**

Bibliography

Akre M, Finkelstein M, Erickson M, et al. Sensitivity of the pediatric early warning score to identify patient deterioration. *Pediatrics.* 2010;125:e763–e769

Brierley J, Carcillo JA, Choong K, et al. Clinical practice parameters for hemodynamic support of pediatric and neonatal septic shock: 2007 update from the American College of Critical Care Medicine. *Crit Care Med.* 2009;37:666–688

Carcillo JA, Kuch BA, Han YY, et al. Mortality and functional morbidity after use of PALS/APLS by community physicians. *Pediatrics.* 2009;124:500–508

Han YY, Carcillo JA, Dragotta MA, et al. Early reversal of pediatric-neonatal septic shock by community physicians is associated with improved outcome. *Pediatrics.* 2003;112:793–799

Kissoon N, Orr RA, Carcillo JA. Updated American College of Critical Care Medicine—pediatric advanced life support guidelines for management of pediatric and neonatal septic shock: relevance to the emergency care clinician. *Pediatr Emerg Care.* 2010;26:867–869

Dermatology

CHAPTER 10

Erythema Multiforme and Stevens-Johnson Syndrome

Introduction

Erythema multiforme (EM) and Stevens-Johnson syndrome (SJS) are relatively uncommon disorders of the skin and mucous membranes. The previous terminology of EM minor and EM major have fallen out of favor as recent evidence suggests that EM and SJS/toxic epidermal necrolysis (TEN) have distinct precipitating factors and clinical features, and therefore are separate entities.

Classic EM involves the skin only, whereas SJS always affects the skin as well as mucous membranes. EM is thought to be a postinfectious process, with herpes simplex virus (HSV) being the most well-documented trigger.

Drugs are the cause of most non-idiopathic SJS cases, although infections and autoimmune diseases may also be triggers. Many drugs have been implicated, but the most common are sulfonamides, anticonvulsants, β-lactam antibiotics, and nonsteroidal anti-inflammatory drugs. The most frequently identified infectious etiology is *Mycoplasma pneumoniae.* SJS typically resolves over a 4- to 6-week period, but the mortality rate is 10% to 30% if untreated.

Clinical Presentation

History

Patients with EM typically present with a mildly pruritic rash in association with a prodrome of mild, nonspecific systemic symptoms such as fever, cough, and rhinorrhea.

A patient with SJS will present with pronounced constitutional symptoms, such as high fever and malaise, along with cutaneous rash and discomfort/poor oral intake related to mucous membrane lesions. The disease typically develops within 2 to 8 weeks of exposure to the offending agent.

Physical Examination

The prototypic EM lesion is a 1- to 3-cm erythematous, edematous plaque that develops a dusky vesicular, purpuric, or necrotic center. Often there is also an edematous ring of pallor surrounded by an erythematous outer ring (the target lesion). In many cases the typical target is not seen, and only the first 2 zones are present. The lesions are typically distributed symmetrically and acrally, predominantly on extensor surfaces. They may also be present on the trunk, palms, soles, and face. The patient may have a low-grade fever, as well as mild extremity and/or facial edema.

A patient with SJS is typically highly febrile and ill-appearing. The cutaneous lesions are more likely to occur on the face and trunk than in classic EM, and they are more often reported as painful or burning. They also tend to be macular, predominate on the trunk, may be coalescent, and often exhibit the Nikolsky sign, which is positive when slight rubbing of the skin causes exfoliation of the outermost layer. Epidermal detachment may occur but does not typically involve more than 10% of body surface area; if it does, consider a diagnosis of TEN. Mucosal lesions (≥2 sites) are requisite for a diagnosis of SJS and are characterized by erythema and bullae that become confluent with pseudomembrane formation. The mucous membrane lesions are typically hemorrhagic in appearance, which is not the case in EM. Oral lesions may extend to the respiratory mucosa, and complications may include pneumonitis and respiratory failure. Ophthalmologic findings include conjunctivitis, keratitis, and uveitis. Less commonly there may be urethritis or acute renal failure.

Laboratory

Both EM and SJS are clinical diagnoses. If SJS is suspected, obtain a complete blood cell count, erythrocyte sedimentation rate and/or C-reactive protein, and a comprehensive metabolic panel. The patient may have a leukocytosis or leukopenia and thrombocytosis, while eosinophilia is common in drug-related cases. Chemical abnormalities include hypoalbuminemia, elevated liver transaminases (75% of patients), and electrolyte imbalances, including hyper-/hyponatremia, acidosis, and elevated blood urea nitrogen and creatinine. The clinical picture is usually clear, but if there is diagnostic uncertainty, arrange a skin biopsy to rule out other diagnoses. In EM there is more dermal inflammation and individual keratinocyte necrosis compared to SJS/TEN, which has minimal inflammation and sheets of epidermal necrosis. Send serologic testing for *Mycoplasma* if that is a likely organism.

Differential Diagnosis

EM is most often confused with urticaria. Other common diagnostic possibilities include drug eruptions, urticarial vasculitis, and viral exanthems. The diagnosis of SJS is usually evident and not confused with other entities. SJS may be confused with DRESS (drug reaction with eosinophilia and systemic symptoms), although a patient with DRESS often has dramatic facial edema and more internal organ involvement (liver, kidney, lungs), without significant mucous membrane involvement. Other entities to consider in the differential diagnosis include Kawasaki disease, bullous pemphigoid, bullous drug eruption, linear immunoglobulin A dermatosis, erythema annulare, staphylococcal scalded skin syndrome, serum sickness, herpetic gingivostomatitis, bullous drug eruption, and Behçet syndrome (Table 10-1).

Treatment

Treatment of EM is supportive and course is usually self-limited over 1 to 2 weeks. Treat the underlying cause (if identified) and discontinue nonessential medications. Topical treatments are typically not helpful. Recurrences may occur, particularly with HSV-associated EM.

The treatment of SJS is also primarily supportive, including meticulous skin care, intravenous hydration and nutrition, and monitoring for complications, such as fluid or electrolyte abnormalities, secondary bacterial infection, and ocular and/or airway involvement. Provision of adequate nutrition in the form of enteral feeds and/or total parenteral nutrition can prevent a catabolic state and may improve outcome. Clear treatment guidelines are lacking due to the infrequency of the disease and the absence of large controlled studies. Systemic corticosteroids, intravenous immune globulin, plasmapheresis, cyclosporine, and immunomodulators have all been used but their effectiveness has not been proven. Consult a dermatologist to determine if any medication is indicated. Reserve antibiotics for identified infections.

Table 10-1. Differential Diagnosis of Stevens-Johnson Syndrome

Diagnosis	Clinical Features
Behçet syndrome	Uncommon in children More discrete genital ulcers Recurrences common
Bullous drug eruption	No systemic symptoms
DRESS	Facial edema Limited mucous membrane involvement Eosinophilia Lesions predominate on extremities and face
Herpetic gingivostomatitis	Fever and oral lesions only No cutaneous eruption
Kawasaki disease	Discrete oral lesions uncommon Non-exudative conjunctivitis, strawberry tongue Edema of the hands and feet
Serum sickness	Arthralgias common No bullae or Nikolsky sign
Staphylococcal scalded skin syndrome	Diffuse painful erythroderma No discrete oral lesions Fissuring and crusting of perioral area

Indications for Consultation

- **Dermatology:** All patients with SJS
- **Ophthalmology:** All patients with SJS

Disposition

- **Intensive care unit transfer:** Extensive body surface area affected or if the respiratory mucosa is involved (risk of respiratory failure and loss of airway)
- **Burn unit:** Extensive disease or more than 10% epidermal detachment
- **Discharge criteria:** Improving clinical condition, adequate oral intake

Follow-up

- **Dermatology:** 3 to 5 days
- **Primary care:** 1 to 2 weeks
- **Ophthalmology:** 3 to 5 days (if ocular involvement present)

Pearls and Pitfalls

- Discontinue any suspected etiologic agent.
- A patient with SJS is at risk for long-term, severe ophthalmic sequelae (corneal ulceration and blindness).

Coding

ICD-9

- EM minor **695.11**
- EM major **695.12**
- SJS **695.13**

Bibliography

French LE, Trent JT, Kerdel FA. Use of intravenous immunoglobulin in toxic epidermal necrolysis and Stevens-Johnson syndrome: our current understanding. *Int Immunopharmacol.* 2006;6:543–549

Hughey LC. Approach to the hospitalized patient with targetoid lesions. *Dermatol Ther.* 2011;24:196–206

Koh MJ, Tay YK. An update on Stevens-Johnson syndrome and toxic epidermal necrolysis in children. *Curr Opin Pediatr.* 2009;21:505–510

Léauté-Labrèze C, Lamireau T, Chawki D, Maleville J, Taïeb A. Diagnosis, classification, and management of erythema multiforme and Stevens-Johnson syndrome. *Arch Dis Child.* 2000;83:347–352

Metry DW, Jung P, Levy ML. Use of intravenous immunoglobulin in children with Stevens-Johnson syndrome and toxic epidermal necrolysis: seven cases and review of the literature. *Pediatrics.* 2003;112:1430–1436

Rashes Associated With Serious Underlying Disease

Introduction

Rashes associated with acute illnesses are very common in children. However, there are a few that are associated with serious diseases that can have significant morbidity and mortality. These include erythroderma, some cases of cellulitis, petechiae/purpura, target lesions, and vesicles/bullae.

Clinical Presentation

History

It is essential to obtain a thorough description of the evolution of the rash. Specifically, determine when and where it started, the initial appearance and any change, and the pattern of spread (from head down to trunk, from hands up to trunk, etc). Note if the rash is painful or pruritic.

Ask about associated symptoms, such as the duration and intensity of any fever, fatigue, irritability, headache, sore throat, myalgia, arthralgia, abdominal pain, vomiting, and diarrhea. Document whether the patient is currently or was recently taking a medication and whether there has been any travel or sick contacts.

Physical Examination

Determine the size and morphology of the rash. Flat lesions smaller than 0.5 cm are called macules; raised lesions of similar size are papules. Vesicles are lesions filled with clear fluid; if the fluid is purulent, the lesions are pustules. Lesions that do not blanch suggest bleeding into the skin and are called petechiae, purpura, or ecchymoses depending on the size.

Document the distribution of the rash. Assess for desquamation and the Nikolsky sign (separation of the epidermis from the dermis with light pressure), which occurs in scalded skin syndrome, toxic epidermal necrolysis, Stevens-Johnson syndrome (SJS), and various bullous disorders.

Also examine all of the mucous membranes (throat, lips, buccal mucosa, conjunctiva, urethra, and anus), looking for vesicles, crusting, erythema, or other abnormalities. Specifically note if there is any eye involvement, such as conjunctival injection, purulent discharge, and abnormalities of the cornea or iris.

Look for edema of the face and/or extremities and check for lymphadenopathy and hepatosplenomegaly.

Laboratory

Obtain a complete blood cell count (CBC) with differential as well as a complete metabolic panel to assess renal and liver function. A urinalysis is helpful to look for hematuria, pyuria, and proteinuria, if suspected. In an ill-appearing patient, obtain a C-reactive protein and/or erythrocyte sedimentation rate, blood culture, coagulation panel, d-dimer, and fibrinogen. In addition, collect cultures from any suspected sites of infection, such as skin, cerebrospinal fluid, and urine. Further bacterial or viral testing may be necessary depending on the clinical picture. If lupus is suspected, order a rheumatologic panel including antinuclear antibodies, anti–double stranded DNA, anti–Smith antibodies, and antiphospholipid antibodies.

In some cases a skin biopsy can be diagnostic.

Radiology

If Kawasaki disease (page 305) is suspected, order an echocardiogram.

Differential Diagnosis

Classify the rash according to its morphology and distribution (Table 11-1).

The differential diagnosis includes infectious exanthems, which often have characteristic features. For example, measles typically presents with a red maculopapular rash that begins on the face and moves down the body, subsequently becoming confluent ("morbilliform" = "measles-like"), in association with fever, cough, coryza, and conjunctivitis. Scarlet fever is characterized by a red, diffuse, sandpapery rash with accentuation in the flexor creases (Pastia lines), fever, and pharyngitis. Epstein-Barr virus may have a maculopapular rash that is predominantly truncal, along with fever, lymphadenopathy, pharyngitis, and splenomegaly. The differential diagnosis is summarized in Table 11-2.

Treatment

Institute contact and/or droplet precautions if an infectious etiology is being considered in an ill-appearing patient.

The treatment of erythema multiforme (page 71), Henoch-Schönlein purpura (page 407), Kawasaki disease (page 305), and SJS (page 71) are detailed elsewhere.

Table 11-1. Serious Rash Morphology		
Rash Type	**Description**	**Possible Diagnoses**
Erythema: Areas of Significant Redness		
Erythroderma	Diffuse erythema (looks like sunburn) Pruritus, desquamation Large portion of body surface involved	TSS Drug reaction Viral or bacterial sepsis Kawasaki disease
Painful erythema	Localized erythema that spreads rapidly Severe pain	Necrotizing fasciitis
Bleeding Into the Skin		
Petechiae	Pinpoint (<2 mm) non-blanching round macules Not palpable	*Infectious:* sepsis (meningococcal, staph, strep), RMSF, other viral, bacterial and fungal *Vasculitis:* HSP, SLE *Trauma:* Accidental, inflicted *Hematologic/oncologic:* ITP, leukemia
Purpura	2 mm–1 cm non-blanching May be palpable	
Ecchymoses	>1 cm non-blanching May be palpable	
Target Lesions: Round or Oval Macules With Red Edge and Clearing or Dusky Center		
	Circular/ovoid macules with erythematous periphery and clearing center, which can become vesicular or dusky Symmetrical eruption Can involve the palms and soles Minimal epidermal detachment (<10% BSA)	EM
Vesicobullous: Blisters Filled With Clear Non-purulent Fluid (Vesicle <1 cm Diameter; Bullae >1 cm Diameter)		
	Characteristically on face and/or trunk Mucosal involvement of lips, mouth, nose, conjunctiva, genitals, rectum (+) Nikolsky sign May become pustular	SJS TEN
	Initial erythema progressing to fragile bullae Prominent on flexural surfaces No mucosal involvement (+) Nikolsky sign May become pustular	SSSS
	Erythroderma or morbilliform rash, progressing to vesicles, bullae, and/or purpura Head-to-toe progression May involve the mucous membranes Prominent facial and periorbital edema	DRESS
	Similarly sized, clustered vesicles on an erythematous base Become hemorrhagic erosions and/or pustules History of eczema	Eczema herpeticum

Abbreviations: BSA, body surface area; DRESS, drug reaction with eosinophilia, systemic symptoms; EM, erythema multiforme; HSP, Henoch-Schönlein purpura; ITP, idiopathic thrombocytopenic purpura; RMSF, Rocky Mountain spotted fever; SJS, Stevens-Johnson syndrome; SLE, systemic lupus erythematosus; TEN, toxic epidermal necrolysis; TSS, toxic shock syndrome.

Table 11-2. Differential Diagnosis of Serious Rashes	
Clinical Features	**Differential Diagnosis**
DRESS Syndrome	
Eruption begins 2–6 weeks after starting inciting drug (antiepileptics, sulfonamides) Symmetrical erythroderma or morbilliform rash becomes vesicular and/or purpuric Triad: fever, rash, internal organ involvement May have lymphadenopathy and pharyngitis Eosinophilia, atypical lymphocytosis May have abnormal LFTs, TFTs, renal function	Infectious mononucleosis Leukemia Lymphoma Viral syndrome
Eczema Herpeticum	
History of eczema or other skin disease Fever Uniform-sized papulovesicles on an erythematous base, progresses to erosions and crusting Lab: Tzanck smear, DFA testing for herpes, HSV-1 and HSV-2, PCR May have keratoconjunctivitis or secondary bacterial infection	Suprainfected eczema
Erythema Multiforme	
May follow a herpes simplex infection Symmetrical distribution of target lesions Usually involves palms and soles in a symmetrical distribution Maximal involvement of only one mucosal surface	Drug reaction Kawasaki syndrome Other hypersensitivities SJS TEN Urticaria Vasculitis Viral syndrome
Henoch-Schönlein Purpura	
Usually <7 years old Initial maculopapular or urticarial rash Progresses to palpable purpura of lower extremities and buttocks Afebrile May have arthralgia/arthritis, hematuria, and/or abdominal pain May develop ileo-ileal intussusception	Acute abdomen Drug reaction EM ITP Meningococcemia SLE Juvenile idiopathic arthritis Other vasculitis RMSF
Idiopathic Thrombocytopenic Purpura	
2–5 years of age History of viral infection or viral immunization 1–6 weeks prior Petechiae and ecchymoses (nonpalpable) Bleeding and bruising with minimal or no trauma No generalized lymphadenopathy or hepatosplenomegaly ↓Platelets with ↑MPV; normal WBC and Hgb	Aplastic anemia Collagen vascular disease Drug reaction Epstein-Barr virus HIV Inflicted trauma Leukemia

Table 11-2. Differential Diagnosis of Serious Rashes, continued	
Clinical Features	**Differential Diagnosis**
Kawasaki Disease	
Usually <5 years old Fever >5 days with marked irritability Polymorphic eruption with late desquamation Cracked lips, strawberry tongue, edema of dorsum of hands/feet, nonpurulent conjunctivitis, cervical lymph node(s)	Adenovirus Drug reaction Juvenile idiopathic arthritis
Meningococcemia	
Fever with rapid progression to toxicity and possible vascular collapse Petechiae and palpable purpura, particularly of distal extremities	Bacterial sepsis HSP Kawasaki disease RMSF Vasculitis
Necrotizing Fasciitis	
Rapidly progressing cellulitis Becomes edematous, with bullae, areas of hemorrhage, necrosis, and/or erythroderma Fever, marked toxicity, hypotension, altered mental status Severe pain and worsening despite antibiotics	Severe cellulitis Other soft tissue infection
Rocky Mountain Spotted Fever	
Erythematous macules beginning on wrists, ankles, palms, and soles Rash spreads centrally becoming petechial and purpuric Illness may begin with headache, myalgia, malaise, GI complaints Classic triad: fever, severe headache, rash May have history of tick bite (60%) Hyponatremia	Enterovirus Kawasaki disease Meningococcemia Mycoplasma Secondary syphilis Streptococcus Viral syndrome
Staphylococcal Scalded Skin Syndrome	
Initial erythema progressing to fragile bullae, especially prominent on flexors Fever Fissures around eyes, nose and mouth *without mucous membrane involvement* (+) Nikolsky sign	Epidermolysis bullosa Nutritional deficiency Scalding burn TEN
Systemic Lupus Erythematosus	
Erythema over the nose and cheeks spreading in a butterfly distribution Fever, myalgia, fatigue, headache, arthralgia, behavioral changes Arthritis, pleuritis, pericarditis (+) ANA, Anti-double stranded DNA, Anti-phospholipid antibodies, Anti-Smith antibodies	Fibromyalgia Lymphoma Malignancies Rheumatologic diseases Viral syndrome

Table 11-2. Differential Diagnosis of Serious Rashes, continued	
Clinical Features	**Differential Diagnosis**
Toxic Epidermal Necrolysis/Stevens-Johnson Syndrome	
New medication in past month: antiepileptics, sulfonamides, β-lactams, macrolides Symmetrical purpuric/erythematous/targetoid macules and bullae that coalesce Rapidly progress to detachment of the epidermis exposing the underlying raw red skin Epidermal detachment <10% in SJS, 10%–30% in SJS/TEN overlap, >30% in TEN Hemorrhage, crusts, and erosions on multiple mucosal surfaces (lips, tongue, buccal mucosa, rectum, genital mucosa) Conjunctivitis, keratitis, uveitis (+) Nikolsky sign ↑Liver transaminases, CRP/ESR; hematuria/proteinuria	Bullous disorder Burns Epidermolysis bullosa EM Graft vs host disease Kawasaki syndrome SSSS
Toxic Shock Syndrome	
May be staphylococcal or streptococcal Prodrome of malaise and myalgia, followed by vomiting, diarrhea, altered mental status Diffuse macular erythroderma Fever, hypotension, tachycardia, multi-organ failure Mucous membrane involvement Desquamation 1–2 weeks later, especially of palms and soles ↑Platelets, fibrinogen, albumin ↓Liver transaminases, d-dimer, CRP/ESR, CPK, BUN/Cr	Drug reaction Kawasaki disease Leptospirosis Meningococcemia RMSF SJS/TEN SSSS Viral syndrome

Abbreviations: BUN/Cr, blood urea nitrogen/creatinine; CPK, creatine phosphokinase; CRP, C-reactive protein; DFA, direct fluorescent antibody; DRESS, drug reaction with eosinophilia systemic symptoms; EM, erythema multiforme; ESR, erythrocyte sedimentation rate; GI, gastrointestinal; Hgb, hemoglobin; HSP, Henoch-Schönlein purpura; HSV, herpes simplex virus; ITP, idiopathic thrombocytopenic purpura; LFTs, liver function tests; MPV, mean platelet volume; PCR, polymerase chain reaction; RMSF, Rocky Mountain spotted fever; SJS, Stevens-Johnson syndrome; SLE, systemic lupus erythematosus; SSSS, staphylococcal scalded skin syndrome; TEN, toxic epidermal necrolysis; TFTs, thyroid function tests; TSS, toxic shock syndrome; WBC, white blood cell count.

Drug Reaction With Eosinophilia Systemic Symptoms (DRESS) Syndrome

Immediately discontinue any medication that could be a possible etiology and treat with prednisone (1–2 mg/kg/day) for at least a few weeks, followed by a slow taper. Transfer the patient to an intensive care unit (ICU) if there is significant hepatic, renal, or other systemic involvement.

Eczema Herpeticum

Give the patient acyclovir, 5 to 10 mg/kg every 8 hours intravenously.

Idiopathic Thrombocytopenic Purpura (ITP)

Avoid medications that affect platelet function, such as nonsteroidal anti-inflammatories and salicylates. If the platelet count is less than 20,000/mm^3, consult a hematologist to discuss treatment options.

Meningococcemia

Immediately obtain a blood culture and treat with intravenous (IV) antibiotics, either ceftriaxone (100 mg/kg/day divided every 12 hours) or cefotaxime (200 mg/kg/day divided every 12 hours). Give antibiotic prophylaxis to household and nursery/child care contacts, as well as persons having contact with the patient's secretions. Options include ciprofloxacin (500 mg orally once), rifampin (10 mg/kg orally twice a day for 2 days), or a single dose of intramuscular ceftriaxone (125 mg <12 years of age; 250 mg >12 years of age).

Necrotizing Fasciitis

Immediately consult a surgeon to perform debridement. Give broad-spectrum antibiotics to cover for aerobic and anerobic organisms. Begin treatment with piperacillin/tazobactam, basing the dose on the piperacillin (<6 months of age: 150–300 mg/kg/day divided every 6–8 hours; >6 months of age and <40 kg: 300–400 mg/kg/day divided every 6–8 hours; >40 kg: 3 g/day divided every 6 hours) *plus* vancomycin (40 mg/kg/day divided every 6 hours, 2 g/day maximum).

Rocky Mountain Spotted Fever (RMSF)

For any age patient, treat with doxycycline (4 mg/kg/day divided twice a day, 100 mg/dose maximum). Transfer the patient to an ICU if unstable or if close monitoring is required.

Staphylococcal Scalded Skin Syndrome (SSSS)

Obtain a CBC, blood culture, electrolytes, and polymerase chain reaction for the toxin. Admit the patient to an ICU or burn unit and treat with clindamycin (40 mg/kg/day divided every 6 hours, 2.7 g/day maximum) or vancomycin (40 mg/kg/day divided every 6 hours, 2 g/day maximum).

Systemic Lupus Erythematosus (SLE)

Defer treatment decisions to a rheumatologist.

Toxic Epidermal Necrolysis (TEN)

Admit the patient to a burn unit and treat like a severe burn with meticulous skin care and aggressive fluid resuscitation. Place the patient in reverse isolation if the rash is extensive. Discontinue any medication that could be a possible cause.

Toxic Shock Syndrome (TSS)

Obtain a CBC, blood cultures, electrolytes, liver function tests, blood urea nitrogen/creatinine, and prothrombin time/partial thromboplastin time. Admit the patient to an ICU and provide fluid resuscitation as needed. Treat with clindamycin (40 mg/kg/day divided every 6 hour, 2.7 g/day maximum) *and*, depending on the prevalence of methicillin-resistant *Staphylococcus aureus* in the community, nafcillin (150 mg/kg/day divided every 6 hours) *or* vancomycin (40 mg/kg/day divided every 6 hours, 2 g/day maximum). Remove any possible foreign bodies (tampons) and drain any infected wounds.

Indications for Consultation

- **Burn service:** TEN/SJS
- **Cardiology:** Kawasaki disease
- **Dermatology:** DRESS syndrome, eczema herpeticum, SLE, SSSS, TEN/SJS
- **Hematology:** ITP
- **Infectious diseases:** Meningococcemia, necrotizing fasciitis, RMSF, TSS
- **Ophthalmology (if eyes are involved):** Eczema herpeticum, SLE, TEN/SJS
- **Rheumatology:** Henoch-Schönlein purpura (severe), SLE
- **Surgery:** Necrotizing fasciitis

Disposition

- **Burn unit:** TEN/SJS
- **Pediatric ICU:** Meningococcemia, TSS
- **Discharge criteria:** Nontoxic appearance, adequate oral hydration, no need for IV medication

Pearls and Pitfalls

- The distribution of the rash and the presence of mucosal involvement are often key features for making the correct diagnosis.
- Rapid diagnosis and treatment are important. If the patient appears seriously ill, consult and treat early.
- Some causes of rashes require notification of local departments of health.

Coding

ICD-9

- DRESS syndrome **995.27**
- Eczema herpeticum **054.0**
- Erythema multiforme **695.1**
- ITP **287.31**
- Kawasaki disease **446.1**
- Meningococcemia **036.2**
- SJS **695.13**
- SJS/TEN overlap **695.14**
- SLE **710.0**
- TEN **695.15**
- TSS **040.82**

Bibliography

Berk DR, Bayliss SJ. MRSA, staphylococcal scalded skin syndrome, and other cutaneous emergencies. *Pediatr Ann.* 2010;39:627–633

Burkhart CN, Morrell DS. *VisualDx: Essential Pediatric Dermatology*. Philadelphia, PA: Wolters Kluwer Lippincott, Williams & Wilkins; 2010:34–35, 186–189, 195–211

Leaute-Labreze C, Boralevi F, Taleb A. Life-threatening dermatoses and emergencies in dermatology: the case of the paediatric patient. In: Revuz J, Roujeau JC, Kerdel FA, Laurence VA, eds. *Life-Threatening Dermatoses and Emergencies in Dermatology*. Berlin: Springer-Verlag; 2009:189–197

Paller A, Mancini AJ. *Hurwitz Clinical Pediatric Dermatology.* 3rd ed. Philadelphia, PA: Elsevier Saunders; 2006:372–378, 400–401, 442–443, 534–541, 557–561, 566–570

Tas S, Simonart T. Management of drug rash with eosinophilia and systemic symptoms (DRESS syndrome): an update. *Dermatology.* 2003;206:353–356

Treat J. Stevens-Johnson syndrome and toxic epidermal necrolysis. *Pediatr Ann.* 2010;39:667–674

Valencia IC, Kerdel FA. Severe staphylococcal cutaneous infections and toxic shock syndrome. In: Revuz J, Roujeau JC, Kerdel FA, Laurence VA, eds. *Life-Threatening Dermatoses and Emergencies in Dermatology*. Berlin: Springer-Verlag; 2009:67–78

CHAPTER 12

Skin and Soft Tissue Infections

Introduction

Skin and soft tissue infections (SSTIs) encompass a variety of disease processes that affect the dermis and subcutaneous layer of the skin. Most cases are caused by either *Staphylococcus aureus* or *Streptococcus pyogenes* (group A streptococcus), and most admitted patients will present with a cellulitis or an abscess. Recently, there has been an increase in SSTI admissions, particularly those caused by methicillin-resistant *S aureus* (MRSA). Additionally, there are emerging erythromycin resistance patterns among *S pyogenes*. As a result, knowledge of local antibiotic susceptibilities is critical for proper evaluation and management of SSTIs.

Usually an SSTI can be managed as an outpatient. Admitted patients generally have an atypical history, rapidly progressing infection, an extensive area or serious site of involvement, are unable to tolerate or are not responding to oral antibiotics, or have signs of sepsis/systemic infection.

Clinical Presentation

History

Important considerations in SSTIs are immune status, previous hospitalization history, animal exposure, bite wounds, marine exposures, foreign body penetrating injuries, trauma, surgery, previous antimicrobial use, travel history, and current/recent country of residence.

Physical Examination

SSTIs present with a combination of erythema, warmth, induration, and pain/tenderness, and may be accompanied by fever, lymphangitis, or lymphadenitis. Cellulitis is specifically characterized by erythema, warmth, and tenderness with poorly defined borders. It involves the deeper dermis and subcutaneous fat and lacks the fluctuance of an underlying suppurative focus. However, it may be a sentinel for a deeper or more complicated pyogenic infection, such as an abscess, fasciitis, or boney involvement.

A skin or subcutaneous abscess involves the dermis and deeper tissues. The superficial skin will usually have a warm, erythematous, tender nodule or mass, often with underlying fluctuance and, in some cases, a central superficial pustule may be seen.

Laboratory

No laboratory tests are necessary if the patient is well-appearing and not immunocompromised. If there is a concern about sepsis, obtain a complete blood cell count (CBC) and blood culture, but do not get a blood culture in an otherwise well-appearing patient. Send an erythrocyte sedimentation rate or C-reactive protein if an underlying fasciitis or associated osteoarticular infection is possible. Send a culture of a draining abscess if not already performed prior to admission. Do not obtain a superficial swab for culture on intact skin or perform a needle aspirate for culture when there is no detectable abscess.

Radiology

In general, imaging is not needed. However, if the patient has a rapidly spreading cellulitis, order an ultrasound to determine whether there is a deeper abscess. If there is concern for foreign body, obtain a screening ultrasound or plain film, but if the object is deep, the patient will likely need magnetic resonance imaging (MRI). Also obtain an MRI when there is a concern about fasciitis, pyomyositis, osteomyelitis, more extensive infection, or the site of involvement is near a vital structure.

Differential Diagnosis

Generally, making the diagnosis of a skin and soft tissue infection is straightforward. However, there are a number of conditions with similar appearances that are either more serious or require different therapy (Table 12-1).

Treatment

General principles of management include closely monitoring the extent and progression of the infection by marking the margins of the affected area.

First-line treatment for a fluctuant abscess is incision and drainage. Depending on the size of the wound and local practice, keep the abscess cavity open with either a drain or packing. Treat with clindamycin or alternatives (see below) while awaiting culture identification and susceptibility results. Use warm compresses if an underlying abscess has not been drained.

The microbiology of SSTI is of particular importance in guiding specific antimicrobial management. There are a number of treatment options for a community-acquired SSTI in a patient without a concerning medical history, a significant exposure, or signs of sepsis.

If MRSA is unlikely, initiate intravenous (IV) treatment with a semi-synthetic penicillin (nafcillin 100–150 mg/kg/day divided every 6 hours, 12 g/day maximum) or a first-generation cephalosporin (cefazolin 100 mg/kg/

Table 12-1. Differential Diagnosis of Skin and Soft Tissue Infections	
Diagnosis	**Differentiating Features**
Abscess	Well-demarcated, overlying erythema May be fluctuant or spontaneously draining
Cellulitis	Poorly demarcated macular or raised Erythematous and warm
Erysipelas	Well-demarcated or raised edges Extremely painful (St Anthony's fire)
Fungal infection (deep)	Superficial crusted lesion (papule, pustule, plaque) May have history of foreign body at the same site
Hydradenitis suppurativa	Affects apocrine sweat glands or sebaceous glands Superficial pustules and deep follicular rupture May cause scarring and tract formation
Local allergic reaction (insect bite)	Pruritus Central punctum within the swelling Usually seen in skin not covered by clothing
Necrotizing fasciitis	Superficial progressive destruction of fascia and fat Leaves a "wooden-hard" feel Painful edges with an anesthetic center
Necrotizing skin and soft tissue infection	Deeper and more devastating than cellulitis Constant pain, bullae, ecchymosis, systemic signs
Panniculitis	Inflammation of subcutaneous fat tissue Tender skin nodules or papules
Pyoderma gangrenosum	Pustule or lesion with surrounding edema Progresses to ulcerated lesion Associated with systemic disorders (leukemia)
Pyomyositis	Purulent foci within individual muscle groups Severe localized pain
Staphylococcal scalded skin syndrome	Diffuse erythematous rash with wrinkled appearance Positive Nikolsky sign

day divided every 8 hours, 6 g/day maximum). Otherwise, where there is a significant rate of MRSA but a low prevalence of clindamycin-resistant strains, use IV clindamycin (40 mg/kg/day divided every 6–8 hours, 900 mg/dose or 2.7 g/day maximum). However, if there is a significant rate of clindamycin resistance in the community (>20 %), or the patient has a history of frequent hospitalizations or clindamycin-resistant MRSA, give trimethoprim-sulfamethoxazole (10 mg TMP/kg/day IV divided every 12 hours), *and* a first-generation cephalosporin or semi-synthetic penicillin (as above) for adequate *S pyogenes* coverage.

If an apparent focal cellulitis or abscess fails to respond to the above choices for empiric antimicrobial coverage or the patient is initially seriously ill or toxic, use vancomycin (40–60 mg/kg/day divided every 6 hours). The goal is to maintain trough values at 10 to 15 mcg/mL. In serious staphylococcal infections, add empiric bactericidal coverage for methicillin-susceptible *S aureus* using nafcillin or cefazolin (see dosing above), particularly if the involved site is near a vital structure.

For a septic-appearing patient add ceftriaxone or cefepime (100 mg/kg/day divided every 12 hours, 4 g/day maximum) to the staphylococcal coverage if there are concerns for gram-negative rod involvement (eg, environmental contamination or immunocompromised host). If any patient does not respond to vancomycin, obtain an infectious diseases consult for consideration of other antimicrobials such as daptomycin.

Another option for MRSA is linezolid. The dosing is age-dependent (<5 years old: 10 mg/kg/dose every 8 hours; 5–11 years: 10 mg/kg/dose every 12 hours; ≥12 years: 600 mg/dose every 12 hours, oral or IV). Linezolid may cause bone marrow suppression as early as the second week of therapy, so monitor the CBC weekly. Doxycycline (2–4 mg/kg/day oral or IV divided every 12–24 hours; 100 mg/dose or 200 mg/day maximum) is an alternative in a patient older than 8 years who does not have severe or disseminated staphylococcal disease.

When a patient does not respond appropriately to antibiotics, obtain imaging to look for a deeper source of infection or an adjacent deep venous thrombosis. Start with an ultrasound.

Indications for Consultation

- **Infectious disease:** Unusual exposures, immunocompromised patient, failure to respond to therapy, severe illness, institutional approval of certain antimicrobial agents
- **Pediatric surgery or interventional radiology:** Abscess drainage

Disposition

- **Intensive care unit transfer:** Sepsis or a severe disease, such as necrotizing skin and soft tissue infection, necrotizing fasciitis, or staphylococcal scalded skin syndrome
- **Discharge criteria:** Afebrile, stable or receding margins of involvement, tolerating oral antibiotics or home IV therapy arranged

Follow-up

- **Primary care:** 2 to 3 days to evaluate continued response to treatment and removal of packing/drain (if placed)

Pearls and Pitfalls

- A streptococcal cellulitis may be caused by a nephritogenic strain, placing the patient at risk for subsequent acute glomerulonephritis.
- Recent or concurrent varicella infection is a risk factor for the development of streptococcal necrotizing fasciitis, as is concurrent ibuprofen use.
- Clindamycin has good enteral bioavailability, but has an unpleasant taste. Ask the pharmacy to flavor it to improve patient compliance.

Coding

ICD-9

- Carbuncle and furuncle, unspecified site **680.9**
- Cellulitis and abscess, unspecified site **682.9**
- Fasciitis, necrotizing **728.86**

Bibliography

Blankenship RB, Baker T. Imaging modalities in wounds and superficial skin infections. *Emerg Med Clin North Am.* 2007;25:223–234

Hankin A, Everett WW. Are antibiotics necessary after incision and drainage of a cutaneous abscess? *Ann Emerg Med.* 2007;50:49–51

Klevens RM, Morrison MA, Nadle J, et al. Invasive methicillin-resistant *Staphylococcus aureus* infections in the United States. *JAMA.* 2007;298:1763–1771

Liu C, Bayer A, Cosgrove SE, Daum RS, et al. Clinical practice guidelines by the Infectious Diseases Society of America for the treatment of methicillin-resistant *Staphylococcus aureus* infections in adults and children: executive summary. *Clin Infect Dis.* 2011;52:285–292

Paintsil E. Pediatric community-acquired methicillin-resistant *Staphylococcus aureus* infection and colonization: trends and management. *Curr Opin Pediatr.* 2007;19:75–82

Ear, Nose, Throat

CHAPTER 13

Acute Bacterial Sinusitis

Introduction

Acute bacterial sinusitis is an inflammation of the mucosal lining of one or more of the paranasal sinuses. While acute viral sinusitis is a normal accompaniment of an upper respiratory infection, in approximately 1 out of 15 cases it may be followed by acute bacterial sinusitis. Outpatient treatment will suffice for most cases of bacterial sinusitis, although a patient may require inpatient therapy if there is evidence of toxicity, failure of outpatient treatment, or an underlying immunodeficiency. Serious complications of bacterial sinusitis can occur secondary to the spread of infection. The most common are periorbital and orbital cellulitis. Less often, intracranial extension can cause a brain abscess, meningitis, or cavernous venous sinus thrombosis. Uncommonly, cranial vault involvement may result from a frontal sinusitis (Pott puffy tumor), most commonly in a teenaged male.

A history of recurrent bacterial sinusitis raises the possibility of an underlying chronic allergic condition, immunodeficiency, or a defect (anatomical or mechanical) causing poor sinus drainage (cystic fibrosis, immotile cilia, sinonasal polyps).

The most common causes of acute bacterial sinusitis are *Streptococcus pneumoniae*, nontypable *Haemophilus influenzae*, and *Moraxella catarrhalis*. However, with severe, complicated, and chronic infections, *Staphylococcus aureus* (including methicillin-resistant strains), anaerobic bacteria, and fungi may be involved.

Clinical Presentation

History

Uncomplicated acute bacterial sinusitis typically presents with persistent or worsening signs and symptoms for 10 or more days, although rarely it can be rapidly progressive, severe, and even fulminant. Symptoms can include low-grade fever, nasal discharge of any quality, daytime cough (which may be worse at night), headache (which can be severe and positional), or facial pain or pressure. A more severe form of acute bacterial sinusitis presents with 3 or 4 days of a temperature of at least 39°C (102.2°F) and purulent nasal discharge in an ill-appearing child. There may be other complaints that are related to complications, such as vomiting and severe headache (intracranial spread) or eye pain and visual disturbances (orbital cellulitis).

Physical Examination

Perform a thorough ear, nose, and throat and neurologic examination. The patient may appear toxic, with swelling of the forehead, face, or eyelids. There may be pain with eye movements and/or decreased visual acuity. Nasal speculum examination of the nasopharynx may reveal a purulent discharge material from under the middle turbinate. With intracranial spread there may be bradycardia, hypotension, nuchal rigidity, and VIth nerve palsy secondary to increased intracranial pressure.

Laboratory

No specific laboratory testing is needed other than aerobic and anaerobic cultures if sinus drainage is performed. Obtain a blood culture if the patient appears toxic. If there is a concern for intracranial extension, perform a lumbar puncture (to evaluate for increased intracranial pressure and pleocytosis) after obtaining a head computed tomography (CT) with contrast or magnetic resonance imaging (MRI).

Radiology

The clinical presentation of acute bacterial sinusitis is usually sufficient to make the diagnosis, so that routine imaging of the sinuses is unnecessary. If the patient has a clinical picture consistent with a complication, obtain a CT with contrast or an MRI of the orbits (preseptal or orbital cellulitis) or head (Pott puffy tumor, venous thrombosis).

Differential Diagnosis

The presentation of the complications of acute bacterial sinusitis is summarized in Table 13-1.

Treatment

Treat acute bacterial sinusitis with either cefotaxime (150 mg/kg/day divided every 6 hours, 6 g/day maximum), ceftriaxone (100 mg/kg/day divided every 12 hours, 4 g/day maximum), or ampicillin-sulbactam (100 mg/kg/day divided every 6 hours, 8 g/day maximum). Add vancomycin (60 mg/kg/day divided every 6 hours, 4 g/day maximum) if there is a complication (orbital or periorbital cellulitis, cavernous sinus thrombosis, or Pott puffy tumor) or a failure of appropriate inpatient therapy (as above). Tailor the antibiotic choices based on clinical response, culture results (if any), and community patterns of antimicrobial resistance. Continue the intravenous antibiotics until the symptoms are improving, then change to oral antibiotics to complete at least

Table 13-1. Complications of Sinusitis

Diagnosis	Clinical Features
Brain abscess	Headache Altered mental status
Cavernous sinus thrombosis	Toxicity, headache Altered mental status Ophthalmoplegia (III, IV, VI) Signs of ↑ICP
Meningitis	Headache Photophobia Meningismus
Orbital cellulitis	Proptosis, chemosis Limited EOMs
Pott puffy tumor	Marked forehead swelling May have signs of ↑ICP
Preseptal cellulitis	May have a break in the skin integrity No ophthalmoplegia

Abbreviations: EOMs, extraocular movements; ICP, intracranial pressure.

a 14-day course. In a more severe or complicated case the patient may require antibiotic therapy for up to 4 weeks.

Consult an otolaryngologist and/or infectious diseases specialist for consideration of sinus drainage if the patient has a clinical deterioration, does not improve after 48 hours of adequate empiric therapy, or presents with signs or symptoms of a complication. In addition, consult a neurosurgeon if the clinical picture suggests intracranial extension.

Despite being commonly used, there are little data to support the use of adjunctive therapies such as nasal saline irrigation, antihistamines, or decongestants.

Indications for Consultation

- **Allergy and immunology:** Suspicion of an immunodeficiency or recurrent episodes of sinusitis that may be allergic in nature
- **Infectious disease:** Recurrent sinusitis, isolation of rare or resistant pathogen, complication of sinusitis, sinusitis unresponsive to standard antimicrobial therapy
- **Neurosurgery:** Possible intracranial extension
- **Ophthalmology:** Possible orbital or intracranial extension
- **Otolaryngology:** Recurrent or chronic sinusitis, complication of sinusitis, need for sinus aspiration

Disposition

- **Intensive care unit transfer:** Intracranial extension, sepsis
- **Discharge criteria:** Afebrile for 24 to 48 hours, clinical improvement, good oral intake including able to take appropriate antibiotic

Follow-up

- **Primary care:** 1 week, to assess the need for an extended antibiotic course
- **Otolaryngology (if involved):** 1 week

Pearls and Pitfalls

- If the patient is asymptomatic, do not treat an incidental finding of sinus inflammation that is seen on CT.
- If the patient has recurrent bacterial sinusitis or chronic sinusitis, consider an evaluation for allergic rhinitis, cystic fibrosis, immunodeficiency, Kartagener syndrome and other immotile-cilia syndromes, and polypoid disease.
- Both transillumination and ultrasound of the sinuses are unreliable, especially in a patient younger than 10 years.

Coding

ICD-9

- Acute frontal sinusitis **461.1**
- Acute sinusitis, unspecified **461.9**
- Chronic sinusitis, unspecified **473.9**

Bibliography

Anzai Y, Paladin A. Diagnostic imaging in 2009: update on evidence-based practice of pediatric imaging. What is the role of imaging in sinusitis? *Pediatr Radiol.* 2009;39 (suppl 2):S239–S241

Hicks CW, Weber JG, Reid JR, Moodley M. Identifying and managing intracranial complications of sinusitis in children: a retrospective series. *Pediatr Infect Dis J.* 2011;30:222–226

Shaikh N, Wald ER, Pi M. Decongestants, antihistamines and nasal irrigation for acute sinusitis in children. *Cochrane Database Syst Rev.* 2010;(12):CD007909

Soon VT. Pediatric subperiosteal orbital abscess secondary to acute sinusitis: a 5-year review. *Am J Otolaryngol.* 2011;32:62–68

Wald ER. Acute otitis media and acute bacterial sinusitis. *Clin Infect Dis.* 2011;52 (suppl 4):S277–S283

CHAPTER 14

Cervical Lymphadenopathy

Introduction

Cervical lymphadenopathy is a common, and generally benign, finding among many preschool and school-aged children. There are 3 types of cervical lymphadenopathy.

1. Reactive adenopathy secondary to a nearby viral or bacterial illness
2. Adenitis, an infection of the node itself (most commonly *Staphylococcus aureus* or group A streptococcus, although viral, anaerobic, atypical *Mycobacterium,* and *Mycobacterium tuberculosis* can also result in cervical adenitis)
3. Adenitis secondary to systemic disease (especially Epstein-Barr virus [EBV], cytomegalovirus [CMV], autoimmune diseases, and malignancies).

Clinical Presentation

History

Ask about exposure to sick contacts and cats (especially kittens or puppies for *Bartonella henselae*), recent travel (tuberculosis or bubonic plague), dental history (caries, abscess), and ingestions of medications (especially antiepileptic), unpasteurized animal products (brucellosis, *Mycobacterium bovis*), or raw meat (toxoplasmosis). Assess the patient's immunization status, especially focusing on mumps vaccination.

With reactive adenopathy there is usually a history of preceding or concurrent viral or bacterial infection in the head or neck. The onset of adenitis may be insidious in nature or there may be a history of exposure to such an illness. A patient with a systemic disease may have symptoms such as fever, weight loss, and fatigue. With a malignant process, there may be a history of increasing size of the node, weight loss, weakness, pallor, night sweats, fever, and easy bruisabilty.

Physical Examination

Perform a thorough examination of the head, neck, oral cavity, skin, and respiratory tract looking for infections that may be draining into the affected node(s). Check for generalized lymphadenopathy and hepatosplenomegaly.

Reactive lymph nodes typically are multiple, shotty, discrete, non-tender, mobile, non-fluctuant, and less than 2 cm in diameter. The overlying skin is intact, with normal texture and color.

Adenitis presents as a tender enlarged node, initially firm, but becoming more fluctuant with time. The node may be erythematous with warm, adherent overlying skin. The physical examination is different for an atypical *Mycobacterium* infection, in which the node is often non-tender, without warmth, but with a violet or purplish color, while the patient is well-appearing without fever. A tuberculous node typically has overlying erythema and often suppurates, and the patient usually presents with systemic signs and symptoms (fever, weight loss, fatigue).

A malignant node is fixed, hard, and matted and most often located in the supraclavicular region.

A systemic disease may have associated diffuse lymphadenopathy and/or hepatosplenomegaly.

Laboratory

No laboratory testing is necessary for adenitis, although obtain a culture if the node is drained. If a systemic disease is a concern (generalized lymphadenopathy, hepatosplenomegaly, weight loss, night sweats, hard or irregular-shaped node), obtain a complete blood cell count (CBC), erythrocyte sedimentation rate or C-reactive protein, liver function tests, EBV and CMV serology, blood culture (if febrile and toxic-appearing), and if a malignancy is suspected, lactate dehydrogenase (LDH), uric acid, and chest x-ray. Send *Bartonella,* brucellosis, and HIV testing if indicated based on the history and physical examination. Place a purified protein derivative if the patient has persistent cervical lymphadenopathy, especially if the node is firm, rubbery, or matted.

In general imaging studies are not indicated, although an ultrasound can be helpful to assess for abscess formation and to determine when to perform surgical drainage. Obtain computed tomography of the neck if there are signs of airway compromise.

Differential Diagnosis

Determine whether the node is infected, versus reactive to a local infection or secondary to a systemic disease (Table 14-1). See page 115 for the differential diagnosis of neck masses.

Treatment

Treat suspected bacterial adenitis parenterally. Start with clindamycin (40 mg/kg/day divided every 6 hours, 2.7 g/day maximum) if methicillin-resistant *Staphylococcus aureus* is a concern. Otherwise, use nafcillin or oxacillin (150 mg/kg/day divided every 6 hours), ceftriaxone (100 mg/kg/day divided every

REPUBLIC BANK

It's just easier here.[sm]

RepublicBank.com Member FDIC

```
ACCOUNT#  ***********0039
AMOUNT                  4,818.00
DDA DEPOSIT                TLR#     84 AM
TR#      129  12:44:46  5/18/2015   ON
```

Checks and other items received for deposit or payment are subject to the rules and regulations of this bank and are subject to verification.

Table 14-1. Differential Diagnosis of Cervical Lymphadenitis

Diagnosis	Clinical Features
Adenitis (staph, strep)	Node is erythematous, warm, and tender Unilateral
Atypical *Mycobacterium*	Afebrile Node is nonerythematous and non-tender Evolves over weeks to months
Bartonella	Kitten or puppy scratch 1–8 weeks prior Well-appearing May have conjunctivitis
Branchial cleft cyst	Found at the lower border of the sternocleidomastoid May be draining
Epstein-Barr virus or cytomegalovirus	Fatigue Generalized lymphadenopathy Hepatosplenomegaly
Kawasaki disease	≥5 days of fever Mucous membrane changes Non-purulent conjunctivitis Edema of hands and feet Polymorphic rash Lymphadenitis: a single matted area >1.5 cm
Malignancy	Weight loss, fever, fatigue, hepatosplenomegaly Node is firm, fixed, matted, increasing in size
Parotitis	Obscures the angle of the jaw Drainage from Stensen duct
Tuberculosis	Fever, fatigue, weight loss Overlying erythema May drain spontaneously

12 hours), cefazolin (75 mg/kg/day divided every 8 hours), or ampicillin-sulbactam (100 mg/kg/day divided every 6 hours). If the patient deteriorates or does not respond after 48 hours, add vancomycin (45 mg/kg/day divided every 8 hours). Also order warm compresses every 4 hours. If the node becomes fluctuant, arrange for incision and drainage by a general surgeon or otolaryngologist. Obtain an ultrasound if it is unclear whether the node is ready for drainage. Switch to an equivalent oral antibiotic once the patient responds.

If bartonellosis (cat scratch disease) is suspected treat the patient as above with adequate staphylococcal and streptococcal coverage. Although azithromycin, rifampin, trimethoprim-sulfamethoxazole, or gentamicin may offer some advantage, it is not necessary to specifically treat an immunocompetent patient who is not acutely or severely ill.

If an atypical mycobacterial infection is suspected, surgical excision and culture are recommended. Avoid incision and drainage, which can result in a chronic draining fistula. If complete excision is not possible, arrange for curettage and give antimycobacterial therapy with azithromycin (5 mg/kg every day) or clarithromycin (15 mg/kg/day divided every 12 hours) plus rifampin (20 mg/kg/day divided every 12 hours) or ethambutol (15 mg/kg every day).

If a malignancy is suspected, obtain a CBC with reticulocyte count, LDH, uric acid, complete metabolic profile, and chest x-ray and consult a hematologist/oncologist. The treatment of Kawasaki disease is discussed on page 308.

The treatment for EBV, CMV, and other mononucleosis-like syndromes is supportive. However, if the patient has significant upper airway obstruction, insert a nasopharyngeal tube (nasal trumpet) and give methylprednisolone (1 mg/kg every day).

Indication for Consultation

- **General surgery or otolaryngology:** Incision and drainage or surgical excision needed
- **Infectious disease:** Suspected mycobacterium infection
- **Oncology:** Suspected malignancy
- **Rheumatology:** Suspected collagen vascular disease

Disposition

- **Intensive care unit transfer:** Airway compromise or a rapidly progressing infection that is not responsive to parenteral therapy
- **Discharge criteria:** Afebrile for more than 24 hours with improvement in adenitis, no respiratory distress, tolerating adequate oral intake

Follow-up

- **Primary care:** 2 to 3 days
- **Hematology/oncology (malignancy suspected):** Immediate
- **Infectious diseases:** 1 week (suspected *Mycobacterium* infection)

Pearls and Pitfalls

- Adenopathy persisting for more than 3 weeks requires further workup, including tuberculosis and possible biopsy for malignancy.
- Incision and drainage of a suspected *Mycobacterium* node can lead to chronic draining sinus tract or disseminated disease.
- Posterior cervical adenopathy is almost always reactive or viral.

- A well-appearing patient with an adenitis can be discharged on oral antibiotics and warm compresses, with follow-up for incision and drainage if the node becomes fluctuant.

Coding

ICD-9

• Bartonellosis	**088.0**
• Lymphadenitis, acute	**683**
• Lymphadenitis, chronic	**289.1**
• Mycobacterial disease, unspecified	**031.9**

Bibliography

Dulin MF, Kennard TP, Leach L, Williams R. Management of cervical lymphadenitis in children. *Am Fam Physician.* 2008;78:1097–1098

Gosche JR, Vick L. Acute, subacute, and chronic cervical lymphadenitis in children. *Semin Pediatr Surg.* 2006;15:99–106

Leung AK, Davies HD. Cervical lymphadenitis: etiology, diagnosis, and management. *Curr Infect Dis Rep.* 2009;11:183–189

Papadopouli E, Michailidi E, Papadopoulou E, et al. Cervical lymphadenopathy in childhood epidemiology and management. *Pediatr Hematol Oncol.* 2009;26:454–460

Tracy TF Jr, Muratore CS. Management of common head and neck masses. *Semin Pediatr Surg.* 2007;16:3–13

CHAPTER 15

Infectious Croup

Introduction

Croup is a disorder of the upper airway, usually of infectious origin, that causes subglottic mucosal inflammation and edema. Croup is also referred to as laryngotracheitis or laryngotracheobronchitis because the larynx, trachea, and bronchi may all be involved. Parainfluenza I and II are the primary pathogens, but many other respiratory viruses cause a similar clinical picture. In a child, the subglottic area, specifically within the cricoid cartilage, is the narrowest part of the upper airway. In this region, 1 mm of mucosal edema can decrease airflow by 80%.

Croup commonly occurs in children between 3 months and 3 years of age, with a peak incidence at 2 years. There is a slight male predominance, and a strong family history exists in 15% of cases. It occurs more frequently in the fall and winter months.

Clinical Presentation

History

Usually the patient experiences a gradual onset of nonspecific cold symptoms, including coryza, cough, sore throat, and low-grade fever. Usually on the second or third night, the illness progresses and the child develops the characteristic hoarse voice, barky or seal-like cough, and in some cases inspiratory stridor and tachypnea. Caregivers often report that the symptoms are worse at night.

Physical Examination

Stridor is primarily inspiratory (airway obstruction below the glottis), but occasionally is expiratory (airway obstruction above the glottis) or a combination of both. Mild disease is characterized by minimal retractions, normal air entry, and either the absence of stridor or stridor only occurring with agitation. In a moderate case, stridor is present at rest and worsens with agitation. Other findings include mild to moderate suprasternal retractions and decreased lung aeration. Severe disease and impending respiratory failure are characterized by agitation, decreased mental status, cyanosis, continuous stridor, severe retractions, markedly decreased lung aeration, and/or hypoxemia.

Radiology

Croup is a clinical diagnosis and imaging is not required. If performed, subglottic narrowing (steeple sign) may be seen on an anterior-posterior neck radiograph. However, this finding may be absent and therefore is not required to make the diagnosis. False-positive radiographs may be seen if the infant is crying or poorly positioned.

If a congenital or acquired anatomical airway abnormality is suspected (<3 months of age, recurrent croup, unusually persistent or severe disease), order a 2-view chest x-ray. Consult an otolaryngologist to discuss additional diagnostic workup, such as laryngoscopy or an esophagram.

Differential Diagnosis

The history or the presence of the barking cough usually suggests the diagnosis. However, the differential diagnosis is summarized in Table 15-1.

Table 15-1. Differential Diagnosis of Croup

Diagnosis	Clinical Features
Angioedema	History of allergies or exposure to offending substance Swelling of lips/tongue Urticarial rash
Bacterial tracheitis	Abrupt onset of upper airway obstruction in patient recovering from a viral illness (croup, influenza) Toxic appearance with high fever Copious, purulent secretions on suctioning
Epiglottitis (very rare)	Abrupt onset with fever and toxicity Rapid progression to respiratory obstruction Patient prefers a "sniffing" posture
Foreign body aspiration	History of choking/gagging Sudden onset of cough, stridor, and dyspnea No upper respiratory infection prodrome or fever
Peritonsillar abscess	Older children and adolescents Severe sore throat, muffled voice, and trismus Exudative tonsillitis with uvula deviation
Retropharyngeal abscess	Fever, toxicity, and dysphagia with drooling Muffled stridor without barking cough Limited neck extension
Spasmodic croup	Recurrent episodes of nighttime barky cough and stridor No upper respiratory infection or fever May have history of allergies

Treatment

Systemic steroids are the mainstay of treatment. Dexamethasone is preferred because of its long half-life, low cost, and ease of administration. A single dose of 0.3 mg/kg (range 0.15–0.6 mg/kg, maximum 10 mg) orally, intravenously, or intramuscularly is safe and effective, regardless of disease severity. Since the oral, intravenous (IV), and intramuscular (IM) routes are equally efficacious, reserve IM or IV administration for a patient who is unable to tolerate oral medication or has severe respiratory distress. While the benefit of continued steroid therapy is unclear, give a second dose of dexamethasone if the patient is still requiring epinephrine after 24 to 48 hours of hospitalization.

In addition to steroids, administer nebulized racemic epinephrine (0.05 mL/kg, 0.5 mL maximum, diluted in 3 mL of normal saline) to a patient with moderate to severe disease. The effect of racemic epinephrine lasts for just a few hours, so repeat every 2 to 4 hours, as needed. Since symptom rebound may occur, monitor the patient prior to discharge for 4 to 6 hours following the last dose.

If there is severe airway obstruction with signs of impending respiratory failure, intubate the patient and transfer to an intensive care unit (ICU). Because the edema is within the narrowest part of the upper airway (cricoid cartilage), use an endotracheal tube that is 0.5 mm smaller than typically calculated for the patient's age. Call anesthesiology if a difficult intubation is anticipated.

Avoid agitating the patient, as crying significantly increases negative intrathoracic pressure and worsens airway collapse. Do not administer humidified oxygen, unless the patient is hypoxic, as it does not improve the symptoms and forcing a mask on an agitated patient will only exacerbate the respiratory distress. Similarly, do not attempt to obtain a blood gas prior to intubation, as it will only serve to agitate the patient.

Indications for Consultation

- **Anesthesia:** Emergent airway management required
- **Otolaryngology:** Significant airway compromise, long duration of symptoms (>1 week), recurrent croup episodes (>2 episodes/season), concern for epiglottitis, bacterial tracheitis, or foreign body aspiration, or evaluation for congenital or acquired airway narrowing

Disposition

- **ICU transfer:** Severe respiratory distress and hypoxemia
- **Discharge criteria:** Mild respiratory distress, no nebulized epinephrine treatment in 6 hours, oxygen saturation greater than 94% on room air, adequate oral intake

Follow-up

- **Primary care:** 1 to 3 days
- **Otolaryngology:** 1 to 2 weeks if the patient has an underlying airway anomaly

Pearls and Pitfalls

- Reserve nebulized epinephrine for patients with moderate to severe respiratory distress.
- The cricoid cartilage is the narrowest part of the pediatric upper airway.
- When intubating a croup patient, use an endotracheal tube size that is 0.5 mm smaller than calculated for the patient's age.

Coding

ICD-9

Croup	**464.4**

Bibliography

Cherry JD. Clinical practice. Croup. *N Engl J Med.* 2008;358:384–391

Chun R, Preciado DA, Zalzal GH, Shah RK. Utility of bronchoscopy for recurrent croup. *Ann Otol Rhinol Laryngol.* 2009;118:495–499

Dobrovoljac M, Geelhoed GC. 27 years of croup: an update highlighting the effectiveness of 0.15 mg/kg of dexamethasone. *Emerg Med Australas.* 2009;21:309–314

Moore M, Little P. Humidified air inhalation for treating croup. *Cochrane Database Syst Rev.* 2006;3:CD002870

Russell KF, Liang Y, O'Gorman K, Johnson DW, Klassen TP. Glucocorticoids for croup. *Cochrane Database Syst Rev.* 2011;1:CD001955

CHAPTER 16

Mastoiditis

Introduction

Mastoiditis is a bacterial infection of the mastoid bone and air cells. It is a complication of acute otitis media (AOM), secondary to spread of the infection beyond the middle ear via boney erosion or through the emissary vein of the mastoid. Although the incidence has decreased dramatically as a result of antibiotic therapy for AOM and vaccinations, there has recently been an increase in the number of severe cases, including subperiosteal abscesses. The most common pathogen remains *Streptococcus pneumoniae*, although gram-negative bacilli (*Pseudomonas aeruginosa*, nontypable *Haemophilus influenzae*) are also implicated. There has been an increase in the amount of disease due to *Staphylococcus aureus* (including methicillin-resistant *S aureus*) and *Streptococcus pyogenes*, while *Moraxella catarrhalis* and *Aspergillus* are rarely involved.

Clinical Presentation

History

Usually there is a history of AOM during the preceding 2 weeks. Typical complaints include fever (>38.3°C; 101°F) along with headache, otalgia and/or otorrhea, and pain over the mastoid process. A younger patient may have nonspecific complaints such as irritability, anorexia, and fatigue.

Chronic mastoiditis may occur and can be either subclinical or present with prolonged otorrhea and otalgia.

Physical Examination

The mastoid process is swollen, erythematous, tender (can be severe), and occasionally fluctuant. The auricle is displaced both anteriorly and inferiorly (or down and outward in a patient <2 years of age), while the ipsilateral tympanic membrane frequently, but not always, shows the signs of AOM (erythema, bulging, loss of landmarks). Usually the neurologic examination is nonfocal, although with more severe disease cranial nerve involvement may occur (most frequently VI, VII, or the ophthalmic branch of V). As a result, the patient may have a facial palsy or double vision.

Laboratory

If mastoiditis is suspected, obtain a computed tomography (CT) scan of the temporal bones, as plain mastoid radiographs are unreliable. Typical findings include clouding of the mastoid air cells and loss of the intermastoid cell septa secondary to the osteomyelitic process. Fluid in the middle ear and mastoid without the loss of bony septa can be seen with AOM and is not diagnostic of acute mastoiditis. Other findings may include abscess formation and intracranial extension. Persistent infection in the mastoid cavity can lead to coalescent mastoiditis, or empyema of the temporal bone. This is divided into the following 5 stages (increasing in severity):

- Stage 1: Hyperemia to mucosal lining of mastoid air cells
- Stage 2: Transudate and/or exudates within the cells
- Stage 3: Necrosis of the bone
- Stage 4: Cell wall loss with abscess formation
- Stage 5: Extension

Obtain a complete blood cell count, erythrocyte sedimentation rate (ESR) and/or C-reactive protein (CRP), and a blood culture. Typically the patient has a leukocytosis with a left shift, as well as elevated CRP and ESR. The blood culture will be positive in about 5% of cases.

Differential Diagnosis

Usually the diagnosis is clear, based on fever, ipsilateral AOM, and displacement of the pinna with swelling, erythema, and tenderness of the posterior auricular area. Distortion or swelling of the pinna may also be seen with an insect bite reaction or a chondritis. The differential diagnosis of mastoiditis is summarized in Table 16-1.

Treatment

Obtain an otolaryngology consult. Surgical drainage is indicated if a subperiosteal or intracranial abscess is seen on CT scan or if the patient does not improve clinically after 24 to 48 hours of intravenous (IV) antibiotics. Other surgical interventions may include myringotomy and tympanocentesis, as well as simple or radical mastoidectomy. In addition, tympanocentesis fluid sent for Gram stain and culture will help to guide the choice of antibiotics.

After the CT is obtained, a lumbar puncture is indicated if the patient presents with altered mental status or signs of intracranial extension. If there is a cerebrospinal fluid pleocytosis, request a neurosurgery consult.

Treat with IV ceftriaxone (100 mg/kg per day divided every 12 hours, 4 g/day maximum) or cefotaxime (200 mg/kg per day divided every 6–8 hours,

Table 16-1. Differential Diagnosis of Mastoiditis	
Diagnosis	**Clinical Features**
Acute otitis media	No erythema, tenderness, or swelling over mastoid Pinna not displaced
Basilar skull fracture	No fever or ipsilateral AOM Pinna not displaced Ecchymoses over mastoid, which may be bilateral
Chondritis	Erythema and swelling contiguous with break in the skin No ipsilateral AOM
Insect bite reaction	No fever Punctum may be evident No ipsilateral AOM
Langerhans cell histiocytosis	Recurrent AOM Seborrheic rash
Otitis externa	Otorrhea and otalgia No erythema, tenderness, or swelling over mastoid Pinna not displaced

Abbreviation: AOM, acute otitis media.

12 g/day maximum), *and* clindamycin (40 mg/kg per day divided every 6–8 hours, 2.7 g/day maximum). Add vancomycin (40–60 mg/kg divided every 6 hours, 4 g/day maximum) if intracranial spread is suspected or there is no response within 24 hours of initiation of therapy. Add cefepime (50 mg/kg divided every 8 hours, 2 g/day maximum) if *Pseudomonas* is implicated. For stages 3 to 5 disease, a minimum of 6 weeks of IV or parenteral antibiotics is necessary, tailored to the specific organism (if identified). Add a topical antimicrobial for chronic mastoiditis (ciprofloxacin otic drops 0.25 mL twice a day for 7 days).

For stages 1 and 2, give a shorter IV course (7–10 days), followed by oral therapy (to complete a 4-week course) once the patient has been afebrile for 24 hours and there is improvement in the inflammatory markers and physical examination.

Indications for Consultation

- **Neurology and neurosurgery:** Signs of intracranial extension
- **Otolaryngology:** All patients

Disposition

- **Intensive care unit transfer:** Intracranial spread or associated meningitis
- **Discharge criteria:** Afebrile for 48 hours, with significant clinical improvement and downward trending of the inflammatory markers

Follow-up

- **Primary care:** 1 week
- **Otolaryngology:** 2 weeks

Pearls and Pitfalls

- An infant may not have the classic displacement of the pinna.
- Not every case of mastoiditis is associated with an ipsilateral AOM.
- A patient with mastoiditis is at risk for hearing loss, so audiology follow-up is necessary.

Coding

ICD-9

• Acute mastoiditis with other complications	**383.02**
• Chronic mastoiditis	**383.1**
• Mastoiditis without complications	**383.00**
• Subperiosteal abscess of mastoid	**383.01**

Bibliography

Agrawal S, Husein M, MacRae D. Complications of otitis media: an evolving state. *J Otolaryngol.* 2005;34 (suppl 1):S33–S39

Choi SS, Lander L. Pediatric acute mastoiditis in the post-pneumococcal conjugate vaccine era. *Laryngoscope.* 2011;121:1072–1080

Pang LH, Barakate MS, Havas TE. Mastoiditis in a paediatric population: a review of 11 years experience in management. *Int J Pediatr Otorhinolaryngol.* 2009;73:1520–1524

van den Aardweg MT, Rovers MM, de Ru JA, Albers FW, Schilder AG. A systematic review of diagnostic criteria for acute mastoiditis in children. *Otol Neurotol.* 2008;29: 751–757

CHAPTER 17

Neck Masses

Introduction

The etiologies of pediatric neck masses include inflammatory, congenital, and neoplastic processes. Most are benign and inflammatory in nature, either reactive cervical lymphadenopathy or lymphadenitis (page 99). Thyroglossal duct cysts (TDCs) and branchial cleft anomalies (BCAs) are the most common congenital neck masses. Malignant processes account for a small minority of neck masses, but must always be considered in the differential diagnosis.

TDCs are the most common midline neck masses and present during the first 5 years of life. Ectopic thyroid glands are commonly associated with TDCs, and the cysts themselves may contain thyroid tissue. Consequently, the patient may be hypothyroid. Branchial cleft anomalies are the most common lateral neck masses, with anomalies of the second branchial cleft accounting for 95% of cases. Branchial cleft sinuses and fistulas present during infancy and early childhood, whereas cysts present later on in life.

Clinical Presentation

History

Determine the rate of growth. Generally, a benign process is characterized by rapid growth (with the exception of non-Hodgkin's Lymphoma), whereas slow growth is more typical of a malignancy. Ask about systemic symptoms, such as fever, fatigue, weight loss, and night sweats, which suggest a malignant process over an infectious one. Cysts often fluctuate in size, increasing with upper respiratory tract infections. Chronic, intermittent drainage is consistent with a sinus tract and fistula.

Physical Examination

Perform a thorough examination of the mass, paying particular attention to the location, consistency, mobility, and whether there is an orifice. Most masses located anterior to the sternocleidomastoid muscle are benign, but consider a thyroid mass to be malignant until proven otherwise. In general, masses located in the supraclavicular region, posterior triangle, and both the anterior and posterior triangles are more likely to be malignant. Other clues to a malignancy include a single, dominant lymph node that persists for more than 6 weeks and firm, painless masses that are matted or fixed to underlying structures. A fluctuant mass is usually an abscess or cyst, while an orifice suggests a sinus tract or fistula.

Perform a complete physical examination. Cranial nerve deficits, stridor, and tracheal deviation suggest mass impingement on surrounding structures. Pay particular attention to generalized lymphadenopathy and hepatosplenomegaly, which suggest a malignancy. Skin findings are often clues to the etiology (viral exanthema).

Non-inflamed TDCs are painless, cystic, midline masses that move with tongue protrusion and swallowing. Although primarily located below the hyoid bone, they may be found anywhere from the base of the tongue to the thyroid gland. Infected cysts are painful, erythematous, and fluctuant.

Non-inflamed branchial cleft cysts are painless, fluctuant, lateral masses. Second branchial cleft cysts are commonly located along the anterior boarder of the sternocleidomastoid muscle, while first branchial cleft cysts can be anywhere from the external auditory canal to the angle of the mandible. Cysts often become inflamed during upper respiratory tract infections and become erythematous and painful.

Laboratory

Benign Masses

For cystic lesions, discuss with the surgeon if a fine-needle aspiration (FNA) is recommended (not when mycobacterial infection is a concern). If performed, order a Gram stain, routine anaerobic and aerobic cultures, histopathology, and cytology. For TDCs, obtain thyroid studies.

Malignant Masses

If a malignant process is suspected, order a complete blood cell count with differential and peripheral blood smear, chemistries, lactate dehydrogenase, uric acid, and liver function tests.

Radiology

Benign Masses

If the diagnosis remains uncertain after clinical assessment, order an ultrasound to evaluate cystic masses such as a TDC or BCA. For a TDC, obtain the ultrasound and/or thyroid scan to look for thyroid tissue prior to any surgical excision. If a sinus tract and fistula are present, consult with the surgeon regarding the need for a computed tomography (CT) to completely visualize the tract.

Malignant Masses

Prior to ordering imaging, discuss the case with the radiologist and consulting oncologist and/or surgeon. CT and magnetic resonance imaging allow for better visualization of soft tissue structures and delineation of anatomical boundaries than ultrasound.

Differential Diagnosis

The priorities are to rule out a neoplasm and address a life-threatening complication, such as airway compression. The differential diagnosis is summarized in Tables 17-1 and 17-2.

Treatment

Benign Cystic Masses

If there are no signs of airway compromise, treat an infection, if present, before arranging surgery. If possible, perform an FNA to obtain fluid for Gram stain and routine aerobic and anaerobic culture. Use clindamycin (40 mg/kg/day intravenous [IV] divided every 8 hours, 2.7 g/day maximum) or ampicillin-sulbactam (150 mg/kg per day of ampicillin IV divided every 6 hours, 8 g/day ampicillin maximum) to cover oropharyngeal flora. When the patient is afebrile and clinically improved, change to an oral antibiotic such as clindamycin (30 mg/kg/day oral divided every 8 hours) or a narrow-spectrum antibiotic if the sensitivities are known, to complete at 10- to 14-day course.

For TDC and BCA, the mass must be fully excised or it may reoccur. Consult a surgeon (otolaryngology or general surgery) to discuss the timing of surgery, which usually can be scheduled as an outpatient procedure.

Table 17-1. Congenital Neck Masses

Diagnosis	Clinical Features
Cystic hygroma	Soft, painless compressible mass that transilluminates
Dermoid cyst	Midline painless, doughy, or rubbery mass Moves with overlying skin Does not move with tongue protrusion or swallowing
Hemangioma	Present at birth or shortly thereafter Rapid growth phase followed by slow involution Red to blue soft mass
Teratoma	Common cause of neonatal airway obstruction Firm mass with irregular boarders Imaging: bulky heterogeneous mass with solid and cystic component
Thymic cyst	Painless, unilateral cystic mass

Table 17-2. Neoplastic Neck Masses	
Diagnosis	**Clinical Features**
Benign Neoplastic Masses	
Lipoma	Soft, painless subcutaneous mass Golf ball–sized
Neurofibromas	Soft, skin-colored cutaneous or subcutaneous nodules
Thyroid nodule	Midline nodule that moves with the thyroid gland Consider to be malignant until proven otherwise
Malignant Neoplastic Masses	
Hodgkin's lymphoma	Slow-growing neck mass Painless, rubbery or firm lymph node Anterior or posterior cervical, preauricular, supraclavicular lymph nodes Fever, night sweats, weight loss, hepatosplenomegaly
Neuroblastoma	*Metastatic Disease (Primary Abdomen or Thorax Tumor)* Proptosis, periorbital swelling, and ecchymoses Acute cerebellar ataxia (opsoclonus-myoclonus and nystagmus) *Primary Cervical Disease* Lateral or retropharyngeal neck mass Symptoms of mass impingement on surrounding organs (cranial nerve palsies, Horner syndrome, cough, stridor, dysphagia)
Non-Hodgkin's lymphoma	Rapidly enlarging neck mass Painless, firm to hard lymph node Spinal accessory, supraclavicular lymph nodes Fever, weight loss, bone and joint pain
Rhabdomyosarcoma	Painless, hard mass Anterior and posterior cervical areas Symptoms of mass impingement on surrounding organs (hoarseness)
Thyroid carcinoma	Firm mass that feels different from other thyroid tissue History of irradiation

Malignant Masses

If a malignant mass is suspected, consult an oncologist for recommendations about additional imaging, blood work, and biopsy (FNA versus excisional). Also discuss which surgical service is most appropriate for managing the patient, as well as whether to transfer the patient to an oncology or surgical service.

Indications for Consultation

- **Oncology:** Malignant neck masses
- **Otolaryngology or general surgery:** TDC, BCA, or any other neck mass that requires biopsy or surgical excision

Disposition

- **Intensive care unit transfer:** Airway obstruction
- **Discharge criteria:** Stable on room air and tolerating oral intake, including any antibiotics; appropriate diagnostic and treatment plan in place (surgical intervention or oncologic consultation if indicated)

Follow-up

- **Primary care:** 3 to 4 days
- **If surgery was performed:** 1 to 3 days with the surgical service

Pearls and Pitfalls

- About 1% of patients with a preoperative diagnosis of TDC will actually have a median ectopic thyroid gland containing all of the functional thyroid tissue.
- If a patient is hypothyroid, have a high suspicion for an ectopic thyroid gland.

Coding

ICD-9

• Branchial cleft cyst	**44.42**
• Branchial cleft sinus or fistula	**44.41**
• Enlargement of lymph nodes	**785.6**
• Neck mass	**784.2**
• Thyroglossal duct cyst	**759.2**

Bibliography

Dickson PV, Davidoff AM. Malignant neoplasms of the head and neck. *Semin Pediatr Surg.* 2006;15:92–98

Foley DS, Fallat ME. Thyroglossal duct and other congenital midline cervical anomalies. *Semin Pediatr Surg.* 2006;15:70–75

Tracy TF Jr, Muratore CS. Management of common head and neck masses. *Semin Pediatr Surg.* 2007;16:3–13

Waldhausen JH. Branchial cleft and arch anomalies in children. *Semin Pediatr Surg.* 2006;15:64–69

Wetmore RF, Potsic WP. Differential diagnosis of neck masses. In: Flint PW, Haughey BH, Lund VJ, et al, eds. *Cummings Otolaryngology—Head and Neck Surgery.* 5th ed. Philadelphia, PA: Mosby Elsevier; 2010:2812–2821

CHAPTER 18

Orbital Cellulitis

Introduction

Orbital (postseptal) cellulitis and periorbital (preseptal) cellulitis are the major infections of the orbital tissues. There has been a notable increase in cases of both in recent years, possibly as a consequence of the increase in multi-drug-resistant organisms. Orbital cellulitis is an ocular emergency, as there is significant morbidity and mortality, including intracranial extension, in up to 5% of patients. A rare complication is osteomyelitis of the frontal bone (Pott puffy tumor).

The orbital septum is a fibrous membrane running from the periosteum of the orbital bones to the tarsal plates. It functions as a barrier between the skin/subcutaneous tissues and the intraorbital structures, preventing superficial (ie, periorbital/preseptal) infections from extending inward.

Orbital cellulitis is most often secondary to extension of sinusitis (most often chronic ethmoid) through the thin and porous medial orbital wall (lamina papyracea), although it can also occur via hematogenous spread or from direct trauma or surgery. As a consequence of the association with sinusitis, it is most common during the winter months, secondary to group A streptococcus, *Streptococcus pneumononiae,* and *Staphylococcus aureus. Pseudomonas, Klebsiella, Eikenella,* and *Enterococcus* are less common, while fungal pathogens are a concern in an immunocompromised patient. A poly-microbial infection with both aerobic and anaerobic bacteria can occur in an older adolescent.

Clinical Presentation

History

Ask about recent sinus infections, facial trauma, or dental surgery. In addition, confirm that the patient has normal immune status.

Physical Examination

The patient typically presents with fever; malaise; regional adenopathy; and warm, tender, erythematous lid swelling. The cardinal signs are proptosis, conjunctival chemosis, pain with eye movement, and ophthalmoplegia, which may be noted by the patient despite severe lid swelling preventing direct observation of the extraocular movements. However, all of these signs are not always present. Increased intraocular pressure and a purulent nasal discharge may also be seen. Decreased visual acuity or visual field defects, which may be present initially or later in the course, is an ophthalmologic emergency secondary to involvement of the optic nerve. Unremitting headache and altered mental status suggest intracranial extension, while forehead swelling occurs with Pott puffy tumor.

Laboratory

Obtain a computed tomography (CT) scan of the orbits and sinuses (not a head CT) to confirm the diagnosis and look for an orbital abscess, subperiosteal abscess, or intracranial extension. Also obtain a complete blood cell count, erythrocyte sedimentation rate and/or C-reactive protein, and a blood culture. A lumbar puncture is indicated if there is concern for cerebral or meningeal involvement without evidence of increased intracranial pressure.

Differential Diagnosis

It is essential to distinguish orbital cellulitis from periorbital cellulitis, as more aggressive medical and surgical intervention is required with the former. Passively open the eyelids and examine the eyes for conjunctival injection, discharge, proptosis, chemosis, pain with eye movement, and ophthalmoplegia, and check the visual acuity. With an orbital cellulitis the erythema and edema might be limited to the orbit and may not extend onto the face and forehead, as may be seen with a periorbital infection. However, the swelling of Pott puffy tumor may be mistaken for a periorbital infection. The differential diagnosis is summarized in Table 18-1.

Treatment

If orbital cellulitis is suspected or confirmed, promptly consult both an otolaryngologist and an ophthalmologist for possible surgical intervention. Treat intravenously with

1. Ampicillin-sulbactam (200 mg/kg per day divided every 6 hours, 8 g/day maximum) *or* ceftriaxone (100 mg/kg per day 4 g/day maximum) *or* cefotaxime (200 mg/kg per day divided every 6 to 8 hours, 12 g/day, maximum)

plus

2. Clindamycin (40 mg/kg divided every 6 hours, 2.7 g/day maximum) *or* vancomycin (40 mg/kg per day divided every 6 hours, 4 g/day maximum)

Table 18-1. Differential Diagnosis of Orbital Cellulitis	
Diagnosis	**Clinical Features**
Eyelid Edema	
Conjunctivitis	May be bilateral No fever or toxicity
Insect bite	Punctum may be evident May have history of a bite No fever or toxicity
Allergic reaction	No fever or toxicity May have urticarial or swelling elsewhere
Nephrotic syndrome	No fever or toxicity May have swelling in dependent areas Proteinuria
Trauma	May have history or evidence (ecchymoses) of trauma No fever or toxicity
Exophthalmos	
Orbital neoplasm	Slowly progressive "swelling" May have visual changes No fever or toxicity
Hyperthyroidism	Tachycardia, palpitations, lid lag, heat intolerance Goiter may be palpated
Forehead Swelling	
Preseptal cellulitis	May have a history of trauma or a break in the skin No limitation of extraocular movement, proptosis, or chemosis
Pott puffy tumor	Adolescent History compatible with frontal sinusitis No/limited orbital swelling

Indications for Consultation

- **Ophthalmology:** All patients
- **Otolaryngology:** All patients

Disposition

- **Intensive care unit transfer:** Intracranial extension
- **Interinstitutional transfer:** Ophthalmology or otolaryngology service not immediately available
- **Discharge criteria:** Afebrile for 48 hours, with significant clinical improvement, including normal visual acuity and extraocular movements as well as a downward trending of the inflammatory markers; continue oral antibiotics for minimum of 2 weeks

Follow-up

- **Otolaryngology and/or ophthalmology:** Weekly during the antibiotic course

Pearls and Pitfalls

- A subperiosteal abscess may respond to intravenous antibiotics and not require drainage.
- There is a 10% risk of residual loss of visual acuity.
- 90% of cases of orbital cellulitis result from direct spread of sinusitis (most commonly of the ethmoid).

Coding

ICD-9

• Orbital cellulitis	**376.01**
• Orbital osteomyelitis	**376.03**
• Orbital periostitis	**376.02**

Bibliography

Botting AM, McIntosh D, Mahadevan M. Paediatric pre- and post-septal peri-orbital infections are different diseases. A retrospective review of 262 cases. *Int J Pediatr Otorhinolaryngol.* 2008;72:377–383

Goodyear PW, Firth AL, Strachan DR, Dudley M. Periorbital swelling: the important distinction between allergy and infection. *Emerg Med J.* 2004;21:240–242

Hennemann S, Crawford P, Nguyen L, Smith PC. Clinical inquiries. What is the best initial treatment for orbital cellulitis in children? *J Fam Pract.* 2007;56:662–664

Nageswaran S, Woods CR, Benjamin DK Jr, Givner LB, Shetty AK. Orbital cellulitis in children. *Pediatr Infect Dis J.* 2006;25:695–699

Yang M, Quah BL, Seah LL, Looi A. Orbital cellulitis in children—medical treatment versus surgical management. *Orbit.* 2009;28:124–136

CHAPTER 19

Parotitis

Introduction

As a result of mumps immunization, parotitis is now uncommon in children. Risk factors include dehydration, poor oral hygiene, medications (antihistamines, anticholinergics), immunosuppression, and glandular anatomical abnormalities. Most cases are caused by infection (viral or bacterial) or by juvenile recurrent parotitis (JRP).

Bacterial parotitis occurs in infants younger than 2 months (particularly in premature infants in the neonatal intensive care unit) and sporadically in children older than 10 years. The most common pathogen is *Staphylococcus aureus*, but streptococci, gram-negative bacilli, and anerobic bacteria can also be involved, while *Bartonella henselae* can cause a chronic infection. Complications of bacterial parotitis are rare, but if the infection spreads to contiguous structures the patient is at risk for mandibular and tempormandibular joint osteomyelitis, jugular vein thrombophlebitis, mediastinitis, aspiration pneumonia, sepsis, and airway obstruction.

Viral parotitis occurs in children aged 3 to 10 years, either secondary to mumps (in both immunized and unimmunized patients) or other viruses, such as Epstein-Barr virus, enteroviruses, parainfluenza viruses, influenza viruses, cytomegalovirus, HIV, lymphocytic choriomeningitis virus, herpes simplex viruses, and coxsackievirus. With the exception of HIV infection, viral parotitis is self-limited over 7 to 10 days. HIV infection of the parotid gland(s) can be either recurrent or chronic.

JRP presents at a mean age of 6 years. The etiology is unknown, but occasionally cases are associated with an underlying immunodeficiency or autoimmune process. If bacterial superinfection occurs, *Streptococcus pneumoniae* is the most common pathogen. Most episodes resolve spontaneously within a few days to weeks, and the disease itself disappears by puberty.

Sjögren syndrome, which is an autoimmune chronic inflammatory disorder, can also present with parotid swelling. It is characterized by decreased salivary and lacrimal production and classically presents with dry mouth and dry eyes. Swelling of the parotids is gradual and typically bilateral.

Clinical Presentation

History

Bacterial parotitis presents with acute, unilateral swelling and intense tenderness of the parotid gland with overlying skin erythema and warmth. High fever and toxicity are common.

Viral parotitis presents with several days of fever, malaise, and headache before parotid gland swelling develops. The swelling and pain are initially unilateral, but eventually become bilateral with one gland affected more than the other. Other symptoms include ipsilateral ear pain, trismus, and dysphagia.

Recurrent parotitis primarily presents with unilateral parotid gland swelling that occurs every 3 to 4 months. It is usually accompanied by fever and pain.

Physical Examination

The patient will have fever and parotid gland pain and swelling that obscures the angle of the jaw. Examine the mass carefully to ensure that the swelling originates from the parotid gland itself and not surrounding structures such as lymph nodes.

Bacterial, viral, and recurrent parotitis may be differentiated by examining the skin overlying the parotid gland and applying external pressure to the parotid gland and observing the Stensen duct (located in the buccal mucosal opposite the upper second molar). In bacterial parotitis, the overlying skin is extremely tender and erythematous. The duct opening is inflamed and prominent, and the secretions are purulent. In viral parotitis, there is significant skin and soft tissue swelling over the gland, but erythema and warmth are absent. The duct appears erythematous and has clear secretions. In JRP, overlying skin findings are rare and duct secretions are clear or purulent.

Laboratory

If viral parotitis is suspected, no further workup is required unless HIV is suspected. If clinically indicated and available, send specific virus polymerase chain reaction (PCR) studies.

If bacterial parotitis is suspected, express pus from the Stensen duct and send for Gram stain and routine aerobic and anaerobic cultures, as well as fungal and mycobacterial cultures if the patient has an immunodeficiency or chronic disease. However, to avoid culture contamination with intraoral flora, it is optimal to perform a fine-needle aspiration via the intraoral route. Also obtain a blood culture if the patient is severely ill or appears toxic. If there is no improvement after several days of antibiotics, order an ultrasound to look for an abscess. To evaluate for *B henselae,* send either a PCR or, more commonly, *Bartonella* serology.

If JRP is diagnosed, obtain serum immunoglobulins (including IgA) and an ANA. Arrange an ultrasound to look for the hallmark finding of sialectasis (cystically dilated intraglandular ducts). Order a sialogram if there is concern for additional anatomical abnormality, such as stones or strictures.

Differential Diagnosis

The differential diagnosis is summarized in Table 19-1.

Treatment

Manage viral parotitis conservatively with analgesics such as acetaminophen (15 mg/kg orally [PO] every 4–6 hours) or ibuprofen (10 mg/kg PO every 6 hours), hydration, gland massage (frequency per provider discretion), sialogogues (lemon drops/candy), and good oral hygiene.

Table 19-1. Differential Diagnosis of Parotitis

Diagnosis	Clinical Features
Bartonella	Tender, swollen lymph node Overlying erythema, can be suppurative Enlarged lymph nodes proximal to inoculation site
Bulimia	Adolescent females Painless bilateral parotid swelling Dental enamel erosion
Granulomatous parotitis	Painless enlarging parotid mass without surrounding inflammation Pathogens: cat scratch disease, *Mycobacterium tuberculosis,* atypical mycobacteria, *Acintomyces, Francisella tularensis,* and *Brucella* species
HIV	Parotitis can be the first sign of HIV Bilateral tender parotid enlargement
Lymphadenitis	Tender, swollen lymph node Overlying erythema and swelling Angle of jaw is not obscured
Neoplasm (lymphoma, leukemia, MALT tumor)	Constitutional or systemic symptoms Cervical adenopathy rather than parotid inflammation
Pneumoparotid	Unilateral/bilateral parotid swelling Increased intraoral pressure (musical instruments, anesthesia) forces air into Stensen duct.
Sjögren syndrome	History of autoimmune disease Bilateral parotid swelling Xerophthalmia, xerostomia, and conjunctivitis

Treat bacterial parotitis with clindamycin (40 mg/kg/day intravenous [IV] divided every 8 hours, 2.7 g/day maximum) to cover *S aureus*. If there is a high prevalence of clindamycin-resistant methicillin-resistant *S aureus,* treat with vancomycin (45 mg/kg/day IV divided every 8 hours, 4 g/day maximum). Clinical improvement typically occurs within the first 48 hours of IV treatment. Switch to oral antibiotics once the patient is afebrile with decreased swelling and pain, and complete a 7- to 14-day course.

If there is no response to antibiotics, replace clindamycin (if it was the initial antibiotic) with vancomycin (as above) and add a third-generation cephalosporin such as cefotaxime (50 mg/kg/day IV divided every 8 hours, 6 g/day maximum) to cover gram-negative pathogens. Order an ultrasound to evaluate for abscess formation and consult otolaryngology if surgical drainage is indicated. Also involve otolaryngology for severe, refractory, or recurrent parotitis to ascertain whether other treatment options (sialography, surgery) are required. If saliva or pus is not expressed from the Stensen duct, cannulation, and dilation may be required to establish patency.

The management of JRP is similar to that for viral parotitis. In addition, sialography or endoscopy and ductal dilation may be therapeutic. Antibiotics are not required unless there is concern for a superimposed bacterial infection. Prophylactic antibiotics are ineffective in preventing recurrences.

Indications for Consultation

- **Immunology:** JRP, HIV
- **Infectious diseases:** HIV
- **Otolaryngology:** Bacterial parotitis, JRP
- **Rheumatology:** Sjögren syndrome

Disposition

- **Intensive care unit transfer:** Sepsis, shock, spread of infection to surrounding tissues with airway compromise
- **Discharge criteria:** Afebrile, tolerating oral intake, improvement in parotid gland swelling and pain, pus no longer expressed from Stensen duct

Follow-up

- **Primary care:** 2 to 3 days.
- **Otolaryngology (if involved):** 1 to 2 weeks, during the outpatient antibiotic course

Pearls and Pitfalls

- If Stensen duct obstruction occurs, secretions will not be present.
- The keys to diagnosis are the appearance of the skin overlying the parotid gland and duct secretion composition.

Coding

ICD-9

• Mumps without complication	**072.9**
• Parotid abscess	**527.3**
• Sialoadenitis	**527.2**

Bibliography

Al-Dajani N, Wootton SH. Cervical lymphadenitis, suppurative parotitis, thyroiditis, and infected cysts. *Infect Dis Clin North Am.* 2007;21:523–541

Clark JR, Campbell JR. Parotitis. In: Feigin RD, Cherry JD, Demmler-Harrison GJ, Kaplan SL, eds. *Textbook of Pediatric Infectious Diseases.* 6th ed. Philadelphia, PA: Saunders; 2009:197–200

Leerdam CM, Martin HC, Isaacs D. Recurrent parotitis of childhood. *J Paediatr Child Health.* 2005;41:631–634

McMillan, J, Feigin, RD, DeAngelis, C, Douglas, JM. Parotitis. In: McMillan JA, Feigin RD, DeAngelis C, Jones DM, eds. *Oski's Pediatrics.* 4th ed. Philadelphia, PA: Lippincott, Williams & Wilkins; 2006:1519–1523

Nahlieli O, Shacham R, Shlesinger M, Eliav E. Juvenile recurrent parotitis: a new method of diagnosis and treatment. *Pediatrics.* 2004;114:9–12

Peritonsillar Abscess

Introduction

Peritonsillar abscess (PTA) or quinsy is a collection of pus located in the space between the tonsil and the superior pharyngeal constrictor muscle. It is the most frequent deep neck infection in older children and adolescents, but is uncommon in young children.

Infections are polymicrobial. The most common pathogens are *Streptococcus pyogenes* (group A streptococcus) and mixed oropharyngeal anaerobes (including *Fusobacterium, Prevotella, Bacteriodes, Porphyromonas,* and *Peptostreptococcus* species). Other pathogens include S*taphylococcus aureus* (including methicillin-resistant *S aureus* [MRSA]) and *Haemophilus influenzae.*

One of the most feared complications of PTA is spontaneous rupture of the abscess with subsequent aspiration pneumonia. Other rare complications include abscess extension into adjacent structures causing airway obstruction, ipsilateral vocal cord paralysis, coronary artery erosion, internal jugular vein thrombosis, mediastinitis, sepsis, and cervical vertebrae osteomyelitis.

Clinical Presentation

History

There is usually a history of a recent infection, such as tonsillitis, streptococcal pharyngitis, or viral respiratory illness (especially mononucleosis). Typical complaints include fever, severe sore throat, drooling, dysphagia, a muffled or "hot potato" voice, and trismus (inability to fully open the mouth secondary to irritation and reflex spasm of the internal pterygoid muscle). Other symptoms include odynophagia, neck pain, and ipsilateral ear pain.

Physical Examination

The classic findings are trismus, a bulging tonsil covered with exudate, and deviation of the uvula away from the affected side. Other findings include halitosis, pooling of saliva in the floor of the mouth, palpation of a fluctuant tonsil, and tender ipsilateral cervical lymphadenopathy.

Laboratory

No laboratory testing is needed. Although empiric antibiotic coverage is often successful, if a drainage procedure is performed, send the specimens for Gram stain and both aerobic and anaerobic cultures.

Radiology

Imaging is also not necessary to make the diagnosis of PTA and is contraindicated in a patient with airway compromise. However, obtain a computed tomography scan of the neck with intravenous (IV) contrast if it is impossible to differentiate PTA from other deep neck space infections on clinical grounds. The surgeon may request intraoral ultrasonography to distinguish PTA from peritonsillar cellulitis and to guide needle aspiration.

Differential Diagnosis

See Table 20-1.

Treatment

Immediate surgical drainage is indicated if the patient presents with airway compromise. Otherwise, arrange for either a needle aspiration or incision and drainage. The type of initial drainage procedure varies, based on the availability of a pediatric emergency medicine physician trained in needle aspiration or the otolaryngologist's preference.

A quinsy tonsillectomy (tonsillectomy with simultaneous abscess drainage) is indicated if the initial abscess drainage is inadequate as evidenced by abscess recurrence or no improvement in the symptoms. It is also the preferred approach by otolaryngology if the patient has a history of severe or recurrent pharyngitis or obstructive sleep apnea.

Table 20-1. Differential Diagnosis of Peritonsillar Abscess

Diagnosis	Clinical Features
Angioedema	History of allergies or exposure to offending substance Swelling of lips/tongue, urticarial rash Stridor and respiratory distress
Bacterial tracheitis	Abrupt onset of upper airway obstruction in patient recovering from a viral illness (croup, influenza) Copious, purulent secretions on suctioning
Epiglottitis (very rare)	Abrupt onset with fever and toxicity Rapid progression to respiratory obstruction Patient prefers a "sniffing" posture
Retropharyngeal abscess	Occurs in preschool-aged children No peritonsillar swelling or uvula deviation Limited neck extension
Uvulitis	Swelling and erythema of the uvula No peritonsillar swelling

Medical management includes analgesia (avoid nonsteroidal anti-inflammatory drugs until discussed with otolaryngology), fluid hydration, and antibiotics. Treat with clindamycin (40 mg/kg/day divided every 8 hours IV, 2.7 g/day maximum). IV ampicillin-sulbactam (150 mg/kg/day of ampicillin divided every 6 hours, 8 g/day maximum) is an alternative choice if the prevalence of MRSA is low. Add vancomycin (45 mg/kg/day IV divided every 8 hours, 4 g/day maximum) or linezolid (<12 years: 10 mg/kg every 8 hours IV; ≥12 years: 10 mg/kg every 12 hours IV, 1.2 g/day maximum) if the patient does not respond to clindamycin after surgical drainage, there is locally a high MRSA prevalence, or the patient presents with severe disease. Continue IV therapy until the patient is afebrile and clinically improved, at which time change the patient to oral therapy, such as empiric clindamycin (30 mg/kg/day divided every 8 hours, 4.8 g/day maximum) or a narrow-spectrum antibiotic based on known sensitivities to complete a 14-day course. Once the acute illness is over, the surgeon may schedule a tonsillectomy for 1 to 3 months in the future, particularly if the course was complicated or the patient has recurrences.

Do not use corticosteroids in the treatment of PTA.

Indications for Consultation

- **Anesthesia:** Signs of airway compromise including stridor, increased work of breathing, and hypoxemia
- **Otolaryngology:** No response to antibiotics, drainage procedure needed, or recurrent abscess formation

Disposition

- **Intensive care unit transfer:** Signs of airway compromise or complications such as severe aspiration pneumonia, coronary artery erosion, internal jugular vein thrombosis, or mediastinitis
- **Discharge criteria:** Afebrile, improved neck range of motion, adequate pain control on oral medication, adequate oral intake

Follow-up

- **Primary care:** 3 to 5 days
- **Ear, nose, and throat (ENT) (if surgery was performed):** During the outpatient antibiotic course

Pearls and Pitfalls

- If there are signs of airway compromise, promptly consult both ENT and anesthesia and move the patient to a setting where an emergent artificial airway can be secured.
- PTA recurs in 5% to 15% of patients.

Coding

ICD-9

- Peritonsillar abscess (quinsy) **475**
- Tonsillitis (acute or NOS) **463**
- Tonsillitis (chronic) **474.00**

Bibliography

Galioto NJ. Peritonsillar abscess. *Am Fam Physician*. 2008;77:199–202

Goldstein NA, Hammerschlag MR. Peritonsillar, retropharyngeal, and parapharyngeal abscesses. In: Feigin RD, Cherry JD, Demmler-Harrison GJ, Kaplan SL, eds. *Textbook of Pediatric Infectious Diseases*. 6th ed. Philadelphia, PA: Saunders; 2009:177–185

Johnson RF, Stewart MG. The contemporary approach to diagnosis and management of peritonsillar abscess. *Curr Opin Otolaryngol Head Neck Surg*. 2005;13:157–160

Khayr W, Taepke J. Management of peritonsillar abscess: needle aspiration versus incision and drainage versus tonsillectomy. *Am J Ther*. 2005;12:344–350

Millar KR, Johnson DW, Drummond D, Kellner JD. Suspected peritonsillar abscess in children. *Pediatr Emerg Care*. 2007;23:431–438

CHAPTER 21

Retropharyngeal Abscess

Introduction

Retropharyngeal abscess is a suppurative bacterial infection of the retropharyngeal space. This is the area between the pharynx and cervical vertebrae that extends from the skull into the superior mediastinum. It most often occurs in children younger than 6 years with a peak incidence at 4 years. Recently there has been an increase in the number of cases.

Retropharyngeal lymph nodes drain the nasopharynx, adenoids, posterior paranasal sinuses, and middle ear structures. These nodes are prominent in young children, but begin to atrophy before puberty, accounting for the increased incidence in younger children and relatively rare occurrence in adolescents, except following posterior pharyngeal wall trauma. A preceding oropharyngeal infection leads to a retropharyngeal cellulitis that organizes into a phlegmon and then into an abscess.

Most infections are polymicrobial, with a recent increase in the incidence of group A streptococcus. Other common pathogens include *Staphylococcus aureus* (including methicillin-resistant *S aureus* [MRSA]) and respiratory anaerobes (*Fusobacterium*, *Prevotella*, *Bacteriodes*, *Porphyromonas*, and *Peptostreptococcus* species).

The morbidity and mortality of retropharyngeal abscesses result from extension into adjacent structures. Complications include airway obstruction, abscess rupture and subsequent aspiration, mediastinitis, internal jugular vein thrombosis (Lemierre disease), carotid artery aneurysm, and sepsis. These complications are very rare due to early diagnosis and treatment.

Clinical Presentation

History

A younger child presents with an antecedent history of ear, nose, throat, or nonspecific upper respiratory tract infection, while an older patient will often have a history of preceding pharyngeal trauma (penetrating foreign body, endoscopy, intubation, dental procedure).

The most common presenting symptoms are fever, neck pain, neck swelling, sore throat, dysphagia, and odynophagia. Other complaints may include irritability, decreased oral intake, muffled voice, or drooling. Stridor and upper airway obstruction are uncommon presenting symptoms in children.

Physical Examination

Typical findings include neck tenderness, limitation of neck movements (especially neck extension), and torticollis. Cervical lymphadenopathy is common, with the nodes located deep to the sternocleidomastoid muscle. Inspection of the oropharynx may reveal midline or unilateral posterior pharyngeal swelling, but this is absent in more than 50% of younger children.

Laboratory

No laboratory testing is needed. If the patient is toxic-appearing or does not respond to empiric antibiotic therapy, attempt to make a definitive microbial diagnosis by arranging surgical incision and drainage and sending specimens for Gram stain and both aerobic and anerobic cultures.

Radiology

If the diagnosis of retropharyngeal infection is equivocal and the patient has no signs of airway obstruction, obtain a screening lateral neck radiograph. This will confirm retropharyngeal swelling, but will not differentiate between cellulitis, phlegmon, or abscess. Proper x-ray technique is important to avoid an artificially thickened appearance of the retropharyngeal soft tissues. Ensure that it is performed during inspiration, with the neck extended and the patient in a true lateral position. Widened prevertebral soft tissues, exceeding the anteroposterior diameter of the adjacent vertebral body, is consistent with retropharyngeal inflammation.

If a retropharyngeal abscess is suspected based on clinical assessment or soft tissue swelling noted on x-ray, obtain a neck computed tomography (CT) scan with intravenous (IV) contrast. The study will then identify the location of the infection as well as any extension into other adjacent neck or chest spaces. Findings suggestive of an abscess include ring enhancement and irregular abscess border (referred to as scalloping).

Differential Diagnosis

See Table 21-1.

Treatment

Immediate surgical drainage is indicated for any patient with airway compromise. Otherwise, treat medically for 24 to 48 hours and obtain an otolaryngology consult if there is no improvement. Findings associated with drainable

Table 21-1. Differential Diagnosis of Retropharyngeal Abscess

Diagnosis	Clinical Features
Anaphylaxis	Swelling of lips/tongue Urticarial rash Stridor and respiratory distress
Bacterial tracheitis	Abrupt onset of upper airway obstruction in patient recovering from croup Toxic appearance Copious, purulent secretions on suctioning
Croup	Harsh, barky cough; stridor; and drooling No limited neck movement No posterior pharyngeal swelling
Epiglottitis (rare)	Abrupt onset with fever, toxicity, and drooling Rapid progression to respiratory obstruction Patient prefers a "sniffing" posture
Meningitis	Ill-appearing, irritable, photophobia Limited neck flexion and other meningeal signs
Peritonsillar abscess	Older children and adolescents Severe sore throat, muffled voice, and trismus Exudative tonsillitis with uvula deviation
Uvulitis	Swelling and erythema of the uvula

fluid at surgery include symptoms for more than 2 days, prior antibiotic therapy, and a fluid collection with a cross-sectional area greater than 2 cm^2 on CT scan.

Treat with clindamycin (40 mg/kg/day IV divided every 8 hours, 2.7 g/day maximum). Ampicillin-sulbactam (150 mg/kg/day IV divided every 6 hours, 8 g/day maximum) is an alternative choice if there is a low prevalence of MRSA. Add vancomycin (15 mg/kg IV every 8 hours, 4 g/day maximum) or linezolid (<12 years: 10 mg/kg IV every 8 hours; ≥12 years: 10 mg/kg IV every 12 hours, 1.2 g/day maximum) if the patient does not respond to clindamycin after surgical drainage, there is a high MRSA prevalence locally, or the patient presents with severe disease. Continue IV therapy until the patient is afebrile and clinically improved, at which time change to oral therapy with empiric clindamycin (10 mg/kg every 8 hours) or a narrow-spectrum antibiotic based on known sensitivities to complete a 14-day course.

If there is no clinical improvement after 24 to 48 hours of antibiotic therapy, obtain a neck CT with IV contrast to evaluate for the presence of a drainable fluid collection.

Indications for Consultation

- **Anesthesia:** Signs of airway compromise including stridor, increased work of breathing, and hypoxemia
- **Otolaryngology:** Surgical drainage needed

Disposition

- **Intensive care unit transfer:** Signs of airway compromise or complications such as mediastinitis, internal jugular vein thrombosis, or coronary artery aneurysm
- **Discharge criteria:** Afebrile with significant clinical improvement, including increased neck range of motion, decreased pain, and good oral intake

Follow-up

- **Primary care:** 2 to 3 days
- **Otolaryngology (if surgery was performed):** During the outpatient antibiotic course

Pearls and Pitfalls

- If there are signs of airway compromise, promptly consult both ear, nose, and throat and anesthesia specialists and move the patient to a setting where an emergent artificial airway can be secured.
- Stridor and other signs of airway compromise are uncommon presenting findings.

Coding

ICD-9

Retropharyngeal abscess	**478.24**

Bibliography

Elsherif AM, Park AH, Alder SC, et al. Indicators of a more complicated clinical course for pediatric patients with retropharyngeal abscess. *Int J Pediatr Otorhinolaryngol.* 2010;74:198–201

Goldstein NA, Hammerschlag MR. Deep neck abscesses. In: McMillan JA, Feigin RD, DeAngelis C, Jones DM, eds. *Oski's Pediatrics.* 4th ed. Philadelphia, PA: Lippincott, Williams & Wilkins; 2006:1492–1496

Goldstein NA, Hammerschlag MR. Peritonsillar, retropharyngeal, and parapharyngeal abscesses. In: Feigin RD, Cherry JD, Demmler-Harrison GJ, Kaplan SL, eds. *Textbook of Pediatric Infectious Diseases.* 6th ed. Philadelphia, PA: Saunders; 2009:177–185

Grisaru-Soen G, Komisar O, Aizenstein O, et al. Retropharyngeal and parapharyngeal abscess in children—epidemiology, clinical features and treatment. *Int J Pediatr Otorhinolaryngol.* 2010;74:1016–1020

Schuler PJ, Cohnen M, Greve J, et al. Surgical management of retropharyngeal abscesses. *Acta Otolaryngol.* 2009;129:1274–1279

Endocrinology

CHAPTER 22

Diabetes Insipidus

Introduction

Diabetes insipidus (DI) is caused by a deficiency (central DI) of antidiuretic hormone (ADH) or insensitivity to ADH in the kidneys (nephrogenic DI). Both causes prevent water from being reabsorbed in the kidneys and lead to increased urine production. Central DI is caused by genetic defects, congenital abnormalities (septo-optic-dysplasia, holoprosencephaly), disruptions in the hypothalamic-pituitary ADH production (trauma, neoplasms, infections, autoimmune disorders), or idiopathic causes. Nephrogenic DI may be genetic, idiopathic, or acquired, including kidney disease (chronic renal failure, pyelonephritis, obstructive uropathy, polycystic kidney disease), medications (amphotericin B, gentamicin, lithium), and electrolyte disorders (hypokalemia, hypercalcemia).

Clinical Presentation

History

The patient may present with nonspecific findings such as irritability, intermittent fever, vomiting, seizures, hypotonia, or failure to thrive. Obtain a detailed history to assess fluid intake, urine output, and the voiding pattern. The parents may report polydipsia and polyuria (>2 L/m^2/day). Extreme thirst and nighttime fluid intake can also lead to sleep disturbances and daytime tiredness. However, polydipsia may be absent if the patient does not have an intact thirst mechanism. Enuresis in a previously toilet-trained child is also common. A patient with known DI may present with some other cause for a disruption of the homeostasis, such as an intercurrent illness.

Physical Examination

The initial priority is to assess for evidence of severe dehydration or shock (dry mucous membranes, delayed capillary refill, skin tenting, weak peripheral pulses). Also, look for other sequelae of pituitary dysfunction (adrenocorticotropic hormone or growth hormone deficiency), visual and central nervous system dysfunction (headache, visual field changes), and craniofacial midline defects (septo-optic dysplasia).

Laboratory

If DI is suspected, obtain serum for osmolality and electrolytes, and urine for osmolality, specific gravity, and glucose. If intracranial pathology is suspected, arrange for magnetic resonance imaging (MRI) with gadolinium, as computed tomography lacks the detail necessary to properly evaluate the hypothalamus and pituitary gland. The characteristic "bright-spot" of the posterior pituitary seen on T1-weighted MRI images is often decreased or absent in patients with central DI.

The key laboratory findings in DI are

- Urine output greater than the upper limit of normal (150 mL/kg/day for infants; 110 mL/kg/day for toddlers; 40 mL/kg/day for older children)
- Urine specific gravity remains low (<1.005)
- Urine osmolality less than serum osmolality
- Urine osmolality less than 300 mOsm/kg (often remains <150 mOsm/kg)
- Serum hyperosmolality (>300 mOsm/kg)

To confirm the diagnosis of DI, consult a pediatric endocrinologist to perform a water deprivation test followed by a vasopressin test. The differential diagnosis of polyuria is summarized in Table 22-1.

Treatment

Fluid Replacement

- **Resuscitation.** The initial priority is fluid resuscitation with 0.9% normal saline if the patient presents in hypovolemic shock (page 63). Then, correct the hypernatremia and dehydration after calculation of fluid deficit, using 0.45% normal saline over 48 hours to prevent a rapid drop in serum sodium and cerebral edema.

Table 22-1. Differential Diagnosis of Polyuria

Diagnosis	Clinical Features
Primary polydipsia Psychogenic (compulsive) Dipsogenic (abnormal thirst)	Serum and urine osmolality normal to low-normal
Osmotic diuresis (diabetes)	Hyperglycemia ↑serum osmolality Serum sodium normal or decreased
Post-obstructive diuresis	Serum sodium/osmolality normal Urine osmolality normal or decreased
Cushing syndrome	Hyperglycemia Characteristic physical findings: round face, upper body fat, striae
Fanconi syndrome	Acidosis, hypokalemia, hyperchloremia Rickets, osteomalacia Growth failure
Urinary tract infection	Urinary symptoms: dysuria, urgency

- **Free water deficit.** The free water deficit = 4 mL/kg x weight (kg) × (concentration Na^+ measured – concentration Na^+ desired [145mEq/L])
- **Maintenance and ongoing urine losses.** Calculate maintenance fluids (1,600 mL/m^2/day) and ongoing fluid loss from urine output and replace these amounts with 0.45% normal saline.
- **Closely monitor the serum sodium.** The goal is a rate of correction of less than 0.5 mEq/L/hour or 10 mEq/L/day or less to prevent cerebral edema.

Central DI

Treat central DI with desmopressin (DDAVP), which is available as oral, intranasal, and subcutaneous preparations. DDAVP decreases urine output by causing increased water reabsorption in the renal collecting ducts. The doses are

- **Oral:** 50 mcg twice a day (bid), titrate to desired response (100–800 mcg/day <12 years; 100–1200 mcg/day divided bid or 3 times a day [tid] >12 years)
- **Intranasal:** 5 to 30 mcg/day divided bid (3 months–12 years); 5 to 40 mcg/day divided every day tid (>12 years)
- **Subcutaneous:** 2 to 4 mcg/day divided bid

Nephrogenic DI

Manage patients with nephrogenic DI with a low-sodium diet (300–500 mg/day) and diuretics.

- Hydrochlorthiazide: 4 mg/kg/day divided bid (<6 months); 1 to 2 mg/kg/day divided bid (>6 months)
- Amiloride: 0.3 mg/kg/day

Indications for Consultation

- **Endocrinology:** All patients
- **Neurology, neurosurgery, and/or oncology:** Abnormal MRI findings

Disposition

- **Intensive care unit transfer:** Severe dehydration and hypovolemic shock requiring fluid resuscitation, will be receiving the water deprivation and vasopressin tests
- **Discharge criteria:** Clinical improvement, electrolyte abnormalities corrected, a pharmacologic regimen in place, and the family educated about measuring urine output and giving doses of DDAVP

Follow-up

- **Primary care:** 1 to 2 weeks
- **Endocrinologist:** 2 to 3 days

Pearls and Pitfalls

- Surgical or accidental trauma may cause central DI in a previously healthy child if the pituitary is damaged.
- Central DI may be the initial presentation of a brain tumor (germinoma, craniopharyngioma).

Coding

ICD-9

- Central DI **253.5**
- Nephrogenic DI **588.1**
- Primary polydipsia **783.5**

Bibliography

Chang Y. Diabetes insipidus. In: Perkin R, Swift J, Newton D, Anas N, eds. *Pediatric Hospital Medicine Textbook of Inpatient Management.* 2nd ed. Philadelphia, PA: Lippincott, Williams & Wilkins; 2008:534–537

Ghirardello S, Garrè ML, Rossi A, Maghnie M. The diagnosis of children with central diabetes insipidus. *J Pediatr Endocrinol Metab.* 2007;20:359–375

Makaryus AN, McFarlane SI. Diabetes insipidus: diagnosis and treatment of a complex disease. *Cleve Clin J Med.* 2006;73:65–71

Ranadive SA, Rosenthal SM. Pediatric disorders of water balance. *Endocrinol Metab Clin North Am.* 2009;38:663–672

Diabetic Ketoacidosis

Introduction

Diabetic ketoacidosis (DKA) is the leading cause of morbidity and mortality in a child with diabetes. DKA occurs when there is a disruption in the balance between insulin and the counterregulatory hormones, either from a lack of circulating insulin (type 1 diabetes mellitus [T1DM]) or increased counterregulatory hormones in response to stress (trauma, acute gastroenteritis, sepsis). This imbalance leads to a catabolic state, which precipitates the hallmarks of DKA: hyperglycemia, hyperosmolality, increased lipolysis, ketonemia, and metabolic acidosis. An osmotic diuresis ensues, causing dehydration and the production of more counterregulatory hormones, further disrupting the balance.

DKA is the initial presentation of T1DM in about one-quarter of patients, primarily children younger than 5 years and those whose families do not have easy access to medical care. In a patient with known T1DM, DKA tends to occur when there is missed insulin dosing, mismanagement of insulin during illness, or in the setting of a severe febrile or gastrointestinal illness. While DKA is a more common presentation in T1DM, as many as 25% of children with T2DM initially present with DKA.

A young patient (<5 years old) with severe DKA (severe acidosis, low bicarbonate, high blood urea nitrogen) is at increased risk for cerebral edema (CE). This potentially fatal complication of DKA, whose pathogenesis remains unclear, can manifest 4 to 12 hours after treatment is initiated.

Clinical Presentation

History

A patient with DKA often presents with a history of polyuria, polyphagia, polydipsia, and weight loss, sometimes accompanied by nausea, vomiting, or severe abdominal pain. However, nocturia, enuresis, or nonspecific systemic complaints (lethargy or fatigue) can be the initial symptoms. The family or patient may also present complaining of glucosuria or ketonuria because they used urine dipsticks at home.

Physical Examination

The patient presents with signs of dehydration (delayed capillary refill, dry mucous membranes, tachycardia, skin tenting), Kussmaul breathing (rapid, deep sighing), and possibly a fruity breath odor. In severe cases, there may be evidence of hypovolemic shock (hypotension, oliguria, weak pulses, cool extremities) and weight loss. In addition, the patient may have an altered mental status or be obtunded, which is very worrisome for CE. Other signs of CE are inappropriate slowing of the heart rate and rising blood pressure.

Laboratory

Use the following laboratory criteria to confirm the diagnosis of DKA:

- **Diabetic:** Hyperglycemia (blood glucose >200 mg/dL)
- **Keto:** Ketonemia and ketonuria
- **Acidosis:** Venous pH less than 7.3 and bicarbonate less than 15

For any patient with suspected DKA, send a complete blood cell count, serum comprehensive metabolic panel and osmolality, HbA1c and β-hydroxybutyrate levels, venous or arterial blood gas, and urinalysis to check for ketones. If DKA is the initial presentation in a child with new onset diabetes, also obtain a C-peptide, insulin level, insulin autoantibody, ICA512 and GAD65 antibodies, tissue transglutaminase antibody, total IgA (to evaluate for celiac disease), and thyroid peroxidase antibody and thyroglobulin antibody (to evaluate for autoimmune thyroid disease). If infection is suspected, obtain appropriate cultures (urine, blood, throat, wound, etc).

The serum sodium may be low because of dilutional/pseudohyponatremia. The excess glucose is confined to the extracellular space and this causes the osmotic movement of water into the space, thus resulting in a relatively lowered sodium concentration. As the hyperglycemia is corrected with treatment and the osmotic movement of water is reversed, the serum sodium will rise.

There is a total body depletion of potassium as intracellular stores are lost from transcellular shifts (exchange of K^+ for extracellular H^+; glycogenolysis and proteolysis from insulin deficiency causes potassium efflux from cells); osmotic diuresis, which leads to increased urinary losses; and gastrointestinal losses from vomiting. However, the serum potassium may be normal, high, or low. If timely measurement of serum potassium is not available, obtain an electrocardiogram to look for evidence of hypokalema (flat T waves, appearance of U waves, widened QT interval) or hyperkalemia (peaked T waves, short QT interval). Once correction of electrolyte abnormalities is started, the serum potassium will fall. Very close monitoring and replacement, as needed, is essential.

Differential Diagnosis

While there are a number of different causes for metabolic acidosis, polyuria, and hyperglycemia, only DKA causes all 3. The differential diagnosis is summarized in Table 23-1.

Table 23-1. Differential Diagnosis of Diabetic Ketoacidosis	
Diagnosis	**Clinical Features**
Metabolic Acidosis, Ketosis	
Salicylate poisoning	Metabolic acidosis (+/- respiratory alkalosis) No ketosis Serum glucose↓ or ↑ (usually <300 mg/dL)
Sepsis	Fever, toxic appearance, source of infection Serum glucose normal or increased No Kussmaul breathing or fruity breath odor
Severe gastroenteritis/dehydration	May have diarrhea Lactic acidosis → metabolic acidosis Serum glucose mildly increased, decreased, or normal
Starvation	No hyperglycemia or glycosuria Bicarbonate usually >18 mEq/L
Polyuria	
Post-surgical/relief of obstructive uropathy	No glucosuria/ketonuria Serum glucose normal No metabolic acidosis
Urinary tract infection	(+) Urinary symptoms: dysuria, urgency No metabolic acidosis Serum glucose normal
Hyperglycemia	
Corticosteroid administration	↑Serum glucose No metabolic acidosis
Nonketotic hyperosmolar state	↑↑Serum glucose and osmolality No/minimal ketosis; no metabolic acidosis Stupor or coma
Stress	↑Serum glucose No ketonuria No metabolic acidosis

Treatment

Consult with a pediatric endocrinologist and/or pediatric intensivist early in the course. Obtain a height and weight (compare to premorbid weight) after assessing the severity of the dehydration and level of consciousness. The goals of therapy are restoring circulating volume, correcting metabolic derangements, avoiding treatment complications (CE), and identifying and treating the underlying cause (infection, insulin pump malfunction, etc).

Initial Management

The total fluid goal is 2,500 mL/m²/day, which is approximatey maintenance fluids plus 7% to 10% deficit. Give an initial normal saline (NS) or lactated Ringer (LR) fluid bolus, 10 mL/kg over 1 hour, and subtract this amount from the total fluid goal. Repeat once if clinically indicated. Exercise caution when administering initial fluids so as not to potentiate CE. However, if there is evidence of shock, give supplemental oxygen and fluid resuscitation as indicated.

If CE is suspected, elevate the head of the bed, reduce the intravenous (IV) fluid rate by one-third, and give mannitol (0.5–1 g/kg IV) or hypertonic (3%) saline (5–10 mL/kg). Consider intubation if there is impending respiratory failure. After the patient is stabilized, order a head computed tomography to confirm the diagnosis and look for other intracranial pathology (eg, thrombosis or hemorrhage).

After the fluid bolus(es), begin a regular insulin drip (0.1 units/kg/hour) to counteract the ongoing catabolic state. Use the 2-bag system to efficiently correct metabolic derangements (Box 23-1).

Monitoring

Successful management of DKA requires meticulous monitoring and frequent adjustments in treatment based on the patient's response. Monitor the vital signs, neurologic status, and intake and output. Obtain fingerstick glucose measurements every hour to adjust the fluid infusion to prevent hypoglycemia. Add dextrose to the infusion earlier if the rate of fall of glucose is greater than 90 mg/dL/hour or the patient develops hypoglycemia. The goal is a blood glucose in the range of 150 mg/dL. Check electrolytes and blood gases every 2 hours times 3 then every 6 hours until metabolic derangements have normalized. Test the urine for ketones every void until the ketones are cleared.

Box 23-1. 2-Bag System

Use fingerstick glucose measurements to adjust IV rate.

Potassium

- K^+ ≤5.5 mEq/L
  - Bag A: LR/NS + 1.5 mEq KCl/100 mL + 2 mmol KPO_4/100 mL
  - Bag B: D10 LR/NS + 1.5 mEq KCl/100 mL + 2 mmol KPO_4/100 mL
- K^+ ≥5.5 mEq/L
  - Bag A: LR/NS
  - Bag B: D10LR/NS

IV rate

Use the blood glucose to determine the ratio between the Bag A and Bag B IV rates.

Total IV rate (mL/h) = Bag A rate (mL/h) + Bag B rate (mL/h)

Glucose

- ≥300 mg/dL: Use only Bag A
- 251–300 mg/dL: 75% Bag A and 25% Bag B
- 201–250 mg/dL: 50% Bag A and 50% Bag B
- 151–200 mg/dL: 25% Bag A and 75% Bag B
- ≤150 mg/dL: Use only Bag B

Abbreviations: IV, intravenous; LR, lactated Ringers; NS, normal saline.

Chapter 23: Diabetic Ketoacidosis

Transition

Clinical improvement occurs as the metabolic derangements are corrected and the clinical signs of DKA resolve. Transition to oral fluids and appropriately reduce IV fluids when there is substantial clinical improvement. The most convenient time to transition to a subcutaneous (SC) insulin regimen is prior to a meal. Give rapid-acting SC insulin approximately 15 to 30 minutes or regular SC insulin 1 to 2 hours before stopping the insulin infusion. If an intermediate or long-acting SC insulin preparation is used, be sure to allow a longer overlap time with the insulin infusion and taper the infusion. This overlap period prevents rebound hyperglycemia. Continue to monitor finger-stick glucose hourly while the patient remains on the insulin infusion. Once the infusion is stopped, monitor the blood glucose every 2 to 4 hours and, if stable, transition to monitoring before meals, mid-afternoon, at bedtime, and at 2:00 am.

Indications for Consultation

- **Endocrinologist:** All patients in DKA
- **Nutritionist:** For discharge planning, once the DKA is resolved

Disposition

- **Intensive care unit transfer:** Severe DKA (pH <7.10), insulin drip, new onset DKA in a patient younger than 5 years, altered mental status, signs of sepsis
- **Discharge criteria:** Maintaining euglycemia on a carbohydrate-consistent diet and an appropriate insulin regimen; instructing the family/patient on monitoring glucose and managing hypo-/hyperglycemia; and arranging necessary follow-up

Follow-up

- **Primary care physician:** 1 to 2 weeks
- **Endocrinologist:** 2 to 3 days

Pearls and Pitfalls

- The measured sodium rises during treatment and does not indicate worsening hypertonicity. Moreover, failure of the corrected sodium to rise or declining sodium are risk factors for CE.
- In DKA, the anion gap is usually 20 to 30 mmol/L. A gap greater than 35 mmol/L suggests concurrent lactic acidosis.

- The serum pH may initially decrease as hydration mobilizes peripheral lactic acid. However, once renal perfusion improves, the excretion of organic acids increases. If biochemical derangements are not being corrected, reassess the patient, consider other potential causes of impaired insulin response (infection, errors in insulin preparation), and adjust insulin therapy if warranted.
- There is no evidence to support the routine use of bicarbonate to correct metabolic acidosis.

Coding

ICD-9

- CE **348.5**
- T1DM, uncontrolled **250.03**
- DKA, type I **250.13**
- Hyperosmolar nonketotic state, type II **250.22**

Bibliography

Cooke DW, Plotnick L. Management of diabetic ketoacidosis in children and adolescents. *Pediatr Rev.* 2008;29:431–435

Harris G, Flordalisi I. Diabetic ketoacidosis: a physiologic approach to management. In: Perkin R, Swift J, Newton D, Anas N, eds. *Pediatric Hospital Medicine Textbook of Inpatient Management.* 2nd ed. Baltimore, MD: Lippincott, Williams & Wilkins; 2008:528–537

Klein M, Sathasivam A, Novoa Y, Rapaport R. Recent consensus statements in pediatric endocrinology: a selective review. *Endocrinol Metab Clin N Am.* 2009;38:811–825

Koul PB. Diabetic ketoacidosis: a current appraisal of pathophysiology and management. *Clin Pediatr (Phila).* 2009;48:135–144

Rewers A. Current controversies in treatment and prevention of diabetic ketoacidosis. *Adv Pediatr.* 2010;57:247–267

Wolfsdorf J, Craig ME, Daneman D, et al. Diabetic ketoacidosis in children and adolescents with diabetes. *Pediatr Diabetes.* 2009;10 (suppl 12):118–133

Equipment and Procedures

Intravenous Lines

Introduction

Peripheral intravenous (IV) catheter placement is a very common, but challenging procedure in pediatrics. The small caliber of the vessels, the anxious and often uncooperative patient, and the worried parents add to the complexity of this procedure.

Informed Consent/Patient Preparation

Written consent is not needed in order to place an IV. However, prior to beginning, inform the parents of the procedure and its indications. Also explain it to the patient in developmentally appropriate language. It is often helpful to show an anxious child the IV catheter beforehand and demonstrate that only a "thin straw" will be placed in the vein. Be sure to explain each step to the patient during the procedure and emphasize that staying still will make the process easier. Avoid using phrases like "this will not hurt" or "you will not feel a thing," as these are misleading to the patient. If possible, perform the procedure in a treatment room or other area, and not a young child's bed.

Supplies and Setup

The following supplies are necessary when preparing for IV placement:

- IV catheters (18 gauge to 24 gauge)
- T-connector set
- 3- to 5-mL normal saline flushes
- 3-mL and/or 5-mL syringes (if concomitant blood sampling is needed)
- Tourniquet (or rubber band)
- Gloves
- Alcohol swabs (iodine swabs if blood cultures will be obtained)
- Gauze
- Tape/Tegaderm
- Appropriately sized arm board/footboard

Choosing the correct IV catheter size is integral to proper IV placement and depends on the patient's age, caliber of the veins visualized, and indication for IV placement. In emergent situations where fluid resuscitation is necessary, insert a large-bore IV to facilitate the rapid delivery of large volumes. In most other scenarios, use the smallest IV possible (<1 year of age: 22 or 24 gauge; 1–8 years of age: 20 or 22 gauge; older patient: 20 gauge or larger). Note that the smaller the gauge, the larger the diameter of the catheter.

Prior to IV insertion, apply warm packs or blankets to the patient's extremities to assist with vasodilation and make it easier to visualize potential IV sites. It is helpful to work with an assistant who can restrain the extremity at the joints above and below the intended insertion site and reach for supplies as needed. Attach a saline flush to the T-connector and flush normal saline through the tubing prior to connecting the T-connector to the IV. Attach the T-connector to an empty syringe if obtaining a blood specimen is intended after the IV insertion. Cut the tape in advance into the desired sizes for securing the IV site.

Sometimes the parents, patient, or physician will request a topical anesthetic prior to IV insertion. In order to provide anesthesia, these creams must be placed on the predetermined IV insertion site 30 to 60 minutes prior to the procedure, so they cannot be used in emergent situations, but can be very helpful when time permits. Other distracting techniques, either by a child life specialist or other care providers, can also help alleviate some of the pain and anxiety of this procedure.

Procedure

The most common sites for IV insertion in an infant or child are the dorsum of the hand or foot and the antecubital fossa. Place a tourniquet proximal to the IV insertion site. Clean the area with an alcohol swab for better visualization and look for the optimal vein for IV insertion. Start with the most distal vessel possible, leaving the more proximal ones for subsequent attempts or for future central catheter insertion, if needed. If possible, avoid inserting an IV into the patient's dominant hand. If finding a vessel proves difficult, use a transilluminating or ultrasound device, which may help localize a vein.

When a vein is localized, clean the area thoroughly with alcohol or with iodine if blood cultures will be obtained. Use your nondominant hand to hold the skin taut distal to the IV insertion site. Hold the IV catheter bevel up at an angle of 10 to 20 degrees from the skin. Slowly advance the needle through the skin and into the vein until you see blood return in the hub of the catheter. At that point, hold the needle steady and using your index finger, advance just the plastic catheter over the needle into the vein until the hub is abutting the skin. Retract the needle while applying pressure to the vein so that blood will not pour out when the needle is removed.

Quickly attach the T-connector to the hub of the IV catheter. Secure the hub of the IV with a short piece of tape placed perpendicular to the IV hub near the skin insertion site. Use more tape or a piece of Tegaderm to secure the IV site. If blood samples are needed, connect the T-connector to an empty syringe and aspirate blood. When the desired amount of blood is obtained, attach a sterile saline flush to the T-connector and flush slowly into the vein. The saline should easily flush through the catheter. If it does not, readjust the hub of the IV as it may be positioned near a valve.

While flushing the T-connector inspect the site for signs of infiltration, such as redness, warmth, induration, pain, and swelling. If an IV infiltration is suspected, remove the catheter immediately. Apply a warm pack to the skin to help with the induration and pain. Blanching during the saline flush suggests that an artery, rather than a vein, has been cannulized. Remove the catheter and apply pressure to the site.

After flushing the IV with saline, remove the syringe from the T-connector and lock the catheter. Secure the T-connector tubing to the patient's skin with another piece of tape. Finally, secure the extremity to an arm board or footboard to minimize potential movement and manipulation.

Extravasation of caustic substances or vesicants, such as total parenteral nutrition, chemotherapeutic agents, certain antiepileptics, and antibiotics, can cause serious damage and necrosis to the surrounding tissues. If extravasation of such an agent occurs, stop the infusion immediately and remove the IV. Consultation with plastic surgery may be indicated.

Difficult Intravenous Access (DIVA) Score

Use the DIVA to identify a patient for whom it may be challenging to obtain IV access. A total score of 4 or higher predicts a greater than 50% failure rate during the first attempt to place an IV. Therefore, if the DIVA score suggests a difficult IV insertion, arrange for the most skilled person to be present.

- Vein not visible: 2 points
- Vein not palpable: 2 points
- Premature birth (<38 weeks' gestation): 3 points
- 1 to 2 years of age: 1 point
- Younger than 1 year: 3 points

Pearls and Pitfalls

- Rarely, cellulitis of the IV site or bacteremia can occur with peripheral IV placement. Changing IV sites every 3 to 5 days will help reduce the risks.

Coding

CPT

- Peripheral IV placement **36000**
- Scalp IV placement (patient <3 years of age) **36405**

Bibliography

Dougherty L. IV therapy: recognizing the differences between infiltration and extravasation. *Br J Nurs.* 2008;17:896–901

Haas NA. Clinical review: vascular access for fluid infusion in children. *Crit Care.* 2004;8:478–484

Rauch DA, Dowd D, Eldridge D, et al. Peripheral difficult venous access in children. *Clin Pediatr.* 2009;48:895–901

Lumbar Puncture

A lumbar puncture (LP) is most commonly performed to evaluate potential central nervous system infections. It is also used to measure intracranial pressure and to obtain cerebrospinal fluid (CSF) during the evaluation of other conditions, such as demyelinating diseases, tumors, and other neurologic diseases. An LP is sometimes necessary to drain CSF, although this is usually performed by a neurosurgeon or pediatric intensivist. Proper positioning and a "good hold" are the keys to a successful LP attempt.

When performing an LP, communicate clearly with consulting specialists to ensure that all of the requested samples are obtained and sent for the correct laboratory studies. In addition, make a habit of saving in the laboratory an extra tube with 1 to 2 mL of refrigerated or frozen CSF, in the event that additional tests are needed.

Risks and Contraindications

- Potential airway and cardiovascular difficulties when a patient with cardiorespiratory compromise is positioned for the procedure. If this is a concern, give intravenous (IV) antibiotics after a blood culture has been obtained (if the LP is being performed to diagnose an infection) and perform the procedure in a controlled, monitored situation after initial resuscitation and stabilization.
- Potential herniation in a patient with known increased intracranial pressure or a mass lesion.
- Infected tissue overlying the entry site of the spinal needle. This might result in iatrogenic introduction of flora into the CSF space.
- Potential for uncontrolled bleeding. Ensure that the platelet count is greater than 50,000/mL^3 prior to performing an LP.
- An uncooperative patient who cannot remain still. Sedation may be required so that the LP can be performed under controlled circumstances. However, the person performing the LP *cannot also provide the sedation*.

Consent

Use simple and reassuring terms to explain the risks of a "spinal tap" to the parents: "There is always a chance of infection and bleeding whenever the skin is broken, but this risk is not much different than when an IV is inserted. Many babies fall asleep during the procedure."

Parents are often worried that somehow their child might become paralyzed from an LP. It is therefore helpful to raise this issue concretely, even if the parents do not ask: "The needle is being inserted only into the outermost portion of the fluid around the spinal cord. I will take out less than a teaspoon of fluid and that will be replaced within one hour. I have never heard of a child being paralyzed after an LP."

An appropriate layperson's description for a written consent form that parents sign is, "Insert a needle into the lower back to remove spinal fluid for analysis." Offer the parents the option of staying in the room for the procedure if they are confident that they are unlikely to faint and their presence does not cause performance anxiety.

Procedure

1. Apply EMLA or LMX over the interspaces as soon as an LP is being considered to minimize delays and maximize analgesia.
2. Consent: Obtain written informed consent (if required by the institution). Prepare relevant paperwork (universal time-out).
3. Equipment: Prepare the equipment and holder. Include a fourth collection tube, at least 2 spinal needles, oxygen, suction, pulse oximetry, and other monitors as indicated. Use a 22-gauge 1.5-inch spinal needle for an infant or toddler younger than 2 years, 22-gauge 2.5-inch needle for a child aged 2 to 12 years, and a 20- or 22-gauge 3.5-inch needle for an adolescent.
4. Choose position: Review restraint and positioning with the holder. Select either the lateral decubitus or sitting positioning, which expands the intravertebral space and may allow easier and more reliable identification of the midline of the vertebral column. In either position, identify the L4-5 interspace in the midline at the level of the iliac crests.
5. Sterile field: Position the patient and prepare draping. Ensure the surface is clean, flat, and relatively firm. Apply sterile gloves.
6. Time-out. Identify the patient and follow other institution-specific procedure protocols.
7. Prepare and drape the patient.
8. Position: Have the holder restrain the patient in the optimal position. In the lateral decubitus position, apply pressure to the shoulders to get the patient into a fetal position with a C-shaped kyphosis, while avoiding compressing the head. For the seated position, place a rolled-up towel anterior to the patient's chest/abdomen to facilitate the desired maximal kyphosis of the fetal position.

9. *Do not compromise on positioning.* Identify landmarks and midline structures and give the holder feedback about the patient's 3-dimensional space. Maximize kyphosis without inducing a lateral scoliosis. In the lateral decubitus position, to facilitate midline insertion in the sagittal plane, maintain the patient's back perpendicular to the plane of the bed. Also maintain the patient's back parallel/tangential to the edge of the bed at the skin entry to facilitate a consistent cephalad approach toward the umbilicus.
10. Anesthesia. If local anesthesia is given, raise an intradermal wheel over the L4-5 site either before or immediately after prepping and drying of the skin. For a toddler or older child, inject additional local anesthesia gradually and sequentially into the deeper layers of soft tissue and ligaments, taking care not to inject any into the CSF itself.
11. Insert. Use the smallest gauge spinal needle available to reduce potential pressure shifts and minimize the risk of post LP headache. Insert the spinal needle, with the trocar in place, through the skin, midline at L4-5 with the bevel pointing cephalad or parallel to the spine. In either position, angle the needle toward the umbilicus. Keep the trocar in the needle until a pop is felt or a reasonable depth is reached. Then remove the trocar and gently manipulate (advance, withdraw, rotate) the needle. Observe the hub for CSF return. The needle may be held a number of different ways.
    a. 1-handed technique: Hold the needle between the index and middle finger of the dominant hand and advance with the thumb.
    b. 2-handed technique: Advance the needle with both thumbs, guiding the direction with the index fingers braced against the patient's back.

    If a firm surface is felt, it is likely to be bone, often the bottom of L4. Remove the needle to the level of the outermost ligamentous tissues, and re-angle somewhat more caudally. If a bright gush of red blood is obtained, the needle is probably lateral of the midline in one of the paravertebral veins. Withdraw the needle completely, and try again at L3-4. If there is no fluid return at all, the needle is probably still within ligamentous tissues. Slowly advance and manipulate the needle; for an infant, 1 to 2 cm will suffice. During the initial LP attempt, in the absence of streaming of blood at the needle hub, homogenously red, translucent CSF that does not clear as additional fluid is collected may be evidence of an intracranial bleed. Collect 1 mL (0.5 mL minimum) of CSF into each of 4 tubes and send as indicated below. If the tap is traumatic, the culture is still valid and is the priority when insufficient CSF is collected for all of the routine, but immediate, studies. Turbid fluid is presumptive evidence of bacterial meningitis, while clear fluid is reassuring, but not a guarantee of a normal cell count or protein level.

a. Tube 1:Gram stain, culture and sensitivity
b. Tube 2: glucose and protein
c. Tube 3: additional studies (herpes simplex virus or enterovirus polymerase chain reaction, myelin basic protein, serology)
d. Tube 4: cell count

12. Opening pressure. To measure opening pressure, perform the LP in the lateral decubitus position. Prepare the manometer, stopcock, and flexible tubing in advance. As soon as CSF flows from the hub, attach the male end of the flexible tubing to the hub with the stopcock in the off to drainage position. Keep the stopcock at the level of the spinal column and gently straighten the legs and back. The opening pressure is equal to the height of the column in centimeters of water once respiratory variation is observed. Open the stopcock to drainage (off to the needle) to collect CSF. Turn the stopcock off to the manometer to complete CSF collection.
13. Remove the needle. After the 4 specimens are obtained, reinsert the trocar and withdraw the needle.
14. Notify. Tell the parents of the preliminary findings (clear, traumatic, or turbid) and how their child tolerated the procedure.
15. Write a procedure note: "LP performed to rule out meningitis in a febrile 6-week-old. After obtaining informed consent, identifying patient, and a time-out, patient was prepped and draped in the customary sterile fashion and a 22-gauge 1.5-inch spinal needle was inserted into the L4-5 interspace on the first attempt. 5 mL of clear CSF was obtained and sent for the usual studies. Patient tolerated the procedure well; no complications."
16. Post-procedure. While the traditional recommendation is to keep older children and adolescents flat in bed for 4 to 6 hours to avoid a post-LP or spinal headache, there is little evidence to support this practice. Treatment options for a severe spinal headache include narcotic analgesics, IV caffeine (500 mg) or, for persistent symptoms, an epidural blood patch performed by an anesthesiologist.

Pearls and Pitfalls

- Place EMLA or LMX in the lumbar area as soon as an LP is being considered.
- Spend time making sure positioning is optimal, with the patient in the ideal position and the operator comfortably seated.
- If the LP is part of a rule out sepsis workup in an infant, get the urine first, as the patient may urinate during the manipulation and undressing for the LP.

Coding

CPT

LP diagnostic **62270**

Bibliography

Boon JM, Abrahams PH, Meiring JH, Welch T. Lumbar puncture: anatomical review of a clinical skill. *Clin Anat.* 2004;17:544–553

Cronan KM, Wiley JF. Lumbar puncture. In: King BR, Henretig FM, eds. *Textbook of Pediatric Emergency Procedures.* 2nd ed. Philadelphia, PA: Lippincott, Williams & Wilkins; 2008:505–514

Gibson T. Lumbar puncture. In: Zaoutis LB, Chiang VW, eds. *Comprehensive Pediatric Hospital Medicine.* Philadelphia, PA: Mosby Elsevier; 2007:1240–1242

Turnbull DK, Shepherd DB. Post-dural puncture headache: pathogenesis, prevention and treatment. *Br J Anaesth.* 2003;91:718–729

CHAPTER 26

Noninvasive Monitoring

Collection and monitoring of objective data such as vital signs and pulse oximetry are essential in the clinical assessment of pediatric patients. Noninvasive monitoring techniques provide continuous measurement of physiological function, allowing early recognition of changes in clinical status. Caregivers must remain attentive to the monitors, recognize significant physiological changes, and respond with appropriate measures. Excessive alarms may result in nurse desensitization and delayed response to subsequent alarms. Therefore, it is important to set appropriate, individualized alarm parameters to prevent alarm fatigue.

Temperature Monitoring

There is considerable controversy regarding the appropriate thermometer and ideal site for temperature measurement. Precise and accurate temperature measurements are most important in a young infant, since the presence of fever frequently triggers a laboratory evaluation for sepsis. Rectal temperatures are the most accurate with the least variability and therefore the standard of care for infants. However, avoid using a rectal thermometer if the patient is immunocompromised or has had recent anorectal surgery. While oral temperatures are reliable estimates of core temperature, they may be inaccurate due to improper placement or recent intake of fluids. Axillary temperatures are lower than core temperature and more variable due to environmental factors. Otic (tympanic) and temporal artery thermometers use infrared thermal detection to provide quick estimates of the core temperature, but both are less sensitive than oral or rectal temperatures in detecting fever. Whichever method is used, document serial temperatures to establish a trend.

Cardiorespiratory Monitors

Cardiorespiratory (CR) monitors use 3 chest leads to continuously measure the pulse (via electrocardiography) and respirations (via impedance pneumography), with preset alarms for high and low rates. False alarms are common due to loose leads, patient movement, and poor detection of respiratory movements in small infants.

Use CR monitoring for a patient at risk of cardiac or respiratory decompensation. Discuss age-appropriate alarm limits with the care team and family, and investigate alarm events with prompt clinical assessment of the child. Document the patient assessment and interventions for all significant events. Basic CR monitoring may detect bradycardia, tachycardia, and simple arrhythmias, but telemetry and electrocardiogram-trained nurses are required to detect more sophisticated arrhythmias.

However, do not rely on CR monitors for the detection of apnea. Pneumography can only detect central apnea, which is characterized by a lack of respiratory effort. Apnea is commonly due to airway obstruction, in which chest wall movements persist and continue to be detected by pneumography. Bradycardia is delayed until profound hypoxia develops.

Pulse Oximetry

Pulse oximetry (O_2 sat) is commonly used as a noninvasive method to monitor the oxygenation of a patient's hemoglobin. A sensor placed on a finger, toe, hand, foot, or ear uses light to detect the percentage of hemoglobin that is oxygenated, which is an accurate estimate of O_2 sat for a patient breathing room air who has a normal hemoglobin type and a relatively normal hematocrit. Pulse oximetry provides continuous assessment of circulating oxygen levels, but falsely low levels are commonly encountered. Incorrect sensor placement, patient movement, skin abnormalities, fingernail polish, ambient light interference, and distal hypoperfusion may all cause falsely low O_2 sat levels. To ensure accuracy, verify the presence of a steady pulse and/or waveform on the pulse oximetry monitor. Pulse oximetry may also be inaccurate when hemoglobin binding is altered, as in carbon monoxide or cyanide poisoning, or methemoglobinemia.

Indications for continuous O_2 sat monitoring include a patient who requires significant supplemental oxygen or frequent assessment, or is at risk of deterioration. Order intermittent O_2 sat monitoring for a patient with a more stable respiratory illness. Use a spot check of O_2 sat for making decisions to wean oxygen or change the patient's respiratory care plan. Although continuous pulse oximetry is a sensitive tool, it may detect transient decreases in oxygen saturation that are not clinically significant and do not indicate a need for supplemental oxygen. This is especially true for mild desaturations that occur at night during sleep.

Pulse oximetry does not assess for adequate ventilation. In addition, the detection of apnea and/or airway obstruction may be delayed, as arterial oxygenation decreases gradually during such events. Use capnography or blood gas analysis to assess for hypercarbia or respiratory acidosis. Finally, O_2 sat does not equal partial pressure of arterial oxygen (PaO_2), so that a high saturation while on supplemental oxygen may mask a significant alveolar-arterial gradient.

Capnography

The gold standard for assessing ventilation is arterial blood gas analysis; however, this requires a painful procedure and laboratory time, while providing only intermittent data. In contrast, capnography is the measurement of carbon dioxide levels in expired air. Recent technological improvements allow the analysis of smaller gas samples, enabling its use in a child who is breathing via face mask or nasal cannula.

Capnography is indicated for the assessment of ventilation in a patient with respiratory, cardiac, or neurologic diseases. It provides continuous surveillance of end-tidal carbon dioxide, which is an accurate estimate of the partial pressure of arterial carbon dioxide ($PaCO_2$). Capnography is also useful as an instantaneous apnea monitor. While traditional pneumography often fails to detect obstructive apnea (since chest wall movements continue), the dramatic fall in expired carbon dioxide will be immediately detected by capnography. Order capnography for confirming successful endotracheal intubation and continuously monitoring endotracheal tube placement and patency in a critically ill patient.

Applications

Sedation

The use of procedural sedation in pediatrics has increased significantly in the last decade. However, sedation carries significant risks, such as hypoventilation, apnea, airway obstruction, laryngospasm, and cardiopulmonary impairment. Continuous observation of the patient and monitoring of vital signs, pulse oximetry, and capnography are essential to ensure that complications are immediately recognized and interventions rapidly instituted. In particular, use capnography for prompt detection of airway obstruction or hypoventilation during sedation and recovery.

Transport

Noninvasive monitoring is critical during the transport of a patient, as assessment becomes more difficult in an ambulance or aircraft. Rely on continuous noninvasive CR, pulse oximetry, and capnography monitoring to detect clinical changes.

Bibliography

American Academy of Pediatrics, American Academy of Pediatric Dentistry, Coté CJ, Wilson S, Work Group on Sedation. Guidelines for monitoring and management of pediatric patients during and after sedation for diagnostic and therapeutic procedures: an update. *Pediatrics*. 2006;118:2587–2602

Eipe N, Doherty DR. A review of pediatric capnography. *J Clin Monit Comput*. 2010;24:261–268

Graham KC, Cvach M. Monitor alarm fatigue: standardizing use of physiological monitors and decreasing nuisance alarms. *Am J Crit Care*. 2010;19:28–34

Paes BF, Vermeulen K, Brohet RM, van der Ploeg T, de Winter JP. Accuracy of tympanic and infrared skin thermometers in children. *Arch Dis Child*. 2010;95:974–978

CHAPTER 27

Suprapubic Bladder Aspiration

Suprapubic bladder aspiration is indicated to obtain a specimen in a patient who is younger than 6 months. After that, catheterization or clean catch is preferred. It is best to wait for at least 1 hour after the patient's last void and/or 45 minutes after a feed before attempting a suprapubic aspiration. Suprapubic aspiration is the gold standard and is preferable to catheterization in a male with a tight foreskin and a female when the urethral meatus cannot be visualized. Prior to inserting the needle, bladder ultrasound can be useful for visualizing the presence of urine in the bladder.

Contraindications

Do not perform a suprapubic bladder aspiration if the patient has a coagulopathy or intestinal obstruction, or if there is an infection of the overlying skin. Obtain urine via catheterization instead.

Complications

Complications from the procedure include cellulitis, hematuria, and intestinal perforation.

Procedure

1. Explain the procedure to the parents, including the potential complications. Obtain consent for the procedure if required by institutional policy.
2. Gather all necessary equipment, including sterile gloves, a 22-gauge 1½-inch straight needle, alcohol pads, povidone-iodine swabs, and a 3- to 5-mL syringe.
3. Open the package of gloves. Use the interior as the sterile field and place the needle, syringe, alcohol pads, and povidone-iodine swabs on it.
4. Have an assistant restrain the patient in a supine, frog-leg position. Also have an assistant occlude the urethra in a male to prevent urination during preparation.
5. Clean the suprapubic area with the povidone-iodine solution 3 times. Then wipe with alcohol pads. Put on the sterile gloves.
6. Palpate the symphysis pubis. Insert the needle 1 to 2 cm above it, puncturing the skin at a 10- to 20-degree angle aiming slightly caudad. Exert suction on the syringe while advancing the needle, but do not go deeper than 1 inch. Aspirate the urine into the syringe.
7. Remove the needle once the aspiration is complete. Clean the remaining povidone-iodine from the patient.

8. Transfer the urine in the appropriately labeled containers.
9. If urine is not obtained either perform a catheterization or wait 1 to 2 hours and repeat the suprapubic aspiration.
10. Write a post-procedure note in the medical record.

Pearls and Pitfalls

- Perform the procedure at least 1 hour after the last void or 45 minutes after a feed.
- The success rate of the procedure may be improved by ultrasound guidance, which allows confirmation of a full bladder and visualization of the puncture

Coding

CPT

Aspiration of bladder with needle **51100**

Bibliography

Chu RW, Wong YC, Luk SH, Wong SN. Comparing suprapubic urine aspiration under real-time ultrasound guidance with conventional blind aspiration. *Acta Paediatr.* 2002;91:512–516

Karacan C, Erkek N, Senel S, et al. Evaluation of urine collection methods for the diagnosis of urinary tract infection in children. *Med Princ Pract.* 2010;19:188–191

Loiselle JM. Ultrasound-assisted suprapubic bladder aspiration. In: King C, Henretig FM, eds. *Textbook of Pediatric Emergency Procedures.* 2nd ed. Philadelphia, PA: Lippincott, Williams & Williams; 2008:1220–1226

Tracheostomies

Introduction

A child with medical complexity is often dependent on technology, such as a tracheostomy tube (TT). In the immediate postoperative period, any problems associated with such equipment are best managed by the surgical team who performed the insertion procedure. However, once this period has passed, the patient may present to the hospitalist with malfunctions or infections associated with these devices.

A TT is maintained for chronic respiratory insufficiency or inability to protect the airway. Common complications include inappropriate fit (due to growth or weight gain), partial or complete obstruction, mechanical failure (uncommon), and infection (tracheitis, cellulitis, or abscess). Other complications include pressure necrosis, tracheal granuloma, tracheal stenosis, and fistulae to the esophagus or innominate artery. The benefit of the tracheostomy is that it allows for assisted airway clearance, but since the site is a more direct entry into the tracheobronchial tree it is a portal for infection.

Clinical Presentation

History and Physical Examination

A patient with a TT may present with local skin breakdown caused by inadequate stoma care, an inappropriately sized tube, or overly tight tracheostomy ties. Partial obstruction is not uncommon, although a suction catheter can usually still be passed, giving the misleading impression that the lumen is clear. Sometimes, secretions may obstruct the entire lumen, except for the diameter of the suction catheter.

Ask about the routine care of the TT, including the frequency and what materials are used for daily skin care. Typically this involves half-strength hydrogen peroxide (mixed with sterile water). Determine when the TT was last exchanged (TTs are usually changed monthly), whether it was up- or downsized, and when the most recent direct laryngoscopy and bronchoscopy was performed to assess the health of the stoma site. Evaluate the integrity of the balloon by using a 5-mL syringe to deflate the balloon, then remove it and refill it outside of the patient's body to check for leaks.

Laboratory

A simple set of anteroposterior and lateral neck radiographs can confirm the position of a TT, although it cannot assess functionality. If indicated, order a bedside endoscopy or a direct laryngoscopy and bronchoscopy, performed by an otorhinolaryngologist, to assess for any tracheal granuloma or stenosis.

If infection is a concern, obtain a Gram stain of secretions suctioned from the TT. However, this must be interpreted with care to properly distinguish between colonization and actual infection. The hallmark of infection is an increased number of white blood cells along with a predominant organism, in the setting of fever and cough. During infections, TT secretions are usually described as thick, green, and foul smelling.

Differential Diagnosis

The diagnosis of common complications is summarized in Table 28-1.

Treatment

If a patient is unable to effectively clear their secretions, use the following formula to choose a flexible suction catheter that is slightly less than half the diameter of the TT (Table 28-2):

$$\text{Diameter of TT (mm)} \times 1.5 = \text{French gauge for suction catheter}$$

$$\text{(Example: 4 mm TT} \times 1.5 = \text{6F suction catheter)}$$

In general, do not insert the suction catheter any deeper than the length of the TT to avoid mucosal injury. It may sometimes be necessary to gently advance the catheter further, until a cough is stimulated or resistance is met. Apply suction only while the catheter is being removed and never during the insertion process. Use the lowest amount of pressure required to effectively

Table 28-1. Common Acute Complications of Tracheostomies

Diagnosis	Clinical Features
Accidental decannulation	Absent TT at stoma site
Infection (vs colonization)	Fever Increased cough Change in color/odor of tracheal aspirate WBCs on Gram stain of aspirate
Minor bleeding	Suctioning depth, frequency, or pressure is excessive Insufficient humidification of airway Infection (hemoptysis)
Obstruction: complete or partial	Respiratory distress or failure Falling PO_2, rising PCO_2

Abbreviations: PCO_2, partial pressure of carbon dioxide; PO_2, partial pressure of oxygen; TT, tracheostomy tube; WBC, white blood cell.

Chapter 28: Tracheostomies

Table 28-2. Equivalency of Common Sizes of Tracheostomy Tubes and Suction Catheters									
Bivona					**Shiley**				
Size	**ID**	**OD**	**Length (mm)**	**Suction Catheter**	**Size**	**ID**	**OD**	**Length (mm)**	**Suction Catheter**
2.5 NEO	2.5	4.0	30	6					
3.0 NEO	3.0	4.7	32	6 or 8	3.0 NEO	3.0	4.5	30	6
3.5 NEO	3.5	5.3	34	6 or 8	3.5 NEO	3.5	5.2	32	6 or 8
4.0 NEO	4.0	6.0	36	6 or 8	4.0 NEO	4.0	5.9	34	6 or 8
					4.5 NEO	4.5	6.5	36	6 or 8
2.5 PED	2.5	4.0	38	6					
3.0 PED	3.0	4.7	39	6 or 8	3.0 PED	3.0	4.5	39	6
3.5 PED	3.5	5.3	40	6 or 8	3.5 PED	3.5	5.2	40	6 or 8
4.0 PED	4.0	6.0	41	6 or 8	4.0 PED	4.0	5.9	41	6 or 8
4.5 PED	4.5	6.7	42	6 or 8	4.5 PED	4.5	6.5	42	6 or 8
5.0 PED	5.0	7.3	44	8 or 10	5.0 PED	5.0	7.1	44	8 or 10
5.5 PED	5.5	8.0	46	10 or 12	5.5 PED	5.5	7.7	46	10 or 12

Abbreviations: ID, internal diameter; NEO, neonatal; OD, outer diameter; PED, pediatric.

clear the airway (50–100 mm Hg for a child). Individual institutions have policies that require the use of sterile, modified sterile, or clean technique for suctioning TT.

When in doubt, remove the TT and replace it promptly. The patient should always have 2 spare tubes immediately available for emergencies, one of the same size and one of a size smaller than the one currently in use. If no spare TT is available, inspect the current one for any occlusion. In an emergency, use an endotracheal tube of the same diameter; trim the length after insertion.

Many respiratory therapists are knowledgeable about the mechanics of TT exchange, and this skill is easily mastered by hospitalists. To change a TT, the required supplies include a pair of gloves and the availability of suction, oxygen, and lubricant. Place the patient in the supine position with a neck roll to extend the cervical spine. Gently remove the TT using an upward and outward movement. Insert the new TT following the same arc in reverse, inward and downward. Immediately remove the obturator and hold the TT securely in place until new tracheostomy ties are applied. If the procedure proves to be difficult, insert a suction catheter, then advance the new TT over it (similar to a modified Seldinger technique).

If there is an abscess adjacent to the stoma site, arrange for an incision and drainage, send a specimen for Gram stain and culture, and select antibiotics that treat both skin and respiratory flora, including methicillin-resistant *Staphylococcus aureus* (clindamycin 15–25 mg/kg/day intravenous divided every 6–8 hours, 4.8 g/day maximum).

Indications for Consultation

- **Wound or stoma team:** Difficult wound
- **Pediatric otolaryngology:** Clinical or radiographic evidence of tracheostomy tube malfunction, dislodgment, or inappropriate fit

Disposition

- **Intensive care unit transfer:** Difficult TT replacement
- **Discharge criteria:** Stable tube and clean site

Follow-up

- **Primary care:** 1 to 2 weeks
- **Surgical subspecialist (if involved):** 1 week

Pearls and Pitfalls

- The patient must have 2 spare, new tracheostomies available at all times. One must be of the current size (diameter and length), and one a size smaller.
- It is important to note the difference in neonatal- and pediatric-sized tubes when selecting a TT. The numerical sizes appear the same; however, there are significant differences in how they fit (Table 28-2).
- When selecting items for home care, a portable suction machine is preferable.
- Teach family members safe techniques for changing a TT.

Coding

ICD-9

- Attention to tracheostomy **V55.0**
- Tracheostomy complication, unspecified **519.00**
- Tracheostomy infection **519.01**
- Tracheostomy mechanical complication **519.02**
- Tracheostomy status **V44.0**

Bibliography

Al-Samri M, Mitchell I, Drummond DS, Bjornson C. Tracheostomy in children: a population-based experience over 17 years. *Pediatr Pulmonol.* 2010;45:487–493

Eber E, Oberwaldner B. Tracheostomy care in the hospital. *Paediatr Respir Rev.* 2006;7:175–184

Hess DR. Tracheostomy tubes and related appliances. *Respir Care.* 2005;50:497–510

Kremer B, Botos-Kremer AI, Eckel HE, Schlöndorff G. Indications, complications, and surgical techniques for pediatric tracheostomies—an update. *J Pediatr Surg.* 2002;37:1556–1562

Mahadevan M, Barber C, Salkeld L, Douglas G, Mills N. Pediatric tracheotomy: 17 year review. *Int J Pediatr Otorhinolaryngol.* 2007;71:1829–1835

Urinary Bladder Catheterization

Urinary bladder catheterization is indicated for diagnosis of a urinary tract infection or pyelonephritis in an infant or young child who cannot give a reliable clean catch specimen. It is also used to relieve urinary retention.

Contraindications

Do not perform a bladder catheterization if the patient has a pelvic fracture or suspected trauma to the urethra (blood at the meatus).

Complications

Potential complications of catheterization include urethral trauma, bladder trauma, vaginal catheterization, urinary tract infection, and an intravesical knot (rare).

Procedure

Explain the procedure to the parents, including the potential complications. Obtain consent for the procedure if required by institutional policy. Once the procedure is completed, write a post-procedure note in the medical record.

Males

1. Gather all equipment needed for the procedure, including sterile gloves, an appropriate-sized catheter (8F in newborns, 10F in most children, and 12F in older children), syringe (at least 10 mL), sterile gloves, sterile lubricant, povidone-iodine swabs, and a urine collection cup/tube.
2. Open the package of gloves. Use the interior as the sterile field and place the catheter, syringe, lubricant, and povidone-iodine swabs on it.
3. Once all the equipment is arranged, open the diaper and quickly, but gently, grab the penis mid-shaft and squeeze to prevent spontaneous urination. Use light, persistent pressure to retract the foreskin and expose the meatus. Prepare the urethral meatus and penis by gently cleaning with the povidone-iodine solution.
4. Have an assistant hold the patient's legs in a frog-leg position.
5. Put on the sterile gloves and lubricate the catheter. Attach the syringe to the catheter. Have an opened urine cup within reach in case the patient urinates during the preparation, in essence providing a true clean catch.

6. Gently grasp and extend the penile shaft to straighten the urethra. Hold the lubricated catheter near the meatus and insert the catheter into the urethra. Slowly advance the catheter and apply continued pressure to get past the resistance that is typically felt at the external sphincter.
7. Once urine is visualized in the tubing pull back on the syringe. Remove the catheter once the collection is completed. Do not pull back on the syringe while manipulating the catheter.
8. If a Foley catheter is being placed, use the same technique. In addition, test the integrity of the balloon prior to inserting the catheter. Once the catheter is well inserted into the bladder, inflate the balloon with the recommended amount of saline, then gently retract the catheter until slight resistance is met. Attach the catheter to the collection container using sterile technique.
9. Place the specimen in the appropriate labeled container (eg, for urinalysis or urine culture). A trace amount of urine (≤1 mL) is adequate for a culture.
10. Clean off the povidone-iodine solution with water and gauze.
11. Rapidly transport the specimen to the laboratory. Place it on ice if there is any potential for delay.

Females

For females the principles are similar to catheterization in males. Have an assistant spread the labia. The urethral orifice is anterior to the vaginal orifice and the catheter needs to be advanced just a few centimeters to reach the bladder in females.

Pearls and Pitfalls

- Obtain the urine first if the catheterization is part of a sepsis workup in an infant.
- Always have the urine collection cup open while performing the procedure in case the patient spontaneously voids.
- If urine is not obtained, leave the catheter in, as the patient will eventually void. There is no need to re-catheterize.

Coding

CPT

- Insertion of temporary bladder catheter **51701**
- Complex insertion of temporary catheter **51703**

Bibliography

Beno S, Schwab S. Bladder catheterization. In: King C, Henretig FM, eds. *Textbook of Pediatric Emergency Procedures.* 2nd ed. Philadelphia, PA: Lippincott, Williams & Williams; 2008:888–894

Karacan C, Erkek N, Senel S, et al. Evaluation of urine collection methods for the diagnosis of urinary tract infection in children. *Med Princ Pract.* 2010;19:188–191

Ethics

Do Not Resuscitate/Do Not Intubate

Introduction

Do not resuscitate/do not intubate (DNR/DNI) orders are a part of advanced directives for patients with life-limiting illnesses and/or when they (or their surrogates) believe that resuscitation would not be in the patient's best interests. Also known as do not attempt resuscitation (DNAR) or allow natural death (AND), these orders are not to be used in isolation, but as part of an overall discussion with the patient (if appropriate) and the parents/guardians as to the overall goals of treatment. DNR/DNI orders can be instituted while the patient is receiving other intensive therapies, such as chemotherapy, if resuscitation is not desired should an arrest occur. DNR/DNI orders can be specific for inpatients, outpatients, or apply to both settings, as a part of a comprehensive end-of-life plan. They may differ from state to state.

Use DNR and DNI orders to help convey the wishes of a patient, parents, or guardians in the event of a cardiorespiratory arrest. As part of a comprehensive care plan, related orders (eg, advance directives/advance care plans) can also describe the preferred responses to a deteriorating clinical situation before the point of an arrest. These orders, and the documented discussions that generated them, can also address pain control, palliative care, medically provided fluids and nutrition, and the social needs of the family.

Most hospitals have DNR/DNI policies or guidelines as well as forms or order sets. As a child ages toward adolescence, there may be guidelines related to obtaining the patient's assent in addition to the consent of the parents or guardians. In general, always consider the wishes of the adolescent when making decisions about limiting life-sustaining medical treatments.

Process

When a child or adolescent either has a terminal illness/condition and/or is nearing the end of life, arrange for the attending physician and pertinent consultants, along with the patient (if appropriate) and family, and possibly the primary care provider, to discuss the nature and direction of the patient's care. This dialogue is best accomplished when the child or family is *not in a crisis.* For a patient cared for by hospitalists, it is especially important to include physicians from the child's medical home in the process. If the child is a ward of the state, involve the designated medical decision-maker(s). Once the overall goals are identified, develop and institute the plans to help accomplish them. Resuscitation options are varied and may be as comprehensive as no intervention in the event of an arrest (no intubation, CPR, cardiac medications, or intravenous medications). In other cases, a "limited DNR/DNI" order can be created by defining which therapies can be initiated. For example, positive pressure ventilation with bag and mask and suctioning might be permitted, while chest compressions, intubation, mechanical ventilation, and cardiac medications are not. The more specific the delineation of the plan, the more effectively it can be performed according to the patient's and family's wishes. In addition to the specific details, it is essential to document the discussion that occurred and the goals of care that were identified.

Have an attending physician, and not a trainee, write the orders in the paper chart or electronic medical record. Avoid verbal orders, which are appropriate only in rare situations, as with a well-known patient whose previous DNR/DNI orders may have lapsed and need to be reinstituted prior to the attending arriving on site. Parental "signing" of DNR/DNI orders is not required in most states and should generally be avoided. In addition, as soon as the DNR/DNI plan is ordered, discuss and review it with the health care team, including the bedside nurse, so that it is clearly understood by all who are responsible for its implementation. If there is a lengthy hospitalization, review the DNR/DNI orders periodically to ensure that the patient and family continue to support the goals of care. Some hospitals may have policies that define how frequently the orders must be reviewed or rewritten, and some facilities may allow a home DNR/DNI order to remain in effect after hospitalization, although it may need prompt renewal. Others may require new orders be instituted on admission, so it is useful to become familiar with a given hospital's policies in this area.

DNR/DNI orders are typically rescinded, and then need to be reinstituted, when a patient goes to surgery, since surgery and anesthesia increase the chance that a patient may require some type of "resuscitation." Some institutions are now recommending an approach called "required reconsideration" prior to surgery to help clarify the situation. Under this policy, the anesthesiologist and surgeon will meet with the patient/family and attending physician to discuss the goal(s) of the DNR order and how to incorporate it into the overall surgical plan.

DNR/DNI orders may be used at home and may therefore stay in effect for longer periods (60–90 days). However, this regulation will vary among states, so providers should become familiar with their state regulations and forms. In some states, an outpatient form, the POLST or MOLST (Physician, or Medical, Orders for Life-Sustaining Treatment), may be helpful to communicate goals of care. In such a case, provide copies of the orders to the home care agency involved, as well as local emergency departments, law enforcement, and ambulance companies as appropriate.

Follow-up

- DNR/DNI orders are generally time limited and may require renewal (eg, every 3–5 days for inpatient orders or when the patient changes service). Be aware of various hospital policies and state and local laws.
- DNR/DNI orders can be rescinded at any time.

Pearls and Pitfalls

- A delay in initiating discussions about the overall goals and possible resuscitation for a patient with a life-limiting condition is the major obstacle to having a clear plan in place.
- Clearly and concisely document the plan.

Coding

ICD-9

DNR status **V49.86**

Bibliography

American Academy of Pediatrics Committee on Bioethics. Guidelines on foregoing life-sustaining medical treatment. *Pediatrics.* 1994;93:532–536

Fallat ME, Deshpande JK; American Academy of Pediatrics Section on Surgery, Section on Anesthesia and Pain Medicine, and Committee on Bioethics. Do-not-resuscitate orders for pediatric patients who require anesthesia and surgery. *Pediatrics.* 2004;114:1686–1692

Hastings Center. *Guidelines on the Termination of Life-Sustaining Treatment and the Care of the Dying.* Briarcliff Manor, NY: the Hastings Center: 1987:46–52

Minnesota Emergency Medical Services Regulatory Board. Provider orders for life sustaining treatment. http://www.emsrb.state.mn.us/docs/POLST_Minnesota_Form.pdf

President's Commission for the Study of Ethical Problems in Medicine and Biomedical and Behavioral Research. *Deciding to Forego Life-Sustaining Treatment.* Washington, DC: US Government Printing Office; 1983:231–255

CHAPTER 31

Informed Consent: Permission, Assent, and Confidentiality

The principle of autonomy requires physicians to obtain informed consent from adult patients. Some exceptions to this rule exist, mostly involving emergencies and surrogate decision-making for those who lack decisional capacity. Similarly, physicians who treat children are generally required to obtain informed permission from the parent(s) or legal guardian, although there are exceptions to this rule. When caring for a developmentally capable older child or adolescent, it is appropriate to also obtain informed assent, an affirmative action agreeing to the treatment.

Informed consent is a process, not a document. Rather than mere disclosure, it involves communicating, in language the patient or surrogate can understand, the various risks and benefits of a course of treatment, including any alternative therapies. While this does not mean discussing every imaginable outcome, it does require conveying the information that a reasonable person would want and need in order to make a wise decision.

Consent may be obtained verbally, implied from the cooperation of the parent, or documented and signed on a form. Use written consent for invasive procedures or if the patient will be sedated. Use developmentally appropriate language and concepts to obtain assent from older children. When a language barrier exists, use a professional translator rather than a family member, and document that person's name in the medical record. When the process is finished, have the patient/parent teach-back the information to confirm their comprehension.

Disputes

Sometimes there will be disagreements during the informed consent process. Parents have the presumptive authority to grant permission for medical care for their child, as well as a duty to make beneficent decisions for the child. The courts, in *Troxel v Granville,* "have recognized the fundamental right of parents to make decisions concerning the care, custody, and control of their children," although there are limits to this parental authority. For example, to protect the child, the law requires that physicians, nurses, and other medical personnel be mandatory reporters of neglect and abuse. Per American Academy of Pediatrics policy (1995), "Although physicians should seek parental permission in most situations, they must focus on the goal of providing appropriate care and be prepared to seek legal intervention when parental refusal places the patient at clear and substantial risk."

Counseling, mediation, and obtaining a second opinion are preferred first-line methods for dealing with conflict, rather than embarking on legal intervention. Social workers and ethics committees are useful resources in these situations, but if a decision is made to overrule the parent there are due process requirements, typically using the state child protective services hotline and appearing before a judge. The local expert in child abuse, hospital security personnel, the hospital attorney, and social workers may have experience with this process. Finally, if the child is in imminent danger, law enforcement agents may take immediate custody.

Harm Threshold

Medical personnel may draw erroneous conclusions when relying solely on their own personal judgment about what is "in the best interests of the child." They must recognize that parents can, and must, balance the many competing needs of all family members when making decisions. There is a threshold of harm below which society generally does not intervene and overrule parents. For example, while it is not in the best interests of a child to be driven through a blizzard so that the parent can buy cigarettes, it would be legally imprudent and procedurally impractical for society to intervene. This harm threshold is dependent on the risk of harm (probability), the exposure (severity of the injury), and the immediacy of the danger. This threshold varies significantly among jurisdictions. Some judges are activists, while others are more deferential to familial authority, setting a threshold that "no reasonable parent would decline treatment." In addition, accommodating cultural and religious diversity is an endorsed virtue, but one with limits. There will be situations where parents may legally act against medical advice. Proper documentation is essential in these circumstances.

Custody

Family and guardianship laws vary by state and local jurisdiction. With the usual joint custody, either parent may have the authority to give permission for medical care. After a divorce, the authority to give permission may be specifically granted to just one of the parents, even if the other continues to have visitation rights. However, a noncustodial parent may still have a right to disclosure of medical information. Clarify the social situation, particularly before invasive medical procedures. A grandmother may provide most day-to-day care without having legal guardianship. She may bring the child to the emergency department for a fever and her permission, by custom, may be sufficient agency to permit an examination and simple treatment. In contrast, very invasive procedures warrant efforts to obtain formal consent from the true legal parent and guardian. When the patient is in imminent danger, the appropriate action is to protect the child's health.

Special Situations

There are many exceptions that modify the general principles outlined above. Family law, guardianship law, child protection law, mental health law, and the law of medical practice vary among jurisdictions. Knowledgeable local attorneys can provide guidance on legal principles when drafting hospital policies. Obtain legal counsel for specific circumstances, since in many situations a state may not have guiding precedents.

Consent Directly From a Minor

The age of majority for health care decisions is generally 18 years, but there are some differences among a few states. Patients younger than 18 years may have the authority to give informed consent, without regard to parental permission, if they are mature minors. That legal definition also varies among the states, involving factors such as emancipation, military service, marriage, or being the minor parent of a child herself. In some states, a parent younger than 18 years may give consent for her own general medical treatment. In others, while the minor parent can give consent for the treatment of her own child, she remains under parental authority.

Exceptions Based on Disease

A minor has authority to give informed consent for medical care for certain disorders. Treatment of sexually transmitted infections is almost always allowed based solely on the minor's consent, although some states set a minimum age for this. Rules for contraception, abortion, and prenatal care are more varied. The Guttmacher Institute has an online table that is updated monthly. In some localities, a minor may give consent for drug and alcohol treatment and for outpatient mental health services.

Confidentiality and Parental Notification

Confidentiality requirements also vary by jurisdiction, status of the minor, and the medical procedure involved. State law determines most of this, but federal law, federal funding rules, and clinic policies may further regulate confidentiality. Be circumspect when making promises of confidentiality, and inform the adolescent that there are situations, such as suicidal/homicidal ideation or abuse, in which the physician is required by law to take action. In addition, billing statements, explanation of benefits, and medical records available to the parent are potential leaks of information that can compromise any promised confidentiality. In general, encouraging the minor to inform the parent may help ensure compliance with the treatment plan.

Bibliography

American Academy of Pediatrics Committee on Bioethics. Informed consent, parental permission, and assent in pediatric practice. *Pediatrics.* 1995;95:314–317

Diekema DS. Parental refusals of medical treatment: the harm principle as threshold for state intervention. *Theor Med Bioeth.* 2004;25:243–264

Diekema DS; American Academy of Pediatrics Committee on Bioethics. Responding to parental refusals of immunization of children. *Pediatrics.* 2005;115:1428–1431

Guttmacher Institute. Minors' right to consent to health care and to make other important decisions. http://www.guttmacher.org/graphics/gr030406_f1.html

Guttmacher Institute. An overview of minors' consent law. http://www.guttmacher.org/statecenter/spibs/spib_OMCL.pdf

McCullough LB, Chervenak FA. Informed consent. *Clin Perinatol.* 2007;34:275–285

Gastroenterology

CHAPTER 32

Gallbladder Disease

Introduction

There is a wide spectrum of gallbladder disease in children, including cholelithiasis (gallstones), choledocholithiasis (stones in the common bile duct), calculous or acalculous cholecystitis (inflamed gallbladder with or without stones), and hydrops of the gallbladder (acute distension without inflammation). Gallstones occur in less than 1% of children, but the incidence may be increasing because of the rising rates of obesity and the diagnosis of asymptomatic gallstones via ultrasound. Patients with risk factors (chronic hemolytic disorders, obesity, cystic fibrosis, postpartum, recent weight loss) have a higher incidence of gallbladder disease, with a prevalence of 40% among adolescents with sickle cell disease. However, in about 80% of patients the gallstones are asymptomatic, although pancreatitis can occur in 5% to 10%.

Historically, up to 50% of the cases of cholecystitis in children were acalculous, developing from biliary dyskinesia or acquired biliary stasis secondary to compression of the cystic duct by edema, lymph node, or congenital malformation. Recently, more cases have been secondary to gallstone disease.

Hydrops of the gallbladder occurs in up to 20% of children with Kawasaki disease, as well as in patients with other infections or conditions (staphylococcal or streptococcal infection, leptospirosis).

Clinical Presentation

The presentation of biliary tract disease is summarized in Table 32-1.

History

A patient with gallbladder inflammation, distension, or biliary colic from gallstones presents with complaints of nausea, vomiting, anorexia, and abdominal pain. The biliary colic may be described as a constant right upper quadrant pain that radiates to the shoulder. There may also be a history of previous episodes of cholecystitis. An older child or adolescent may describe the pain as postprandial, especially if the meal was fatty, but this history is not reliable. The patient may also report light-colored stools and dark urine, which raises a suspicion for obstructive jaundice. The presentation of hydrops is similar to cholecystitis.

Inquire about predisposing risk factors, including hemolytic disease, obesity, family history of gallstones, Native American descent, artificial heart valve, pregnancy or recent delivery, cystic fibrosis, bowel resection or ileal

Table 32-1. Presentation of Biliary Tract Diseases	
Diagnosis	**Clinical Features**
Acalculous cholecystitis	Fever and pain Leukocytosis with normal liver function tests Ultrasound: inflamed gallbladder with no gallstones
Asymptomatic gallstones	No pain, nausea, or vomiting Incidental finding on ultrasound
Calculous cholecystitis	Fever and pain Leukocytosis with normal liver function tests Ultrasound: gallstones in gallbladder
Cholangitis	Charcot triad: fever, jaundice, right upper quadrant pain May have acholic stools and dark urine (infants) Leukocytosis
Choledocholithiasis	Jaundice (↑direct bilirubin) and pain Ultrasound: no gallstones ↑alkaline phosphatase and gamma-glutamyl transferase
Hydrops	Normal gallbladder wall but dilated lumen
Pancreatitis	Pain may radiate to the back ↑amylase and lipase

disease, Down syndrome, bronchopulmonary dysplasia, recent total parenteral nutrition (TPN), ceftriaxone, cyclosporine, or furosemide use. Acalculous cholecystitis risk factors include prolonged fasting, infective endocarditis, TPN or opiate use, and infection (streptococcal and gram-negative sepsis, leptospirosis, Rocky Mountain spotted fever, typhoid fever, ascariasis, and *Giardia lamblia*). Other parasitic, candidal, and viral infections can also cause acalculous cholecystitis in an immunocompromised host.

Further history can suggest symptoms of complications of gallstones. Pain that radiates to the back occurs with pancreatitis. Fever and malaise may suggest cholecystitis or cholangitis, if associated with jaundice.

Physical Examination

With calculous or acalculous cholecystitis, there will be right upper quadrant abdominal pain with a positive Murphy sign (pain during inspiration while palpating the right upper quadrant). The gallbladder may be palpable, but hepatosplenomegaly is uncommon in primary gall bladder disease. Hepatomegaly may be present if there has been longstanding obstructive cholestasis causing cirrhosis. If a gallstone is obstructing the common bile duct, there may be jaundice and scleral icterus. With bacterial cholangitis or cholecystitis there will be fever, tachycardia, and tachypnea. Perforation of the gallbladder presents with peritoneal signs, such as guarding, rebound tenderness, and a firm or distended abdomen.

Laboratory

If gallbladder disease is suspected, obtain a complete blood cell count with differential, liver function panel with alkaline phosphatase, amylase, lipase and, if the patient is febrile, a blood culture.

Radiology

Order an abdominal ultrasound to look for stones, sludge, or a thickened gallbladder. However, make the patient NPO at least 4 hours before the study. The ultrasound may be normal if the stone is in the common bile duct or the diagnosis is gallbladder dyskinesia.

Cholescintigraphy is helpful when there are no gallstones in the gallbladder on ultrasound but there is still concern for extrahepatic biliary disease or obstruction of the common bile duct. In the latter case, there will be good hepatic uptake but no, or delayed, gallbladder filling.

If a patient has signs of cholecystitis or cholangitis, but there are no stones in the gallbladder on ultrasound, arrange magnetic resonance cholangiopancreatography (MRCP) or endoscopic retrograde cholangiopancreatography (ERCP) if available. These can demonstrate stones in the common bile duct as well as assess the biliary tree anatomy for congenital malformations.

Differential Diagnosis

There are a number of common and/or serious diseases that can present with right upper quadrant pain (Table 32-2).

Treatment

Acute Cholecystitis

Make the patient NPO, give maintenance intravenous hydration with D5 ½ normal saline + 20 mEq KCl, and correct any additional electrolyte or fluid deficit. Although cholecystitis is typically an inflammatory disease, secondary infection can occur, so empiric antibiotic is usually indicated. Give antibiotic coverage for gram-negative bacilli and anaerobes, with ampicillin/sulbactam (200 mg/kg/day divided every 6 hours, 8 g ampicillin/day maximum), piperacillin/tazobactam (300 mg/kg/day divided every 8 hours, 16 g piperacillin/day maximum), or the combination of ceftriaxone (50–75 mg/kg/day divided every 12–24 hours, 4 g/day maximum) *and* metronidazole (30 mg/kg/day divided every 6 hours, 4 g/day maximum).

Analgesia is a priority. Start with a nonsteroidal anti-inflammatory drug, such as ketorolac (0.5 mg/kg every 6 hours for 5 days, 120 mg/day maximum),

Table 32-2. Differential Diagnosis of Right Upper Quadrant Pain

Diagnosis	Clinical Features
Appendicitis	Atypical location of appendix (especially in pregnancy)
Fitz-Hugh-Curtis syndrome	Sexually active female ↑CRP/ESR Possible vaginal symptoms/culture positive
Gastroenteritis	May have diarrhea
Hepatitis	↑ALT and AST (SGPT and SGOT)
Musculoskeletal pain	Afebrile May have point tenderness Normal LFTs, ESR, ultrasound
Peptic ulcer disease	Guaiac positive stool Pain relieved by meals, antacids, H_2 blockers
Pleural effusion	Decreased breath sounds Positive chest x-ray
Pneumonia	Decreased breath sounds or rales Positive chest x-ray

Abbreviations: ALT, alanine transaminase; AST, aspartate transaminase; CRP, C-reactive protein; ESR, erythrocyte sedimentation rate; H_2, histamine 2; LFTs, liver function tests; SGOT, serum glutamic-oxaloacetic transaminase; SGPT, serum glutamic-pyruvic transaminase.

which may prevent progression of the cholecystitis. However, the patient may require an opiate, such as morphine sulfate (0.05–0.1 mg/kg/dose every 2–4 hours; maximum 2 mg/dose infant, 4–8 mg/dose child, 15 mg/dose adolescent).

Consult with a surgeon, as an acute cholecystectomy may be necessary if supportive care does not relieve the pain or there are signs of peritonitis, sepsis, or worsening distress. Otherwise, if the patient improves quickly, elective surgery (preferably a laparoscopic cholecystectomy) is indicated 6 to 12 weeks after resolution of the symptoms. However, instruct the patient to return to the hospital immediately for an urgent cholecystectomy if the symptoms of cholecystitis recur.

Cholelithiasis

Manage asymptomatic cholelithiasis on an outpatient basis with a follow-up ultrasound in 6 months. However, if the patient has a hemolytic disease, consult with a surgeon to plan a cholecystectomy.

Choledocholithiasis

In addition to supportive care, consult a gastroenterologist and surgeon to arrange an MRCP or ERCP to look for, and possibly remove, the obstructing stone. However, if a cholecystectomy is planned, a cholangiography is usually also performed to confirm the presence or absence of a stone.

Acalculous Cholecystitis

Treat the underlying condition, such as discontinuing the implicated medication or giving antibiotics for the inciting infection.

Hydrops of the Gallbladder

This is usually self-limited, so no specific treatment is necessary.

Indications for Consultation

- **Gastroenterology or surgery (depending on the availability of ERCP):** Choledocholithiasis
- **Hematology or other subspecialists:** As needed for underlying disease
- **Surgery (urgent):** Cholecystitis or hydrops of the gallbladder with perforation, empyema, or necrosis

Disposition

- **Intensive care unit transfer:** Sepsis or peritonitis
- **Discharge criteria:** Afebrile, adequate oral hydration and pain control

Follow-up

- **Primary care:** 1 week
- **Surgery:** 3 to 5 days (if the patient had a cholecystectomy); 1 to 2 weeks to arrange for an elective cholecystectomy in next 2 to 3 months

Pearls and Pitfalls

- Consider cholangitis and consult surgery if fever and jaundice accompany cholecystitis

Coding

ICD-9

• Acute cholecystitis	**575.0**
• Cholelithiasis with acute cholecystitis without obstruction	**574.00**
• Gallstones without mention of obstruction	**574.20**
• Gallstones with biliary obstruction	**574.21**
• Hydrops of the gall bladder	**575.3**
• Obstructive jaundice	**576.8**

Bibliography

Bogue CO, Murphy AJ, Gerstle JT, Moineddin R, Daneman A. Risk factors, complications, and outcomes of gallstones in children: a single-center review. *J Pediatr Gastroenterol Nutr.* 2010;50:303–308

Broderick A. Gallbladder disease. In: Kleinman R, Goulet O-J, Mieli-Vergani G, Sanderson I, eds. *Walker's Pediatric Gastrointestinal Disease.* 5th ed. Hamilton, Ontario: BC Decker; 2008:1173–1182

Kurbegov AC. Pediatric biliary disease. In: Perkin RM, Swift JD, Newton DA, Anas NG, eds. *Pediatric Hospital Medicine.* 2nd ed. Baltimore, MD: Lippincott, Williams & Williams; 2008:605–611

Poddar U. Gallstone disease in children. *Indian Pediatr.* 2010;47:945–953

CHAPTER 33

Gastroenteritis

Introduction

Gastroenteritis is an intraluminal inflammation of the gastrointestinal (GI) tract involving any region from the stomach to the colon. Infectious gastroenteritis may be caused by bacteria, viruses or parasites, or by preformed toxins produced by bacteria. Viral causes are most common, with rotavirus being the most frequent agent necessitating hospitalization. The most common causes of inflammatory bacterial gastroenteritis in the United States are *Salmonella* and *Campylobacter*.

Clinical Presentation

History

Complete a thorough history to help determine the possible etiology, assess the severity of dehydration, and rule out other serious illnesses that can present as vomiting and/or diarrhea. Determine the character of the vomiting and/or diarrhea, including the number of episodes and whether there was any bile or blood in the vomitus or blood or mucus in the stools. Ask about fever, abdominal pain, other illnesses, injuries, medications, recent sick contacts, animal contacts (specifically farm animals or reptiles), travel history, and potential exposure to contaminated food or water. In addition, to assess the hydration status and severity of the illness, determine recent oral intake, urine output, acute weight loss (if known), and any change in mental status.

Viral Gastroenteritis

Symptoms of rotavirus typically manifest 2 to 4 days after exposure, usually beginning with fever and vomiting followed by frequent loose or watery diarrhea. However, diarrhea may be the only symptom. Complete resolution of symptoms typically occurs within 7 days. Other viral agents, including norovirus, produce similar symptoms, but typically are less severe, of a shorter duration, and often without fever. Enteric adenovirus may also mimic rotavirus, but may be more common in summertime, and can be more prolonged, lasting up to 7 to 10 days.

Bacterial Gastroenteritis

Signs and symptoms typically overlap with viral gastroenteritis but may cause a more significant colitis associated with diarrhea with gross blood, mucus, and pus (dysentery); fever; myalgia; abdominal pain; and tenesmus. Extraintestinal manifestations may accompany specific bacterial infections, such as

Campylobacter (erythema nodosum, glomerulonephritis, reactive arthritis), *Escherichia coli* (hemolytic uremic syndrome [HUS]), *Salmonella* (erythema nodosum, reactive arthritis), *Shigella* (encephalopathy, glomerulonephritis, reactive arthritis, Reiter syndrome, seizures), and *Yersinia* (erythema nodosum, glomerulonephritis, hemolytic anemia, reactive arthritis).

Non-typhi *Salmonella*-associated gastroenteritis typically causes fever and watery diarrhea and may result in a more severe inflammatory colitis. The illness may also be complicated by bacteremia, especially in a patient who is immunocompromised or younger than 1 year. Ask about exposure to potential sources of *Salmonella*, including reptiles and contaminated food products, such as eggs and milk products.

Salmonella (typhi/paratyphi) is usually acquired outside the United States and causes a systemic infection, with remitting fever that becomes sustained. Other complaints include abdominal pain and other constitutional symptoms such as headache, malaise, anorexia, and lethargy. The patient may progress to have a blanching macular rash on the trunk and an altered mental status. *S typhi* can also cause intestinal perforation that presents as peritonitis or septic shock, although this is rare in a child.

Shigella infection ranges from mild watery stools to dysentery. Certain species of the bacteria may also produce the Shiga toxin that causes endothelial damage and HUS, as well as seizures. *Shigella* bacteria are more resistant to acid compared with other bacteria and can transmit disease through the stomach. Since only 10 to 100 organisms may cause disease, it is therefore highly contagious.

Gastroenteritis caused by *Yersinia* infection is relatively uncommon in the United States. A known risk factor is cooking chitterlings (pig intestines). In a younger child it may present as a mild, self-limited disease, whereas an older patient may have more prominent symptoms including abdominal pain and tenderness due to mesenteric adenitis.

Campylobacter-associated infection is characterized by fever, chills, crampy abdominal pain, and bloody mucoid diarrhea. It can also cause frank rectal bleeding. The source of *Campylobacter* infection is primarily food, such as poultry and eggs.

E coli, which has several identified classes, can cause the full spectrum of diarrheal illness. The enterohemorrhagic *E coli* 0157:H7 organism, in particular, produces the Shiga toxin that may cause HUS. Other classes of the bacteria include enterotoxigenic, which causes watery diarrhea in developing countries, and enteroinvasive, which typically results in food-borne outbreaks of dysentery due to undercooked ground beef, raw milk, and occasionally raw vegetables. The enteropathogenic form of the bacteria causes acute and chronic diarrhea in infants and the enteroaggregative form causes acute and chronic watery diarrhea.

Clostridium difficile is found in cases of antibiotic-associated diarrhea, particularly after treatment with β-lactams and clindamycin. As with other bacterial sources of diarrhea, symptoms can range from mild diarrhea to life-threatening enterocolitis.

Parasitic Gastroenteritis

Protozoan gastroenteritis most often presents with persistent diarrhea lasting 2 to 4 weeks. *Giardia lamblia* is the leading cause of waterborne disease in the United States. Typical infections are characterized by explosive, foul-smelling, watery diarrhea with abdominal cramps and bloating. *Entamoeba histolytica* causes a range of symptoms, including amebic dysentery, which is characterized by bloody or mucoid diarrhea, prolonged watery diarrhea, and hepatic abscesses.

Physical Examination

The priority is an accurate assessment of the patient's hydration status. Clinical scoring systems have been validated, which factor in some combination of the patient's general appearance, mental status, subjective thirst, heart rate, pulse rate and quality, respiratory effort, potentially sunken eyes, tear production, mucous membrane moistness, skin turgor, capillary refill, mottled appearance of extremities, and urine output. Categorize the dehydration status as minimal (<3% of body weight), moderate (3%–9% of body weight), or severe (>9% of body weight), which will then guide rehydration. As noted above, extraintestinal manifestations noted on the physical examination may provide clues to the etiology of infection.

Laboratory

Per Centers for Disease Control and Prevention and American Academy of Pediatrics guidelines, laboratory testing for uncomplicated acute gastroenteritis with mild or moderate dehydration is not needed. Laboratory evaluation is indicated for patients who exhibit severe dehydration or excessive losses predisposing to electrolyte imbalance. If there is concern for certain extraintestinal manifestations, such as HUS, obtain a complete blood cell count (CBC), peripheral smear, electrolytes, and blood urea nitrogen (BUN) and creatinine. If the patient has dysentery (blood, pus, and mucus in the stools) send stool samples for blood, leukocytes, and culture. Routine stool cultures will typically recover *Shigella*, *Salmonella*, *Campylobacter*, and *Yersinia*, but if the stools are bloody, specifically order testing for *E coli* 0157:H7. Evaluation for *C difficile* toxin is indicated if the patient has severe, persistent diarrhea or predisposing conditions such as recent or multiple courses of antibiotics, an underlying GI disorder or immunodeficiency, or has recently been hospitalized. However, do not routinely test a patient younger than 1 year because there are many false-positives. Also, there is no need to test for cure because the toxin can remain after symptoms resolve.

Send a stool sample for ova and parasites if the patient has pertinent travel history, contact with untreated water, or prolonged GI symptoms. Order a direct microscopy of stool to look for parasites, eggs, and cysts, although many laboratories now use an ELISA test for *Giardia* and *Cryptococcus.*

Obtain a CBC and blood culture if there is concern for a serious bacterial illness. If there is suspicion for a urinary tract infection also obtain a urine culture.

Differential Diagnosis

While most often the patient will have a viral gastroenteritis, the priority is to ensure that there is not a serious, or even life-threatening, alternative diagnosis (Table 33-1). This is particularly true if the patient presents with unopposed vomiting (no diarrhea), a toxic appearance, or a widened pulse pressure, or required excessive fluid resuscitation.

Suspect myocarditis (page 47) if the patient has insidious signs and symptoms, such as increased tachycardia and development of a new gallop rhythm or murmur without a good clinical response to fluid resuscitation. Similarly, if the patient has an altered mental status that does not respond to fluids, consider a toxic ingestion, encephalitis, intussusception, or increased intracranial pressure.

Treatment

Oral rehydration therapy (ORT) is the mainstay of management for mild and moderate dehydration. Intravenous fluids, such as normal saline or Ringer lactate, are indicated for a patient who is severely dehydrated, persistently vomiting, or unable to tolerate ORT, or has an underlying condition that can be exacerbated by dehydration, such as a metabolic disorder. For mild dehydration, replace the losses based on the patient's weight. For example, if the patient's body weight is less than 10 kg, give 60 to 120 mL of oral rehydration solution (ORS) for each stool or emesis; if the body weight is greater than 10 kg, use 120 to 240 mL of ORS for each stool or emesis. If the patient has moderate dehydration, replace the fluid deficit with 50 to 100 mL/kg over 3 to 4 hours. Afterward, provide maintenance fluids and calories, as well as appropriate replacement of losses, as done with mild dehydration.

Table 33-1. Differential Diagnosis of Gastroenteritis

Diagnosis	Clinical Features
Adrenal insufficiency	Unopposed vomiting (no diarrhea) Weakness, fatigue, anorexia Previous steroid exposure
Appendicitis	Abdominal pain precedes vomiting Minimal or no diarrhea Signs of acute abdomen (guarding, rebound)
Increased intracranial pressure	History of trauma or underlying neurologic disorder Unopposed vomiting May have Cushing triad (↓pulse with ↑blood pressure)
Inflammatory bowel disease	Chronic symptoms and poor growth Extraintestinal symptoms: rash, arthritis, uveitis
Intussusception	Sudden onset of severe, crampy pain and inconsolability Pain associated with drawing up of legs Guaiac (+) or currant jelly (late) stools
Malabsorption syndromes (celiac)	Chronic diarrhea and weight loss Diet related
Metabolic acidosis (diabetic ketoacidosis)	History of weight loss/polydipsia/polyuria but no diarrhea Deep (Kussmaul) breathing Mental status change out of proportion to vomiting
Myocarditis	Usually no diarrhea Tachycardia out of proportion to dehydration Gallop rhythm
Peritonitis	Fever (may be high) Worsening abdominal pain Rebound and guarding on abdominal examination
Small bowl obstruction	Persistent bilious vomiting Abdominal distention History of previous abdominal surgery
Urinary tract infection	Dysuria, urgency, frequency (+) urinalysis

Correct severe dehydration with 1 to 3 20-mL/kg boluses of an isotonic fluid, either normal saline or lactated Ringer solution, until the patient no longer has orthostatic vital sign changes and/or has adequate urine output (1 mL/kg/hour) with improved peripheral perfusion and mental status. Unless the patient has renal disease, sickle cell disease, or diabetes, the urine output is a good gauge as to whether subsequent boluses are needed. At that point, *after the patient has voided*, change to D5 ½ normal saline at 1.5 times maintenance rate, with potassium added (20 mEq/L). If the patient can tolerate oral intake, start ORT and decrease the intravenous (IV) fluid rate as the oral intake improves.

Frequent reassessments, including input and output (stool and urine with specific gravity), vital signs, and physical examination, are crucial for both tracking ongoing losses and diagnosing an underlying illness other than a viral gastroenteritis. Be particularly suspicious of an alternative diagnosis if the patient has an inadequate response to fluid administration, persistent inability to tolerate oral intake, or severe abdominal pain. If myocarditis is suspected (unopposed vomiting and poor response to fluid resuscitation), immediately obtain an electrocardiogram, chest x-ray, and cardiology consult. If altered mental status persists despite the fluid boluses, obtain electrolytes, liver function tests, toxicology screening, and a lumbar puncture, before or after an imaging study of the brain.

If the patient does not void after 3 fluid boluses, insert a bladder catheter and obtain electrolytes, BUN, and creatinine. Poor perfusion despite multiple boluses occurs with distributive shock secondary to sepsis. Treat with broad-spectrum antibiotics and vasopressors and transfer the patient to an intensive care unit (ICU) setting.

There is no indication for gut rest. As soon as oral intake can be tolerated, resume an unrestricted diet, including complex carbohydrates, lean meat, fruits, vegetables, milk products, or breast milk/infant formula. If the patient has persistent nausea and/or vomiting that interferes with resuming oral intake, give a dose of oral (sublingually) or IV ondansetron (0.05–0.1 mg/kg every 6 hours, 4 mg maximum). Do not use ondansetron if there is any concern about a surgical abdomen or other underlying medical problems such as long QTc syndrome.

Treat all patients with culture-positive *Shigella*, as well as those with a high suspicion and severe disease, dysentery, or an underlying immunosuppressive disorder with antibiotics *while awaiting culture results*. Indications for treating culture-positive *Salmonella* include age younger than 3 months, bacteremia, typhoid fever, chronic underlying GI disease, immunocompromised status, or sickle cell disease. Treatment of *Campylobacter* can shorten the duration of illness and prevent relapse when given early during infection.

Options for treatment of *Shigella*, *Salmonella*, and *Campylobacter* include ceftriaxone (50 mg/kg every day, 4 g/day maximum), azithromycin (12 mg/kg/day, 500 mg/day maximum), and trimethoprim-sulfamethoxazole (20 mg/kg/day divided every 6–8 hours, 640 mg/day maximum). Fluoroquinolones, such as ciprofloxacin (20–30mg/kg/day divided every 12 hours, 800 mg/day maximum) are also effective, but not officially approved by the US Food and Drug Administration for a patient younger than 18 years. Treat for 5 days, but prescribe an extended 10- to 14-day course for invasive, nonfocal infections, such as bacteremia or enteric fever, caused by nontyphoidal *Salmonella* or

S typhi. Note that a relapse of enteric fever occurs in up to 15% of patients and requires re-treatment. Due to the highly contagious nature of *Shigella*, treat symptomatic family members and others with close contact with the patient as well.

Upon diagnosis of antibiotic-associated *C difficile*, discontinue the offending antibiotic. If the patient has severe or persistent symptoms, treat with oral metronidazole (30 mg/kg/day divided every 6 hours for 10 days, 1.5 g/day maximum) or oral vancomycin (40–50 mg/kg/day divided every 6 hours for 7–10 days, 2 g/day maximum).

Also use metronidazole for *Giardia* (15 mg/kg/day divided 3 times a day for 5 days, 750 mg/day maximum) and amebiasis (35–50mg/kg/day divided 3 times a day for 10 days, 1.5 g/day maximum). The treatment of choice for cryptosporidium is a 3-day course of nitazoxanide (1–3 years of age: 100 mg twice a day [bid]; 4–11 years of age: 200 mg bid; >11 years of age: 500 mg bid).

Indications for Consultation

- **Gastroenterology:** Persistent diarrhea (>14 days), significant GI bleeding, or suspected inflammatory bowel disease
- **Surgery:** Possible acute abdomen

Disposition

- **ICU transfer:** Decompensated shock, not responsive to fluid boluses, concern for acute adrenal insufficiency, diabetic ketoacidosis, increased intracranial pressure, or myocarditis
- **Discharge criteria:** Dehydration resolved, oral intake adequate to maintain hydration, oral antibiotics (if indicated) tolerated

Follow-up

- **Primary Care:** 2 to 3 days

Pearls and Pitfalls

- Viral gastroenteritis typically presents with vomiting and diarrhea without blood or mucus.
- Bacterial gastroenteritis may present as dysentery, with bloody, mucoid stools.
- Vomiting without diarrhea (unopposed vomiting) may be caused by a non-GI disease.
- The presence of diarrhea does not rule out an appendicitis.

Coding

ICD-9

• Bacterial enteritis, unspecified	**008.5**
• Dehydration	**276.51**
• Enteritis, infectious	**009.0**
• Enteritis, noninfectious	**558.9**
• Rotavirus enteritis	**008.61**
• Salmonella enteritis	**003.0**
• Vomiting	**787.03**

Bibliography

Allen K. The vomiting child—what to do and when to consult. *Aust Fam Physician.* 2007;36:684–687

American Academy of Pediatrics. *Salmonella* infections. In: Pickering LK, Baker CJ, Kimberlin DW, Long SS, eds. *Red Book: 2012 Report of the Committee on Infectious Diseases.* Elk Grove Village, IL: American Academy of Pediatrics; 2012:635–640

Colletti JE, Brown KM, Sharieff GQ, Barata IA, Ishimine P; ACEP Pediatric Emergency Medicine Committee. The management of children with gastroenteritis and dehydration in the emergency department. *J Emerg Med.* 2010;38:686–698

Goldman RD, Friedman JN, Parkin PC. Validation of the clinical dehydration scale for children with acute gastroenteritis. *Pediatrics.* 2008;122:545–549

Hartling L, Bellemare S, Wiebe N, et al. Oral versus intravenous rehydration for treating dehydration due to gastroenteritis in children. *Cochrane Database Syst Rev.* 2006;3:CD004390

Laufer M, Siberry G. Gastrointestinal diseases. In: Zaoutis LB, Chiang VW, eds. *Comprehensive Pediatric Hospital Medicine.* Philadelphia, PA: Mosby; 2007:394–401

Gastrointestinal Bleeding

Introduction

Gastrointestinal (GI) bleeding is a common complaint that requires prompt evaluation. The presentation and differential diagnosis are broad, with a spectrum ranging from an occult, self-limited bleed, to a severe, rapidly progressive, life-threatening hemorrhage that can originate from either the upper GI (UGI) or lower GI (LGI) tract. A systematic approach is critical, beginning with the confirmation of actual blood that originates from the GI tract, an assessment of the severity of the bleeding, and the initiation of appropriate resuscitation, if necessary. Once the patient is stabilized, the priorities are determining the exact cause and site of the bleeding (UGI vs LGI) and planning for subsequent treatment.

Clinical Presentation

History

Ask about the duration of bleeding or symptoms and the estimated amount of blood loss, measured in terms understandable to nonmedical caregivers, such as teaspoons. Document the presence of fever, lethargy, and weight loss, as well as the location, intensity, and pattern of any abdominal pain. Determine if there have been any prior episodes of bleeding or a family history of peptic ulcer, *Helicobacter pylori* infection, or similar symptoms.

Obtain a thorough history regarding the diet, medications, and possible ingestions, as certain foods and drugs can give the false appearance of blood. Any food with a red skin (beets, tomatoes, apples) or anything containing red food coloring (candy, drinks, gelatin) can be mistaken for frank blood if vomited. Likewise, medications containing flavoring syrups (antibiotics, certain preparations of acetaminophen) can resemble hematemesis. Spinach, blueberries, plums, grapes, and medications that contain iron or bismuth can cause melena-like stools.

Aspirin, nonsteroidal anti-inflammatory drugs (NSAIDs), and corticosteroids increase the risk of GI bleeding by directly damaging gastric mucosa. Anticoagulants (heparin, warfarin, aspirin, NSAIDs) can affect coagulation and increase the risk of mucocutaneous bleeding. In addition, some medications (doxycycline, aspirin, NSAIDs) can cause an esophagitis.

UGI Bleeds

By definition, the bleeding originates proximal to the ligament of Treitz and often presents with hematemesis, which can be coffee ground or bright red in appearance, depending on the source, severity, and chronicity of the bleed. A slow UGI bleed may also present with melena or, if the bleeding is brisk enough, hematochezia (bright red or dark blood per rectum). Ask about a history of lesions or active disease in the nose, mouth, pharynx, larynx, or lungs, which can lead to swallowed blood and mimic a UGI bleed. Also ask about a history of prematurity and possible umbilical artery line insertion. Other important symptoms are vomiting and retching (Mallory-Weiss tear) and itching and jaundice (liver disease and portal hypertension). Also ask about a history of abdominal trauma from an automobile or bike accident (handle-bar injury), which can lead to duodenal injury.

LGI Bleeds

Ask about the quality, consistency, and frequency of the stool. A very slow LGI bleed can present with melena, but more commonly presents with hematochezia. Hard stool that is blood-streaked on the outside occurs with bleeding in the rectal vault or anal canal. Bloody diarrhea suggests colitis, most often secondary to an infectious etiology, as does the presence of mucus mixed with the stool, whereas currant jelly stool is a classic finding of intussusception. Ask about weight loss, rash, joint pain, atopy in the family or patient, or tenesmus, which, along with a family history of chronic bleeding, GI, or autoimmune disorders, can suggest inflammatory bowel disease (IBD).

Physical Examination

The patient can appear well or ill as a result of the underlying condition causing the GI bleed, or as a consequence of the bleeding itself. Carefully assess the patient's vital signs (including orthostatic changes), growth parameters, general appearance, peripheral pulses, capillary refill, and mental status to determine if aggressive resuscitation or urgent specialty consultation is needed.

Examine the oral and nasal mucosa for freckles (associated with polyps) or evidence of bleeding or trauma, and the abdomen for distension, bowel sounds, tenderness, ascites, masses, hepatosplenomegaly, or signs of an acute abdomen. Epigastric tenderness is nonspecific but may indicate peptic ulcer disease, gastritis, or esophagitis, while hepatosplenomegaly in conjunction with caput medusae is highly suggestive of portal hypertension with esophageal varices. Cutaneous hemangiomas raise the suspicion for other vascular lesions within the GI tract (upper and/or lower). Perform a careful anal and rectal examination looking for fissures, skin tags, fistulas, occult blood, impacted stool, or polyps.

Laboratory

The goals of the diagnostic evaluation are to first confirm the presence of actual blood, and then to determine the source and severity of the bleed. Obtain a complete blood cell count (CBC) and a stool guaiac for both UGI and LGI bleeds and a Gastroccult for a UGI bleed. If the bleeding is either hemodynamically significant or ongoing, repeat the CBC at least every 6 to 12 hours. If there is evidence of liver dysfunction or a coagulopathy is suspected (easy bruising or a history of recurrent bleeding, liver disease, or anticoagulant use) obtain a comprehensive chemistry profile with liver function tests and a prothrombin time (PT)/partial thromboplastin time/international normalized ratio. Also obtain a C-reactive protein and/or erythrocyte sedimentation rate if the clinical picture suggests an inflammatory process based on findings such as weight loss, fatigue, fever, arthralgias or arthritis, purpura suggestive of Henoch-Schönlein purpura, or a prior history of such symptoms.

If the patient has hematochezia associated with high fever or toxicity, obtain stool for fecal polymorphonuclear leukocytes, bacterial stool culture (common pathogens include *Salmonella*, *Shigella*, *Yersinia enterocolitica*, *Campylobacter jejuni*, *Escherichia coli* 0157:H7), and *Clostridium difficile* toxin A and B. If indicated by a recent travel history to endemic areas, send stool for *Entamoeba histolytica* and *Trichuris trichiura*. Obtain a urinalysis if the initial test results are consistent with hemolytic uremic syndrome (anemia, thrombocytopenia, evidence of hemolysis on peripheral smear, and renal impairment). For hemodynamically significant bleeds, order a type and screen in anticipation of giving blood products.

Nasogastric or orogastric lavage is not routinely indicated, unless the source of a GI bleed is uncertain or the bleeding is clinically significant. If the lavage returns fresh blood, blood-tinged secretions, or coffee-ground secretions, a UGI or nasopharyngeal source of bleeding is confirmed. The lavage may be falsely negative if the bleeding has stopped or if the source is distal to a closed pylorus. A lavage with bilious fluid may indicate an open pylorus and/or a small bowel obstruction. Do not use ice water because it does not slow bleeding and may cause hypothermia in an infant or young child. Repeated lavage may cause electrolyte imbalances.

Radiology

Radiologic tests, such as abdominal imaging with an anteroposterior abdominal x-ray (commonly referred to as KUB), an ultrasound, computed tomography (CT) scan, UGI series with/without small bowel follow-through, or barium enema may be useful for locating the source of the bleeding and determining the appropriate next step in evaluation (ie, upper vs lower endoscopy) and treatment.

Obtain an abdominal ultrasound with Doppler when there is evidence of liver disease suggestive of portal hypertension that may be causing esophageal varices. If esophagogastroduodenoscopy (EGD) is not readily available, a UGI series can identify a radio-opaque foreign body, and gastric and duodenal ulcers. Abdominal CT scan with intravenous contrast, abdominal magnetic resonance imaging, or UGI series can further evaluate for esophageal varices. A UGI series with small bowel follow-through is also the test of choice for a suspected malrotation with midgut volvulus (presents with bilious emesis, not hematemesis). However, defer radiographic imaging until the patient is hemodynamically stable.

If further visualization of the potential bleed site is needed, an EGD, performed by a gastroenterologist, is the next best plan of action if a UGI bleed is suspected. An EGD can identify sites of active bleeding and initiate therapeutic interventions when indicated. Obtain an emergency EGD when bleeding is considered to be life-threatening. Otherwise, an EGD is best performed in a controlled setting under anesthesia.

If an infant or younger child has a lower GI bleed, obtain a KUB with either an upright or a cross-table lateral view looking for intestinal obstruction or pneumatosis intestinalis, or findings consistent with an intussusception or volvulus. If intussusception is strongly suspected request an air contrast enema, which will be both diagnostic and therapeutic. However, obtain an abdominal CT scan or ultrasound if an ischemic process is suspected in an older child. When a Meckel diverticulum is suspected, obtain a Meckel scan with technetium-99 to identify ectopic gastric tissue seen in either the diverticulum or intestinal duplications. In select cases, capsule endoscopy, exploratory laparoscopy, or laparotomy is necessary to identify the source. If the diagnosis remains uncertain, a slow bleed may be identified with a bleeding scan done with technetium-99–labeled red cells, and more active bleeding may be detected with angiography.

Differential Diagnosis

The presence of hematemesis, melena, or hematochezia can help narrow the differential diagnosis when evaluated in the context of the patient's age. Hematemesis reflects bleeding proximal to the ligament of Treitz and melena is secondary to bleeding proximal to the transverse or descending colon with a slow intestinal transit time allowing bacteria to denature the hemoglobin.

Hematochezia usually (but not always) reflects bleeding distal to the transverse colon. Table 34-1 summarizes the most common causes by age group and location of bleed.

Table 34-1. Most Common Causes of Gastrointestinal (GI) Bleeding

Upper GI Bleed	Lower GI Bleed
Neonate	
Coagulopathy (vitamin K deficiency) Milk protein sensitivity Swallowed maternal blood Vascular malformations	Allergic colitis (cow's milk protein allergy) Anorectal fissures Coagulopathy (vitamin K deficiency) Necrotizing enterocolitis Swallowed maternal blood Vascular malformation
1 Month–2 Years	
Esophageal varices Esophagitis Gastritis Ingestion (toxin, foreign body) Stress gastritis or ulcer Vascular malformation	Anorectal fissures Infectious colitis Allergic colitis (cow's milk protein allergy) Intussusception Meckel diverticulum Polyps Lymphonodular hyperplasia Vascular malformations
2–5 Years	
Esophageal varices Esophagitis Gastritis Ingestion (toxin, foreign body) Mallory-Weiss tear Reflux esophagitis Stress ulcer Vascular malformation	Anorectal fissure Henoch-Schönlein purpura Infectious colitis Inflammatory bowel disease Intussusception Lymphonodular hyperplasia Meckel diverticulum Peptic ulcer disease Polyps Vascular lesions
Older Child or Adolescent	
Esophageal varices Gastritis Inflammatory bowel disease Mallory-Weiss tears Reflux esophagitis Ulcers Vascular malformation	Henoch-Schönlein purpura Infectious colitis Inflammatory bowel disease Meckel diverticulum Peptic ulcer disease Polyps Vascular lesion

Treatment

The priority is hemodynamic stabilization including correction of any coagulopathies or blood product deficits. Once stabilization has begun, treat active bleeding with empiric gastric acid-reduction therapy with either an H_2-blocker or a proton-pump inhibitor until a UGI bleed has been ruled out (Table 34-2). If peptic ulcer disease is suspected based on the history, treat with a cytoprotective agent such as sucralfate. If liver disease or a prolonged PT is discovered, or if hemorrhagic disease of the newborn is suspected, treat with vitamin K.

In addition to the above therapies, treatment for cases of severe bleeding requires gastroenterology consultation. Therapeutic options then may include octreotide or vasopressin, vasoactive agents that are infused to control severe bleeds from varices or bleeding ulcers. Furthermore, treatment for specific lesions found on endoscopy or surgical exploration can be accomplished through electrocoagulation, heater probe, multipolar probe, endoscopic hemoclips, band ligation, sclerotherapy (injection or laser), or ligation and resection of the lesion. Biologic therapies, such as monoclonal antibodies to tumor necrosis factor-α, may be needed for treatment of GI hemorrhage due to IBD.

Table 34-2. Initial Treatment of Active Gastrointestinal Bleeding

Indication	Drug Name (Class)	Dose
Active bleeding	Cimetidine (H_2-blocker)	20–40 mg/kg/day PO divided q 6 h (800 mg/day maximum)
	Famotidine (H_2-blocker)	0.5 mg/kg/day PO or IV either q hs or divided bid (40 mg/day maximum)
	Ranitidine (H_2-blocker)	PO: 1.5–2.5 mg/kg q 12 (600 mg/day maximum) IM or IV: 0.75–1.5 mg/kg q 6–8 h (400 mg/day maximum)
	Lansoprazole (PPI)	≤30 kg: 15 mg q day >30 kg: 30 mg q day
	Pantoprazole (PPI)	<40 kg: 0.5–1 mg/kg/day IV q day >40 kg: 20–40 mg IV q day
Peptic ulcer disease Bleeding ulcer	Sucralfate (mucosal adhesive)	40–80 mg/kg/day PO divided q 6 h (4 g/day maximum)
Liver disease Prolonged PT Hemorrhagic disease of the newborn	Vitamin K	1–2 mg IM, IV, SC q day Preferred route is SC. Severe reactions resembling anaphylaxis or hypersensitivity have rarely occurred after IV or IM administration.

Abbreviations: bid, twice a day; h, hours; H_2, histamine 2; hs, at bedtime; IM, intramuscular; IV, intravenous; PO, oral; PPI, proton-pump inhibitor; PT, prothrombin time; q, every; SC, subcutaneous.

Indications for Consultation

- **Gastroenterology:** Severe bleeding, endoscopy needed, suspicion of liver disease, portal hypertension, or IBD
- **Surgery:** Possible surgical abdomen (volvulus, intussusception, perforation), abdominal trauma, suspicion of a duplication cyst or Meckel diverticulum, exploratory laparotomy needed

Disposition

- **Intensive care unit transfer:** Hemodynamic instability
- **Discharge criteria:** The cause of the bleeding has been identified and controlled, anemia adequately treated, and nutrition optimized

Follow-up

- **Primary care:** 1 to 2 weeks
- **Gastroenterology and/or surgery:** Depending on the source and expected chronicity of the bleed

Pearls and Pitfalls

- Swallowed blood (from cracked nipples in a breastfed infant), coughing, tonsillitis, lost teeth, epistaxis, genitourinary bleeding, or menarche may give the false appearance of GI bleeding.
- Medications (Pepto-Bismol, iron, liquid Tylenol) and foods (red juice, beets) can falsely give the physical and chemical appearance of blood.
- Artificial devices (nasogastric or orogastric tubes; tracheostomy tubes; gastro, gastro-jejunal, or jejunal tubes) in which the device tip is causing mucosal irritation can lead to ulceration and bleeding.

Coding

ICD-9

- Blood in stool **578.1**
- Hematemesis **578.0**
- Hemorrhage of GI tract unspecified **578.9**

Bibliography

Boyle JT. Gastrointestinal bleeding in infants in children. *Pediatr Rev.* 2008;29:2:39–52

Chawla S, Seth D, Mahajan P, Kamat D. Upper gastrointestinal bleeding in children. *Clin Pediatr (Phila).* 2007;46:16–21

Gremse DA. Acute gastrointestinal bleeding. In: Perkin RM, Swify JD, Newton DA, Anas NG, eds. *Pediatric Hospital Medicine.* 2nd ed. Philadelphia, PA: Lippincott, Williams & Wilkins; 2008:304–309

Kamath BK, Manula P. Gastrointestinal bleeding. In: Liacouras C, Piccoli D, eds. *Pediatric Gastroenterology: The Requisites in Pediatrics.* Philadelphia. PA: Mosby Elsevier; 2008:87–97

Murphy MS. Management of bloody diarrhoea in children in primary care. *BMJ.* 2008;336:1010–1015

Inflammatory Bowel Disease

Introduction

Inflammatory bowel diseases (IBD), including ulcerative colitis (UC) and Crohn disease (CD), cause chronic intestinal inflammation characterized by clinical exacerbations and remissions. Specific symptoms are dependent on the extent and location of inflammation, with significant individual variability in disease severity. CD can affect any portion of the gastrointestinal (GI) tract, but commonly involves the colon and terminal ileum. UC affects the rectum and colon in a continuous pattern. Pediatric IBD most commonly presents during adolescence, but it also occurs in younger children.

Clinical Presentation

History

A patient with new-onset or an exacerbation of IBD classically presents with abdominal pain, bloody diarrhea, weight loss, and increased stool frequency, including nocturnal bowel movements. There may also be fever, fatigue, slowed growth velocity, and delayed puberty. However, the onset of IBD may be subtle, presenting solely with growth delay. At some point, about one-third of patients with IBD have extra-intestinal manifestations, including arthritis, arthralgias, skin eruption (erythema nodosum, pyoderma gangrenosum), aphthous stomatitis, and ophthalmologic inflammation. Other extra-intestinal manifestations and complications include cholelithiasis, nephrolithiasis, primary sclerosing cholangitis, and osteoporosis. On occasion, these extra-intestinal manifestations are the sole presenting signs or symptoms of the disease.

Physical Examination

Perform a complete physical examination, including perianal and digital rectal examinations. Plot the height, weight, and body mass index, and assess the Tanner stage. Common findings include abdominal tenderness, inflamed rectal skin tags, perianal fissures, and drainage from enterocutaneous fistulas. A mass is sometimes palpable when there is significant intestinal inflammation or an abscess.

Laboratory

If IBD or an IBD exacerbation is suspected, obtain a complete blood cell count; C-reactive protein (CRP) and/or erythrocyte sedimentation rate (ESR); a comprehensive metabolic panel; and stool for guaiac, culture, ova and parasites, and *Clostridium difficile.* Also check the amylase and lipase if the patient has mid-epigastric pain. Findings can include anemia and thrombocytosis, elevated ESR and CRP, hypoalbuminemia, and guaiac-positive stools, although all of these can be normal. These studies, in addition to fecal calprotectin, may be helpful in differentiating relapse from other causes of abdominal pain, but sometimes imaging and/or endoscopy/colonoscopy is required. Given the lack of diagnostic predictive value and high cost, do not use an IBD serology panel as a screening test. Obtain blood cultures if an IBD patient who is receiving immunosuppressive medications is febrile (>38°C).

Radiology

If the patient presents with severe abdominal pain, order an abdominal x-ray to evaluate for small bowel obstruction or perforation (free air). In severe acute colitis, toxic megacolon can also be identified on a plain film (transverse colon dilatation). If a patient with known or suspected CD presents with persistent or escalating abdominal pain, persistent fever, bilious emesis, cutaneous fistulae, or persistent rectal bleeding without a source on endoscopy, order an upper GI series with small bowel follow-through, computed tomography (CT) enterography, or magnetic resonance (MR) enterography to evaluate for internal disease (stricture, fistula, abscess). If there is concern for extraluminal disease, but both MR and CT enterography are unavailable or the patient is unable to tolerate enteral/rectal contrast or lying still, obtain a CT with contrast, or for perianal disease, MR imaging with contrast.

Diagnostic Procedures

Endoscopy and colonoscopy with biopsies are needed to make a diagnosis of IBD, but defer them until the patient is clinically stable. These procedures may be indicated intermittently to evaluate the extent of relapsing disease before changing therapy. Both upper endoscopy and colonoscopy are required, as CD may affect any site in the GI tract, from the mouth to the anus. Findings that distinguish CD from UC are patchy inflammation and non-caseating granulomas. In UC there is continuous chronic inflammation starting in the rectum and extending proximally. However, in some cases pediatric CD can also present with pancolitis, with or without granulomas.

Differential Diagnosis

Infectious colitis may mimic the acute presentation of IBD. Obtain stool cultures and *C difficile* toxin A and B assay or polymerase chain reaction. However, the presence of *C difficile* does not rule out IBD, as a patient with IBD is at increased risk for nonantibiotic-associated *C difficile* infection. The differential diagnosis of IBD is summarized in Table 35-1.

Complications

GI complications include spontaneous perforations and peritonitis, abdominal and perirectal abscesses, fistulas, strictures, small bowel obstructions, and toxic megacolon. A patient with IBD is at increased risk for thrombosis and thromboembolism due to a hypercoaguable state. In addition, many

Table 35-1 Differential Diagnosis of IBD

Diagnosis	Clinical Features
Bloody Diarrhea	
Allergic colitis	Usually <5 years of age No extra-intestinal manifestations Peripheral eosinophilia
Infectious colitis (*Campylobacter, Clostridium difficile,* CMV, *Entamoeba histolytica, Escherichia coli, Salmonella, Shigella, Yersenia*)	Usually a more acute presentation Extra-intestinal manifestations rare, other than fever and arthritis
Henoch-Schönlein purpura	Usually more acute presentation Purpura on legs and buttocks May have hematuria Extra-intestinal manifestations rare, other than arthritis
Abdominal Pain, Diarrhea, and Weight Loss	
Celiac disease	Non-bloody diarrhea Positive celiac serologies Biopsy shows villous blunting
Constitutional Symptoms (weight loss, fever, fatigue, ↑CRP/ESR)	
Beçhet	Can have genital ulcers Biopsy does not show chronic inflammation
HIV, other immunodeficiencies	Recurrent infections Leukopenia
Juvenile idiopathic arthritis Other connective tissue disorders	GI symptoms are usually less prominent
Malignancy	May have pancytopenia May have tumor lysis
Tuberculosis	Bloody stools rare

Abbreviations: CMV, cytomegalovirus; CRP, C-reactive protein; ESR, erythrocyte sedimentation rate; GI, gastrointestinal; IBD, irritable bowel disease.

medications used to treat IBD cause immunosuppression, leading to risk of community-acquired and opportunistic infections. See Table 35-2 for other important potential side effects of IBD treatment.

Treatment

IBD therapy is individualized and best guided by a gastroenterologist, but it always involves induction and maintenance therapy. The goals of inpatient treatment are to stabilize the patient, treat complications, and improve symptoms while ideally inducing a disease remission. Consult with a gastroenterologist for acute symptoms, but management may include fluid resuscitation, packed red blood cells (10–15 mL/kg) for symptomatic anemia or significant anemia in the setting of continued blood loss, and 25% albumin infusion (1 g/kg, 25 g maximum) if the serum albumin level is less than 2 g/dL. Maximize nutrition, first with a trial of oral feeds, but use tube feedings if the patient is unable to or cannot tolerate oral feedings. If that is not adequate, initiate parenteral nutrition. Try to avoid using opioids for analgesia as they may decrease GI motility and increase the risk of bacterial translocation, as well as mask peritoneal signs in an acutely ill patient. The treatment of IBD complications is summarized in Table 35-3.

Indications for Consultation

- **Gastroenterology:** All patients
- **Hematology:** Suspected complication of hypercoaguable state
- **Infectious diseases:** Immunosuppressed patient with high fever or not improving on appropriate antibiotic therapy
- **Surgery:** Suspected perforation, small bowel obstruction, toxic megacolon; abscess, stricture, or fistula; intractable bleeding; UC that has failed medical management

Table 35-2. Medication Adverse Effects[a]

Medication	Adverse Effects (All Cause Immunosuppression)
6-Mercaptopurine	Hepatotoxicity, lymphoma, pancreatitis
Corticosteroids	Adrenal suppression, glaucoma, hyperglycemia, hypertension, mood disturbance, pseudotumor cerebri, poor wound healing, psychosis, osteopenia, and fractures
Cyclosporine	Hypertension, lymphoma, renal impairment
Infliximab	Anaphylaxis, lymphoma, reactivation of latent diseases (tuberculosis, hepatitis B, histoplasmosis, coccidiomycosis)
Mesalamine	Myocarditis/pericarditis, nephritis, pancreatitis
Methotrexate	Hepatotoxicity, lymphoma, pneumonitis

[a]Severe only; not a comprehensive list.

Table 35-3. Treatment of IBD Complications

Complication	Treatment
Crohn Disease	
Complex fistula	IV antibiotics[a]: Regimen 1a–d[b] Surgery consultation
Intra-abdominal abscess	IV antibiotics[a]: Regimen 1a–d[b] Surgery consultation
Perianal abscess	IV antibiotics[a]: Regimen 2a–b[b] Surgery consultation
Small bowel obstruction	NPO Decompression with NGT Urgent surgical intervention
Complications of Both Crohn Disease and Ulcerative Colitis	
Perforation	IV antibiotics[a]: Regimen 1a–d[b] Urgent surgery consultation NPO Treat DIC, electrolyte abnormalities, and hypotension
Toxic megacolon	IV antibiotics[a]: Regimen 1a–d[b] Urgent surgery consultation NPO Correct electrolyte abnormalities
Sepsis	IV antibiotics[a]: Regimen 1a–d[b] Hemodynamic support
Thrombosis or thromboembolism	Consult with hematology and possibly vascular surgery and neurology Possible anticoagulation, thrombolysis, or surgery

Abbreviations: DIC, disseminated intravascular coagulation; div, divided; h, hours; IV, intravenous; NGT, nasogastric tube; NPO, nothing by mouth; q, every.

[a] Choose empiric antibiotics based on local resistance patterns and likely organism. Use broader coverage for critically ill patients and narrow coverage based on identification and sensitivities, if available.

[b] Regimens

Regimen 1a: Cefoxitin 100–160 mg/kg/day div q 4–6 h *with or without* gentamicin 7.5 mg/kg/day div q 8 h

Regimen 1b: Cefotaxime 100–200 mg/kg/day div q 6–8 h *and* metronidazole 30 mg/kg/day div q 8 h

Regimen 1c: Piperacillin/tazobactam 300 mg/kg/day div q 8 h

Regimen 1d: Meropenem 60 mg/kg/day div q 8 h

Regimen 2a: Metronidazole 30 mg/kg/day div q 8h *and/or* ciprofloxacin 20–30 mg/kg/day div q 12 h

Regimen 2b: Cefotaxime 100–200 mg/kg/day div q 6–8 h *and* metronidazole 30 mg/kg/day div q 8 h

Note: Add clindamycin 30 mg/kg/day div q 8 h or vancomycin 45 mg/kg/day div q 8 h if methicillin-resistant *Staphylococcus aureus* is a concern.

Disposition

- **Intensive care unit transfer:** Shock, impending respiratory failure, peritonitis, life-threatening electrolyte abnormalities, severe postoperative complications, thrombotic complications
- **Discharge criteria:** Tolerating maintenance oral or tube diet, intravenous medications discontinued, pain well-controlled, no or minimal blood in stools, stable hemoglobin with no symptoms of anemia

Follow-up

- **Gastroenterology:** 1 to 2 weeks

Pearls and Pitfalls

- IBD is a risk factor for nonantibiotic-associated *C difficile.*
- Abdominal distension may be caused by obstruction, ileus, perforation, or toxic megacolon.
- A patient with known IBD may have another etiology for acute abdominal symptoms, such as appendicitis or pancreatitis. Pursue a careful differential diagnosis for each presentation.

Coding

ICD-9

- Crohn disease (colitis) **555.1**
- Crohn disease (small intestine and large intestines) **555.2**
- Crohn disease (small intestine) **555.0**
- Crohn disease (unspecified site) **555.9**
- Irritable bowel syndrome **564.1**
- UC (left sided) **556.5**
- UC (pancolitis) **556.6**
- UC (unspecified site) **556.9**
- Colitis, dietetic or noninfectious, unspecified **558.9**

Bibliography

Benor S, Russell GH, Silver M, Israel EJ, Yuan Q, Winter HS. Shortcomings of the inflammatory bowel disease Serology 7 panel. *Pediatrics.* 2010;125:1230–1236

Bousvaros A, Antonioli DA, Colletti RB, et al. Differentiating ulcerative colitis from Crohn disease in children and young adults: report of a Working Group of the North American Society for Pediatric Gastroenterology, Hepatology, and Nutrition and the Crohn's and Colitis Foundation of America. *J Pediatr Gastroenterol Nutr.* 2007;44:653–674

Dotson JL, Hyams JS, Markowitz J, et al. Extraintestinal manifestations of pediatric inflammatory bowel disease and their relation to disease type and severity. *J Pediatr Gastroenterol Nutr.* 2010;51:140–145

Mack DR, Langton C, Markowitz J, et al. Laboratory values for children with newly diagnosed inflammatory bowel disease. *Pediatrics.* 2007;119:1113–1119

Mamula P, Markowitz J, Baldassano R. *Pediatric Inflammatory Bowel Disease.* New York, NY: Springer; 2008

Turner D, Travis SP, Griffiths AM, et al. Consensus for managing acute severe ulcerative colitis in children: a systematic review and joint statement from ECCO, ESPGHAN, and the Porto IBD Working Group of ESPGHAN. *Am J Gastroenterol.* 2011;106:574–588

Meckel Diverticulum

Introduction

A Meckel diverticulum (MD) is often discovered as an incidental finding. However, an MD will come to medical attention acutely if it is the cause of lower gastrointestinal (GI) bleeding (as a result of ectopic gastric mucosa), intestinal perforation, or intestinal obstruction when it serves as a lead point for an intussusception or a focus for a volvulus.

Clinical Presentation

History

The most common presentation is painless rectal bleeding, usually manifesting as the passage of dark red stool, but with massive bleeding it can be bright red. A history of cramping abdominal pain may also be present. Less often, there may be melena and abdominal pain. An intestinal perforation or obstruction is uncommon, presenting with anorexia, severe abdominal pain, and bilious emesis.

Intussusception is the second most common presentation. The patient may have the typical history of intermittent, colicky abdominal pain with drawing up of the legs, vomiting, lethargy, and a late finding of bloody, currant jelly stools.

Physical Examination

Vital signs are usually within normal limits, but there may be hypotension and tachycardia if significant blood loss has occurred. The typical presentation can be unremarkable, except for rectal bleeding without tenderness on rectal examination. A patient with severe GI bleeding may have altered mental status. Hypoactive bowel sounds, abdominal distension, rebound, rigidity, and guarding, if present, suggest an acute abdomen from possible perforation or obstruction. A painful, right lower quadrant mass may be noted with an intussusception.

Laboratory

There is no specific laboratory test that can confirm MD (see Gastrointestinal Bleeding, page 205). Perform a stool guaiac to confirm the presence of blood, and obtain a complete blood cell count, coagulation profile, and type and screen. Order an abdominal x-ray, which may demonstrate evidence of obstruction, perforation, or a mass, suggestive of intussusception.

The gold standard for diagnosis is the Meckel scan, technetium-99m pertechnetate scintigraphy. It is indicated for a hemodynamically stable patient with painless lower GI bleeding. The technetium-99 is absorbed by ectopic gastric mucosa (if present), producing an increased area of uptake. Prior to the scan, administer pentagastrin (6 mcg/kg) or an H_2 receptor antagonist, such as cimetidine (20 mg/kg/day divided every 6 hours) in order to increase the sensitivity.

Differential Diagnosis

The differential diagnosis is summarized in Table 36-1.

Table 36-1. Differential Diagnosis of a Meckel Diverticulum

Diagnosis	Differentiating Features
Rectal Bleeding or Melena	
Anal fissure	History of constipation or diarrhea Fissure noted on rectal examination
Bacterial enteritis	Fever, abdominal pain May be associated with vomiting and diarrhea
Coagulopathy	Other bleeding manifestations Petechiae, purpura, ecchymoses
Irritable bowel disease	Fever, weight loss, oral ulcers, clubbing Perianal skin tags/fissures
Milk protein allergy	Usually neonates and young infants May have vomiting and/or eczematous rash
Peptic disease	Abdominal pain relieved by eating or antacids
Abdominal Pain With Bilious Vomiting	
Ileocolic intussusception	Intermittent abdominal pain with drawing up of legs Currant jelly stools (late finding)
Inflicted trauma	Bruising on abdomen Other signs of trauma
Midgut volvulus	Ill appearing, sudden onset bilious emesis May have abdominal distension
Necrotizing enterocolitis	Feeding intolerance Fever, vomiting, abdominal distension Progressive lethargy

Treatment

Consult a surgeon to plan an expeditious resection. However, the priority is the treatment of hypovolemia and/or shock (page 59). Insert 2 large-bore intravenous lines and give 2 to 3 20-mL/kg normal saline boluses. If the patient remains unstable or the hemoglobin is less than 7 g/dL, arrange for a packed red blood cell transfusion.

If there is a concern for an intestinal obstruction, make the patient NPO, place a nasogastric tube to continuous wall suction, consult surgery, and order an upper GI series. If the patient has an intussusception, make the patient NPO and consult surgery for a probable resection as pneumatic reduction is typically ineffective in the setting of an MD as a lead point.

Indications for Consultation

- **Surgery:** Confirmed MD, rectal bleeding associated with signs of shock, concern about an intestinal perforation

Disposition

- **Intensive care unit transfer:** Hypovolemic shock
- **Discharge criteria:** No GI bleeding and tolerating maintenance oral fluids

Follow-up

- **Primary care:** 1 week
- **Surgery (if resection performed):** 2 to 3 days

Pearls and Pitfalls

- An inflamed MD may present with right lower quadrant pain and fever, mimicking appendicitis.
- Because MD-associated intussusception is ileoileal, the patient may present with bilious vomiting. Also, an air enema is usually ineffective.

Coding

ICD-9

MD	**751.0**

Bibliography

Liang HH, Wei PL, Hung CS, Wang W, Huang CS. Acute abdomen in infant. Meckel's diverticulum and ileo-ileocolic intussusception. *Ann Emerg Med.* 2011;57:24, 28

Louie JP. Essential diagnosis of abdominal emergencies in the first year of life. *Emerg Med Clin North Am.* 2007;25:1009–1040

Villalva VM. Gastrointestinal bleeding. In: Zaoutis LB, Chiang VW, eds. *Comprehensive Pediatric Hospital Medicine*. Philadelphia, PA: Elsevier; 2007:161–166

Yuan HC, Kamat D, Ashraf A. Index of suspicion. *Pediatr Rev.* 2005;26:68–74

Zani A, Eaton S, Rees CM, Pierro A. Incidentally detected Meckel diverticulum: to resect or not to resect? *Ann Surg.* 2008;247(2):276–281

Pancreatitis

Introduction

Pancreatitis is an acute, recurrent, or chronic inflammatory condition of the pancreas. Acute pancreatitis is generally secondary to systemic viral or bacterial infections, structural abnormalities, medications, toxic ingestions, metabolic disorders, trauma, autoimmune disorders, and occasionally cholelithiasis, although 25% of pediatric cases are idiopathic. Rarely, pancreatitis can progress to necrotizing pancreatitis with potential insufficiency.

Pancreatitis can lead to abnormal endocrine or exocrine function, which usually resolves completely. However, a relapse of acute pancreatitis, especially if there are recurring episodes, may cause persistent inflammation and ultimately result in chronic pancreatitis and chronic inflammatory changes within the ductal system. Progression to pancreatic insufficiency and insulin-dependent diabetes occurs in severe cases of chronic pancreatitis and in hereditary pancreatitis, an autosomal dominant condition.

Clinical Presentation

History

The patient presents with acute abdominal pain, vomiting, fever and, rarely, shock. The abdominal pain is continuous, typically epigastric or in the upper quadrants, occasionally radiating to the back or shoulders, and worsened by oral intake. The patient may report relief when leaning or bending forward. Nausea and vomiting tend to occur as the inflammation progresses.

Inquire about predisposing factors including trauma; drug or medication exposure; recent illness; and family history of hyperlipidemia, gallstones, or pancreatitis.

Physical Examination

The patient may appear restless, with abdominal pain as the hallmark symptom. The pain can be in any quadrant, but is commonly in the upper quadrants or epigastrium, with radiation to the back. Abdominal rigidity, guarding, and hypoactive or absent bowel sounds with ileus are common. An epigastric mass secondary to pseudocyst may be palpable. In a severe case, other findings may include diminished breath sounds due to sympathetic pleural effusions, toxic appearance, periumbilical ecchymoses (Cullen sign), and flank ecchymoses (Grey Turner sign).While mild jaundice can be present with any etiology of pancreatitis, moderate to severe jaundice is typically associated with common bile duct obstruction from gallstones or edema of the head of the pancreas.

Laboratory

If pancreatitis is suspected, obtain a serum amylase and lipase. The amylase rises within hours of pain onset (usually >160 U/L), but has a low sensitivity (75%). In contrast, elevation of the lipase typically occurs 72 hours after symptom onset, but it is more sensitive and specific (both 90%) for pancreatic inflammation. However, the degree of elevation of either amylase or lipase does not correlate to disease severity. Also order a complete blood cell count, electrolytes (including calcium and magnesium), glucose, blood urea nitrogen, liver enzymes (aspartate transaminase, alanine transaminase, alkaline phosphatase, gamma-glutamyl transpeptidase) and function tests (albumin, international normalized ratio, total bilirubin), a fasting lipid panel, and coagulation studies.

Radiology

Radiographic studies are not required to diagnose pancreatitis. Rather, they are useful for determining the etiology of the pancreatitis. Obtain an abdominal x-ray series and, if possible, an abdominal ultrasound, which is the optimal radiographic examination. The plain radiographs can show bowel distension, pancreatic calcification, ileus, or a pancreatic pseudocyst. However, an ultrasound can evaluate for many causes of abdominal pain, and in pancreatitis, can demonstrate pancreatic anatomy, gallstones or ductal dilatation, cysts or abscess, and edema. Obtain either an abdominal computed tomography or magnetic resonance imaging if an ultrasound is either unavailable or suboptimal, which is often the case if air is present in the duodenum or the pancreas is already severely injured.

For a patient with recurrent acute or chronic pancreatitis due to obstruction of the pancreatic duct, arrange an evaluation of the biliary system, preferably with magnetic resonance cholangiopancreatography (MRCP) and/or endoscopic retrograde cholangiopancreatography (ERCP). Both can provide diagnostic information, and the ERCP may potentially be therapeutic for ductal abnormalities, as stone removal or stent placement is possible. Contraindications include active inflammation, pseudocyst, and abscess. MRCP is preferable if a therapeutic procedure will not be necessary.

Differential Diagnosis

Elevation of the serum amylase can occur in many other conditions, including salivary gland inflammation, diabetic ketoacidosis, perforated gastric ulcer, gallbladder disease, ruptured fallopian tube, and renal failure. The differential diagnosis of pancreatitis is summarized in Table 37-1.

Treatment

Make the patient NPO and insert a nasogastric tube to suction if the patient has repeated vomiting or has significant abdominal distension. Give maintenance fluid while correcting any electrolyte abnormalities. Start with D5 ½ normal saline (NS) or D5 NS with 20 mEq KCl/L at a maintenance rate. If the patient is dehydrated, replace the volume deficit with an isotonic solution (NS, Ringer lactate). Monitor vital signs every 4 hours and the clinical examination closely, as the patient is at risk for third-spacing fluid (peritoneal or pleural cavity) and intravascular depletion. Follow the electrolytes and urine output until normal and address abnormalities with electrolyte-specific correction and fluid replacement.

If the patient remains NPO for more than 3 to 5 days, provide total parenteral nutrition (TPN), without intra-lipids if hypertriglyceridemia is present. Substitute low-fat elemental jejunal feeds for TPN for a patient with no signs of bowel obstruction or ileus. To minimize the duration of being NPO, resume

Table 37-1. Differential Diagnosis of Pancreatitis

Diagnosis	Clinical Features
Acute gastroenteritis	Diarrhea may be present Pain is mild, not associated with eating, not relieved by leaning forward Pancreatic enzymes normal (may be slightly elevated with emesis)
Viral hepatitis	Pain localized to right upper quadrant Liver enzymes may be normal during acute phase Pancreatic enzymes normal
Appendicitis	Pain is constant and precedes the vomiting Pain can migrate from periumbilical area to right lower quadrant Pancreatic enzymes normal
Intussusception	Pain is cramping and intermittent-associated with drawing up the legs Hematochezia Pancreatic enzymes normal
Peptic ulcer	Epigastric pain, worse before meals, not relieved by leaning forward May improve with antacids Pancreatic enzymes normal (may ↑ with severe ulcer, perforation)
Cholelithiasis	Right upper quadrant colicky pain, which may worsen with meals Pancreatic enzymes normal

no- or low-fat enteral intake cautiously once the patient's pain is resolving and bowel sounds are present. *Normalization of the pancreatic enzymes is not necessary before resuming feedings.* If the diet is tolerated without escalation of pain, slowly advance back to a regular diet.

For analgesia, give morphine (0.05–0.1 mg/kg every 2–4 hours, as needed, 15 mg/dose maximum), as there is no evidence to confirm the concern regarding interference with biliary drainage. Order patient-controlled analgesia if the patient is age-appropriate (page 271). Usually interval dosing without a basal rate will suffice.

Antibiotics are generally not indicated for a patient with acute or chronic pancreatitis. Bacterial superinfection is a common complication of necrotizing pancreatitis, and coverage of enteric gram-negative organisms is indicated with either piperacillin/tazobactam (9–<40 kg: 100 mg/kg of piperacillin every 8 hours; >40kg: 3 g of piperacillin every 6 hours) or imipenem (60–100 mg/kg/day divided every 6 hours, 2–4 g/day maximum). If an enlarging pseudocyst or pancreatic abscess is present, consult with a pediatric surgeon and pediatric gastroenterologist for possible drainage. Treat the primary or underlying cause of the pancreatitis, if possible.

Indications for Consultation

- **Gastroenterology:** Recurrent acute or chronic pancreatitis, pancreatic complications, pancreatic insufficiency, or need for ERCP. Collaboration may be needed for follow-up.
- **Genetics:** Recurrent pancreatitis, hypertriglyceridemia, hereditary pancreatitis
- **Pain service:** Uncontrolled or prolonged pain
- **Surgery:** Pseudocyst, abscess, or necrotizing pancreatitis

Disposition

- **Intensive care unit transfer:** Shock or suspected sepsis
- **Discharge criteria:** Tolerating low-fat diet, electrolyte abnormalities corrected, pain resolved

Follow-up

- **Primary care:** 2 to 3 days
- **Pediatric gastroenterologist:** 2 to 3 weeks if the course was complicated or consultation was required

Pearls and Pitfalls

- Bowel rest, electrolyte correction, and pain control initiated early are the keys of treatment.
- There is no evidence to support the use of trending enzyme levels to monitor clinical progression.
- Pseudocyst is present in 10% of cases that are unrelated to abdominal trauma.

Coding

ICD-9

- Acute pancreatitis **577.0**
- Chronic pancreatitis **577.1**
- Pancreatic cyst or pseudocyst **577.2**

Bibliography

Darge K, Anupindi S. Pancreatitis and the role of US, MRCP and ERCP. *Pediatr Radiol.* 2009;39 (suppl 2):S153–S157

Jolley CD. Pancreatic disease in children and adolescents. *Curr Gastroenterol Rep.* 2010;12:106–113

Lowrey PV, Poley JR. Pancreatitis. In: Zaoutis VW, Chiang LB, eds. *Comprehensive Pediatric Hospital Medicine.* St Louis. MO: Mosby; 2007:641–645

Nydegger A, Couper RT, Oliver MR. Childhood pancreatitis. *J Gastroenterol Hepatol.* 2006;21:499–509

Stringer MD. Pancreatitis and pancreatic trauma. *Semin Pediatr Surg.* 2005;14:239–246

Kandula L, Lowe ME. Etiology and outcome of acute pancreatitis in infants and toddlers. *J Pediatr.* 2008;152:106–110

Gynecology

CHAPTER 38

Dysfunctional Uterine Bleeding

Introduction

Dysfunctional uterine bleeding (DUB) is painless, profuse, and irregular menstrual bleeding of endometrial origin unrelated to any structural or systemic disease. While anovulation due to hypothalamic-pituitary-ovarian axis immaturity is the most common cause of DUB, there are many other etiologies.

Heavy (>80 mL) or prolonged (>7 days) vaginal bleeding that occurs at regular cyclic intervals is known as menorrhagia. Irregular (acyclic) vaginal bleeding is called metrorrhagia. Prolonged or heavy periods that occur at irregular intervals are termed menometrorrhagia.

A patient with DUB will be admitted for hemodynamic instability, inability to tolerate oral intake and medications, severe anemia (hemoglobin <7 g/dL), psychological stress associated with the heavy bleeding, and/or inadequate follow-up.

Clinical Presentation

History

Obtain the history with and without the presence of the patient's parent or legal guardian. Ask about the age of menarche, and whether or not there was heavy bleeding at the first menses. Determine the menstrual cycle interval (normal 3–6 weeks) and the number of days of bleeding. Menstrual loss requiring pad or tampon changes every 1 to 2 hours, with anything longer resulting in "flooding" or "accidents," is excessive, particularly if the menses last 8 days or longer. Ask about the impact of the bleeding on adolescent psychosocial well-being (missed days at school and inability to participate in sporting and social activities). Use the HEADSS assessment as a tool to screen for health risk behaviors. Focus on recent sexual activity, overall number of partners, recent partners, pregnancy, and possibility of sexual abuse. Determine the method of contraception and whether condoms are used.

Ask about associated symptoms, such as lightheadedness, syncope, abdominal or pelvic pain, nausea, vomiting, fever, vaginal discharge, and headaches. Inquire about a history or family history of excessive bleeding with surgical or dental procedures, easy bruising or petechiae, frequent nose bleeds, or gingival bleeding. Review and document the patient's current medications, asking specifically about hormones, nonsteroidal anti-inflammatory drugs, anticoagulants, platelet inhibitors, chemotherapy, androgens, and spironolactone.

Physical Examination

Perform a complete physical examination. Record the weight, height, vital signs, and orthostatic blood pressures. Note the body habitus and palpate the thyroid. For a suspected pituitary adenoma, check the optic fundi and perform visual field testing. Determine Tanner staging of the breasts and assess for galactorrhea. Examine the skin for pallor, petechiae or hematomas, acanthosis nigricans, hirsutism, and rashes. Palpate the abdomen for a uterine or ovarian mass. Examine the genitalia and note the pubertal hair Tanner stage. Look for signs of sexual abuse (abrasions, contusions or punctuate tears of the perineum and perianal areas) and sexually transmitted infections (STIs) (malodorous vaginal discharge, vaginal erythema, vesicular lesions or ulcers).

If the patient is sexually active perform a pelvic examination and obtain samples for testing. A pelvic examination under anesthesia may be necessary for a virginal adolescent with bleeding that cannot be controlled with hormone therapy, significant anemia, or pelvic and abdominal pain.

Laboratory

Order a pregnancy test, complete blood cell count with differential and platelet count, prothrombin time/partial thromboplastin time, and type and screen. If the patient is sexually active, test for STIs, including *Neisseria gonorrhea*, chlamydia, syphilis, HIV, bacterial vaginosis, *Trichomonas,* and yeast. If heavy bleeding has been present since menarche, obtain coagulation studies, including testing for Von Willebrand factor.

Arrange for a pelvic ultrasound if the pregnancy test is positive (to rule out ectopic pregnancy) or a mass is palpated during the pelvic examination.

Other laboratory testing is dictated by the findings on physical examination and may include thyroid function tests (goiter, short stature, obesity, skin dryness, and myxedema); testosterone, free testosterone, dehydroepiandrosterone, luteinizing hormone/follicle-stimulating hormone ratio and dehydroepiandrosterone (obesity, hirsutism, and acne suggestive of polycystic ovarian syndrome [PCOS]); prolactin (galactorrhea, headaches, visual fields defects, papilledema); and 17-hydroxyprogesterone (hirsutism, severe acne, clitoromegaly suggestive of late onset congenital adrenal hyperplasia).

Differential Diagnosis

Most cases of DUB (90%) during the first 2 years after menarche are secondary to physiological anovulation from delayed maturation of the hypothalamic pituitary axis. However, DUB is a diagnosis of exclusion. The differential diagnosis primarily includes pregnancy (either intrauterine or ectopic) and local infections. Systemic etiologies include bleeding disorders, endocrine disorders, and medications. Local causes include trauma, foreign bodies and, rarely, benign and malignant tumors (Table 38-1).

Anovulation and vaginal bleeding can also be seen in PCOS, Turner syndrome, systemic illnesses (cystic fibrosis, inflammatory bowel disease, autoimmune disorders), strenuous exercise, or emotional stress (anorexia nervosa).

Treatment

For severe uterine bleeding, when the patient cannot tolerate oral medication, start intravenous (IV) conjugated estrogen (25 mg every 4–6 hours for up to 24 hours) until the bleeding stops. Then change to an oral contraceptive (such as 30 mcg ethinyl estradiol/0.3 mg norgestrel) 1 pill every 6 hours until bleeding slows down (usually 24–36 hours), then taper by one pill every 3 days.

Start an antiemetic (ondansetron 8 mg 3 times a day) to minimize nausea and vomiting due to high-dose estrogen and initiate iron therapy (60 mg elemental iron divided twice a day to 4 times a day) while in the hospital.

A blood transfusion is indicated for a hemoglobin less than 7 g/dL associated with signs of hemodynamic instability (tachycardia, orthostatic hypotension) or ongoing bleeding, or if the bleeding cannot be controlled. However, intensive care unit (ICU) monitoring and surgical intervention may be necessary if the bleeding does not respond to the above therapy.

Table 38-1. Differential Diagnosis of Dysfunctional Uterine Bleeding

Diagnosis	Clinical Features
Anovulation	Menarche within last 2 years No fever or abdominal/pelvic pain
Ectopic pregnancy	Positive pregnancy test Abdominal pain, nausea, vomiting
Missed abortion	Low back or abdominal pain Tissue or clot-like material passing from the vagina
Sexually transmitted infection/pelvic inflammatory disease	Vaginal discharge Fever, abdominal or pelvic pain, nausea and vomiting Cervical motion/adnexal tenderness
Trauma	Lacerations and/or abrasions Bruising of the perineum and perianal area
Von Willebrand	Heavy vaginal bleeding at the first menses Epistaxis and gum bleeds Family history of excessive bleeding

Indication for Consultation

- **Gynecology:** Severe vaginal bleeding that does not respond within 24 hours to IV conjugated estrogen

Disposition

- **ICU transfer:** Severe bleeding and signs of shock with poor peripheral perfusion and/or hypotension.
- **Discharge criteria:** Hemodynamically stable, the bleeding under control, tolerating oral hormonal therapy

Follow-up

- **Primary care physician and/or gynecologist:** 1 to 2 days

Pearls and Pitfalls

- DUB remains a diagnosis of exclusion. The underlying pathology dictates the treatment.
- High-dose estrogen therapy requires the use of antiemetics.
- The potential exists for patient and/or family resistance to hormonal or contraceptive use.

Coding

ICD-9

DUB	**626.8**

Bibliography

Benjamins LJ. Practice guideline: evaluation and management of abnormal vaginal bleeding in adolescents. *J Pediatr Health Care.* 2009;23:189–193

Emans S. Dysfunctional uterine bleeding. In: Emans SJ. Laufer MR, Goldstein DP, eds. *Pediatric and Adolescent Gynecology.* 5th ed. Philadelphia, PA: Lippincott, Williams & Wilkins; 2005:270–286

Gray SH, Emans SJ. Abnormal vaginal bleeding in adolescents. *Pediatr Rev.* 2007;28:175–182

Grover S. Bleeding disorders and heavy menses in adolescents. *Curr Opin Obstet Gynecol.* 2007;19:415–419

Levine L, Schwartz D. Dysfunctional uterine bleeding. In: Zaoutis LB, Chiang VW, eds. *Comprehensive Pediatric Hospital Medicine.* Philadelphia, PA: Mosby Elsevier; 2007:1083–1086

CHAPTER 39

Sexually Transmitted Infections

Introduction

Chlamydia and gonorrhea are the most common bacterial causes of sexually transmitted infections (STIs) in adolescents. Other STIs include human papillomavirus (HPV), herpes simplex virus (HSV), trichomoniasis, bacterial vaginosis (BV), syphilis, and HIV. Although most cases of STI are managed on an outpatient basis, these infections may coexist with, or be included in, the differential diagnoses of many conditions in hospitalized adolescents. In addition, pelvic inflammatory disease (PID) can have significant long-term consequences, including infertility, ectopic pregnancy, and chronic pelvic pain.

Clinical Presentation

History

Without a parent or partner present, ask about the number of sexual partners, partner history of STIs, and history of sexual assault or abuse. In a female, ask about vaginal discharge, odor, pruritus, irritation, dysuria, heavy bleeding, spotting, abdominal or back pain, nausea or vomiting, fever, and dyspareunia. In a male, ask about testicular pain, penile discharge, dysuria, and pruritus. For all patients elicit any history of arthralgias, malaise, pharyngitis, conjunctivitis, and generalized or localized rashes. However, many STIs are asymptomatic.

Physical Examination

The priority is the genital examination. In a post-pubertal female, note any external lesions or excoriations. Perform a bimanual examination for adnexal tenderness, cervical motion tenderness (CMT), or uterine/lower abdominal pain associated with PID. If a speculum examination is done, examine the cervix for friability, as well as blood or mucopurulent material within the endocervical canal. Note the color, consistency, and malodor of any abnormal discharge. Collect specimens for nucleic acid amplification testing (NAAT) for chlamydia and gonorrhea, and for a KOH and wet preparation, to identify inflammation, clue cells, trichomonads, and yeast forms. Also feel for lower abdominal pain, rebound tenderness, and right upper quadrant abdominal pain, which can occur with perihepatitis (Fitz-Hugh-Curtis syndrome). In a male, examine for lesions, urethral discharge, testicular pain, hydrocele, and swelling of the epididymis. Consider the need for a rectal examination.

In a prepubertal or virginal female, perform a careful external examination of the anogenital region for signs of trauma and sexual abuse, such as abrasions, contusions, and punctate tears of the perineum and perianal areas. While a speculum examination is not routinely indicated, a bimanual rectal examination will allow for evaluation of the uterus and cervix. If abuse is suspected, involve a child protection/abuse specialist.

In addition, note any pustules, especially on extensor surfaces of the extremities, or maculopapular exanthem, including the palms and soles. Look for conjunctivitis, oropharyngeal lesions, and lymphadenopathy (generalized, inguinal). The clinical findings of STIs are summarized in Table 39-1.

Table 39-1. Clinical Presentation of Sexually Transmitted Infections (STIs)

STI	Clinical Features
Bacterial vaginosis	Homogenous gray-white smooth discharge over vaginal walls External mild irritation, malodorous discharge
Candidal vulvovaginitis	Thick, cheesy, white discharge Irritation and pruritus
Condyloma accuminatum (human papillomavirus)	Flesh-colored, painless anogenital warts May be pruritic
Epididymitis	Unilateral testicular pain and swelling Dysuria, urgency
Gonorrhea (disseminated)	Petechial/pustular exanthema Asymmetrical arthralgias, tenosynovitis, septic arthritis
Herpes simplex virus	Painful/pruritic vesicles or shallow ulcerations Vaginal/penile discharge, dysuria Tender inguinal lymphadenopathy
Pelvic inflammatory disease	Dyspareunia, and spotting off-cycle or with intercourse Fever, nausea, vomiting, lower abdominal pain, dysmenorrhea Increased vaginal discharge/bleeding Cervical motion and/or adnexal tenderness
Reiter syndrome (chlamydia)	Conjunctivitis, urethritis, arthritis
Syphilis (primary)	Single painless ulcer (chancre) Non-tender inguinal lymphadenopathy
Syphilis (secondary)	Fever, malaise, myalgias, pharyngitis Salmon-pink macules/copper papules involving palms and soles Condyloma lata (anogenital flesh-colored hypertrophic papules) Generalized painless adenopathy
Trichomonas	Malodorous, frothy yellow-green discharge External irritation

Laboratory

Screen sexually active adolescents for chlamydia and gonorrhea, rapid plasma reagin/Venereal Disease Research Laboratory (RPR/VDRL), and HIV. NAAT of urine, cervical, and vaginal testing is highly sensitive and specific for chlamydia and gonorrhea. The sensitivity of chlamydia and gonorrhea culture is considerably lower, but the specificity is 100%, so for medicolegal reasons it is indicated in cases of suspected sexual abuse. In a prepubertal female, obtain a vaginal/rectal culture (endocervical samples are not necessary). Perform a pregnancy test and, if positive, obtain an ultrasound to rule out an ectopic pregnancy if the patient has abdominal pain.

In suspected PID, order a complete blood cell count and a C-reactive protein and/or erythrocyte sedimentation rate, as well as liver function tests if there are symptoms of hepatitis/cholecysitis (these are often normal in Fitz-Hugh-Curtis syndrome). Send any abnormal vaginal discharge for NAAT, Gram stain, and microscopy for white blood cells (WBCs), *Trichomonas*, candidiasis, and BV.

For a male, send any urethral discharge for microscopy, Gram stain, and NAAT. More than 5 WBCs/high-power field is consistent with urethritis.

Culture the base of any unroofed vesicular lesions for HSV, but do not send a Tzanck preparation, which lacks sufficient sensitivity and specificity. Send darkfield examinations or direct fluorescent antibody for *Treponema pallidum* from ulcerative lesions. Confirm a positive RPR/VDRL with treponemal tests (fluorescent treponemal antibody-absorption, *T pallidum* particle agglutination, enzyme immunoessays).

Radiology

An ultrasound may be helpful for evaluating both gynecologic (ovarian) pathology and a suspected appendicitis. Constipation can be ruled out with an abdominal x-ray.

Differential Diagnosis

It can be challenging to make the correct diagnosis in an adolescent female with abdominal pain (Table 39-2).

Treatment

Treatment of STIs is almost always allowed based solely on the minor's consent, although some states set a minimum age for this. The Guttmacher Institute has an online table that is updated monthly (www.Guttmacher.org). Except for one state, which requires parental notification for a positive HIV

Table 39-2. Differential Diagnosis of Abdominal Pain in the Sexually Active Female	
Diagnosis	**Clinical Features**
Appendicitis	Periumbilical pain → right lower quadrant Vomiting follows onset of pain, anorexia Rebound, guarding, leukocytosis
Ectopic pregnancy	(+) Pregnancy test Missed or late menstruation Vaginal bleeding Abdominal or pelvic pain
Endometriosis	Chronic abdominopelvic or low back pain, may be associated with menstrual cycle Dysmenorrhea, dyspareunia
Ovarian cyst	Pelvic pain Menstrual irregularities Acute pain with rupture
Ovarian torsion	Nausea, vomiting Fever uncommon, except with late presentation Severe acute lower abdominal pain
Nephrolithiasis	Colicky pain (may occur in paroxysms) Nausea, vomiting, dysuria May have hematuria
Pelvic inflammatory disease/ tubo-ovarian abscess	Nausea, vomiting, fever Cervical motion/adnexal tenderness ↑Vaginal discharge ↑C-reactive protein/erythrocyte sedimentation rate/white blood cell
Pyelonephritis	Dysuria, urgency, frequency Costovertebral angle tenderness (+) Urinalysis and urine culture

test, no state requires that physicians notify parents regarding STI evaluation or treatment.

The most common STIs encountered in the hospitalized patient are discussed below. Please refer to the *Red Book: 2012 Report of the Committee on Infectious Diseases* (www.aapredbook.org) for specific treatments of less prevalent infections. Additionally, hold treatment with metronidazole and HIV prophylaxis until the pregnancy test is known to be negative.

PID

Initiate treatment as soon as a presumptive diagnosis is made in order to reduce the chances of long-term sequelae. Indications for inpatient treatment include

- Inability to exclude a surgical emergency as the cause of the symptoms
- Pregnancy

- Outpatient therapy failed or not tolerated
- Tubo-ovarian abscess
- Severe illness with high fever, nausea, and vomiting
- Lack of adequate social or financial support to begin or comply with consistent oral therapy

Treat with intravenous (IV) cefotetan (2 g IV every 12 hours) or cefoxitin (2 g IV every 6 hours) *plus* doxycycline (100 mg oral [PO] every 12 hours). Continue the IV therapy until the patient is improving for 24 to 48 hours but complete a 14-day course of doxycycline. If the patient cannot tolerate PO medications, start clindamycin (900 mg IV every 8 hours) *plus* gentamicin (2 mg/kg IV once [loading dose], then 1.5 mg/kg every 8 hours [maintenance]), since IV administration of doxycycline can be painful. If a tubo-ovarian abscess is present, add metronidazole (500 mg PO/IV twice a day [bid] for 14 days). Cultures/NAAT results do not change empiric coverage and response does not change the total of 14 days of treatment.

If the response to antibiotics (improvement in the pain, CMT, adnexal tenderness, fever) is not prompt (24–72 hours), obtain a pelvic ultrasound looking for a tubo-ovarian abscess or other causes of abdominal pain (appendicitis, ovarian torsion, cysts). If minimal improvement is seen with appropriate antibiotics within 3 to 5 days, consult a gynecologist for further evaluation (laparoscopy) and surgical intervention.

Chlamydia/Gonorrhea (Uncomplicated)

Treat empirically with one dose of azithromycin 1 g PO (*or* doxycycline 100 mg PO bid for 7 days) and one dose of ceftriaxone 250 mg intramuscular (IM) (*or* cefixime 400 mg PO). This covers for potential coinfection and may hinder the development of resistant gonorrhea.

Epididymitis: One dose of ceftriaxone (as above) *plus* doxycycline (100 mg PO bid for 10 days). Also provide bed rest, scrotal elevation, and analgesia.

HSV

Treat with acyclovir 5 to 10 mg/kg IV every 8 hours for 2 to 7 days or until there is clinical improvement. Continue with oral therapy (acyclovir 400 mg PO 3 times a day *or* valacyclovir 1 g PO bid) to complete a minimum of 10 total days of treatment. Adjust the dose for renal impairment.

Syphilis (Primary)

Treat with one dose of IM benzathine penicillin G (50,000 million units/kg, 2.4 million units maximum).

Trichomoniasis

Treat with one dose of metronidazole 2 g PO.

BV

Treat with metronidazole 500 mg PO bid for 7 days *or* metronidazole gel (0.75%) one applicator (5 g) intravaginally daily for 5 days.

Postexposure Prophylaxis (PEP) for HIV

Indications for initiation of PEP include

- Exposure where the risk of transmission is high (exposure to blood, genital secretions, or infected body fluids of a person known to be HIV positive).
- Medical care is sought less than 72 hours after exposure.
- The patient or parent is able to strictly adhere to a 28-day regimen.

PEP is not generally recommended without the presence of all 3, as the efficacy of prophylaxis is unlikely to outweigh the risks and side effects of antiretroviral regimens. Consult a pediatric HIV specialist or, if one is not locally available, the National Clinicians Post-Exposure Prophylaxis Hotline (888/448-4911) for recommendations about PEP in specific situations. Additional information regarding pediatric and adolescent antiretroviral regimens can be found at the US Department of Health and Human Services Web site for HIV/AIDS: http://aidsinfo.nih.gov/contentfiles/PediatricGuidelines.pdf.

Indications for Consultation

- **Infectious diseases:** HIV-positive adolescents with a coexisting STI, new HIV diagnosis or suspected high-risk exposures, complicated disseminated gonococcal infection, complicated HSV
- **Obstetrics/gynecology:** Possible ectopic pregnancy, pregnant female with PID, tubo-ovarian abscess, prolonged symptoms of PID
- **Urology:** Possible testicular torsion or abscess or epididymitis

Disposition

- **Intensive care unit transfer:** Complicated HSV infections (central nervous system or disseminated disease), syphilis with cardiac or neurologic involvement
- **Discharge criteria:** Improved symptoms and tolerating oral medications

Follow-up

- **Primary care:** 48 hours, then 1 to 2 weeks and at 3 to 6 months for chlamydia and gonorrhea retesting

Pearls and Pitfalls

- Maintain high suspicion for PID in a sexually active female and treat, even if testing for chlamydia and gonorrhea is negative (to avoid possible long-term sequelae).
- Notify and treat the partner(s) of an adolescent infected with chlamydia, gonorrhea, or *Trichomonas.* More information regarding expedited partner therapy may be found at www.cdc.gov/std/ept/.
- While all 50 states allow minors to consent for confidential STI screening and treatment, be aware of state-specific differences as reporting and insurance confidentiality measures vary.
- Review contraception options and condom use. Refer to the American Academy of Pediatrics policy statement, "Contraception and Adolescents."

Coding

ICD-9

• BV	**616.10**
• Cervicitis	**616.0**
• Chlamydia, unspecified	**099.50**
• Contact with or exposure to HIV	**V01.79**
• Contact with or exposure to STI	**V01.6**
• Contact with or exposure to *Trichomonas*	**V01.89**
• Epididymitis, unspecified	**604.90**
• Gonorrhea, unspecified	**098.0**
• HIV positive (asymptomatic)	**V08**
• HSV without mention of complication	**054.9**
• Non-gonococcal urethritis, unspecified	**099.40**
• PID	**614.9**
• Primary genital syphilis	**091.0**
• Screen for bacterial and spirochetal STI	**V74.5**
• Screen for chlamydial diseases	**V73.88**
• Screen for HPV	**V73.81**
• Screen for other specified viral diseases	**V73.89**
• Secondary syphilis, unspecified	**091.9**
• Urogenital trichomoniasis, unspecified	**131.00**

Bibliography

American Academy of Pediatrics. Sexually transmitted infections. In: Pickering LK, Baker CJ, Kimberlin DW, Long SS, eds. *Red Book: 2012 Report of the Committee on Infectious Diseases*. Elk Grove Village, IL: American Academy of Pediatrics; 2012:821–827

American Academy of Pediatrics Committee on Adolescence, Blythe MJ, Diaz A. Contraception and adolescents. *Pediatrics.* 2007;120:1135–1148

Centers for Disease Control and Prevention. Sexually transmitted diseases, treatment guidelines, 2010. *MMWR Morb Mortal Wkly Rep.* 2010;59(No. RR-12):1–110. http://www.cdc.gov/std/treatment/2010/STD-Treatment-2010-RR5912.pdf

Guttmacher Institute. State policies in brief. An overview of minor's consent law. http://www.guttmacher.org/statecenter/spibs/spib_OMCL.pdf

Havens PL; American Academy of Pediatrics Committee on Pediatric AIDS. Postexposure prophylaxis in children and adolescents for nonoccupational exposure to human immunodeficiency virus. *Pediatrics.* 2003;111:1475–1489

Straub DM. Sexually transmitted diseases in adolescents. *Adv Pediatr.* 2009;56:87–106

Hematology

CHAPTER 40

Acute Complications of Cancer Therapy

Introduction

The survival rate for children with malignancies continues to improve, although at the cost of associated side effects and toxicities. Chemotherapy, which targets rapidly dividing cells (eg, bone marrow, gut, hair), leads to significant cytotoxic side effects. While the effects of radiation are more localized, there can be profound consequences, including nausea, vomiting, pain, and skin changes. Surgery can lead to issues with wound care, infection, and pain management. Although most pediatric oncology patients are managed at tertiary care centers, the hospitalist will occasionally care for such children.

Clinical Presentation and Diagnosis

Many chemotherapeutic agents share a number of side effects (Table 40-1), which commonly include the following.

Adrenal Insufficiency

Steroids are broadly used in treating pediatric cancers such as acute lymphoblastic leukemia, certain lymphomas, and brain tumors. A patient may receive a prolonged course of high-dose steroids, without tapering. Even months after induction therapy is complete, the patient remains at risk for adrenal insufficiency. A patient may also have significant exposure to steroids as prophylaxis for chemotherapy-induced nausea and vomiting. However, these doses are generally not high enough or prolonged enough to cause adrenal insufficiency.

Signs of adrenal suppression can be subtle and hard to differentiate from most chemotherapy-related toxicities, including dizziness, weakness, poor appetite, muscle aches, and persistent nausea. More commonly, suspect severe adrenal insufficiency in a patient presenting with signs of infection, hypotension, shock, or vital sign instability. Laboratory abnormalities may include hyponatremia, hyperkalemia, and metabolic acidosis with a normal anion gap.

Extravasation

Some chemotherapeutic agents may cause damage if they inadvertently leak from a vein into surrounding tissue. Initially, local reactions may include erythema and pain, but they may progress over days to weeks to blistering, ulcerations, and necrosis. Severe pain and loss of function may result if the necrosis extends to the nerves, ligaments, tendons, and bones.

Fever and Myelosuppression

Bone marrow suppression leads to anemia, thrombocytopenia, and leukopenia. Because granulocytes have the shortest life span and are the first line of defense against bacterial infection, oncology patients are at risk for neutropenia and subsequent infections. A patient with fever and neutropenia (absolute neutrophil count <500/mm^3) deserves immediate attention. Fever is defined differently at many centers, but commonly it is a temperature higher than 101°F (38.3°C), or several low-grade temperatures (100.1–100.9°F; 37.8–38.3°C) in a 24-hour period. However, a patient receiving steroids might not mount a febrile response. It is also critical to assess what type of indwelling catheter the child has (none, peripheral intravenous catheter, peripherally inserted central catheter, Broviac, Port-A-Cath), as these carry various risks of infection and antibiotic coverage may differ.

Determine the date of the most recent chemotherapy to predict the expected direction of the white blood cell (WBC) trend, as most agents cause suppression 7 to 10 days after infusion. Also note the specific agents and doses received, recent blood transfusions (a transfusion reaction can cause fever), and a history of other infections, which may help guide antibiotic choices. Perform a thorough physical examination. Priorities include the oropharynx and perianal region (looking for mucositis and perianal abscesses), as well as central venous line insertion sites, looking for signs of infection, such as erythema, tenderness, or discharge. It is important to note that with a low WBC count or prior steroid use, the patient may not be able to mount the typical signs of infection, including fever, purulence, discharge, or erythema. Carefully evaluate any areas of tenderness and swelling. A neutropenic patient is also at risk for neutropenic colitis (typhlitis), a fatal complication, so perform a thorough abdominal examination and consult with a surgeon if there is any concern. Also, except in an emergency, do not permit rectal interventions (taking temperature or giving medications) in a patient with neutropenia.

Hemorrhagic Cystitis

A patient receiving cyclophosphamide or ifosfamide may present with painless hematuria secondary to bladder wall irritation. The urine will be red, and not tea-colored as is seen with upper tract bleeding.

Mucositis

As chemotherapy affects any rapidly dividing cell, the gastrointestinal mucous membranes are at high risk of becoming inflamed and ulcerated. This can occur anywhere from the mouth to the anus. Signs and symptoms include exquisite pain, drooling, dysphagia, abdominal pain, diarrhea, melena, or hematochezia. This can interfere with adequate oral hydration and also create an entry point for infectious agents. A patient who has received high-dose Ara-C is at particular risk for a mucositis-related infection, including *Streptococcus mitis*, which can cause life-threatening sepsis.

Nausea/Vomiting

Nausea and vomiting can be caused by chemotherapy and radiation, or can occur postoperatively. Chemotherapy-induced nausea vomiting (CINV) is either acute, occurring within the first 24 hours after receiving chemotherapy, or delayed, which occurs more than 24 hours after administration and can persist up to 1 week after therapy. The consequences of CINV include dehydration, electrolyte imbalance, anorexia, weight loss, and increased susceptibility to infections.

Skin Manifestations

A patient undergoing chemotherapy or radiation can have skin changes. For example, methotrexate can cause acrodermatitis in a stocking glove distribution. Abscesses, swelling, and line site swelling can be signs of infection in a neutropenic patient. Skin findings that are especially worrisome include blackened spots or ulcerated/crusted lesions that could be signs of a potentially fatal disseminated mold or fungus infection.

Radiation therapy can induce skin breakdown and maceration, which can also be a significant nidus for infection. Carefully examine crevices and nonobvious skin folds in or near the radiation field. Chronic, diffuse hyperpigmentation may result from radiation.

Tumor Lysis Syndrome

Tumor lysis refers to metabolic derangements caused by the rapid breakdown of tumor cells, with subsequent release of intracellular contents. A patient with leukemia or lymphoma is at particular risk. Tumor lysis syndrome may occur prior to treatment in a patient with a very high white count at presentation or those with very rapidly growing tumors (eg, Burkett lymphoma). Typically however, it begins 12 to 72 hours after the induction of chemotherapy.

Metabolic derangements include hyperuricemia, hyperkalemia, and hyperphosphatemia. Because phosphorus precipitates with calcium, the patient can also develop hypocalcemia. Uric acid crystals and calcium-phosphorus precipitates can obstruct the renal tubules, producing oliguria and, ultimately, renal failure. Other clinical manifestations include nausea/vomiting, seizures, muscle cramping, tetany, and arrhythmias.

Table 40-1. Side Effects of Chemotherapeutic Agents

Onset	Common	Occasional	Rare
PEG-Asparaginase			
Within 1–2 days	Diarrhea Local allergic reaction	Rash	Anaphylaxis Hyperuricemia
Within 2–3 weeks	↑Ammonia Coagulation abnormalities	Hyperglycemia Pancreatitis	DIC/hemorrhage Thromboses
Bleomycin			
Within 1–2 days	High fever	Rash	Anaphylaxis Hypotension
Within 2–3 weeks	Skin hyperpigmentation Raynaud phenomenon		Alopecia Onychloysis
Later		Interstitial pneumonitis	
Carboplatin			
Within 1–2 days	Nausea/vomiting	Hypersensitivity reaction	Metallic taste Mucositis
Within 2–3 weeks	Myelosuppression	Hepatotoxicity Nephrotoxicity	
Later		Ototoxicity	Peripheral neuropathy
Cisplatin			
Within 1–2 days	Nausea/vomiting	Metallic taste	Anaphylaxis
Within 2–3 weeks	↓Mg High frequency hearing loss Nephrotoxicity	↓Ca, ↓K, ↓Na Peripheral neuropathy	Hepatotoxicity Seizures Vestibular dysfunction
Corticosteroids			
Within 1–2 days	Hyperphagia	Gastritis	Hyperuricemia
Within 2–3 weeks	Personality changes Pituitary-adrenal axis suppression	Hyperglycemia Poor wound healing	Hypertension ↑Intraocular pressure Pancreatitis
Cytarabine (Ara-C)			
Within 1–2 days	Conjunctivitis Nausea/vomiting	Fever Flu-like symptoms	Anaphylaxis Cerebral/cerebellar dysfunction
Within 2–3 weeks	Alopecia Myelosuppression Stomatitis	↓Ca, ↓K Diarrhea Pulmonary capillary leak	Hepatotoxicity Sinusoidal obstruction syndrome
Cyclophosphamide			
Within 1–2 days	Nausea/vomiting	Diarrhea	Anaphylaxis Transient blurred vision, SIADH
Within 2–3 weeks	Alopecia Myelosuppression	Hemorrhagic cystitis	Cardiac toxicity

Table 40-1. Side Effects of Chemotherapeutic Agents, continued			
Onset	**Common**	**Occasional**	**Rare**
Doxorubicin/Daunorubicin			
Within 1–2 days	Nausea/vomiting Pink/red body fluid discoloration	Hyperuricemia	Diarrhea
Within 2–3 weeks	Myelosuppression	Mucositis	Conjunctivitis
Later		Cardiomyopathy	
Etoposide			
Within 1–2 days	Nausea/vomiting		Anaphylaxis Hypotension during infusion
Within 2–3 weeks	Alopecia Myelosuppression	Diarrhea Urticaria	Mucositis Peripheral neuropathy Stevens-Johnson syndrome
Ifosfamide			
Within 1–2 days	Nausea/vomiting	CNS toxicity	↓K Encephalopathy
Within 2–3 weeks	Myelosuppression	Cardiac toxicity	Hemorrhagic cystitis Hepatotoxicity
Later			Fanconi-like syndrome Renal failure
Irinotecan			
Within 1–2 days	Cholinergic symptoms Nausea/vomiting	Headache	Anaphylaxis Dyspnea
Within 2–3 weeks	Hepatotoxicity Myelosuppression		Colitis Renal failure
Methotrexate			
Within 1–2 days	Transaminase elevation	Nausea/vomiting	Acral erythema Stevens-Johnson syndrome Toxic epidermal necrolysis
Within 2–3 weeks		Mucositis Myelosuppression	CNS toxicity Renal toxicity
Mercaptopurine (6-MP)			
Within 1–2 days		Diarrhea Nausea/vomiting	Hyperuricemia Urticaria
Within 2–3 weeks	Myelosuppression	Mouth sores	Hepatotoxicity Pancreatitis

Table 40-1. Side Effects of Chemotherapeutic Agents, continued

Onset	Common	Occasional	Rare
Topotecan			
Within 1–2 days	Nausea/vomiting	Hypotension Rash	Anaphylaxis Rigors
Within 2–3 weeks	Myelosuppression	Hepatotoxicity Mucositis	Paresthesias
Vinblastine			
Within 1–2 days			Jaw pain Seizure
Within 2–3 weeks	Alopecia Myelosuppression	Constipation	Hemorrhagic enterocolitis Peripheral neuropathy Ototoxicity/vestibular dysfunction
Vincristine			
Within 1–2 days		Headache Jaw pain	Bronchospasm
Within 2–3 weeks	Alopecia Constipation		Ptosis/diplopia Seizures
Later	Loss of deep tendon reflexes	Peripheral paresthesias	Autonomic neuropathy Sinusoidal obstruction syndrome

Abbreviations: Ca, calcium; CNS, central nervous system; DIC, disseminated intravascular coagulation; K, potassium; Mg, magnesium; Na, sodium; SIADH, syndrome of inappropriate antidiuretic hormone hypersecretion.

Treatment

Adrenal Insufficiency

If acute adrenal insufficiency is suspected, immediately initiate aggressive fluid and steroid replacement. Obtain vital signs as well as serum electrolytes and glucose. If the patient is hypotensive, give 20 mL/kg normal saline (NS) boluses over 30 to 60 minutes until the blood pressure normalizes. Treat hypoglycemia (<60 mg/dL) with 2 to 4 mL/kg of D10 and recheck in 15 minutes. If hyperkalemia is documented, immediately obtain an electrocardiogram, looking for evidence of cardiotoxicity with peaked T waves (T wave greater than one-half the R or S wave), a prolonged PR interval, or QRS widening. If any of these are present, or if the potassium is greater than 7 mEq/L, discontinue the administration of exogenous potassium and use therapeutic agents that can transiently redistribute potassium: 25% dextrose (2 mL/kg over 30 minutes and repeat every 30 minutes) along with regular insulin (1 unit/kg/hour); nebulized albuterol. Also give 10% calcium gluconate

(1 mL/kg = 100 mg/kg/dose every 3–5 minutes) to protect the myocardium. To enhance potassium excretion, use a loop diuretic (furosemide 1–2 mg/kg intravenous [IV] every 6 hours) and polystyrene sulfonate (1 g/kg). Dialysis is indicated for life-threatening hyperkalemia.

Continue with D5NS at 1.5 to 2 times the maintenance rate. Give a bolus of IV or intramuscular (IM) hydrocortisone (infant: 25 mg, toddler: 50 mg, child/adolescent: 100 mg) followed by 25 mg/m^2 or 1 mg/kg every 6 hours.

Extravasation

If suspected, stop the infusion immediately and institute measures to remove as much of the extravasated drug as possible. Apply warm or cold compresses, depending on the agent (Table 40-2). There are also specific antidotes for some medications.

Fever and Myelosuppression

If a neutropenic patient is febrile, obtain a complete blood cell count with differential and blood cultures. Some centers will require culture of all lumens of a central line as well as a peripheral site. If a child is at risk for urinary tract infections (UTIs) (ie, prior history of UTI, presence of nephrostomy tubes or Foley catheter, <2 years of age) obtain a urinalysis and urine culture. Obtain stool cultures if abdominal symptoms or significant diarrhea are present. Culture any suspicious lesions on the skin or near surgical or central line sites. Obtain a chest x-ray if there are respiratory symptoms.

Table 40-2. Treatment for Specific Agent Extravasation

Agent	Local Care	Antidote
Actinomycin-D	Cold compress	Dimethyl sulfoxide[a]
Cisplatin	Cold compress	Sodium thiosulfate[b]
Daunorubicin	Cold compress	Dexrazoxane[c]
Doxorubicin	Cold compress	Dexrazoxane
Etoposide	Warm compress	Hyaluronidase[d]
Idarubicin	Cold compress	Dexrazoxane[c]
Mechlorethamine	None	Sodium thiosulfate[b]
Mitomycin	None or cold compress	Dimethyl sulfoxide[a]
Paclitaxel	Cold compress	Hyaluronidase[d]
Vinblastine	Warm compress	Hyaluronidase[d]
Vincristine	Warm compress	Hyaluronidase[d]

[a]Dimethyl sulfoxide: 4 drops/10 cm^2 of skin surface area topically to twice the area of the site 3–4 times a day for 7–14 days.
[b]Sodium thiosulfate: 2 mL for each 100 mg of cisplatin extravasation or 2 mL for each 1 mg of mechlorethamine extravasation.
[c]Dexrazoxane: 1,000 mg/m^2/dose on days 1 and 2, 500 mg/m^2/dose on day 3, each dose 24 hours apart.
[d]Hyaluronidase (150 units/mL): 5 injections of 0.2 mL each infiltrated around the extravasation.

Treat with broad-spectrum antibiotics that cover both gram-positive and gram-negative organisms, but consult with the oncologist for the preferred regimen. Because neutropenic patients are at very high risk for sepsis with gram-negative rods, many regimens tend to double-cover or emphasize antibiotics with activity against these organisms. If the patient appears toxic, a typical regimen includes cefipime (50 mg/kg IV every 8 hours, 6 g/day maximum), gentamicin (2.5 mg/kg IV every 8 hours, 4 g/d maximum), and vancomycin (15 mg/kg IV every 6–8 hours, 4 g/day maximum). If the patient is stable, typical regimens include cefipime with or without gentamicin or piperacillin/tazobactam (100 mg/kg every 8 hours, 16 g of piperacillin component/day maximum). Add vancomycin (15 mg/kg IV every 6–8 hours, 4 g/day maximum) if mucositis is present and the patient has a history of or is at risk for streptococcal sepsis, has erythema or purulence around a central line site, or is recently post–stem cell transplantation. Some centers add metronidazole if there is concern about perirectal ulcers/abscesses. Ensure that all antibiotic doses are appropriate for the patient's renal status.

Consult with an oncologist as transfusion guidelines vary among treating centers. Typically packed red cell transfusions are indicated if the patient is symptomatic from anemia or the hemoglobin is less than 7 to 8 g/dL. Prior to procedures and radiation, some centers aim for a hemoglobin closer to 9 to 10 g/dL. Ensure that all blood products are leukoreduced and, for a cytomegalovirus-negative or pre–/post–bone marrow transplant patient, irradiated.

Guidelines for platelet transfusions are also center-specific. Generally, a transfusion is indicated if the platelet count falls below 10,000/mm^3. A higher threshold may be maintained for a patient with residual brain tumor or bone marrow transplantation, or if the child is young or highly active. If a patient will shortly be undergoing a procedure, is at risk for intracranial hemorrhage, or is on concomitant anticoagulation for a thrombosis, many centers will maintain the platelet count above 50,000/mm^3.

Hemorrhagic Cystitis

Treatment consists of vigorous hydration (per the specific chemotherapy protocol), correction of hematologic abnormalities (packed red blood cell or platelet transfusions, if indicated), and bladder irrigation following placement of a double-lumen Foley catheter by a urologist, if severe. It is also important to rule out viral infections that may cause hemorrhagic cystitis. Prevention involves vigorous hydration to maintain a urine specific gravity below 1.010 or urinary output of 2 to 3 mL/kg/hour and the use of mesna with cyclophosphamide or ifosfamide administration.

Mucositis

Treat with sponge-tipped applicators soaked in 0.9% sodium chloride for debridement, nystatin swish and swallow (100,000 units/mL) 5 mL oral (PO) 4 times a day, and for analgesia, "magic mouthwash" (2% viscous lidocaine, liquid Maalox, and liquid diphenhydramine) every 4 to 6 hours. For anal involvement, prescribe stool softeners (docusate sodium 50–150 mg/day) and "butt paste" (nystatin cream, zinc oxide, Maalox) for analgesia. The pain associated with mucositis is significant and can often require IV opioid therapy and IV fluids or parenteral nutrition while the patient remains NPO.

Nausea/Vomiting

Check if the patient already has a specific antiemetic regimen prescribed, so that the specific medications can be instituted or augmented. For acute nausea/vomiting, use ondansetron (0.15 mg/kg PO/IV every 8 hours, 8 mg/dose maximum), although a single daily dose can be used. Other 5HT3 antagonists are also available, including granisetron and palonosetron. Dexamethasone can be used as an adjunctive antiemetic, but check with the oncologist as it is contraindicated in many cancers. Scopolamine patches are also helpful, as is diphenhydramine (1 mg/kg PO/IV every 6 hours, 50 mg/dose maximum), phenergan (0.25–1 mg/kg PO/IV/IM every 4–6 hours 25 mg/dose maximum), or hydroxyzine (1 mg/kg PO/IV every 6 hours, 50 mg/dose maximum) when additional relief is needed. If the patient has continued nausea/vomiting, the addition of lorazepam (0.04 mg/kg PO/IV every 6 hours, 2 mg/dose maximum) or diazepam (0.2 mg/kg PO/IV every 6–8 hours 0.6 mg/kg/day maximum) may be helpful.

Skin Manifestations

Aspirate or biopsy (as appropriate) any new circumscribed or focal skin lesion. Perform a Tzanck smear and culture of any vesicular lesion that is suspicious for herpes or varicella. Treat radiation-induced skin changes with a lanolin-based ointment.

Tumor Lysis Syndrome

Obtain serum electrolytes, calcium, phosphorus, blood urea nitrogen, creatinine, uric acid, and lactate dehydrogenase prior to beginning chemotherapy and every 4 to 6 hours thereafter. Closely monitor the urine output and specific gravity, maintaining a specific gravity below 1.010.

The type of IV fluid used varies among institutions. Prior to starting chemotherapy, many centers prefer to alkalinize the urine with D^5 ¼ NS with 50 to 100 mEq/L $NaHCO_3$ at a 2-times maintenance rate to maintain a pH of

7.0 to 7.5. Alkalinization is often discontinued once chemotherapy is started to prevent precipitation of calcium phosphorus stones. Give allopurinol (50 mg/m^2 every 6 hours, 600 mg/day maximum) to decrease production of uric acid. Add rasburicase (50–100 units/kg once, contraindicated in a patient with glucose-6-phosphate dehydrogenase deficiency) if the uric acid level remains elevated and/or is rising rapidly despite allopurinol administration.

Treat hyperkalemia as described above for adrenal insufficiency.

Give an oral phosphate binder (ie, sevelamer) for hyperphosphatemia. Calcium replacement for asymptomatic hypocalcemia is not warranted.

Dialysis is indicated for the persistence of hyperkalemia or hyperphosphatemia despite conservative measures and for renal failure with resulting uremia.

Coding

ICD-9

• Acute cystitis	**595.0**
• Adrenal insufficiency	**255.41**
• Chills without fever	**780.64**
• Extravasation of vesicant chemotherapy	**999.81**
• Fever in preexisting (chronic) condition	**780.61**
• Hemorrhagic cystitis	**595.9**
• Mucositis (ulcerative) due to antineoplastic therapy	**528.01**
• Mucositis, unspecified	**528.00**
• Nausea and vomiting	**787.01**
• Neutropenia, drug induced	**288.03**
• Neutropenia, due to infection	**288.04**
• Neutropenia, unspecified	**288.00**

Bibliography

Cefalo MG, Ruggiero A, Maurizi P, et al. Pharmacological management of chemotherapy-induced nausea and vomiting in children with cancer. *J Chemother.* 2009;21:605–610

Di Martino-Nardi J. Endocrine emergencies. In: Crain EF, Gershel JC, eds. *Clinical Manual of Emergency Pediatrics*. New York, NY: Cambridge University Press; 2010:161–193

Koh AY, Pizzo, PA. Infectious diseases in pediatric cancer. In: Orkin S, Fisher D, Look AT, Lux SE, Ginsburg D, Nathan DG, eds. *Oncology of Infancy and Childhood.* Philadelphia, PA: Saunders; 2009:1099–1120

Schulmeister L. Extravasation management: clinical update. *Semin Oncol Nurs.* 2011;27:82–90

Sparreboom A, Evans WE, Baker SD. Chemotherapy in the pediatric patient. In: Orkin S, Fisher D, Look AT, Lux SE, Ginsburg D, Nathan DG, eds. *Oncology of Infancy and Childhood*. Philadelphia, PA: Saunders; 2009:175–207

Walsh TJ, Roilides E, Groll AH, Gonzalez C, Pizzo PA. Infectious complications in pediatric patients. In: Pizzo PA, Poplack DG, eds. *Principles and Practice of Pediatric Oncology.* 5th ed. Philadelphia, PA: Lippincott, Williams & Williams; 2006:1269–1328

CHAPTER 41

Anemia

Anemia is defined as a reduced hemoglobin concentration or red blood cell (RBC) mass below the reference range for age. Any process that causes increased RBC destruction, failure of RBC production, or blood loss can result in anemia. While mild to moderate anemia will typically be addressed in the outpatient setting, the acute onset of anemia or a chronic anemia that outpaces the body's ability to compensate may require inpatient evaluation and/or management. In addition, anemia can occur in the inpatient setting as a comorbidity with many conditions.

Clinical Presentation

History

Symptoms of anemia include pallor, fatigue, weakness, lethargy, decreased energy, headache, and shortness of breath. Palpitations and a sensation of light-headedness may also occur. A very young or preterm infant may present with apnea.

Obtain a thorough history, including the time course of the onset of symptoms, diet (including milk, iron-rich food, and supplement intake), growth and development, recent illnesses, evidence of chronic disease, recent or recurring blood loss, and family history of anemia. Review the newborn screen results, if available. The patient's ethnicity and the presence of pica are also important to elicit. Ask about dark urine, or a personal or family history of splenectomy or cholecystectomy, which may suggest an underlying hemolytic anemia.

Physical Examination

The priority is to assess for hemodynamic compromise, which requires immediate intervention. This includes hypotension, persistent tachycardia, orthostatic changes, a widened pulse pressure, and bounding pulses. A patient with an uncompensated anemia may also present with hypoxia, signs of congestive heart failure, syncope, and altered mental status. A systolic ejection murmur and increased prominence of the cardiac apical impulse may also be noted.

Although the signs of anemia vary greatly with the patient's age, comorbid conditions, and rapidity of onset, a common physical examination finding is pallor, which is best seen in the nail beds, palmar creases, conjunctivae, and mucosal surfaces. Jaundice, frontal bossing, hepatomegaly, and splenomegaly may be noted with a hemolytic process. Evidence of inflammation or systemic disease may be observed in anemia of chronic disease.

Laboratory

Obtain a complete blood cell count, reticulocyte count, and a peripheral blood smear for any anemic patient. If the patient has a clear source of blood loss, these values will serve as baseline measures. If the blood loss is acute, the hemoglobin may not reflect the true volume deficit. In addition, the reticulocyte count may be normal, as the bone marrow may not have had time to respond. If the cause of anemia is unknown, choose additional studies based on the results of these initial tests. It is important to weigh the value of each diagnostic test in relation to the blood volume needed, so as not to exacerbate the patient's degree of anemia. If the patient will be receiving a transfusion, obtain all blood samples prior, so as to evaluate the patient and the donor.

Elevated Reticulocyte Count

The physiological response to anemia includes an increased reticulocyte count, which usually represents a normal bone marrow response to blood loss or hemolysis. Since the reticulocyte count represents a percentage of the total RBCs, it is important to correct for the anemia:

Corrected reticulocyte count =

(Measured reticulocyte count) X (Measured hematocrit/Normal hematocrit)

To evaluate for hemolysis, or shortened RBC lifespan, order antiglobulin (Coombs) testing. A direct antiglobulin test evaluates for antibodies bound to the RBC membrane and, in general, indicates an autoimmune hemolytic anemia when positive. An indirect antiglobulin test assesses for free anti-erythrocyte antibody in the serum and may be positive in an autoimmune hemolytic anemia if the antibody titer exceeds the antigen-binding capacity. Be aware that certain conditions, such as neonatal ABO incompatibility, are associated with low RBC antigens and will result in a positive indirect antiglobulin. Supportive laboratory findings for a hemolytic process include elevated serum potassium, aspartate transaminase (serum glutamic-oxaloacetic transaminase), total bilirubin, and lactate dehydrogenase. A decreased haptoglobin is also indicative of hemolysis, except in a neonate who may intrinsically have a low haptoglobin level.

Request a microscopic evaluation of the peripheral blood smear, looking for abnormal red cell morphologies, including sickled cells, spherocytes, spiculated cells, poikilocytes, elliptocytes, target cells, and Heinz bodies. Additionally, check the other cell lines, looking at platelet morphology and leukocyte abnormalities, especially for the presence of malignant-appearing cells. Order a hemoglobin electrophoresis when there is no clear etiology for a hemolytic process, newborn screen results are unavailable or abnormal, or the family history supports a hereditary defect.

To evaluate for chronic blood loss, guaiac the stools to rule out a gastrointestinal bleed and obtain a urinalysis to look for evidence of renal pathology. Consider other occult sources of blood loss, such as intra-abdominal and intramuscular bleeding. In the very young infant, intracranial bleeds may be associated with anemia.

Low Reticulocyte Count

A low reticulocyte count is consistent with inadequate production of RBCs from the bone marrow. The peripheral smear may demonstrate red cell microcytosis or macrocytosis, or abnormalities of the other cell lines, including hypersegmented neutrophils or lymphoblasts. Obtain a C-reactive protein, iron and total iron binding capacity (TIBC), ferritin, and liver function tests (Table 41-1). Consider testing for parvovirus to evaluate for an infectious etiology of inadequate bone marrow production.

Table 41-1. Diagnosis of Anemia

Diagnosis	Clinical Features
Blood Loss	
Acute blood loss	Overt bleeding Guaiac-positive stool or gastric output May not have ↑reticulocytes for 1–2 days
Chronic blood loss	May be the presentation of von Willebrand in menstruating girls May have guaiac-positive stool ↓ or ↑ reticulocytes May have ↓ serum iron, TIBC
Decreased Production	
Aplastic anemia	Anemia with neutropenia, thrombocytopenia ↓ reticulocytes
B_{12} deficiency	Vegan diet, or breastfed infant of vegan mother History of terminal ilium resection Hypersegmented neutrophils
Chronic inflammation	History: chronic disease ↑ ESR, CRP, ferritin ↓ serum iron, TIBC
Chronic renal disease	Uremia ↓ erythropoietin
Folate deficiency	Goat milk diet

Table 41-1. Diagnosis of Anemia, continued	
Diagnosis	**Clinical Features**
Decreased Production, continued	
Iron deficiency	History: inadequate iron in diet ↓ MCV, MCHC, serum iron, ferritin, reticulocytes ↑ RDW
Liver disease	Jaundice, hepatomegaly ↑ LFTs
Red cell aplasias (Diamond Blackfan)	First year of life Severe presentation Persistence of fetal hemoglobin
Transient erythroblastopenia of childhood	Age: 6 months–3 years Neutropenia, normal platelets, ↓ reticulocytes
RBC Destruction	
Autoimmune hemolytic anemia	Acute severe presentation Positive Coombs test Hemoglobinuria
Inherited hemolytic anemia	Jaundice, organomegaly ↑ bilirubin, reticulocytes Smear: RBC morphology (sickle cells, spherocytes)
Microangiopathic hemolytic anemia	Associated with HUS/TTP Schistocytes on smear Hemoglobinuria
Thalassemia major	Mediterranean or African descent Presents during infancy Splenomegaly Severe anemia with ↓↓MCV

Abbreviations: CRP, C-reactive protein; ESR, erythrocyte sedimentation rate; HUS, hemolytic uremic syndrome; LFTs, liver function tests; MCHC, mean corpuscular hemoglobin concentration; MCV, mean corpuscular volume; RBC, red blood cell; RDW, RBC distribution width; TIBC, total iron binding capacity; TTP, thrombotic thrombocytopenic purpura.

If iron deficiency anemia is suspected, obtain a ferritin, iron, and TIBC (as above). If the mean corpuscular cell volume is greater than normal, order B_{12} and folate levels. Note that ferritin is also an acute phase reactant and may be normal in a patient with a chronic disease and iron deficiency.

Differential Diagnosis

Use the reticulocyte count to distinguish between anemia due to a failure in bone marrow production (decreased) versus early RBC destruction or blood loss (elevated).

Treatment

The treatment of anemia varies based on the etiology. A significant anemia that has developed slowly can usually be tolerated by the patient and is not necessarily an indication for transfusion. However, in the case of acute blood loss in an unstable patient with hemodynamic compromise, give urgent volume expansion with packed RBCs. Administration of colloids or crystalloids, such as normal saline, lactated Ringer or albumin, may be necessary while awaiting the arrival of the blood product. For a critically ill but hemodynamically stable patient, consider transfusing packed RBCs if the hemoglobin is below 7 g/dL or if there are increasing cardiorespiratory symptoms, regardless of the hemoglobin level. The time course for a transfusion varies based on the clinical situation, but in general, give packed red cells over a 4-hour period to avoid circulatory overload. A patient with cardiovascular instability may require a slower rate.

The treatment of a hemolytic anemia depends on the etiology and severity, and typically involves consultation with a hematologist. In general, a patient with an inherited hemolytic anemia needs careful monitoring over time, and may require occasional transfusions as directed by a hematologist. For life-threatening autoimmune hemolysis, urgently consult with a hematologist, who will determine if treatment with high-dose steroids is indicated. One regimen is to start with methylprednisolone (1–2 mg/kg intravenous [IV] every 6 hours) for the first 24 to 72 hours, then transition to prednisone (1–2 mg/kg/day) once the patient is clinically stable. The hematologist may recommend other acute treatment options, such as IV immunoglobulin, plasmapheresis, and exchange transfusion. Long-term management may include splenectomy or autoimmune suppressing drugs.

Consult with a hematologist if the anemia is associated with abnormalities of other blood cell lines, such as leukopenia, leukocytosis, thrombocytopenia, or pancytopenia. In such cases bone marrow aspirate and/or biopsy may be necessary to evaluate for bone marrow failure or infiltration.

Treat iron deficiency anemia with oral elemental iron, 3 to 6 mg/kg/day. Iron sucrose may be a useful alternative if the patient is having difficulty tolerating oral iron. A satisfactory response to treatment is evidenced by an increase in reticulocyte count within 2 to 4 days and an increase in hematocrit within 2 to 4 weeks. Manage anemia of chronic disease by treating the underlying cause.

Manage postoperative anemia conservatively if the patient is hemodynamically stable. However, a transfusion of packed RBCs may be necessary if the patient is tachycardic, hypotensive, hypoxic, excessively fatigued, in significant respiratory distress, or has ongoing blood loss. Additionally, a transfusion may be indicated to promote postoperative healing of grafts or other injuries, for which the patient may require a higher hematocrit than what is needed for cardiovascular stability.

Indications for Consultation

- **Hematology/oncology:** Diagnosis unclear, intravascular hemolysis, condition refractory to treatment, concern for bone marrow failure, bone marrow aspirate required, long-term management considerations, suspicion of malignancy

Disposition

- **Intensive care unit transfer:** Hemodynamic instability
- **Discharge criteria:** Hemoglobin stable, without acute physiological manifestations of anemia

Follow-up

- **Primary care:** 1 to 2 weeks, depending on condition at discharge
- **Hematology:** 1 to 2 weeks, depending on diagnosis and condition at discharge

Pearls and Pitfalls

- If possible, obtain blood studies prior to transfusion of blood products.
- Be cautious about the volume of blood drawn in the anemic child, as iatrogenic blood loss may acutely worsen the patient's anemia and cause clinical decline.
- Occult sources of internal blood loss are the abdomen, head (neonate), and thigh and the chest (trauma victim). Except for a neonate, it is uncommon for intracranial hemorrhage to cause anemia in the absence of neurologic findings on physical examination.
- Steroid treatment can change the appearance of the bone marrow and alter the subsequent treatment and prognosis of certain malignancies. Therefore, if there is any possibility of a malignancy (generalized lymphadenopathy, hepatosplenomegaly, other cell lines affected, etc), consult with a hematologist before starting steroid therapy for an anemic patient.

Coding

ICD-9

• Acute anemia due to blood loss	**285.1**
• Anemia, unspecified	**285.9**
• Anemia of chronic disease	**285.29**
• Aplastic anemia, unspecified	**284.9**
• Autoimmune hemolytic anemia	**283.0**
• Acquired hemolytic anemia, unspecified	**283.9**
• Iron deficiency anemia, unspecified	**280.9**

Bibliography

Clark SF. Iron deficiency anemia: diagnosis and management. *Curr Opin Gastroenterol.* 2009;25:122–128

Davis IJ. Anemia. In: Zaoutis LB, Chiang VW, eds. *Comprehensive Hospital Medicine.* Philadelphia, PA: Mosby; 2007:721–730

Heeney MM. Anemia. In: Rudolph CD, Rudolph AM, Lister GE, First LR, Gershon AA, eds. *Rudolph's Pediatrics.* 22nd ed. New York, NY: McGraw Hill; 2011:1532–1536

Janus J, Moerschel SK. Evaluation of anemia in children. *Am Fam Physician.* 2010;81:1462–1471

King KE, Ness PM. Treatment of autoimmune hemolytic anemia. *Semin Hematol.* 2005;42:131–136

Kliegman, RM, Stanton, BF, Geme, JW, Schor, NF, Behrman, RE, eds. *Nelson Textbook of Pediatrics.* 19th ed. Philadelphia, PA: Elsevier; 2011:1648–1650

Lacroix J, Hébert PC, Hutchison JS, et al. Transfusion strategies for patients in pediatric intensive care units. *N Engl J Med.* 2007;356:1609–1619

Sickle Cell Disease

Introduction

Sickle cell disease (SCD) is an inherited hematologic disorder characterized by having genes for 2 abnormal hemoglobins that result in the sickling of red cells due to the polymerization of the abnormal deoxyhemoglobin S molecule. The clinical features of the disease then result from chronic hemolysis as well as end organ insult secondary to vasoocclusion and vascular injury. The homozygous hemoglobin SS state is the most common and severe form of SCD, but similar manifestations may occur when the heterozygous hemoglobin S is combined with an alternative hemoglobin abnormality, such as in the conditions of hemoglobin SC (also known as sickle hemoglobin C disease) or hemoglobin S-β-thalassemia.

The common complications of SCD that lead to hospitalization include infection, vasoocclusive crisis (VOC), acute chest syndrome (ACS), stroke, splenic sequestration crisis, aplastic crisis, acute cholecystitis and, rarely, priapism (pain control). A patient with SCD has splenic dysfunction and is therefore at high risk for invasive infection from encapsulated organisms, particularly *Streptococcus pneumoniae*. In addition, there is an increased risk for osteomyelitis from *Salmonella* species and *Staphylococcus aureus*. A patient with SCD is also at increased risk for VOC and ACS after receiving general anesthesia.

Other serious but rare complications include hyperhemolysis, hepatic sequestration, multi-organ failure, ocular compartment syndrome, and subarachnoid hemorrhage.

Clinical Presentation

The presentations of the most common complications of SCD are summarized in Table 42-1 and the serious rare complications in Table 42-2.

History

Ask about the patient's usual blood counts (hemoglobin, white blood cell count, reticulocyte count), chronic medications (penicillin, folate, hydroxyurea), history of ACS, prior transfusions (and the indications), transcranial Doppler results, and the name of the physician (usually a hematologist) managing the SCD.

The patient with an established diagnosis of SCD is often admitted for pain and/or fever. Determine the characteristics of the pain, such as location,

Table 42-1. Presentation of Common Complications	
Diagnosis	**Clinical Features**
Acute chest syndrome	Fever, cough, tachypnea, chest pain Hypoxia New lobar or segmental infiltrate on chest x-ray
Acute cholecystitis Choledocholithiasis	Fever in acute cholecystitis Right upper quadrant abdominal pain Positive Murphy sign
Aplastic crisis	Pallor, fatigue, tachypnea, tachycardia +/- hypotension No increase in spleen size ↓ Hemoglobin (from baseline) with ↓ reticulocytes (<1%–2%)
Bacteremia/sepsis	Fever Toxicity/ill-appearing ↑ White blood cells (compared to baseline)
Osteomyelitis	Fever Bone pain is localized or located at an atypical site
Splenic sequestration	Pallor, fatigue, tachypnea Tachycardia +/- hypotension Left upper quadrant tenderness Increasing palpable splenomegaly from baseline ↓ Hemoglobin (from baseline) with normal or ↑ reticulocytes May also have thrombocytopenia
Stroke	Altered mental status Slurred speech, aphasia Facial droop Unilateral weakness or hemiparesis
Vasoocclusive crisis	Pain at typical or multiple sites +/- Fever (usually <101.5°F)

quality, quantity, radiation, and alleviating and exacerbating factors, and compare to the patient's typical pattern of sickle cell pain. Common locations for VOC pain are the extremities, abdomen, and back, but specifically note the presence of chest pain or any respiratory complaints. In addition, ask about the response to current and previous pain management strategies in both the inpatient and outpatient settings. Note the duration and height of the fever and any measures taken to manage it.

Physical Examination

Priorities on examination are the vital signs, as sepsis is the primary consideration when there is fever higher than 38.5°C. Tachycardia and tachypnea can occur in ACS, aplastic crisis, and splenic sequestration. Look for other signs of ACS (accessory muscle use, adventitious lung sounds), aplastic crisis (heart failure), and splenic sequestration (hypovolemic shock). In addition, tachycardia may be secondary to pain, so recheck the vital signs after appropriate analgesia has been given and reassess the pain frequently.

Table 42-2. Presentation of Rare Serious Complications	
Diagnosis	**Clinical Features**
Hepatic sequestration	Pallor Enlarging liver with right upper quadrant tenderness ↓ Hemoglobin (from baseline) with normal or ↑ reticulocytes
Hyperhemolysis	Causes: RBC transfusion, drugs, infections, G6PD deficiency Pallor Worsening scleral icterus and jaundice ↓ Hemoglobin (from baseline) with normal or ↑ reticulocytes Increased LDH from baseline
Multi-organ failure	Confusion (non-focal encephalopathy) Fever Rapid decrease in hemoglobin and platelet count Increasing AST, ALT, LDH, bilirubin, and creatinine Failure of lungs, liver or kidneys
Ocular compartment syndrome (orbital bone infarct)	Eye pain Proptosis
Subarachnoid hemorrhage	Severe headache Altered mental status

Abbreviations: ALT, alanine transaminase; AST, aspartate transaminase; G6PD, glucose-6-phosphate dehydrogenase; LDH, lactate dehydrogenase; RBC, red blood cell.

Compare the degree of scleral icterus, jaundice, splenomegaly, and location(s) of bone pain to the patient's baseline or typical findings. Examine the abdomen for tenderness, distension, organomegaly (spleen and liver), and tenderness over the gallbladder.

Laboratory

Obtain a complete blood cell count and reticulocyte count and compare to the patient's usual values, looking for leukocytosis (compared to the patient's typical baseline), worsening anemia, or bone marrow suppression. Order electrolytes, creatinine, liver function tests, and C-reactive protein (CRP) if indicated by clinical findings.

If the patient has a temperature higher than 38.5°C, also order a blood culture, urinalysis, and urine culture (all females and males <12 months of age). Obtain a chest x-ray if the patient has lower respiratory symptoms and/or chest pain. When osteomyelitis is a diagnostic consideration, order a CRP and erythrocyte sedimentation rate, and consider magnetic resonance imaging (MRI) of the bone.

If there are concerns for a stroke, arrange an MRI/magnetic resonance angiogram (MRA) emergently if the patient is stable enough to tolerate the procedure. However, do not delay treatment if a stroke is suspected clinically. Consider computed tomography of the head if an MRI/MRA is not available.

When transfusion might be needed (aplastic crisis, splenic sequestration, ACS, stroke), obtain blood typing that includes minor antigens C, D, E, and Kell. Confirm that the blood used for transfusions is sickle negative, leukocyte reduced and, if possible, matched for the selected minor antigens.

Differential Diagnosis

A patient may present with an acute disease that is unrelated to the SCD, such as appendicitis or asthma. Always maintain a broad differential diagnosis and do not assume that the patient's complaints are secondary to the SCD.

The most common diagnostic challenge involves the combination of pain and fever. Depending on location of the pain, the differential diagnosis includes infection, VOC, ACS, and osteomyelitis. While both VOC and osteomyelitis present with pain and swelling in the affected bone(s), the pain of osteomyelitis tends to localize to a single site that may represent an atypical location for the patient.

Chest pain associated with fever, cough, wheezing, and tachypnea suggests ACS. A new lobar or segmental infiltrate is required to confirm the diagnosis.

Rule out other potentially life-threatening complications, such as aplastic crisis, hyperhemolysis, and splenic or hepatic sequestration. Pallor, fatigue, tachycardia, and tachypnea occur with aplastic crisis and splenic sequestration. Left upper quadrant abdominal pain can occur with splenic sequestration, while right upper quadrant is seen with cholelithiasis, choledocholithiasis, pancreatitis (from gallstones), or hepatic sequestration.

Neurologic complaints such as change in mental status, facial droop, lateralized weakness, aphasia, or slurred speech may occur with a stroke.

Treatment

Fever/Presumed Sepsis

For the febrile (>38.5°C) patient, give parenteral antibiotics that cover *S pneumoniae* immediately after blood cultures are obtained. Do not delay initiating therapy while awaiting laboratory results. Treat with cefotaxime (150 mg/kg/day intravenous [IV] divided every 8 hours, 6 g/day maximum) *or* ceftriaxone (100 mg/kg/day IV divided every 12 hours, 4 g/day maximum) *or* ampicillin/sulbactam (100 mg/kg/day of ampicillin divided every 6 hours, 8 mg/day maximum) as per local susceptibilities. If the patient has a known cephalosporin or penicillin allergy use clindamycin (40 mg/kg/day IV divided every 6 hours, 4.8 g/day maximum). If the patient is ill appearing or a central nervous system infection is suspected add vancomycin (10–15 mg/kg IV every 6 hours, 4 g/day maximum).

Vasoocclusive Crisis

Since a patient admitted for VOC has not responded to home and/or outpatient pain management, use IV opioids by patient-controlled analgesia (PCA), continuous infusion, or scheduled interval dosing with rescue doses available for breakthrough pain. Titrate the dose to an adequate therapeutic response, which ideally is a minimum of a 50% reduction in pain on the visual scale. Never initiate as-needed dosing alone for a patient with a VOC. A patient with previous opioid exposure may require higher than usual doses of opiates.

The preferred method is PCA, once a child is able to understand that pushing the button decreases pain. For most patients this is by 6 years of age. A typical morphine PCA regimen starts with a total dose of 0.05 to 0.2 mg/kg/hour. The usual basal (continuous) rate is one-third to one-half of this total hourly dose. Calculate the PCA dose (demand) by using the remainder of the total hourly dose and dividing it by the number of total potential doses (6–10) available over an hour. For example, using 0.1 mg/kg/hour as the hourly dose, start with a basal rate of 0.033 mg/kg/hour with 0.0067 mg/kg PCA dose permitted every 6 minutes. Therefore, for a 25-kg patient, the continuous rate is 0.8 mg/hour with 0.17-mg PCA doses (up to 10 in 1 hour). Note that the PCA dose refers to the patient-controlled dose and has many synonyms, including intermittent dose, interval dose, interval bolus, and demand dose.

Reevaluate the patient frequently. Additional physician-ordered rescue doses (0.05 mg/kg every 30 minutes) may be needed until the pain is adequately controlled. Readjust the basal and PCA doses every 12 to 24 hours, basing any changes on the total amount of morphine given to control the pain over that period. Consider increasing the basal rate if the patient demands more than 3 PCA doses per hour and decreasing the basal rate if the patient appears over-sedated. When the pain is well-controlled for 24 hours and the patient is using less than 3 PCA doses per hour, begin weaning by decreasing the basal dose by 10% to 20% as tolerated.

For a patient unable to use PCA, order either a continuous morphine infusion (0.05–0.1 mg/kg/hour) or scheduled interval dosing (0.05–0.15 mg/kg every 2–4 hours). Treat breakthrough pain with 25% to 50% of the interval dose every 20 to 30 minutes, as needed. Readjust the dose based on the total amount of medication needed to control the pain over time. In some cases a morphine rate greater than 0.1 mg/kg/hour may be needed, but this requires careful monitoring for respiratory depression by assessing the respiratory rate, level of sedation, and pulse oximetry. If possible, manage opioid-associated respiratory failure with ventilatory support (bag-valve-mask). The use of naloxone (0.4 mL/dose) may be life-saving in treating respiratory failure, but it will also reverse pain control. When the pain is well-controlled for 24 hours, begin weaning by decreasing the infusion or scheduled dosing by 10% to 20%.

Aggressively treat the side effects of opioids. Manage nausea with metoclopramide (0.1–0.2 mg/kg every 6–8 hours IV/oral [PO], 10 mg/dose maximum) or ondansetron (0.05–0.1 mg/kg IV or PO every 6 hours as needed, 4 mg/dose maximum). Treat pruritus with either diphenhydramine (5 mg/kg/day divided every 6 hours or 0.5 mg/kg every 2 hours, 300 mg/day maximum) or hydroxyzine (2 mg/kg/day divided every 8 hours; 50 mg/day maximum <6 years, 100 mg/day maximum >6 years, 600 mg/day maximum for adults), or change to hydromorphone (0.015–0.02 mg/kg IV every 3–4 hours). Start a bowel regimen (stool softeners, docusate, polyethylene glycol) if multiple opiate doses are anticipated.

IV ketorolac (0.5 mg/kg IV every 6 hours, 30 mg/dose maximum) is a useful adjunct if there are no contraindications (gastritis, ulcer, coagulopathy, renal impairment). Do not use for more than 5 days.

Begin the transition to oral opioids, at an equianalgesic dosing (See Pain Management, page 661) when the pain is well-controlled, the IV morphine dose has been weaned to 0.25 mg/kg/hour or less, and patient has normal gastrointestinal functioning (able to eat and drink without being nauseated). One approach is to first convert the basal rate to the equivalent dose of a long-acting oral opioid, then 24 hours later convert the PCA dose to an equivalent short-acting oral opioid.

To prevent withdrawal symptoms for a patient whose pain has resolved, but has been receiving opioids for 10 days or more, first taper the opioid dose by 10% to 20% over 5 to 7 days. Then, over the next 3 to 5 days, increase the interval from every 6 hours to every 12 hours to every day.

Supportive therapy includes the correction of any fluid deficit dehydration as well as providing maintenance fluid (IV and/or PO). There is no evidence that the increased hydration is helpful, and over-hydration can lead to fluid overload. Provide oxygen as needed to maintain oxygen saturation at 92% or higher. Also order incentive spirometry (10 breaths every 2 hours when awake) to prevent ACS. Other comfort measures include heating pads and relaxation techniques.

Acute Chest Syndrome

Manage pain aggressively (as above), add azithromycin (10 mg/kg PO day 1 [500 mg maximum]; 5 mg/kg every day for 4 more days [250 mg maximum]) to the antibiotic regimen described for fever (as above), and provide oxygen to maintain oxygen saturation 92% or higher. If there is wheezing or rales, add nebulized albuterol (<30 kg: 2.5 mg, >30 kg: 5 mg, every 4–6 hours), methylprednisolone 1 mg/kg every 12 hours (80 mg/dose maximum), and gastrointestinal prophylaxis with ranitidine (2–6 mg/kg/day intramuscular/IV divided every 6–8 hours, 50 mg/dose maximum). Repeat the hemoglobin every 12 hours until stable.

If the patient has worsening respiratory symptoms, such as decreased air movement, inspiratory and expiratory wheezing, increasing use of accessory muscles, increasing oxygen requirements, and a hemoglobin decrease of 1 g/dL or greater, consult with a hematologist to consider a simple transfusion to a goal hemoglobin of 9 to 10 g/dL and transfer the patient to an intensive care unit (ICU). Continued or rapid changes in respiratory status are indications for an exchange transfusion or erythrocytophoresis.

Acute Stroke

Admit the patient to an ICU and consult with a hematologist to arrange emergent exchange transfusion or erythrocytophoresis. The goal is to increase hemoglobin to about 10 g/dL and decrease the hemoglobin S to less than 30%. Do not delay transfusion therapy while obtaining imaging studies, and give oxygen while awaiting the procedure. See pages 441–444 for the general management of a stroke.

Splenic Sequestration

The goal of treatment is to prevent the rapid progression of hypovolemic shock while awaiting the release of the blood trapped in the spleen. Transfer the patient to an ICU, consult with a hematologist, initiate a fluid resuscitation (if needed), and order a packed red blood cell (RBC) transfusion of 5 to 10 mL/kg over 4 hours. Aim for a posttransfusion hemoglobin of less than 9 g/dL to prevent hyperviscosity, as once the sequestered blood is returned from the spleen the hemoglobin may increase by another 1 to 2 g/L.

Aplastic Crisis

The goal of therapy is to prevent cardiovascular compromise secondary to the worsening anemia. If stable, monitor closely and provide IV and PO hydration at maintenance until blood is available. Transfuse 5 mL/kg of packed RBCs over 4 hours. If the patient is not stable, admit to an ICU and initiate a fluid resuscitation while awaiting the transfusion. Assume that the patient has a parvoviral infection (pending serologies) and institute appropriate isolation policies.

Priapism

The goals of care are to control the pain (as above) and prevent ischemic damage. This requires close consultation with both a urologist and a hematologist. Corporal aspiration, with or without irrigation, is indicated for persistent priapism lasting more than 4 hours.

Acute Cholecystitis

The treatment is the same as for a patient without SCD (page 193). Arrange a surgery consult, provide analgesia, and give antibiotic coverage for gram-negative bacilli and anaerobes. Although urgent surgery may be necessary for worsening pain and fever, cholecystectomy is usually done electively after resolution of the acute episode.

Rare Complications

Immediately consult with a hematologist if the patient has one of the rare complications listed in Table 42-2. The critical challenge for the hospitalist is to recognize these rare problems as they develop in a patient with SCD admitted for another reason.

Patient Requiring General Anesthesia

Order incentive spirometry and perioperative oxygen. Also give a transfusion to raise the hemoglobin to at least 10 g/dL to minimize the risk of VOC or ACS.

Indications for Consultation

- **Hematology:** ACS, splenic sequestration, acute aplastic crisis, hyperhemolysis, priapism, possible cerebral vascular accident
- **Neurology:** Possible cerebral vascular accident
- **Ophthalmology:** Orbital compartment syndrome
- **Surgery:** Consideration of cholecystectomy for gall bladder disease
- **Urology:** Priapism lasting more than 4 hours

Disposition

- **ICU transfer:** Septic shock, ACS requiring respiratory support, ongoing cerebral vascular accident, need for exchange transfusion
- **Discharge criteria:** Septicemia excluded (afebrile and negative blood cultures), pain adequately managed by oral medications, ongoing complications (ACS, cerebral vascular accident, etc) stable and no longer require inpatient interventions.

Follow-up

- **Primary care:** 1 to 2 weeks
- **Sickle cell center:** 1 week

Pearls and Pitfalls

- Care coordination between the inpatient and outpatient setting in conjunction with a sickle cell center is essential for the best long-term outcome in a patient with SCD.
- Be careful with fluid administration, as a patient in a chronic high output state due to anemia is susceptible to fluid overload and pulmonary edema. This can be very difficult to differentiate from ACS.
- As with any immunosuppressed patient, the child's appearance may belie the serious clinical situation.
- If possible, transfuse with minor antigen matched (C, D, E, Kell), sickle negative, leukocyte depleted, packed RBCs.
- A packed RBC transfusion of 10 mL/kg typically raises the hemoglobin by 2 g/dL.
- Do not transfuse to a hemoglobin greater than 11 g/dL, which may then result in hyperviscosity.
- Opioid-induced sedation precedes respiratory depression.

Coding

ICD-9

• ACS	**517.3**
• Hg SS with crisis	**282.62**
• Hg SS without crisis	**282.61**
• Priapism	**607.3**
• Sickle cell/Hg C with crisis	**282.64**
• Sickle cell/Hg C without crisis	**282.63**
• Sickle cell-thalassemia with crisis	**282.42**
• Sickle cell-thalassemia without crisis	**282.41**
• Splenic sequestration	**289.52**

Bibliography

Berger E, Saunders N, Wang L, Friedman JN. Sickle cell disease in children: differentiating osteomyelitis from vaso-occlusive crisis. *Arch Pediatr Adolesc Med.* 2009;163:251–255

Caboot JB, Allen JL. Pulmonary complications of sickle cell disease in children. *Curr Opin Pediatr.* 2008;20:279–287

Crabtree EA, Mariscalco MM, Hesselgrave J, et al. Improving care for children with sickle cell disease/acute chest syndrome. *Pediatrics.* 2011;127:e480–e488

Heeney M, Dover GJ. Sickle cell disease. In: Orkin S, et al, eds. *Nathan and Oski's Hematology of Infancy and Childhood.* 7th ed. Philadelphia, PA: Saunders; 2008:950–1014

Lane PA, Buchanan GR, Hutter JJ, et al. Sickle cell disease in children and adolescents: diagnosis, guidelines for comprehensive care, and care paths and protocols for management of acute and chronic complications. http://www.dshs.state.tx.us/newborn/pdf/sedona02.pdf

New England Pediatric Sickle Cell Consortium. Management of acute pain in pediatric patients with sickle cell disease (vaso-occlusive episodes). http://www.nepscc.org/NewFiles/CPG%20Pain%203-09.pdf

Stuart MJ, Setty BN. Acute chest syndrome of sickle cell disease: new light on an old problem. *Curr Opin Hematol.* 2001;8:111–122

Immunology

CHAPTER 43

Immunodeficiency

Introduction

Infections are the most common diseases in childhood. In fact, a normal infant may have 5 to 10 minor infections per year during the first 2 years of life. Most patients with recurrent or severe infections will have atypical manifestations of common conditions, and a patient with recurrent infections in the same location of the body is most likely to have an anatomical abnormality. However, certain patterns of disease may be markers for primary or secondary disorders of the immune system (Table 43-1).

Primary immunodeficiencies (PI) are genetic diseases that can affect any part of the immune system and predispose a patient to recurrent infections, malignancies, and autoimmune diseases. There are some typical patterns of age of onset, infectious organism(s), and site(s) of infection for each type (Table 43-2). However, disease severity and age of onset may vary substantially within a diagnostic category.

Secondary, or acquired immune deficiencies (Table 43-3), are much more common and must be considered in a patient with frequent infections. They may result from infections, autoimmune disorders, malignancies, immunoglobulin (Ig) loss, leukopenia, suppression of the inflammatory response, malnutrition, asplenia, diabetes, and inborn errors of metabolism.

Clinical Presentation

History

Obtain a thorough history, including the age of onset and locations of the infections, types of organisms, and need for intravenous (IV) antibiotic therapy. Defects in antibody production typically present with sinopulmonary infections once transplacental maternal antibody levels decline in a patient who is otherwise thriving. Combined T and B cell defects present early in infancy with failure to thrive (FTT), diarrhea, rash, opportunistic infections, and pneumonia. Phagocytic defects typically present in infancy to early adulthood as skin, lymph node, and organ abscesses, and pneumonia. C3 deficiencies may present early in life similar to antibody defects, while late component deficiencies (C5–C9) predispose older children and young adults to recurrent *Neisseria* infections.

Table 43-1. Clinical Indications for an Immune Deficiency Evaluation

Indication	Examples
Autoimmune phenomena	Systemic or cutaneous lupus Glomerulonephritis Autoimmune endocrinopathies
Chronic diarrhea	Infectious enteritis *(Cryptosporidium, Giardia)* Protein-losing enteropathy
Complications from live vaccines	Paralytic polio after live oral polio vaccine Disseminated BCG infection
Family history of immune deficiency	Autosomal dominant: hyper-IgE X-linked: SCID, CGD
Frequent infections	>8 infections in 12 months >2 sinus infections or pneumonias in 12 months
Infections refractory to treatment	Persistent thrush after 6 months of age Persistent or recurrent verrucae Poor response to conventional antibiotic therapy
Infections with unusual organisms	Atypical *Mycobacterium, Pneumocystis jiroveci*
Unusual locations of infection	Liver abscess
Unusually severe/invasive infections	Life-threatening disseminated CMV Prolonged and severe molluscum contagiosum, *Cryptosporidium parvum,* and *Candida*

Abbreviations: BCG, bacilli Calmette-Guérin; CGD, chronic granulomatous disease; CMV, cytomegalovirus; Ig, immunoglobulin; SCID, severe combined immunodeficiency.

Assess the patient's growth pattern and document vaccine status, as well as whether there have been any severe or unusual adverse reactions to live vaccines. Check the family history for any recurrent infections or known immunodeficiency. Finally, document all previous culture and serologic results.

A PI can also present with autoimmune disease or malignancy. Some patients with common variable immune deficiency (CVID) develop immune thrombocytopenic purpura prior to any infections. Some PIs, such as autoimmune lymphoproliferative syndrome and X-linked proliferative syndrome, are predominantly immune dysregulation, presenting with fever, adenopathy, and hepatosplenomegaly.

Physical Examination

Perform a complete physical examination (Table 43-4), paying special attention to any rash (including the diaper area); evidence of previous or current skin infections or abscess; thrush; the lack of tonsils or palpable lymph nodes (especially in the neck and groin); and signs of otitis media, sinusitis, or pneumonia. Clubbing can be seen with recurrent pneumonias and subsequent bronchiectasis and respiratory failure. Plot the child's growth curves and review for FTT.

Presentation	Defects	Examples	Organisms	Onset	Initial Laboratory
Recurrent sinopulmonary infections (sinusitis, otitis media, pneumonia), diarrhea	Antibody deficiencies	XLA, IgA deficiency, CVID	Encapsulated bacteria, *Giardia lamblia*	After 6–9 months	Ig levels (IgA, IgG, IgM)
FTT, rash, thrush, pneumonia, opportunistic infections	Combined defects	SCID, DiGeorge, Wiskott-Aldridge, hyper-IgM due to CD40 ligand	Adenovirus, *Candida*, CMV, EBV, *Pneumocystis jiroveci*, parainflu-enza, varicella	Infancy	Ig levels T, B, NK cells
Skin or solid organ abscesses, pneumonia, dental infections	Phagocytic defects	CGD, LAD, hyper-IgE syndrome	*Burkholderia cepacia*, *Aspergillus*, *Nocardia*, *Serratia*, *Staphylococcus*	Infancy to young adult	CBC, IgE, CGD assay
Sinopulmonary infections, glomerulo-nephritis	Complement defects	C3, membrane attack Complex, regulatory components	Encapsulated bacteria, especially *Streptococcus pneumoniae* and *Neisseria*	Infancy to young adult	CH50
Mucocutaneous fungal infections, mycobacterial multifocal osteomyelitis, MAC	Cellular deficiencies	Chronic mucocutaneous candidiasis, IFN-γ/IL-12 receptor deficiency	*Candida*, *Mycobacterium*, *Salmonella*	Young child to adolescent	IFN-γ level, DTH for *Candida*

Table 43-2. Primary Immune Deficiencies

Abbreviations: CBC, complete blood cell count; CGD, chronic granulomatous disease; CMV, cytomegalovirus; CVID, common variable immune deficiency, DTH, delayed type hypersensitivity; EBV, Epstein-Barr virus; FTT, failure to thrive; IFN, interferon; Ig, immunoglobulin; LAD, leukocyte adhesion defect; MAC, *Mycobacterium avium* complex; SCID, severe combined immune deficiency; XLA, X-Linked agammaglobulinemia.

Laboratory

The types of infection(s) guide the initial laboratory testing (Table 43-1). For any patient with a suspected primary immune deficiency, obtain a complete blood cell count (CBC) with differential, HIV screen, comprehensive metabolic panel, and quantitative Ig (IgA, IgG, IgM, and IgE) *prior* to consulting an immunologist. Consider cystic fibrosis testing (sweat chloride) if the patient has had frequent sinopulmonary

Table 43-3. Secondary Causes of Immune Deficiency

Autoimmune diseases	JIA, SLE
Infections	HIV, CMV
Immune suppressants	Corticosteroids, chemotherapy, monoclonal antibodies
Malignancies	Leukemia Lymphoma
Immunoglobulin loss	Nephrotic syndrome Protein-losing enteropathy
Asplenia	Sickle cell disease Post-surgical
Malnutrition	Protein deficiency Vitamins A and D deficiency Zinc deficiency
Other	Cirrhosis Cystic fibrosis Diabetes mellitus Inborn errors of metabolism Primary ciliary dyskinesia Uremia

Abbreviations: CMV, cytomegalovirus; HIV, human immunodeficiency virus; JIA, juvenile idiopathic arthritis; SLE, systemic lupus erythematosus.

infections, especially if newborn screening results are not available. Lymphopenia can be a clue for severe combined immunodeficiency (SCID), so a lymphocyte count lower than 3,000/mm^3 in a newborn must be investigated (see below). A low globulin fraction on a metabolic panel suggests decreased Ig levels. Obtain an immunology consult if there is a high index of suspicion or abnormal initial laboratory values. However, if immunology services are not available, pursue further workup as described below.

For recurrent sinopulmonary infections with encapsulated organisms consistent with a B cell defect, order IgA, IgM, and IgG levels, although IgG subclasses are typically not helpful. If the Ig levels are 2 standard deviations below normal for age, order antibody titers (tetanus, diphtheria, pneumococcus) and promptly consult an immunologist. Most laboratories can determine Ig, but confirm that appropriate age-based normal levels are used when interpreting the results.

Suspect a phagocyte deficiency if there are skin, lymph node, or solid organ abscesses, especially with unusual organisms such as *Klebsiella* or *Serratia;* delayed wound healing; cavitary pneumonias; or infections with *Staphylococcus aureus, Burkholderia cepacia, Serratia, Nocardia,* or *Aspergillus.* Order a CBC, peripheral smear for neutrophils, total IgE, and chronic granulomatous disease assay. The dihydrorhodamine oxidative burst assay is preferred over the classic nitroblue tetrazolium. If

Table 43-4. Physical Examination Findings and Associated Immune Deficiencies	
Physical Examination Findings	**Associated Immune Deficiency**
Apthous ulcers	CGD
Ataxia or telangiectasias	Ataxia-telangiectasia
Clubbing	Any immune deficiency leading to recurrent pneumonia or bronchiectasis
Delayed separation of umbilical cord Severe gingivitis	Leukocyte adhesion defect
Failure to thrive	T cell defects (SCID)
Granuloma formation Lymphoid hyperplasia	CGD CVID
Hypertelorism, heart murmur, low set ears, microcephaly, cleft lip and/or palate	DiGeorge syndrome
Lack of tonsils and palpable lymph nodes (especially in the neck and groin)	XLA SCID
Nonspecific rash	SCID
Otitis media/sinusitis findings (perforated or scarred TMs, purulent nasal discharge)	B cell defects (XLA, IgA deficiency, CVID)
Petechiae	Wiskott-Aldrich
Severe diaper dermatitis Persistent or recurrent thrush	T cell defects (SCID, chronic mucocutaneous candidiasis)
Severe eczema	Hyper-IgE syndrome Wiskott-Aldrich
Skin abscess or adenitis (unusual organisms or severe/recurrent with *Staphylococcus aureus*)	Phagocytic defect (CGD)

Abbreviations: CGD, chronic granulomatous disease; CVID, common variable immune deficiency; SCID, severe combined immune deficiency; TM, tympanic membrane; XLA, X-linked agammaglobulinemia.

there is delayed separation of the umbilical cord (after 4–6 weeks of age) and an elevated white blood cell count, order flow cytometry for CD11/CD18, which will be absent in leukocyte adhesion deficiency. Any of these abnormal tests requires prompt consultation.

If an infant has a lymphocyte count less than 3,000 mm^3, an abnormal SCID newborn screen, or a history of opportunistic infections, check the Ig levels along with flow cytometry for T, B, and NK cell enumeration. If these tests are not available locally, send the specimens to a referral laboratory accredited for flow cytometry assessments. Low age-based lymphocyte levels warrant urgent immunology consultation. In an infant with hypocalcemia and heart defects, FISH for chromosome 22q11 will be diagnostic of the DiGeorge deletion, although a positive result is not required for the diagnosis of DiGeorge syndrome.

In a patient with glomerulonephritis and infections, order a CH50 and C3 level for C3 complement deficiency. With recurrent or persistent *Neisseria* infections, order a CH50 to evaluate for terminal complement deficiencies. If this is normal, an alternate pathway AH50 will assess other defects, such as Factor B, D, or properdin. Make sure the samples are sent on ice to avoid a falsely low CH50.

A patient with a PI can be predisposed to infectious or inflammatory diarrhea. Obtain stool studies for culture, *Clostridium difficile, Giardia,* and other ova and parasites for any PI patient with diarrhea.

Differential Diagnosis

Consider an immune deficiency in any patient with frequent infections, unusually severe infections, or infections with atypical organisms.

A patient can have a secondary immune deficiency or a structural or allergic disease that predisposes to frequent infections. Since new cases of HIV continue to occur, order an HIV screen prior to initiating a complex workup. HIV can present in a similar manner as SCID with FTT, rashes, thrush, pneumonia, and opportunistic infections. However, it will generally manifest later in life, as it may take several years for CD4 counts to drop to levels associated with AIDS.

Recurrent benign viral infections are rarely a presentation of an immune deficiency and do not warrant specialized testing. FTT without associated infections (especially opportunistic infections or pneumonia) is rarely the result of PI. Eczema is typically associated with allergic diseases, so consider PI only if there is associated thrombocytopenia, infections, or ectodermal dysplasia (abnormal shedding of primary teeth, propensity to fractures). Sickle cell disease (SCD; page 267) can mimic PI with osteomyelitis and bacteremia. A patient with asplenia (congenital, due to surgical splenectomy, or as a result of another illness such as SCD) can develop infections with encapsulated organisms with resulting bacteremia and sepsis. A patient with recurrent upper and lower respiratory tract infections could have atopic disease or primary ciliary dyskinesia.

Treatment

A patient with a phagocytic defect, combined T/B cell immunodeficiency, or severe hypogammaglobulinemia (X-linked agammaglobulinemia, hyper-IgM, CVID) will typically require admission and aggressive IV antibiotic therapy for a prolonged course (2–4 weeks or longer). See Table 43-5 for appropriate antibiotic choices, but use doses that are on the high end of the typical regimens as found in *Nelson's Pediatric Antimicrobial Therapy* (www.aaporg/nelsonsabx), or elsewhere in this book. If possible, try to get a definitive diagnosis (via cultures, bronchoscopy, etc) to guide therapy. The patient will often need a central line catheter for several weeks, but avoid permanent indwelling access devices as they significantly increase the long-term infection risk.

Suspected SCID is an emergency. Immediately consult with an immunologist if lymphocyte studies are low (see above). SCID patients are at risk for graft versus host disease and must be given irradiated, cytomegalovirus-negative blood products. For a patient with suspected SCID or complete lack of Ig, give IVIG (400–500 mg/kg) and repeat in 1 to 3 days and then monthly. If possible, obtain the appropriate antibody studies before starting IgG therapy.

A patient with PI is at high risk for malignancies and autoimmune diseases. Autoimmune hemolytic anemia, thrombocytopenia, and neutropenia are frequently seen with CVID, hyper-IgM syndrome, and other PIs. Consult both immunology and hematology as the patient may need steroids, high-dose IVIG, or rituximab.

A patient with complete IgA deficiency may have anti-IgA antibodies, which can rarely lead to anaphylactic reactions to IVIG and other blood products. Order washed red cells and IVIG with a low IgA content, but no other special precautions are required.

Table 43-5. Antibiotic Therapy for Immune-Deficient Patients[a]

Defects	Organisms	Typical Antibiotics
Antibody deficiencies	Encapsulated bacteria	Ceftriaxone or levofloxacin
Combined defects	Adenovirus, *Candida*, EBV, CMV, parainfluenza virus, *Pneumocystis jiroveci*, varicella	TMP/SMX *plus* vancomycin *plus* extended β-lactam (meropenem, piperacillin/tazobactam, cefipime, etc) Consider fluconazole and macrolide
Phagocytic defects	*Aspergillus, Burkholderia cepacia, Nocardia, Serratia, Staphylococcus*	Voriconazole *plus* ([TMP/SMX *plus* fluoroquinolone] *or* meropenem) Add vancomycin if *Staphylococcus* likely
Complement	Encapsulated bacteria, *Neisseria*	Same as antibody defects
Cellular deficiencies	*Candida, Mycobacterium, Salmonella*	Ceftriaxone Fluconazole Triple therapy for *Mycobacterium*

Abbreviations: CMV, cytomegalovirus; EBV, Epstein-Barr virus; SMX, sulfamethoxazole; TMP, trimethoprim.
[a]See specific chapters on infectious diseases for dosing guidelines.

Indications for Consultation

- **Immunology:** Abnormal immune laboratory tests or opportunistic infection
- **Infectious diseases:** Complex or opportunistic infection
- **Pulmonologist:** Chronic pulmonary infections, bronchiectasis

Disposition

- **Intensive care unit transfer:** Septic shock, respiratory failure
- **Discharge criteria:** Afebrile 48 hours or longer with appropriate treatment of acute infection underway

Follow-up

- **Primary care:** 1 week
- **Immunology or infectious diseases (if involved):** 2 to 4 weeks

Pearls and Pitfalls

- Admit a patient with severe immune deficiency and temperature of 101°F (38.3°C) or obvious infection and promptly initiate IV antibiotics. A much longer than typical course of IV antibiotics will be necessary.
- Obtain appropriate cultures as quickly as possible.
- Evaluate a patient presenting with parotitis for HIV.
- Complete the laboratory evaluation (quantitative Ig, vaccine and isohemagglutinin titers, and T/B cell testing) prior to treatment with Ig.
- Initiate proper isolation precautions, especially for a patient with suspected SCID.
- If a patient with IgA deficiency is given Ig, monitor closely for anaphylaxis.
- Suspect SCID in an infant with a lymphocyte count lower than 3,000/mm^3.

Coding

ICD-9

- Chronic granulomatous disease **288.1**
- Common variable immunodeficiency **279.06**
- Complement deficiency **279.8**
- DiGeorge syndrome **279.11**
- Hypogammaglobulinemia **279.00**
- IgA deficiency **279.01**
- Immune deficiency unspecified **279.3**

- SCID **279.2**
- XLA **279.04**

Bibliography

Ballow M. Approach to the patient with recurrent infections. *Clin Rev Allergy Immunol.* 2008;34:129–140

Buckley RH, ed. *Diagnostic and Clinical Care Guidelines for Primary Immunodeficiency Diseases.* 2nd ed. Towson, MD: Immune Deficiency Foundation; 2009:1–23. http://209.251.35.238/publications/book_diag/IDFDiagnosticandClinicalCare Guidelines_2ndEdition.pdf

Cassimos DC, Liatsis M, Stogiannidou A, Kanariou MG. Children with frequent infections: a proposal for a stepwise assessment and investigation of the immune system. *Pediatr Allergy Immunol.* 2010;21:463–473

Chinen J, Shearer WT. 6. Secondary immunodeficiencies, including HIV infection. *J Allergy Clin Immunol.* 2008;121(2 suppl):S388–S392

Notarangelo LD. Primary immunodeficiencies. *J Allergy Clin Immunol.* 2010;125: S182–S194

Oliveira J, Thomas A. Fleisher T. Laboratory evaluation of primary immunodeficiencies. *J Allergy Clin Immunol.* 2010;125:S297–S305

Slatter MA, Gennery AR. Clinical immunology review series: an approach to the patient with recurrent infections in childhood. *Clin Exp Immunol.* 2008;152:389–396

Subbarayan A, Colarusso G, Hughes SM, et al. Clinical features that identify children with primary immunodeficiency diseases. *Pediatrics.* 2011;127:810–816

Infectious Diseases

Fever in Infants Younger Than 60 Days

Introduction

In an infant younger than 60 days, fever is defined as a rectal temperature of 38°C (100.4°F) or higher. In this age group, fever may be the only sign of a serious bacterial infection (SBI). Meningitis, bacteremia, and urinary tract infections (UTIs) (most common SBI) are traditionally classified as SBIs, while some studies include other infections such as pneumonia, bacterial gastroenteritis, osteomyelitis, and skin and soft tissue infections. The prevalence of SBI in this age group is estimated to be 5% to 10%, although an infant younger than 28 days is at particular risk. Common organisms encountered in the first 60 days of life include group B *Streptococcus* (GBS), *Escherichia coli* and, uncommonly, *Listeria monocytogenes*.

Clinical Presentation

History

Ask about temperature at home and how it was taken; birth history; maternal infection risks (including herpes simplex virus [HSV] and GBS); underlying medical conditions; level of fussiness or irritability; feeding habits; lethargy; change in respiratory status; vomiting and bowel habits; urine output; rashes; immunization history; exposure to ill contacts; the use of antipyretics; and history of recent travel, immigration, or homelessness.

Of note, axillary and tympanic membrane temperatures are unreliable. However, consider a patient who reportedly had a documented fever at home, but is afebrile on presentation, to be febrile to the degree reported by history.

Physical Examination

The physical examination may be unremarkable, but always evaluate the vital signs and overall appearance. Concerning signs include irritability, lethargy, hypotonia, grunting, bulging fontanelle, tachypnea, apnea, mottled skin, cyanosis, poor capillary refill, and jaundice. Meningeal signs are typically absent in an infant younger than 2 months. Vesicular lesions involving the skin, eye, or mouth can be seen in HSV.

Laboratory

The extent of laboratory workup is age-based and somewhat controversial. Several criteria sets (Boston, Philadelphia, Rochester) have been developed to risk-stratify febrile infants (Table 44-1), but all have important limitations. Choose the guideline to follow *before* performing the laboratory tests and not after the results are obtained. For example, the Boston and Philadelphia criteria require cerebrospinal fluid (CSF) studies, so if the lumbar puncture is unsuccessful, the patient must be classified as high risk.

For *all* febrile patients younger than 60 days, obtain a complete blood cell count with differential; blood culture; and catheterized or suprapubic urinalysis, urine Gram stain, and culture. Obtain a chest radiograph if the patient has a respiratory rate greater than 60 breaths per minute or respiratory signs or symptoms. If there is persistent watery, mucoid, or bloody stool, order a stool for culture and white blood cell count. If HSV is a concern send liver function tests; HSV CSF polymerase chain reaction (PCR); and oropharyngeal, conjunctival, and rectal swabs as well as urine for culture.

Table 44-1. Summary of Low-Risk Criteria

	Rochester	Philadelphia	Boston
Age	≤60 days	29–60 days	28–89 days
Appearance	Well	Well	Well
WBC	5–15,000	<15,000	<20,000
CSF	N/A	<8 WBC/hpf	<10 WBC/hpf
Urine	≤10 WBC/hpf	<10 WBC/hpf Urine Gram stain negative	UA <10 WBC/hpf
Stool	≤5 WBC/hpf (if indicated)	No blood or few/no WBC (if indicated)	N/A
Chest x-ray	N/A	Negative (if obtained)	Negative (if obtained)
Other		Band-neutrophil <0.2	

Abbreviations: hpf, high-power field; N/A, not applicable; UA, urinalysis; WBC, white blood cell count.

Differential Diagnosis

The differential diagnosis includes both infectious and noninfectious etiologies. Viral, bacterial, and fungal infections may be acquired vertically or horizontally. The most common etiologies include viruses such as enteroviruses, rhinoviruses, and respiratory syncytial virus.

Of note, approximately three-quarters of infants who contract HSV infection were born to women who had no history or clinical findings suggestive of genital HSV infection during or preceding pregnancy. Consider HSV in a patient with CSF pleocytosis (Table 44-2). Elevated CSF protein may also suggest HSV infection.

Table 44-2. 95th Percentile for Cerebrospinal Fluid (CSF) White Blood Cell Count (WBC)[a]	
Age	**CSF WBC**
0–28 days	19/mcL
29–56 days	9/mcL

[a]Adapted from Kestenbaum LA, Ebberson J, Zorc JJ, et al. Defining cerebrospinal fluid white blood cell count reference values in neonates and young infants. *Pediatrics*. 2010;125:257–264.

Other rare, infectious etiologies in this population include focal abscesses, cellulitis, omphalitis, osteomyelitis, pertussis, malignancy, and non-accidental trauma.

Treatment

0 to 28 Days of Life

This age group generally requires inpatient admission and empiric intravenous (IV) antibiotics, since low-risk criteria are not as reliable in this age group. Treat with the combination of IV ampicillin (50 mg/kg/dose every 6 hours) *and either* IV gentamicin (full-term neonates 0–7 days of age with normal renal function: 2.5 mg/kg every 12 hours, >7 days 2.5 mg/kg every 8 hours) *or* a third-generation cephalosporin (cefotaxime 50 mg/kg IV every 12 hours <7 days every 6–8 hours >7 days *or* ceftriaxone 50 mg/kg IV/intramuscular every 12 hours). Ceftriaxone is contraindicated if the patient has hyperbilirubinemia or is receiving an IV calcium-containing solution. If the patient has either a CSF pleocytosis or evidence of a soft tissue infection in a community with a significant prevalence of methicillin-resistant *Staphylococcus aureus* (MRSA), give vancomycin (15–20 mg/kg IV every 8–12 hours) *and* a third-generation cephalosporin (as above).

If the clinical presentation is concerning for HSV infection (mucocutaneous vesicles, focal neurologic symptoms, apnea, seizures, lethargy, irritability, hypothermia, CSF pleocytosis, and/or elevated liver transaminases), treat empirically with IV acyclovir (20 mg/kg IV every 8 hours) pending diagnostic studies.

29 to 60 Days of Life

Treat a high-risk patient with a third-generation cephalosporin (as above) pending results of the blood, CSF, and urine cultures. Carefully observe a low-risk infant and start antibiotics if the clinical picture deteriorates (worsening lethargy, irritability, or respiratory distress). Add IV ampicillin (as above) if the patient is ill-appearing or has findings suggestive of a UTI to ensure coverage for *Enterococcus*. As with infants 29 days of age or younger, use vancomycin *and* a third-generation cephalosporin to treat a CSF pleocytosis or evidence of a soft tissue infection in a community with a significant prevalence of MRSA.

Although a patient with clinical bronchiolitis and/or a positive respiratory virus test is at reduced risk for SBI, the risk is not zero. For such a patient 29 to 60 days of age, obtain at least a urine culture, as concurrent UTIs do occur. If the patient is ill-appearing, perform a full sepsis workup regardless of the pulmonary findings and positive respiratory viral testing.

Indications for Consultation

- **Infectious diseases:** Meningitis, HSV infection, abscess, or atypical presentation and/or clinical course

Disposition

- **Intensive care unit transfer:** Hemodynamic instability despite IV fluids and antibiotics or significant respiratory distress, apnea, or seizures
- **Discharge criteria:** Well-appearing, good oral intake, and negative cultures for at least 48 hours.

Follow-up

- **Primary care:** 2 to 3 days

Pearls and Pitfalls

- Birth via cesarean section does not eliminate the risk of neonatal HSV.
- HSV CSF PCR may be negative during the first few days of the illness. Treat empirically and obtain serial CSF testing if there is a high degree of clinical suspicion for HSV.
- Consider enterovirus testing if the patient has a CSF pleocytosis during the warmer months.
- The presence of blood in the CSF is not significantly associated with the rate of HSV meningoencephalitis.
- Persistent fever despite standard empiric antibiotic coverage is most likely secondary to a viral infection and not an atypical bacterial disease.
- Non-accidental trauma can be a cause of fever.

Coding

ICD-9

- Fever (after 29th day of life) **780.60**
- Neonatal fever **778.4**
- Neonatal bacteremia **771.83**
- Neonatal sepsis **771.81**
- Neonatal UTI **771.82**
- Other infections of the neonatal period **771.89**

Bibliography

Gómez B, Mintegi S, Benito J, et al. Blood culture and bacteremia predictors in infants less than three months of age with fever without source. *Pediatr Infect Dis J.* 2010;29:43–47

Hui C, Neto G, Tsertsvadze A, et al. *Diagnosis and Management of Febrile Infants (0–3 Months).* Rockville, MD: Agency for Healthcare Research and Quality; 2012. Evidence Report/Technology Assessments, No. 205

Huppler AR, Eickhoff JC, Wald ER. Performance of low-risk criteria in the evaluation of young infants with fever: review of the literature. *Pediatrics.* 2010;125:228–233

Mintegi S, Benito J, Astobiza E, et al. Well appearing young infants with fever without known source in the emergency department: are lumbar punctures always necessary? *Eur J Emerg Med.* 2010;17:167–169

Olaciregui I, Hernández U, Muñoz JA, et al. Markers that predict serious bacterial infection in infants under 3 months of age presenting with fever of unknown origin. *Arch Dis Child.* 2009;94:501–505

Schwartz S, Raveh D, Toker O, et al. A week-by-week analysis of the low-risk criteria for serious bacterial infection in febrile neonates. *Arch Dis Child.* 2009;94:287–292

Fever of Unknown Origin

Introduction

Fever of unknown origin (FUO) is defined as a temperature higher than 38.3°C (101.0°F) for at least 2 weeks during which a cause has not been identified after thorough clinical evaluation. The duration essentially rules out sepsis and florid bacterial meningitis. There are a vast number of causes of FUO, with infections (especially in a patient <6 years) and rheumatologic diseases (older children) accounting for up to 60% of the diagnoses. More often than not, FUO represents a common disease process presenting in an uncommon fashion, such as an occult bacterial (osteomyelitis, urinary tract infection, missed appendicitis with abdominal abscess) or viral (Epstein-Barr virus [EBV], cytomegalovirus [CMV]) infection. Although exotic etiologies are sometimes entertained and diagnosed (see the following text and tables for clinical clues), first consider common illnesses. However, in approximately one-third of patients, a definitive diagnosis is never confirmed.

Clinical Presentation

History

The diagnosis of the etiology of FUO relies on an exhaustive, and often repeated, history obtained from the patient (if verbal) as well as all caregivers. Focus on associated complaints (cough, vomiting, diarrhea, pain, myalgias, arthralgias, etc), sick contacts, and new and chronic medications. Specifically ask about exposure to kittens (bartonellosis), reptiles or amphibians (salmonellosis), and farm animals (brucellosis, Q fever, leptospirosis), as well as drinking unpasteurized milk or cheese (*Mycobacterium bovis*), ingesting squirrel or rabbit meat (tularemia), pica (*Toxocara,* toxoplasmosis), camping (Lyme disease, ehrlichiosis, anaplasmosis), and travel both outside (malaria, tuberculosis) and within (Lyme disease, histoplasmosis, coccidioidomycosis, blastomycosis) the United States.

In the medical history, look for HIV risk factors, frequent or unusual infections suggesting an immunodeficiency, genetic background (nephrogenic diabetes insipidus, periodic fever syndromes, familial dysautonomia), and abdominal symptoms and poor growth consistent with inflammatory bowel disease (IBD). The pattern, height, and duration of the fever may provide some clues, as in juvenile idiopathic arthritis (JIA) and the periodic fever syndromes, but otherwise rarely lead to a diagnosis.

Physical Examination

Perform a thorough and extensive physical examination and, most importantly, repeat it on a regular basis for new clues to aid in the diagnosis. Ensure that a consistent provider performs a thorough evaluation of all systems, beginning with the skin/scalp and culminating with the neurologic examination, so as to consistently recognize changes. Evaluate the child in both the febrile and non-febrile state, as physical examination findings may be different (the evanescent rash of JIA often occurs only with fever and the heart murmurs of acute rheumatic fever [ARF] or endocarditis will be accentuated). The absence of sweating during fever occurs with dehydration, familial dysautonomia, or atropine exposure.

Assess the child's growth parameters, including height, weight and, when appropriate, head circumference. While growth retardation may be a nonspecific finding of any chronic disease, its presence suggests a highly inflammatory process, such as IBD or perhaps immunodeficiency. Other priorities of the examination include the skin (malar or discoid rash of lupus; petechiae, Janeway lesions, and splinter hemorrhages associated with endocarditis) and an assessment for lymphadenopathy and hepatosplenomegaly suggesting EBV, CMV, or lymphoma. Examine each joint of the skeletal system for evidence of arthritis and tenderness, which may represent osteomyelitis or malignancy. However, severe pain involving multiple joints that is out of proportion to the swelling may represent leukemia rather than JIA. Listen carefully for heart murmurs (ARF, endocarditis), rales (pneumonia), and rubs (pleuritis, pericarditis).

Perform a thorough examination of the head, eyes, ears, nose, and throat looking for signs of sinusitis, such as facial tenderness, and signs of rheumatologic or autoimmune disease, such as mucosal ulcerations. Closely examine the eyes for icterus (liver dysfunction, hemolytic anemia); red, weeping eyes (connective tissue disease, especially polyarteritis nodosa); palpebral conjunctivitis (measles, coxsackievirus, tuberculosis, EBV, bartonellosis, lymphogranuloma venereum); bulbar conjunctivitis (often purulent with infection; non-purulent with Kawasaki disease and leptospirosis); uveitis (sarcoidosis, systemic lupus erythematosus [SLE], Kawasaki disease, Behçet, vasculitis, JIA); chorioretinitis (CMV, toxoplasmosis, syphilis); and proptosis (tumor, infection, thyrotoxicosis, Wegener granulomatosis).

Ensure that the child is relaxed in order to obtain a reliable abdominal examination while palpating for masses (neuroblastoma, abscess) and hepatosplenomegaly. An abnormal gait may represent infection or malignancy of the lower extremities, or a problem with the back or spine (discitis, vertebral osteomyelitis, tumor). Generalized muscle tenderness suggests dermatomyositis, trichinosis, or arboviral infection. Thoroughly examine the neurologic system. Failure of pupillary constriction can be associated with hypothalamic dysfunction, hyperactive reflexes with thyrotoxicosis, and absence of fungiform papillae with familial dysautonomia.

Discuss each examined organ system with the family. They may fear a particular diagnosis, such as cancer or HIV, or equate a detailed, prolonged examination of certain organs with pathology.

Laboratory

Choose laboratory investigation based on the history and physical examination. Personally review all laboratory and radiologic evaluation undertaken in the outpatient setting and use appropriate consultants for interpretation of biopsies, radiographs, or other data. Obtain a complete blood cell count (CBC) with differential, C-reactive protein (CRP)/erythrocyte sedimentation rate (ESR), comprehensive metabolic panel, EBV and CMV titers, blood cultures, and urinalysis and urine culture. Obtain other tests in tier 1 (Box 45-1) if indicated (*Bartonella* titers if there is contact with a kitten; immunoglobulins if there is a history of frequent sinopulmonary infections). If fever persists without a diagnosis despite tier 1 evaluation and observation for several days in the hospital, repeat the CBC with differential, CRP/ESR, and any tests from tier 1 that were abnormal, and perform tier 2 tests if there are specific indications (hepatitis viral panel if liver functions are elevated).

Box 45-1. Laboratory Tiers
Tier 1
CBC with differential, CRP/ESR, comprehensive metabolic panel, serologies (EBV, CMV, *Bartonella*), quantitative serum immunoglobulins, blood cultures, urinalysis and urine culture, stool for blood/leukocytes/culture[a], upper and/or lower GI endoscopy[a], chest x-ray, and TST (INF-γ release assay for a patient >6 years)
Tier 2
Repeat selected tier 1 tests; syphilis[b], toxoplasma[b], hepatitis viruses, brucella[b], Lyme[b], and tularemia titers[b], multiple blood cultures, CT of the sinuses, abdominal ultrasound, lumbar puncture[c], echocardiogram, and bone marrow biopsy[d]

Abbreviations: CBC, complete blood cell count; CRP, C-reactive protein; CT, computed tomography; EBV, Epstein-Barr virus; ESR, erythrocyte sedimentation rate; GI, gastrointestinal; INF, interferon; TST, tuberculin skin test.

[a] If the patient has suspicious symptoms, such as loose stools, mucus or blood in stools, and abdominal pain.

[b] In endemic areas or with exposure.

[c] In an infant or toddler with significant headache, abnormal neurologic examination, or bulging fontanel.

[d] With unexplained hematologic abnormalities such as bi- or pancytopenias, blasts or other abnormal cells on peripheral smear, or underlying conditions that predispose to malignancy, such as Down syndrome.

Differential Diagnosis

First, differentiate FUO from fever without source, pseudo-FUO, factitious fever, and deconditioning. Fever without source is an acute (<3–5 days) febrile illness, in which the origin of the fever is not initially apparent after a careful history and physical examination.

In pseudo-FUO there are serial infections in which the fevers abate and recur, but vague symptoms persist. Have the parents record symptoms, maximum temperature, and route and method of obtaining temperature on a calendar or in a diary. True fevers taken with a thermometer that persist are more likely to represent FUO, while the pattern for pseudo-FUO is high fevers for several days followed by low fevers or "felt warm" with mild persistent symptoms (slight congestion, improving cough) for several days. Then the pattern repeats.

Deconditioning is often seen in the adolescent. After a well-defined, self-limited acute illness the patient develops the "dwindles," characterized by low-grade or subjective fevers, inactivity, and increasing concern from extended family members. Vitality and stamina decrease, but true fevers do not persist.

Next, assess for life-threatening/severe diseases such as Kawasaki disease and acute rheumatic fever. The severity of the disease, and not the anxiety of the family or referring physician, dictates the appropriate pace of the evaluation.

Use the ESR to stratify the likely etiologies: An ESR greater than 30 mm/hour often indicates infectious, autoimmune, or malignant disease; an ESR greater than 100 mm/hour suggests tuberculosis, Kawasaki disease, malignancy, or autoimmune disease. The differential diagnosis is summarized in Table 45-1.

Treatment

Most often the hospitalization is to expedite the evaluation. Therefore, reserve empiric antibiotic therapy for a patient who is toxic or has a compromising underlying condition and a deteriorating clinical course. Unfortunately, up to 80% of patients will have received one dose of antibiotics prior to admission, making the diagnosis more challenging. Nonsteroidal anti-inflammatory drugs can be helpful in symptomatic care, especially in rheumatologic disease, but may mask clues to diagnosis.

Specific treatment depends on the final diagnosis: antibiotics, plus or minus drainage for bacterial disease; steroids and rheumatologic referral for SLE or JIA; steroids and gastroenterology referral for IBD; drug withdrawal for drug fever; and education and psychological or psychiatric referral for factitious fever.

Table 45-1. Differential Diagnosis of Fever of Unknown Origin	
Diagnosis	**Clinical Features**
Bacterial Infections	
Bartonella	Kitten exposure Lymphadenopathy Cranial nerve palsy
Lyme disease	Erythema migrans Oligoarticular arthritis (especially the knee) Cranial nerve palsy (especially VIIth)
Occult abscess	History of antibiotic use Daily fever spike Pain
Osteomyelitis	Refusal to bear weight Bony point tenderness Elevated CRP/ESR
Salmonellosis	Relative bradycardia (pulse doesn't increase with fever) Vomiting and diarrhea (may be bloody) Rose spots and cough (typhoid)
Sinusitis	Cough and postnasal drip Facial erythema or tenderness Swollen erythematous nasal turbinates
Fungal Infections (all can have influenza-like illness, hilar adenopathy, pulmonary infiltrates, and dermatologic and CNS involvement, usually in an immunocompromised patient)	
Blastomycosis	Southeast and Central United States
Coccidioidomycosis	Southwest United States
Histoplasmosis	Mississippi, Ohio and Missouri river valley, Hepatosplenomegaly in toddlers Erythema nodosum in adolescents
Parasitic Infections	
Malaria	Travel to endemic area Rigors, hepatosplenomegaly Hemolytic anemia
Toxoplasmosis	Lymphadenopathy, especially cervical Pharyngitis, myalgias
Tickborne Infections (all can have headache, myalgias, thrombocytopenia)	
Babesiosis	Hemolytic anemia
Ehrlichiosis/anaplasmosis	Nausea Variable rash (or no rash) in a truncal distribution Leukopenia, ↑ liver transaminases

Table 45-1. Differential Diagnosis of Fever of Unknown Origin, continued	
Diagnosis	**Clinical Features**
Viral Infections	
Epstein-Barr virus, CMV	Pharyngitis Generalized lymphadenopathy, hepatomegaly Atypical lymphocytosis
Hepatitis viruses	Blood/body fluid exposure ↑ Liver transaminases and bilirubin
Collagen Vascular Diseases	
Acute rheumatic fever	History of streptococcal infection Migratory polyarthritis Carditis (new murmur)
Juvenile idiopathic arthritis	Quotidian fever spikes alternating with subnormal temperatures Lymphadenopathy, evanescent rash Arthritis (may not be present initially)
Systemic lupus erythematosus	Alopecia, arthritis, malar rash Cytopenias Hematuria
Hereditary	
Anhidrotic ectodermal dysplasia	Lack of sweating with fever Dental defects, abnormal facies, sparse hair
Fabry disease	Angiokeratomas (flat or raised red-black telangiectasias) Burning pain and paresthesias of feet and legs
Familial Mediterranean fever	Serositis, especially peritonitis Arthritis or arthralgia
Malignancy	
Leukemia	Bruising, pallor Bone pain ↑ LDH and uric acid
Neuroblastoma	Proptosis, abdominal mass Opsoclonus-myoclonus (dancing eyes, dancing feet) ↑ Urine catecholamines
Other	
Drug fever	Consider all medications, even eyedrops Lack of other symptoms; relative bradycardia CRP/ESR not elevated
Factitious fever	Thermometer manipulation or injection of pyrogens May need video surveillance
Hemophagocytic lymphohistiocytosis	Splenomegaly Cytopenias, ↓ fibrinogen ↑ Ferritin and triglycerides

Table 45-1. Differential Diagnosis of Fever of Unknown Origin, continued	
Diagnosis	**Clinical Features**
Other, continued	
Inflammatory bowel disease	Growth retardation Abdominal pain Arthritis, erythema nodosum, uveitis
Kawasaki disease	Nonpurulent bulbar conjunctivitis Erythematous polymorphic rash Swollen hands and feet Oral changes

Abbreviations: CMV, cytomegalovirus; CNS, central nervous system; CRP, C-reactive protein; ESR, erythrocyte sedimentation rate; LDH, lactate dehydrogenase.

If the etiology is not determined or is a virus other than a treatable one such as HIV, construct a detailed follow-up plan for the family. This must include symptomatic treatments, both pharmacologic and non-pharmacologic; activity restrictions (heat illness precautions while fever persists, avoidance of abdominal trauma with splenomegaly); routine follow-up with the primary care pediatrician, and indications for emergent visits (severe abdominal pain with EBV that could represent splenic rupture, new signs or symptoms such as arthritis).

Indication for Consultation

- **Infectious diseases:** Uncertain diagnosis in a patient who appears toxic or has been exposed to suspicious foods, animals, places, or activities that are associated with infections; immunocompromised patient
- **Ophthalmology:** If endocarditis, uveitis, IBD, chorioretinitis, or JIA are a concern
- **Various subspecialists:** Based on "most likely" diagnosis information obtained from repeated history and physical examination findings

Disposition

- **Intensive care unit transfer:** Respiratory distress, hypotension, parental monitoring to rule out factitious fever
- **Discharge criteria:** Afebrile for 48 hours or more or diagnosis is confirmed and continued fever is expected, nontoxic appearance, lack of a diagnosis after critical inpatient testing has been performed and appropriate consultation obtained with close outpatient follow-up arranged

Follow-up

- **Primary care:** 1 week
- **Various subspecialists:** Based on the ultimate diagnosis

Pearls and Pitfalls

- The key to the ultimate diagnosis of FUO lies in repeated assessment of both the history and physical examination, not in increasing laboratory workup.
- More often than not, FUO represents a common disease process presenting in an uncommon fashion.

Coding

ICD-9

Fever unspecified	**780.60**

Bibliography

Akpede GO, Akenzua GI. Management of children with prolonged fever of unknown origin and difficulties in the management of fever of unknown origin in children in developing countries. *Paediatr Drugs.* 2001;3:247–262

Ishimine P. Fever without source in children 0 to 36 months of age. *Pediatr Clin North Am.* 2006;53:167–194

McCarthy PL. Fever without apparent source on clinical examination. *Curr Opin Pediatr.* 2003;15:112–120

Pickering LK, Baker CJ, Kimberlin DW, Long SS, eds. *Red Book: 2012 Report of the Committee on Infectious Diseases.* Elk Grove Village, IL: American Academy of Pediatrics; 2012

Powell KR. Fever without a focus. In: Kleigman RM, Behrman RB, Jenson HB, Stanton BF, eds. *Nelson Textbook of Pediatrics.* 18th ed. Philadelphia, PA: Saunders; 2007:1087–1094

Tolan RW Jr. Fever of unknown origin: a diagnostic approach to this vexing problem. *Clin Pediatr (Phila).* 2010;49:207–213

CHAPTER 46

Kawasaki Disease

Introduction

Kawasaki disease (KD) is an acute, self-limited, multi-organ vasculitis of small and medium-sized arteries. It predominantly affects young children, with a peak incidence at 13 to 24 months of age, although it can occur in infants younger than 6 months. The etiology of KD is unknown, although epidemics are most common in the spring and fall.

The most significant complication of KD is vasculitis of the coronary arteries leading to aneurysm formation. This occurs in about 25% of untreated patients, but is seen in less than 10% if treated appropriately with intravenous immune globulin (IVIG) early in the disease course. Risk factors for the development of coronary artery aneurysms include age younger than 6 months or older than 9 years, male gender, duration of fever more than 7 days prior to treatment, and lack of response to initial IVIG dose. Certain laboratory abnormalities also indicate a higher risk: low hematocrit, low albumin, hyponatremia, and elevated alanine transaminase.

Clinical Presentation

History

There are 3 distinct stages of the illness. Most patients will present during the acute stage (first 10–14 days), which is characterized by the abrupt onset of high fever (38.9°C–40°C; 102°F–104°F) for at least 5 days associated with crankiness or irritability. Within 2 to 5 days of the onset of fever, the patient develops other characteristic features of the illness, including a polymorphous erythematous rash in 90% (may involve the palms and soles), nonpurulent conjunctivitis (80%–90%), erythema and cracking of the lips or a strawberry tongue (75%–90%), and swelling of the dorsum of the hands and feet. Less common complaints are abdominal pain, vomiting, and arthralgias.

The subacute phase (approximately 2–6 weeks) is characterized by resolution of the classic complaints (fever, lymphadenopathy, rash, mucositis, extremity changes, conjunctivitis). Periungual desquamation may occur during the second to third week of the illness. Cardiac complications, including coronary artery aneurysms, coronary obstruction and thrombosis, and myocardial and endocardial inflammation, can develop during this time, if not already present. The risk of sudden death is greatest during this phase.

In the final stage, physical findings are no longer apparent. Cardiac complications may either resolve or progress to myocardial ischemia or infarction.

Physical Examination

Perform a thorough head, eyes, ears, nose, and throat examination. Typical findings in the acute stage include conjunctival injection with perilimbic sparing and without exudate; erythema of the mouth and pharynx; a strawberry tongue; dry, cracked lips; and a unilateral cervical lymph node greater than 1.5 cm. Other findings include swelling of the dorsum of the hands and feet and a polymorphic, erythematous rash that may involve the palms and soles. In many cases, within a few days of the appearance of the rash, desquamation of the perineal/diaper region occurs.

Findings with cardiac involvement include tachycardia, a flow murmur, muffled heart sounds, or a gallop.

Less common features are arthritis, involving the small joints during the acute phase, and later the large, weight-bearing joints. Myringitis, urethritis with sterile pyuria, aseptic meningitis (nuchal rigidity) and, rarely, hydrops of the gallbladder (right upper quadrant abdominal mass) may also occur.

During the subacute phase there can be desquamation of the hands and feet. Cardiac manifestations during this stage, if present, are more severe and may reveal signs and symptoms of congestive heart failure, valvular regurgitation, ventricular arrhythmias (premature ventricular contractions, ventricular tachycardia), or myocardial ischemia. Young children with a myocardial infarction rarely present with chest pain, but with shock, vomiting, abdominal pain, and excessive crying instead.

Laboratory

If KD is suspected, obtain a complete blood cell count with differential, erythrocyte sedimentation rate (ESR) and/or C-reactive protein (CRP), chemistries with liver function tests including gamma-glutamyl transferase and alkaline phosphatase, and a urinalysis. Leukocytosis with neutrophil predominance, anemia, elevation of liver enzymes and alkaline phosphatase (seen in hydrops of the gall bladder), decreased albumin and serum sodium, and sterile pyuria may all be present. The ESR and CRP are elevated early in the clinical course, whereas thrombocytosis (>500,000/mm^3) may not occur until the second or third week of the illness. Laboratory abnormalities may persist for 6 to 10 weeks, and normalization of these values coincides with resolution of the disease, although a steady decline in the CRP promptly occurs after successful treatment with IVIG.

If KD is strongly suspected, obtain an electrocardiogram (ECG) and a chest x-ray (unless an echocardiogram will be performed immediately) to screen for cardiac involvement. Although cardiac imaging is critical, do not delay treatment while awaiting these studies. In KD the ECG may reveal tachycardia, prolongation of the PR interval, abnormal Q waves, and nonspecific ST wave changes.

Once a diagnosis of KD is made, consult a cardiologist and arrange a baseline echocardiogram. Coronary abnormalities may be found at presentation.

Blood, throat, and viral cultures may be helpful in differentiating KD from other infectious causes with prolonged fever.

Differential Diagnosis

Strongly suspect KD if a patient between 6 weeks and 12 years of age has fever for more than 5 days in association with 4 of the following 5 major manifestations:

- Conjunctival injection without exudate
- Erythema of the mouth and pharynx; a strawberry tongue; and cracked, red lips
- Erythematous rash of almost any pattern
- Induration of the hands and feet with erythematous palms and soles
- Isolated, unilateral cervical lymphadenopathy greater than 1.5 cm

An atypical presentation, often termed incomplete KD, is increasingly common, especially among infants younger than 12 months. These young infants have the highest risk of coronary artery abnormalities and often are misdiagnosed initially with pyelonephritis or partially treated meningitis. The patient has prolonged fever and fewer than 4 of the principle diagnostic features. However, while the physical examination may not be clearly diagnostic, the laboratory abnormalities follow a similar pattern to what is seen in classic disease. Given that infants and patients with delayed diagnosis of KD are at increased risk for the development of coronary artery abnormalities, it is critical to diagnose KD when the clinical picture is "incomplete" but the abnormal laboratory values and echocardiogram are consistent with the diagnosis.

A number of infectious diseases (toxic shock syndrome, rheumatic fever, scarlet fever, staphylococcal scalded skin syndrome, Rocky Mountain spotted fever, leptospirosis, adenovirus, Epstein-Barr virus, influenza, measles) and noninfectious (Stevens-Johnson syndrome, drug reaction, juvenile idiopathic arthritis, mercury toxicity) etiologies may resemble KD (Table 46-1).

Table 46-1. Differential Diagnosis of Kawasaki Disease	
Diagnosis	**Clinical Features**
Acute rheumatic fever	History of strep infection No conjunctivitis Migratory polyarthritis and/or carditis (regurgitation)
Adenovirus	Exudative pharyngitis Purulent conjunctivitis Mild elevation of inflammatory markers
Juvenile idiopathic arthritis	May have (+) antinuclear antibodies or rheumatoid factor Lack conjunctival and oral findings Lymphadenopathy more generalized
Measles	Exanthem progresses cephalocaudad Purulent conjunctivitis Lack of swelling of hands and feet
Stevens-Johnson syndrome	Purulent conjunctivitis More severe desquamation of mucosal surfaces Sudden onset with progression to shock if untreated
Toxic shock syndrome	Presence of inciting bacterial agent Signs of shock including hypotension Renal involvement with ↑ blood urea nitrogen/creatinine

Treatment

Management in the acute phase is aimed at reducing inflammation in the myocardium and coronary artery wall, as well as preventing thrombosis. The mainstay of inpatient therapy is high-dose IVIG (2 g/kg IVIG over 10–12 hours). During the first 7 to 10 days of the illness also give high-dose aspirin (80–100 mg/kg/day divided every 3 days), but switch to low-dose (3–5 mg/kg/day as a single daily dose) after the patient has been afebrile for 48 hours. Continue the low-dose aspirin until the inflammatory markers (CRP, ESR) normalize and the patient has had a follow-up appointment with cardiology to confirm that no coronary artery abnormalities have developed.

Many patients will become afebrile, with dramatic improvement in the symptoms, during the IVIG infusion. However, the fever can persist for up to 24 hours after the end of the infusion, so do not consider a patient to be IVIG nonresponsive until there is a documented fever more than 36 hours after the end of the infusion. Approximately 10% to 20% of patients with KD will ultimately be IVIG nonresponsive and remain febrile beyond 36 hours. These patients are at increased risk for coronary artery abnormalities. Consult with a KD expert to determine the best course of action. Options include a second course of IVIG (2 g/kg), pulse methylprednisolone (30 mg/kg/day) for 3 days, or infliximab, a tumor necrosis factor inhibitor.

Indications for Consultation

- **Cardiology:** All patients
- **Infectious diseases:** The diagnosis of KD is unclear or there is concern for other infectious etiologies
- **KD expert, if available (may be a cardiologist, rheumatologist, infectious diseases specialist):** Fever persists for more than 36 hours after first immunoglobulin dose

Disposition

- **Intensive care unit transfer:** Cardiac involvement with compromised function
- **Discharge criteria:** Afebrile with improvement of clinical symptoms and decreased inflammatory markers (minimum 24–36 hours after completion of IVIG treatment)

Follow-up

- **Primary care:** 1 to 3 days
- **Cardiology:** 1 to 2 weeks

Pearls and Pitfalls

- Incomplete KD may be more common than a classic presentation, especially at the extremes of the age spectrum.
- Siblings of patients with KD are at higher risk for developing the disease.
- KD can present with an acute abdomen, resulting in admission to a surgical service or with "lymphadenitis," resulting in admission to the ear, nose, throat service.

Coding

ICD-9

KD	**446.1**

Bibliography

Ashouri N, Takahashi M, Dorey F, Mason W. Risk factors for nonresponse to therapy in Kawasaki disease. *J Pediatr.* 2008;153:365–368

Baker AL, Newburger JW. Kawasaki disease. *Circulation.* 2008;118:e110–e112

Ogata S, Bando Y, Kimura S, et al. The strategy of immune globulin resistant Kawasaki disease: a comparative study of additional immune globulin and steroid pulse therapy. *J Cardiol.* 2009;53:15–19

Rowley AH, Shulman ST. Pathogenesis and management of Kawasaki disease. *Expert Rev Anti Infect Ther.* 2010;8:197–203

Satou GM, Giamelli J, Gewitz MH. Kawasaki disease: diagnosis, management, and long-term implications. *Cardiol Rev.* 2007;15:163–169

Uehara R, Yashiro M, Oki I, Nakamura Y, Yanagawa H. Re-treatment regimens for acute stage of Kawasaki disease patients who failed to respond to initial intravenous immunoglobulin therapy: analysis from the 17th nationwide survey. *Pediatr Int.* 2007;49:427–430

Ingestion

CHAPTER 47

Esophageal Foreign Body

Introduction

Coins are the most common foreign bodies ingested by children in the United States. Coins that remain in the esophagus tend to lodge in 3 areas of anatomical narrowing: 60% to 70% are at the thoracic inlet at the upper esophageal sphincter, 10% to 20% in the mid-esophagus at the level of the aortic notch, and about 20% just above the lower esophageal sphincter.

Other less common objects include toys or toy parts, needles and pins, chicken or fish bones, and other food. Batteries and sharp, long objects require special consideration due to a higher risk for complications. Button batteries can conduct electricity in the esophagus, causing liquefaction necrosis and perforation that can develop within hours. There is a high risk for perforation with sharp objects, which can get trapped anywhere in the esophagus. If there is an esophageal abnormality, a foreign body can lodge in an atypical location.

Clinical Presentation

History

The presenting symptoms depend on the type and size of foreign body, as well as the location and duration of impaction. The most common symptoms are drooling, dysphagia, substernal discomfort or a sensation of a foreign body, retching, vomiting, coughing, and difficulty breathing. The presence of fever is concerning because it suggests deep ulceration or perforation. There may be a history of a choking episode, the caregiver may have witnessed the ingestion, or the patient may self-report it. However, up to one-third of patients are asymptomatic and in as many as 40% of cases there is no history of ingestion. If possible, determine the time since the ingestion, as a longer duration (>24 hours) is associated with greater risk for complications.

Physical Examination

The physical examination may be normal, or there may be a range of findings from drooling to respiratory distress secondary to tracheal compression. Neck swelling, erythema, or crepitus is concerning for esophageal perforation. Rarely, a patient presents with massive gastrointestinal bleeding as a result of a foreign body that causes an aortoesophageal fistula.

Laboratory

Obtain anteroposterior and lateral radiographs of the neck and chest to visualize coins or other radio-opaque foreign bodies. Coins appear as a circle on frontal views and as a line on the lateral view. This is in contrast to coins in the trachea, which would have the opposite findings. A radiolucent object will not be visualized on plain x-rays, but its presence may be suggested by compression or displacement of adjacent structures. If the history and physical examination are consistent with an esophageal foreign body but the radiographs are normal, obtain a contrast esophagography to rule out a radiolucent foreign body. Arrange a chest computed tomography if the patient has significant respiratory distress that may be secondary to erosion or extra-luminal extension. A handheld metal detector is another option for identifying and localizing coins and other metallic objects.

Differential Diagnosis

The differential diagnosis is summarized in Table 47-1.

Table 47-1. Differential Diagnosis of an Esophageal Foreign Body

Diagnosis	Clinical Features
Drooling/Dysphagia	
Epiglottitis	Fever, toxicity Sniffing dog position
Peritonsillar abscess	Trismus, hot potato voice Uvula deviated to contralateral side
Retropharyngeal abscess	Fever, drooling Anterior bulging of posterior pharyngeal wall Limited neck hyperextension
Mediastinal mass	Difficulty breathing Recurrent lung infections
Cough/Choking/Cyanosis	
Bronchiolitis	Upper respiratory infection prodrome followed by respiratory distress and wheezing
Gastroesophageal reflux	Intermittent regurgitation Sandifer syndrome
Pneumonia	Fever, cough, tachypnea Infiltrate on chest x-ray
Stridor/Wheezing	
Croup	Hoarseness, barking cough Stridor
Laryngotracheomalacia	Positional inspiratory stridor Presents early in life

Treatment

Management of esophageal foreign bodies depends on the type, location, and size of the object, as well as the patient's size and symptoms. In up to 80% to 90% of cases, the object will pass spontaneously, whereas 10% to 20% must be removed endoscopically and less than 1% will require a surgical procedure.

If the patient is asymptomatic, has no history of esophageal or tracheal abnormality, and less than 24 hours has elapsed since the ingestion, permit a period of observation (up to 24 hours). Make the patient NPO, provide continuous cardiac monitoring with pulse oximetry, and give maintenance intravenous fluids. If the patient remains asymptomatic, repeat the radiograph in 12 to 24 hours. Discharge the patient if the object spontaneously passes into the stomach. However, if drooling, substernal chest pain, vomiting, difficulty swallowing, or respiratory distress develop, or the coin does not progress after 24 hours, consult with otolaryngology, gastroenterology, or surgery to coordinate a removal procedure.

Arrange for immediate removal of a button battery that has lodged in the esophagus. The same is true for large, long, and/or sharp objects. Arrange for emergent endoscopic removal for any patient who has symptoms and cannot manage secretions or exhibits acute respiratory symptoms. Do not prescribe motility agents, such as glucagon.

Depending on institutional skills and preferences, removal options include rigid esophagoscopy, flexible endoscopy (especially for sharp objects and esophageal batteries), a balloon-tipped catheter, or bougienage. Regardless of the technique used, the success rate for removal of an esophageal foreign body is 95% to100%. If several hours have passed to coordinate the removal procedure, repeat the radiograph just prior to the procedure to confirm the position of the foreign body.

During the post-removal period, observe for risks from the procedures, such as bleeding, vomiting, stridor, respiratory distress, or hypoxia. If there are no signs of difficulty breathing or drooling, start a trial of clear liquids to ensure that the patient can tolerate liquids.

Indications for Consultation

- **Gastroenterology, otorhinolaryngology, surgery, or radiology:** Depending on who performs the procedure at a given institution

Disposition

- **Intensive care unit transfer:** Impending respiratory failure or signs of shock
- **Discharge criteria:** Normal respiratory status, no oxygen requirement, no drooling, adequate oral intake.

Follow-up

- **If object required removal:** 1 to 2 weeks with the physician that performed the procedure

Pearls and Pitfalls

- If the foreign body passes into the stomach, instruct the caregivers to watch for signs of abdominal pain, bleeding, or vomiting.
- The patient may continue to complain of a foreign body sensation for several days after removal.

Coding

ICD-9

• Foreign body in esophagus	**935.1**
• Perforation of esophagus	**530.4**

Bibliography

Arms JL, Mackenberg-Mohn MD, Bowen MV, et al. Safety and efficacy of a protocol using bougienage or endoscopy for the management of coins acutely lodged in the esophagus: a large case series. *Ann Emerg Med.* 2008;51:367–372

Kay M, Wyllie R. Pediatric foreign bodies and their management. *Curr Gastroenterol Rep.* 2005;7:212–218

Lee JB, Ahmad S, Gale CP. Detection of coins ingested by children using a handheld metal detector: a systematic review. *Emerg Med J.* 2005;22:839–844

Little DC, Shah SR, Peter SD, et al. Esophageal foreign bodies in the pediatric population: our first 500 cases. *J Pediatr Surg.* 2006;41:914–918

Popel, J, El-Hakim H, El-Matary W. Esophageal foreign body extraction in children: flexible versus rigid endoscopy. *Surg Endosc.* 2011;25:919–922

Waltzman ML, Baskin M, Wypij D, et al. A randomized clinical trial of the management of esophageal coins in children. *Pediatrics.* 2005;116:614–619

Toxic Exposures

Introduction

Toxic exposures are common among children. In 2009, 65% of the total calls to poison centers and 6.8% of the fatalities involved patients young than 20 years. Younger patients (<6 years) tend to have a better outcome because, in general, they present more promptly to a health care facility, have fewer comorbid conditions, are exposed to a single substance, and are not trying to purposely harm themselves. However, some products are so toxic that a very small amount can be fatal (Box 48-1).

Clinical Presentation

History

Ask about the timing and onset of any concerning symptoms, timing and amount of any known exposure, and available sources of exposure in the house, including prescription and over-the-counter medications, household/cosmetic products, illicit drugs, and herbal/alternative and traditional/cultural medications. Determine if there were any recent occupational exposures, venomous/poisonous animal encounters, or plant exposures. Use this historical data and available pharmacy information to determine possible maximum exposures. Assess the patient's intent regarding exposure. Ask about any underlying medical conditions that may affect drug metabolism, such as renal or liver disease.

Physical Examination

Be aware that some toxins have a delayed onset (Table 48-1). Potential physical examination findings are summarized in Table 48-2.

Box 48-1. Toxins That Are Potentially Fatal With Small Doses	
Antidysrhythmics	Diphenoxylate-atropine
Antimalarials (chloroquine, hydroxychloroquine, quinine)	Ethylene glycol
β-antagonists	Methanol
Bupropion	Methylsalicylate
Calcium channel antagonists	Opioids
Camphor	Phenothiazines
Clonidine	Sulfonylureas
Clozapine	Theophylline
	Tricyclic antidepressants

Table 48-1. Toxins With Potential for Delayed Toxicity	
Toxin	**Toxicity**
Acetaminophen	Hepatic and renal failure
Amanita species mushrooms	Hepatic failure
Broudifacoum	Bleeding
Buprenorphine-suboxone	Respiratory failure
Bupropion	Seizures
Colchicine	Gastrointestinal toxicity, multi-organ failure
Diphenoxylate-atropine	Respiratory failure
Diquat	Renal failure, multi-organ failure
Iron	Hepatic, multi-organ failure
Lead	Encephalopathy, seizures, anemia
Paraquat	Pulmonary fibrosis, multi-organ failure
Salicylates	Encephalopathy, seizures, arrhythmias, renal failure, multi-organ failure
Sulfonylureas	Hypoglycemia
Sustained-release β-antagonists	Hypotension, bradycardia
Sustained-release calcium channel antagonists	Hypotension, bradycardia

Table 48-2. Physical Examination Findings	
Symptom	**Substance/Syndrome**
Vital Signs	
Hyperthermia	Anticholinergics, sympathomimetics, uncoupling, serotonin syndrome, malignant hyperthermia, neuroleptic malignant syndrome, gamma-aminobutyric acid (GABA) agonist withdrawal (ethanol, benzodiazepines, barbiturates, baclofen, gamma-hydroxybutyrate)
Hypothermia	Opioids, hypoglycemic agents, carbon monoxide, β-blockers
Tachycardia	Sympathomimetics, anticholinergics, serotonin syndrome, GABA agonist withdrawal, tricyclic antidepressants
Bradycardia	Cholinergics, β-blockers, calcium channel blockers, digoxin, opioids, sedatives, clonidine
Hypertension	Sympathomimetics, elemental mercury, serotonin syndrome GABA agonist withdrawal
Hypotension	Calcium channel blockers, β-blockers, digoxin, clonidine, opioids, tricyclic antidepressants (TCAs)
Tachypnea	Sympathomimetics, anticholinergics, salicylates, hydrocarbons
Bradypnea	Opioids, sedatives, clonidine, cholinergics
Neurologic/Mental Status	
Agitation	Sympathomimetics, anticholinergics, serotonin syndrome
Hallucinations/ delusions	Sympathomimetics, anticholinergics, dextromethorphan, LSD, cannabinoids, PCP, psilocybin, *Salvia divinorum*
Sedation	Opioids, sedatives, carbon monoxide, hydrocarbon inhalants
Seizures	Sympathomimetics, anticholinergics, TCAs, antipsychotics, caffeine, isoniazid, propoxyphene, tramadol, theophylline

Table 48-2. Physical Examination Findings, continued

Symptom	Substance/Syndrome
Head, Eyes, Ears, Nose, Throat	
Dry mucosal membrane	Anticholinergics
Miosis	**C:** carbamates, clonidine, **O:** opioids, organophosphates, olanzapine, **P:** phenothiazines **S:** sedatives
Mydriasis	Sympathomimetics, anticholinergics
Sialorrhea/ drooling	Cholinergics, caustics
Visual loss	Methanol
Cardiopulmonary	
Myocarditis	Ipecac (chronic exposure)
Pulmonary edema (noncardiogenic)	Salicylates, opioids, organophosphates
Torsades de pointes (prolonged QT)	TCAs, methadone, antipsychotics, erythromycin, cisapride, diphenhydramine (See list at azcert.org.)
Ventricular tachycardia (prolonged QRS)	Cocaine, TCAs, anticholinergics, halogenated hydrocarbons, propranolol, propoxyphene
Wheezing/ dyspnea	Hydrocarbons
Gastrointestinal	
Constipation	Anticholinergics, opioids
Diarrhea	Caustics, cholinergics, ipecac, iron, cathartics
Emesis	Caustics, cholinergics, ipecac, ethanol, plants, mushrooms, iron
Hepatotoxicity	Acetaminophen, *Amanita* species mushrooms, phenytoin, ethanol, iron, valproic acid, *Mentha pulegium* (pennyroyal)
Pancreatitis	Ethanol, salicylates, valproic acid
Hematologic and Renal	
Bleeding/bruising	Coumadin, broudifacoum (found in certain rat poison)
Nephrotoxicity	Ethylene glycol, nonsteroidal anti-inflammatory drugs, aminoglycosides

Laboratory

If a toxic exposure is suspected, order a bedside blood glucose, basic metabolic panel (Table 48-3), 12-lead electrocardiogram, and continuous pulse oximetry. Obtain acetaminophen and salicylate levels if the patient has an unknown exposure or suicidal intent. Order neuroimaging, chest x-ray, creatine phosphokinase, liver enzymes, and liver function tests if there is a suspicion of hypoxic injury, such as a patient who is found unconscious. Base all other

Table 48-3. Metabolic Findings Associated With Certain Toxins

Electrolyte Abnormality	Possible Toxins
Hypernatremia	Sodium salts, baking soda, sodium phosphate, drug-induced diabetes insipidus
Hyponatremia	Lithium, diuretics, drug-induced syndrome of inappropriate antidiuretic hormone
Hyperkalemia	Digoxin
Hypokalemia	Sympathomimetics, toluene, insulin, albuterol
Hyperchloremia	Sodium chloride, bromide (spurious)
Metabolic alkalosis	Baking soda
Anion gap metabolic acidosis	Methanol, metformin, iron, isoniazid, ethylene glycol, salicylates, carbon monoxide, cyanide, toluene
Normal anion gap metabolic acidosis	Topiramate, toluene
Hyperglycemia	Sympathomimetics, calcium channel blockers
Hypoglycemia	Insulin, sulfonylureas, β-blockers, ethanol

testing on suspected toxin, and the history, physical examination, and initial laboratory findings.

Confirm urine drug screen results that are indicated for medical, social, or psychiatric management with gas chromatography/mass spectrometry.

Send urine and blood samples to the laboratory for storage on all patients with suspected malicious poisoning with an unknown substance, then use these samples for future testing with guidance of subsequent clinical course, history, and consultant expertise.

Differential Diagnosis

There are many toxic exposures that can present in the same way as common pediatric illnesses. Seizures from sympathomimetics or bupropion can be indistinguishable from generalized seizures. Sympathomimetics, anticholinergics, lead encephalopathy, and serotonin syndrome can mimic infectious meningitis. Consider carbon monoxide poisoning in the evaluation of new-onset migraine or tension headaches. Hydrocarbon ingestion can be confused with an asthma exacerbation. Ipecac administration, early acetaminophen or iron poisoning, and viral gastroenteritis will present with similar symptoms. Viral hepatitis and acetaminophen toxicity will also have similar presentations. Dehydration from poor oral intake and sodium chloride toxicity will present with similar clinical symptoms and laboratory findings. Some poisons present with a consistent constellation of signs and symptoms called toxidromes (Table 48-4).

Table 48-4. Common Toxidromes

	Sympathomimetic	Opioid	Anticholinergic	Cholinergic
Toxins	Cocaine, amphetamines, pseudoephedrine	Heroin, morphine, codeine, fentanyl methadone	Diphenhydramine, TCA, atypical antipsychotics, carbamazepine, *Datura* species	Organophosphates, carbamates
Temperature	Hyperthermia	Hypothermia	Hyperthermia	
Pulse	Tachycardia	Bradycardia	Tachycardia	Bradycardia
Blood pressure	Hypertension	Hypotension		
Respiratory rate	Tachypnea	Bradypnea, apnea		Dyspnea (pulmonary edema)
Skin	Diaphoresis		Dry	Diaphoresis
Neurologic	Agitation, seizures	Sedation, coma	Agitation, seizures	
Eye	Mydriasis	Miosis	Mydriasis	Miosis
Gastrointestinal		Constipation	Constipation	Emesis, diarrhea
Genitourinary	Urinary retention		Urinary retention	Enuresis
Mnemonic	Mimics "fight-or-flight" response		"Mad as a hatter, hot as a hare, blind as a bat, red as a beet, dry as a bone"	**S**alivation **l**acrimation **U**rination **D**efecation **G**astrointestinal upset **E**mesis

Treatment

The initiation of Pediatric Advanced Life Support (if necessary) and supportive care are the mainstays of treatment. Discuss treatment decisions with a regional poison center (1-800-222-1222). Reserve gastrointestinal decontamination (activated charcoal, gastric lavage, whole-bowel irrigation) for select cases:

- Activated charcoal (1–2 g/kg, maximum 50 g): Patient ingested a potentially life-threatening toxin (calcium channel blocker, tricyclic antidepressant), presents within 1 hour after ingestion, and is not an aspiration risk
- Gastric lavage: Patient ingested a potentially life-threatening toxin that can be withdrawn through a gastric tube (liquid), presents within 1 hour of the ingestion, and is not an aspiration risk
- Whole-bowel irrigation (polyethylene glycol 3350 and electrolyte lavage solution, 25 mL/kg/hour, 2 L/hour maximum, until desired effect achieved): Patient ingested a potentially life-threatening toxin (iron, lead, arsenic) and is not an aspiration risk

Treat toxin-induced agitation or seizures with intravenous (IV) lorazepam (0.05–0.1 mg/kg/dose, 2–4 mg maximum). Treat seizures refractory to lorazepam with IV phenobarbital (15–20 mg/kg/dose, 1 g maximum) as phenytoin may be ineffective in treating toxin-induced seizures.

Treat ventricular tachycardia or a QRS interval greater than 100 msec with an IV sodium bicarbonate bolus (1–2 mEq/kg/dose). For Torsades de pointes or a QTc interval greater than 500 msec, give IV magnesium sulfate (25–50 mg/kg/dose, 2 g maximum) and correct any hypokalemia.

Use naloxone (0.1 mg/kg repeat every 2 minutes as needed, 2 mg/dose maximum) to reverse respiratory failure from opioids and to reverse opioid-induced hypotension, particularly in a patient whose hypotension is refractory to standard therapies. Do not use flumazenil in a non–life-threatening benzodiazepine ingestion, as it can cause seizures or precipitate a serious benzodiazepine withdrawal. Reserve flumazenil for a patient with confirmed benzodiazepine ingestion and respiratory failure, without co-ingestion of substances that will lower their seizure threshold, and without a history of previous benzodiazepine use. The dose is (0.01 mg/kg/dose, 0.2 mg maximum).

Give IV N-acetylcysteine (150 mg/kg/hour for 1 hour, then 12.5 mg/kg/hour for 4 hours, then 6.25 mg/kg/hour for a minimum of 16 hours) if the patient has an acute ingestion of acetaminophen and a serum level that is above the toxicity line on the acetaminophen toxicity nomogram (Figure 48-1), a chronic acetaminophen ingestion, and a detectable acetaminophen level or with evidence of liver injury/decreased function or hepatotoxicity and an unknown ingestion (until the etiology is determined). Discontinue the N-acetylcysteine after the 21-hour infusion if the acetaminophen level is undetectable and there is no increase in the patient's aspartate transaminase (AST) and alanine transaminase (ALT). If there has been an increase in AST and ALT, continue IV N-acetylcysteine at 6.25 mg/kg/hour until there is a clinical improvement, decreases in both AST and ALT, and when AST and ALT are both less than 1,000 IU/L.

To enhance elimination of salicylates, initiate serum alkalinization for a patient with a salicylate level of 40 mg/dL or greater or a detectable salicylate level and metabolic acidosis, altered mental status, seizures, vomiting, and/or tinnitus. Put 100 to 150 mEq of sodium bicarbonate in 1 L D5W and run the IV at 1 to 2 times maintenance requirements. The goals are a serum pH of 7.4 to 7.45 and a urine pH of 7.5 to 8, while monitoring the fluid status and potassium (risk of hypokalemia) carefully. The elimination of salicylates, ethylene glycol, methanol, caffeine, and theophylline can be enhanced by hemodialysis.

Institute suicide precautions and consult psychiatry to evaluate a patient with suicidal or unclear intent.

Figure 48-1. Acetaminophen Nomogram

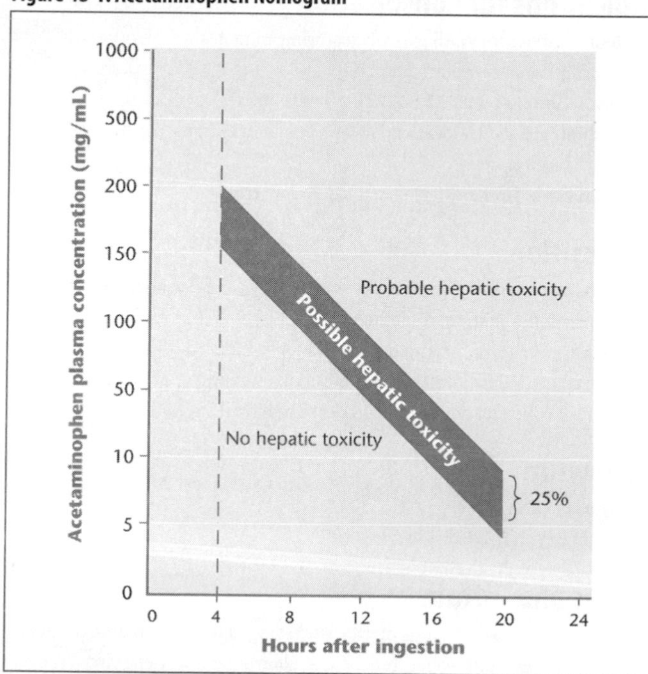

From Fine JS, Auerbach MA, Ching KY, Fullerton KT, Weinberg ER. Poisoning. In: McInerny TK, Adam HM, Campbell DE, Kamat DM, Kelleher KJ, eds. *American Academy of Pediatrics Textbook of Pediatric Care.* Elk Grove Village, IL: American Academy of Pediatrics; 2008:2771

Table 48-5. Select Antidotes

Toxin	Antidote
Acetaminophen	N-acetylcysteine
Carbon monoxide	Oxygen
Cyanide	Cyanocobalamin
Ethylene glycol, methanol	Fomepizole
Heparin	Protamine
Iron	Deferoxamine
Isoniazid	Pyridoxine
Lead	Succimer, CaNa2EDTA (edetate), dimercaprol
Local anesthetics (cardiotoxicity)	Intravenous lipid emulsion (info at lipidrescue.org)
Toxin-induced methemoglobinemia	Methylene blue
Sulfonylureas	Octreotide
Warfarin, broudifacoum	Vitamin K, fresh frozen plasma

Indications for Consultation

- **Medical toxicology:** All patients requiring antidotes, with symptoms, requiring enhanced elimination
- **Poison center (1-800-222-1222):** All patients
- **Psychiatry:** Suicidal ideation, unclear intent, drug abuse, or suspected Munchausen
- **Social work:** Home-safety or self-safety concerns

Disposition

- **Intensive care unit transfer:** Status epilepticus, cardiac arrhythmia, hypotension, agitation, respiratory failure
- **Discharge criteria:** Asymptomatic and toxin-induced organ injury (if any) resolved; psychiatric and social disposition established; observation period met for toxins that are sustained-release or have delayed toxicity

Follow-up

- **Primary care:** 1 week
- **Psychiatry:** If needed, 1 to 2 weeks

Pearls and Pitfalls

- Avoid premature disposition of patients that ingest toxins with delayed toxicity (salicylates, acetaminophen, bupropion, sulfonylureas, ethylene glycol, methanol, sustained-release (SR) β-blockers and SR calcium channel blockers).
- The acetaminophen toxicity nomogram is useful only for a single acute ingestion of a regular (not extended-release) product.
- Do not discontinue N-acetylcysteine in acetaminophen toxicity when acetaminophen level is undetectable, but hepatotoxicity is worsening.
- Establish a trend using serial serum levels with salicylate or iron ingestion.
- Salicylate levels are often reported as mg% or mg/dL, rather than mg/L.
- Know what drugs are included in a serum or urine drug screen and use caution when relying on these tests to prove toxicity, predict prognosis, or to rule in/rule out drug use.
- A database of available antivenins, including exotic species, is found at www.aza.org/antivenom-index/.
- Do not underestimate the possibility of a multidrug ingestion, especially in an adolescent.

Recommended Additional Resource

Micromedex: Online database of toxins, includes acetaminophen toxicity nomogram (www.micromedex.com)

Coding

ICD-9

(See ftp://ftp.cdc.gov/pub/Health_Statistics/NCHS/Publications/ICD9-CM/2011/Dindex12.zip for a complete list of codes for poisonings and toxic effects.)

- Acetaminophen poisoning **965.4**
- Amphetamine poisoning **969.72**
- Anticholinergic syndrome **971.1**
- Carbon monoxide poisoning **986**
- Ethanol poisoning **980.0**
- Iron poisoning **964.0**
- Opioid poisoning, unspecified **965.00**
- Organophosphate poisoning **989.3**
- Salicylate poisoning **965.1**
- Sympathomimetic syndrome **971.2**
- Toxic effects of venom **989.5**

Bibliography

Bronstein AC, Spyker DA, Cantilena LR, et al. 2009 annual report of the American Association of Poison Control Centers' National Poison Data System (NPDS): 27th annual report. *Clin Toxicol (Phila).* 2010;48:979–1178

Eldridge DL, Van Eyk J, Kornegay C. Pediatric toxicology. *Emerg Med Clin North Am.* 2007;25:283–308

Fine JS. Pediatric principles. In: Flomenbaum NE, Goldfrank LR, Hoffman RS, Howland MA, Lewin NA, Nelson LS, eds. *Goldfrank's Toxicologic Emergencies.* 8th ed. New York, NY: McGraw-Hill; 2006:487–500

Greene S, Harris C, Singer J. Gastrointestinal decontamination of the poisoned patient. *Pediatr Emerg Care.* 2008;24:176–186

Hoffman RJ, Grinshpun G, Paulose DT, Haun I. Pediatric toxicology update: rational management of pediatric exposures and poisonings. *EBMedicine.net.* 2007;9:1–28

Hoffman RJ, Nelson L. Rational use of toxicology testing in children. *Curr Opin Pediatr.* 2001;113:183–188

Shah AS, Eddleston M. Should phenytoin or barbiturates be used as a second-line anticonvulsant therapy for toxicological seizures? *Clin Toxicol (Phila).* 2010;48:800–805

White ML, Liebelt EL. Update on antidotes for pediatric poisoning. *Pediatr Emerg Care.* 2006;22:740–746

Liver Diseases

CHAPTER 49

Acute Liver Failure

Introduction

The definition of acute liver failure (ALF) in children is (1) biochemical evidence of acute liver injury without a history of known chronic liver disease and (2) a coagulopathy not corrected by vitamin K. The coagulopathy is characterized by a prothrombin time (PT) greater than 15 seconds (international normalized ratio [INR] >1.5) with hepatic encephalopathy (HE) or a PT greater than 20 seconds (INR >2) with or without encephalopathy. ALF accounts for 10% to 15% of pediatric liver transplants.

The most common causes vary with age, with metabolic abnormalities and acute viral hepatitis in the first year of life, viruses and drugs in older children, and Wilson disease and acetaminophen toxicity in adolescents (Table 49-1). However, a specific etiology cannot be identified in about 50%.

Table 49-1. Etiologies of Acute Liver Failure

Etiology	Examples
Infectious	
Bacterial	Salmonellas, sepsis, tuberculosis
Viral	Cytomegalovirus, Epstein-Barr virus, herpes simplex virus, varicella, viral hepatitis (A, B, C, D coinfection, and E)
Others	Bartonella, leptospirosis, malaria
Drugs and Toxins	
Dose-dependent	Acetaminophen (most common), halothane
Idiosyncratic reaction	Anticonvulsants: phenytoin, sodium valproate, carbamazepine Antibiotics: amoxicillin/clavulanic acid, erythromycin, penicillin, quinolones, rifampin, sulfonamides, tetracyclines, trimethoprim/sulfamethoxazole Others: allopurinol, amiodarone, antiretrovirals, ketoconazole, nonsteroidal anti-inflammatory drugs, propylthiouracil
Synergistic interactions	Barbiturates/acetaminophen, isoniazid/rifampin
Toxins	*Amanita phalloides* (mushroom), carbon tetrachloride, chlorobenzenes, herbal medicines, industrial solvents
Other	
Metabolic	Acute fatty liver of pregnancy, galactosemia, hereditary fructose intolerance, mitochondrial disorders, Niemann-Pick disease type C, tyrosinemia, Wilson disease
Autoimmune	Type 1 and 2 autoimmune hepatitis, giant cell hepatitis with Coombs positive hemolytic anemia
Vascular/ischemic	Acute circulatory/cardiac failure, Budd-Chiari syndrome, cardiomyopathies, heat stroke
Infiltrative	Hemophagocytic lymphohistiocytosis, leukemia, lymphoma

Clinical Presentation

History

The typical presentation is a flu-like illness rapidly followed by progressive jaundice over days to weeks. An infant may present with irritability, poor feeding, and changes in sleep patterns. Other associated symptoms are fever, anorexia, vomiting, abdominal pain, malaise, and lethargy followed by confusion, somnolence, or altered consciousness. Altered mental status often occurs within 2 weeks of the onset of jaundice.

Ask about possible exposure to viral infections, blood products, drugs, or toxins. A history of developmental delay, failure to thrive, or seizures raises the concern for a metabolic disease. There may be a family history of liver disease, autoimmune conditions, infant death, α-1-antitrypsin deficiency, or Wilson disease. An adolescent making a suicide attempt or gesture will often take an overdose of acetaminophen. In addition, it is important to ask about medication use since acetaminophen toxicity can also occur from dosing errors during prolonged therapeutic use.

Physical Examination

Findings depend on the etiology, underlying pathogenesis, and complications. Priorities include the growth parameters, skin (jaundice, bruises, petechiae), abdomen (liver and spleen size, ascites), and the neurologic examination. Also look for peripheral edema and bleeding from mucous membranes or the gastrointestinal tract. Assess the mental status, which may range from mild confusion (excessive crying in infants) to coma with hyperreflexia and decorticate/decerebrate rigidity (late stages). The patient may also have signs of hypoglycemia (pallor, diaphoresis), cerebral edema, and increased intracranial pressure (ICP), including hypertension, bradycardia, and sluggish papillary response. In contrast, findings not usually present in a child with ALF are Kayser-Fleischer rings of Wilson disease, asterixis, and fetor hepaticus.

Complications

Encephalopathy is a major complication of ALF, as a result of cerebral edema secondary to both cerebral hyperammonemia and increased blood flow due to arteriolar dilatation. Determine the grade of the patient's HE.

- Grade I: Change in behavior with minimal change in level of consciousness; inconsolable crying or not acting self in infants and young children
- Grade II: Gross disorientation, drowsiness, possibly asterixis, inappropriate behavior; inconsolable crying or not acting self in infants and young children

- Grade III: Marked confusion, incoherent speech, sleeping most of the time but arousable to vocal stimuli
- Grade IV: Comatose, responsive to pain (IVa) or no response to pain (IVb), decorticate or decerebrate posturing

Other complications include cerebral edema, sepsis (most often caused by *Staphylococcus aureus*), hypotension, coagulopathy, ascites, gastrointestinal bleeding, and hypoglycemia secondary to depletion of hepatic glycogen storage and impaired gluconeogenesis. Renal failure may develop in the later stages.

Laboratory

In general, the consulting gastroenterologist or liver specialist will guide the workup of ALF. Not all laboratory studies need to be obtained immediately, and a tiered workup is usually appropriate. However, on admission, obtain a complete blood cell count (CBC), electrolytes, glucose, calcium and phosphorous, liver function tests (LFTs) (including gamma-glutamyl transferase and albumin), PT and INR, factors V and VII, fibrinogen, ammonia, uric acid, cholesterol, triglycerides, and amylase.

Other diagnostic tests that may be helpful, depending on the likely diagnoses, include serology for hepatitis A (anti-hepatitis A virus immunoglobulin [Ig] M), B (HBsAg, anti-HBcAg), and C (anti-hepatitis C virus), D (anti-hepatitis D virus RNA). Cytomegalovirus, Epstein-Barr virus, and herpes simplex virus are the next most common viruses, particularly in a post-transplantation or immunosuppressed patient. If indicated, obtain serology for a number of less likely pathogens, including human herpesvirus 6, HIV, varicella, adenovirus, echovirus, parvovirus B19, toxoplasmosis, coxsackievirus, leptospirosis, and listeriosis. If an infectious etiology is possible, consider bacterial cultures of blood, urine, stool, throat, skin lesions, and ascitic fluid, as well as viral cultures of urine and skin lesions.

Immunologic studies include Ig (IgG, IgA, IgM), antinuclear antibody, anti-smooth muscle antigen, liver-kidney microsomal antibodies, and complements (C3 and C4).

Obtain serum acetaminophen level as well as toxicology screens of the serum and urine for every patient with ALF. If the time of ingestion is unknown, the acetaminophen level may be very low despite markedly elevated alanine transaminase (ALT) and aspartate transaminase (AST) (>3,500 IU/L).

The evaluation for a metabolic disorder includes amino acids (serum), organic acids (urine), lactate, pyruvate, α-fetoprotein, acylcarnitine, α-1-antitrypsin, ferritin, succinylacetone, ketones, and reducing substances. If Wilson disease is a consideration, initially obtain a serum ceruloplasmin.

Other diagnostic tests include total serum and urine copper levels, bilirubin/alkaline phosphatase ratio, and hepatic copper if a liver biopsy is performed.

Radiology

Select radiologic tests based on the clinical suspicion.

Abdominal Ultrasound and Doppler

Ultrasound is useful to assess liver size, identify ascites and a liver mass, and establish the patency and flow in the hepatic vein (allowing exclusion of Budd-Chiari syndrome), hepatic artery, and portal vein.

Head Computed Tomography

The findings are usually normal in HE, while early cerebral edema may not be evident. Head computed tomography is also useful for ruling out structural causes of encephalopathy.

Electroencephalogram

Order if there is a concern about seizures in an encephalopathic patient.

Differential Diagnosis

Generally the diagnosis of ALF is clear, based on the definition noted above. However, an abnormal PT or INR may also be caused by factor VII or vitamin K deficiency, warfarin ingestion, and disseminated intravascular coagulation. Elevations of liver transaminases (ALT and/or AST) may be a consequence of hepatitis, hemolysis, infectious mononucleosis, muscle injury or myositis, pancreatitis, myocardial injury, and hepatotoxic drugs.

Treatment

Immediately consult with a pediatric gastroenterologist or liver specialist who will guide patient treatment. The patient must be managed in a setting where there is access to the appropriate subspecialists and an intensive care unit (ICU), preferably with facilities for liver transplantation. ICU admission is indicated if the patient is encephalopathic, has an INR greater than 4, or has any cardiorespiratory compromise.

General treatment includes continuous measurement/evaluation of pulse oximetry, vital signs, urine output, and neurologic status. Repeat the blood glucose every 6 hours, electrolytes and PT/INR every 12 hours, and the CBC daily, with surveillance blood and urine cultures. While the use of prophylactic antibiotics is controversial, consider giving empiric broad-spectrum coverage for rapidly progressive ALF, refractory hypotension, and a significant systemic inflammatory response. More specific management guidelines are summarized in Table 49-2.

Table 49-2. Management of Acute Liver Failure	
Complication	**Management**
Cerebral edema	Transfer to an intensive care unit Elevate head of bed to 30 degrees Fluids: 2/3 maintenance, if no sign of dehydration Mannitol bolus (0.5 g/kg) for intracranial pressure >20 mmHg Maintain the plasma osmolality 310–325 mOsm/L
Coagulopathy	Use fresh frozen plasma (10 mL/kg) or recombinant factor VII (90 mcg/kg) for international normalized ratio >7, active hemorrhage, or prior to invasive procedure Platelet transfusion: Platelets <50,000 mm^3, active bleeding, or prior to invasive procedure Consider vitamin K (5–10 mg intravenous given slowly) although acute liver failure coagulopathy is not responsive
Encephalopathy	Avoid stimulation and sedation Dietary protein restriction (1–1.5 g/kg/day) Provide adequate nutrition Lactulose (oral): <1 year 2.5 mL bid; >1 year 10–30 mL tid Do not use aminoglycoside antibiotics. Analgesia: short-acting opiates (fentanyl; no dose modification) Consider early transfer to a transplant center early (Grade I or II).
Gastrointestinal	Grade I or II encephalopathy: Oral or enteral feeding with a low protein diet (1–1.5 g/kg/day) In pronounced hepatic encephalopathy reduce lipids to 1 g/kg/day. Use a nasogastric tube only if the patient is intubated and sedated. Start parenteral nutrition early for advanced encephalopathy. Use a special formula with branched chain amino acids. Treat ascites causing respiratory symptoms with fluid restriction and diuresis (spironolactone [1–3 mg/kg/day divided bid) or tid] or furosemide [1 mg/kg every 6–8 h]). Give a prophylactic parenteral histamine 2 blocker (ranitidine 2–3 mg/kg bid, 300 mg/dose maximum) or sucralfate 2–4 g/day
Hemodynamic instability	Noradrenaline is the inotropic of choice for persistent hypotension with normal filling N-acetylcysteine (150 mg/kg) to improve oxygen metabolism
Hypoglycemia	$D_{10}W$ at 6–8 mg/kg/min (3.6–4.8 mL/kg/h)
Renal failure	Hemodialysis for urine output <1 mL/kg/h
Sepsis	Cefotaxime (100–200 mg/kg/day divided every 6–8 h) or ciprofloxacin (20–30 mg/kg/day divided every 12 h). Consider antifungals (fluconazole 10 mg/kg loading dose) if there is a marked leukocytosis, persistent fever, renal failure, immunosuppressive therapy or worsening coagulopathy.

Table 49-2. Management of Acute Liver Failure, continued	
Ventilatory support	Mechanical ventilation for Grade III encephalopathy or when a patient with Grade I or II requires sedation Sedation: Morphine (with caution at twice usual dosing interval) and midazolam regular dose Do not use positive end-expiratory pressure >8 cm.
Diagnosis	**Management**
Acetaminophen toxicity	N-acetylcysteine (100 mg/kg/day until INR <1.5)
Acute Budd-Chiari syndrome	Transjugular intrahepatic portosystemic shunt Surgical decompression or thrombolysis
Autoimmune hepatitis	Corticosteroids (prednisone 40–60 mg/day)
Galactosemia	Remove dietary lactose
Hereditary fructose intolerance	Remove dietary fructose
Hepatitis b virus	Antiviral therapy with nucleoside/tide analogue
Herpes simplex virus	Acyclovir 60 mg/kg/day divided every 8 h (neonate)
Tyrosinemia	Nitisinone

Prognosis

Overall, a patient with ALF has a much poorer prognosis than one with chronic liver disease (6 month survival rate of 60% vs 90%). Prognostic factors include etiology, degree of encephalopathy, age, and PT. ALF due to all causes has 40% to 50% spontaneous recovery rate and that can be estimated by level of encephalopathy: Grade 1–II: 65% to 70% recovery, Grade III: 40% to 50%, Grade IV: less than 20%. A patient that does not recovery spontaneously will either receive a liver transplant (30%) or die (20%). A patient with acetaminophen toxicity has a 90% chance of spontaneous recovery.

Pearls and Pitfalls

- Sedation is contraindicated in a non-intubated patient with ALF.
- Always consider acetaminophen poisoning. There may be marked elevation of LFTs with a normal or mildly elevated total bilirubin.
- Coagulopathy is an excellent tool for monitoring status and assessing the prognosis.
- LFTs do not correlate with severity of disease. They will increase terminally and are markedly elevated in metabolic diseases. In contrast, they may be low with a worse coagulopathy.

- Alkaline phosphatase to bilirubin ratio less than 2 differentiates fulminant Wilson disease from other causes of ALF.
- Ammonia must be obtained from free-flowing catheter and placed on ice and rapidly transported to the laboratory.

Coding

ICD-9

- Acute and subacute liver failure **570**
- Cerebral edema/ICP **348.5**
- Defibrination syndrome (consumptive coagulopathy) **286.6**
- Hepatic encephalopathy **572.2**

Bibliography

Devictor D, Tissieres P, Durand P, Chevret L, Debray D. Acute liver failure in neonates, infants and children. *Expert Rev Gastroenterol Hepatol.* 2011;5:717–729

Dhawan A. Etiology and prognosis of acute liver failure in children. *Liver Transpl.* 2008;14(S2):S80–S84

Fontana RJ. Acute liver failure including acetaminophen overdose. *Med Clin North Am.* 2008;92:761–794

Squires RH Jr. Acute liver failure in children. *Semin Liver Dis.* 2008;28:153–166

Stravitz RT, Kramer DJ. Management of acute liver failure. *Nat Rev Gastroenterol Hepatol.* 2009;6:542–553

CHAPTER 50

Neonatal Hyperbilirubinemia

Introduction

While jaundice is a common and mostly benign finding in the neonatal period, there is the potential for neurotoxicity. Jaundice, even after the first week of life, is usually due to unconjugated (indirect) hyperbilirubinemia, resulting from physiological jaundice, breast milk jaundice, or ongoing hemolysis from ABO incompatibility. However, timely identification of conjugated (direct) hyperbilirubinemia (direct >2 mg/dL or >20% of total bilirubin), or cholestatic jaundice, and its underlying pathology is critical. Jaundice that presents or persists at 3 weeks of age or later is suspicious for cholestasis, most often caused by biliary atresia and neonatal hepatitis.

Clinical Presentation

History

Ask about jaundice occurring in the first 24 hours of life, as this is almost never normal and is usually due to hemolysis. Determine if the infant has symptoms of acute bilirubin encephalopathy, including lethargy, high-pitched cry, poor feeding and/or vomiting, and poor weight gain, followed by opisthotonus and seizures.

Obtain feeding and bowel histories, including frequency, amount, source of nutrition, and composition of any formula, and ask about dark urine or light stools. Review the maternal and birth history (including fetal ultrasound results), look for evidence of a congenital viral infection, and determine percent weight loss, if any. Ask about family history of jaundice or consanguinity.

Physical Examination

Obtain vital signs and growth parameters and assess for signs of dehydration. Measure liver and spleen size and document the consistency. Palpate for abdominal masses and ascites. Observe for clay-colored stool or dark urine, if possible. Note the level of jaundice, the presence of bruising, and dysmorphic features associated with syndromes, such as triangular facies in Alagille syndrome, macroglossia in hypothyroidism, and microcephaly in congenital cytomegalovirus (CMV).

Laboratory

Obtain total serum bilirubin (TSB) and direct bilirubin (DB) levels (in some hospitals specifically order a neonatal TSB/DB), complete blood cell count (CBC) with differential and smear, reticulocyte count, blood type, and a direct antibody test (Coombs) if previous results are unavailable. Send blood for type and crossmatch if TSB 25 mg/dL or greater, or 20 mg/dL or greater in a sick or preterm infant. Obtain an albumin if the TSB is approaching the exchange transfusion level or is not responding to phototherapy.

If the history and physical examination suggest sepsis, perform blood culture, urine culture, and cerebrospinal fluid for protein, glucose, cell count, and culture. Also obtain a urine culture for a patient older than 3 weeks with elevated indirect bilirubin.

Obtain a quantitative glucose-6-phosphate dehydrogenase if suggested by ethnic or geographic origin (African American, Mediterranean, Middle Eastern, or Southeast Asian) or if there is a poor response to phototherapy in a patient with evidence of hemolysis.

Check the results of the newborn screen. If clinically suspected, repeat for galactosemia and hypothyroidism, as these require urgent management to prevent serious sequelae. Also check for urine-reducing substances.

If the infant has conjugated or direct hyperbilirubinemia, consult a gastroenterologist and obtain blood for culture, CBC, albumin, hepatic profile, glucose, prothrombin time, partial thromboplastin time, and hepatitis serologies and urine for bacterial and CMV culture, urinalysis, and reducing substances. If the results are negative for sepsis, urinary tract infection (UTI), or other specific disease, obtain an abdominal ultrasound and α-1-antitrypsin levels, and if low, perform Pi typing.

If the abdominal ultrasound does not identify a choledochal cyst or another anatomical abnormality as the cause of cholestasis, consult a gastroenterologist or liver specialist for a possible liver biopsy. This can provide evidence of biliary atresia or findings specific for diseases, such as a periodic acid-Schiff stain positive for granules in α-1-antitrypsin deficiency, ductal paucity in Alagille syndrome, and necroinflammatory duct lesions in sclerosing cholangitis. If further clarification is needed after the biopsy and technical expertise and appropriate support staff are available, arrange for an endoscopic retrograde cholangiopancreatography. If other testing modalities are not immediately available, consider scintigraphy or duodenal aspirate. When the diagnosis remains uncertain after biopsy and available imaging, arrange for a surgical laparotomy for intraoperative cholangiogram.

Differential Diagnosis

The differential diagnosis of unconjugated hyperbilirubinemia is summarized in Table 50-1 and conjugated hyperbilirubinemia in Table 50-2.

Treatment

Unconjugated Hyperbilirubinemia

For a newborn 35 weeks or older, treat with intensive phototherapy as per the American Academy of Pediatrics (AAP) Subcommittee on Hyperbilirubinemia nomogram (Figure 50-1). Monitor the therapeutic effect by repeating the TSB level in 2 to 12 hours, depending on the infant's age and prior levels.

Table 50-1. Differential Diagnosis of Unconjugated Hyperbilirubinemia

Diagnosis	Clinical Features
ABO/Rh incompatibility	Can present in first 24 hours of life Coombs positive ↓ Hemoglobin compared to level in newborn nursery
Breast milk jaundice	Presents after 4 days and may last for weeks Rise in total bilirubin <0.5 mg/dL/h
Crigler-Najjar syndrome	Presents at 1–3 days of life Total bilirubin >15 mg/dL Type I responds to phenobarbital treatment
Dehydration	Often due to poor feeding (breastfeeding jaundice) <3–4 stools/day and <6–7 wet diapers/day
Glucose-6-phosphate dehydrogenase (G6PD) deficiency	African American, Mediterranean, Southeast Asian Poor response to phototherapy Abnormal G6PD enzyme assay
Hypothyroidism	Delayed stooling after birth Macroglossia, large fontanelles May be conjugated
Infection/sepsis	Vomiting, lethargy, temperature instability Suspect urinary tract infection if onset of jaundice after 8 days of life May be conjugated
Other hemolytic disorders	Can present in first 24 hours of life Coombs negative Peripheral smear: abnormally shaped red blood cells
Physiological/breastfeeding jaundice	Presents at 24–72 hours and resolves by 10 days
Polycythemia	Plethora, lethargy/irritability, jitteriness Hematocrit >65%
Sequestered blood	Cephalohematoma, bruising, central nervous system hemorrhage

Table 50-2. Differential Diagnosis of Conjugated Hyperbilirubinemia

Diagnosis	Clinical Features
Obstructive	
Alagille syndrome	Facies: broad forehead, deep-set eyes, pointed chin Congenital heart disease, butterfly vertebrae Liver biopsy: paucity of small bile ducts
Biliary atresia	Presents in first 2 months of life Usually full-term female Associated with congenital heart disease Hepatosplenomegaly
Choledochal cyst	May have palpable RUQ mass Often diagnosed prenatally
Gallstones/biliary sludge	May have history of TPN, hemolysis, or fasting (+) Ultrasound
Hepatocellular	
α-1-antitrypsin deficiency	Positive family history Liver biopsy: PAS-positive granules
Congenital infection	CMV, other TORCH, HIV, parvovirus B19, HBV, HCV IUGR, hepatosplenomegaly, thrombocytopenia, rash Abnormal fundoscopic or slit-lamp exam
Cystic fibrosis	May have (+) family history Delayed stooling, meconium ileus Abnormal newborn screen, positive sweat test
Galactosemia	Poor growth, hypotonia, cataracts, liver dysfunction *Escherichia coli* sepsis or UTI Abnormal newborn screen, quantitative GALT test (+) Urine reducing substances
Hypothyroidism	Delayed stooling after birth, lethargy, hoarse cry Macroglossia, large fontanelles, poor growth May be unconjugated
Idiopathic neonatal hepatitis	Recovery without intervention (most cases) Diagnosis usually requires liver biopsy
Panhypopituitarism	Normal growth parameters, microgenitalia (males) Lethargy, hypotension, temperature instability Hypoglycemia, electrolyte disturbances
TPN cholestasis	Usually after 2 weeks of TPN Reverses when TPN stopped
Tyrosinemia	FTT, vomiting, diarrhea, bleeding, hepatomegaly Cabbage-like odor Abnormal newborn screen and/or plasma amino acid and urine organic acid analyses
UTI/sepsis	Vomiting, lethargy, temperature instability Suspect UTI if onset of jaundice after 8 days of life May be unconjugated

Abbreviations: CMV, cytomegalovirus; FTT, failure to thrive; GALT, gut-associated lymphoid tissue; HBV, hepatitis B virus; HCV, hepatitis C virus; HIV, human immunodeficiency virus; IUGR, intrauterine growth restriction; PAS, periodic acid-Schiff stain; RUQ, right upper quadrant; TORCH, toxoplasmosis, other agents, rubella, cytomegalovirus, herpes simplex; TPN, total parenteral nutrition; UTI, urinary tract infection.

Figure 50-1. Guidelines for Phototherapy in Hospitalized Infants ≥35 Weeks' Gestation[a]

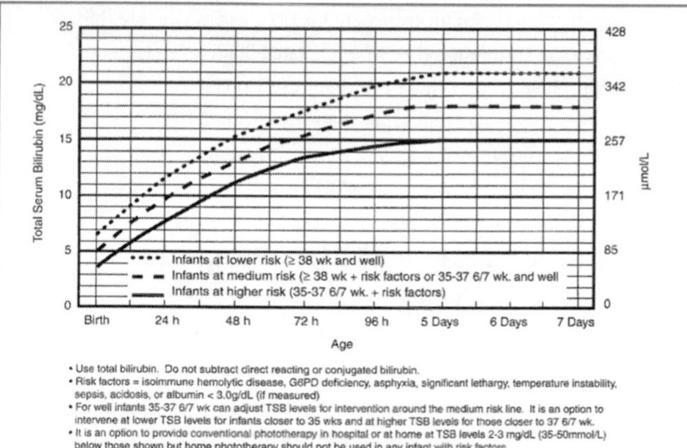
25
20
15
10
5
0
Total Serum Bilirubin (mg/dL)
428
342
257
171
85
0
μmol/L
Infants at lower risk (≥ 38 wk and well)
Infants at medium risk (≥ 38 wk + risk factors or 35-37 6/7 wk. and well
Infants at higher risk (35-37 6/7 wk. + risk factors)
Birth
24 h
48 h
72 h
96 h
5 Days
6 Days
7 Days
Age
• Use total bilirubin. Do not subtract direct reacting or conjugated bilirubin.
• Risk factors = isoimmune hemolytic disease, G6PD deficiency, asphyxia, significant lethargy, temperature instability, sepsis, acidosis, or albumin < 3.0g/dL (if measured)
• For well infants 35-37 6/7 wk can adjust TSB levels for intervention around the medium risk line. It is an option to intervene at lower TSB levels for infants closer to 35 wks and at higher TSB levels for those closer to 37 6/7 wk.
• It is an option to provide conventional phototherapy in hospital or at home at TSB levels 2-3 mg/dL (35-50mmol/L) below those shown but home phototherapy should not be used in any infant with risk factors.

[a]Note: These guidelines are based on limited evidence and the levels shown are approximations. The guidelines refer to the use of intensive phototherapy, which should be used when the TSB exceeds the line indicated for each category.

From American Academy of Pediatrics Subcommittee on Hyperbilirubinemia. Management of hyperbilirubinemia in the newborn infant 35 or more weeks of gestation. *Pediatrics.* 2004;114(1):297–316

Transcutaneous bilirubin measurements are unreliable once treatment is initiated since phototherapy bleaches the skin. The 2004 AAP guidelines recommend treating isoimmune hemolytic disease with intravenous (IV) gammaglobulin (0.5-1 g/kg over 2 hours) if the TSB is rising despite intensive phototherapy or if the TSB level is within 2 to 3 mg/dL of the exchange level. However, newer data do not support the use of IV immunoglobulin in neonates with Rh hemolytic disease.

Encourage more frequent feeding (every 2–3 hours). Offer milk-based formula or expressed breast milk supplementation for a mildly dehydrated infant or if there is more than 12% weight loss. Do not give IV hydration, unless the infant is severely dehydrated or unable to tolerate oral feeds.

If jaundice is due to an acute illness (UTI, sepsis, hypothyroidism), treat the underlying cause.

Conjugated Hyperbilirubinemia

If there is evidence of biliary obstruction, consult with a gastroenterologist and/or a pediatric surgeon for treatment via the Kasai procedure (biliary atresia), liver transplantation (tyrosinemia, late biliary atresia), choledochal cyst excision, cholecystectomy, or bile duct resection.

Ensure adequate nutritional support and medical management of underlying disorders. Consult with a geneticist and experienced nutritionist for dietary guidelines for liver and metabolic diseases.

Discharge Management (Unconjugated Hyperbilirubinemia)

Discontinue phototherapy and discharge home when the TSB level falls to less than 13 to 14 mg/dL. In general, observing for rebound is not necessary if it delays hospital discharge since significant rebound resulting in a readmission is rare. However, obtain a rebound level 6 to 12 hours after discontinuation of phototherapy for a Coombs-positive infant, who is at increased risk for a clinically significant rebound that may require the reinstitution of phototherapy. Offer home phototherapy only if the infant's TSB level is in the "optional phototherapy" range, since home devices, as well as sunlight exposure, are less reliable.

Indications for Consultation

- **Gastroenterology:** Conjugated hyperbilirubinemia
- **Geneticist:** Suspected metabolic disease
- **Pediatric surgery:** Suspected extrinsic/biliary obstruction

Disposition

- **Intensive care unit transfer:** Need for exchange transfusion
- **Discharge criteria (unconjugated hyperbilirubinemia):** TSB level less than 13 to 14 mg/dL, good oral intake

Follow-up

- **Primary care**
  - Patient treated with phototherapy for a hemolytic disease: within 24 hours for a follow-up bilirubin level
  - Patient not requiring phototherapy: 24 hours for clinical assessment with or without a repeat TSB level
  - Jaundice persists beyond 2 to 3 weeks of age: reevaluate for cholestasis

Pearls and Pitfalls

- Some infants with cholestatic jaundice exposed to phototherapy may develop a dark, grayish-brown discoloration of the skin, serum, and urine (the bronze infant syndrome). This is not a contraindication to continued phototherapy.
- Chronic bilirubin encephalopathy (kernicterus) is characterized by severe athetoid cerebral palsy, paralysis of upward gaze, hearing loss, and intellectual impairment.
- Clinical assessment of TSB is particularly inaccurate in a darker-skinned infant.

Coding

ICD-9

- Breast milk jaundice **774.39**
- Perinatal jaundice due to hepatocellular damage **774.4**
- Perinatal jaundice from hereditary hemolytic anemias **774.0**
- Perinatal jaundice from other causes **774.5**
- Perinatal jaundice from other excessive hemolysis **774.1**
- Physiological jaundice **774.6**
- Unspecified fetal and neonatal jaundice **774.6**

Bibliography

Ahlfors CE. Predicting bilirubin neurotoxicity in jaundiced newborns. *Curr Opin Pediatr.* 2010;22:129–133

American Academy of Pediatrics Subcommittee on Hyperbilirubinemia. Management of hyperbilirubinemia in the newborn infant 35 or more weeks of gestation. *Pediatrics.* 2004;114:297–316

Lease M, Whalen B. Assessing jaundice in infants of 35-week gestation and greater. *Curr Opin Pediatr.* 2010;22:352–365

Moyer V. Guideline for the evaluation of cholestatic jaundice in infants: recommendations of the North American Society for Pediatric Gastroenterology, Hepatology and Nutrition. *J Pediatr Gastro Nutr.* 2004;39:115–128

Smits-Wintjens VE. Intravenous immunoglobulin in neonates with rhesus hemolytic disease: a randomized controlled trial. *Pediatrics.* 2011;127:680–686

Miscellaneous Issues

The Economics of Pediatric Hospitalist Medicine

The increasing prevalence of pediatric hospital medicine practices has raised important questions regarding the financial sustainability of these groups at individual institutions. Pediatric hospitalist groups are rarely able to support themselves with professional fees alone, and thus often need to partner with hospitals to establish efficient, profitable, quality models of care.

Is My Group Profitable?

To begin, it is important to note the distinction between hospital charges and physician charges. A hospitalized patient receives one bill from the hospital to cover the bed, the antibiotics, etc, and another from the physician to cover intellectual and procedural services. These latter charges are physician, or professional, fees, which are associated with *Current Procedural Terminology* codes.

Nonacademic Model

The ability of a group to support itself with professional fees depends on the group's structure. Most pediatric hospital medicine programs receive some form of a stipend as they are not financially self-sufficient (ie, professional fee collections do not cover total program costs). A hospitalist group that does not stay in-house 24/7, keeps most of the reimbursed dollar, and has good contracts with insurance companies in a low-competition marketplace may be independently sustainable. In a nonacademic environment there may be fewer outside demands on scheduling, so the group can design shifts that are maximally profitable. However, in such a setting, there will usually be no residents to assist in providing 24/7 coverage if it is requested. This can adversely affect the group's profitability and/or the hospital's expenses. When a hospital does ask the group to provide more extended coverage, perhaps to meet a community need or to attract patients, the hospitalist group can request value-added payments or a stipend from the hospital to increase revenue and meet the program's financial needs.

The priorities of a for-profit nonsupported program will be professional fees and volume of services. In contrast, other for-profit companies may negotiate a stipend from the contractor (typically a hospital), to provide other non-billable services or to meet other quality metrics that are of value to the hospital. For example, a community hospital–supported program may be concerned with having a program that allows the hospital to preserve its newborn services and pediatric market share while providing high-quality care and ensuring the satisfaction of the local primary care providers.

Academic Model

In contrast, an academic model with hospitalists employed by a hospital or medical school faces additional challenges regarding reimbursement and scheduling. Reimbursement is often shared with the medical school and hospital administration, so that only a portion, if any, of the receipts goes to the physicians. In addition, the overall reimbursement rate may be lower at large, urban tertiary academic institutions, which face strong competition, lower market penetration, and possibly weaker strength for negotiating fees. Finally, mandates from outside agencies, such as Accreditation Council for Graduate Medical Education, regarding work hours and resident supervision may require hospitalist presence during low-volume patient hours during which little in the way of professional fees are generated for the hospitalists. Once again, value-added payments may be necessary.

Other potential benefits to an academic department include improved efficiency of subspecialists and surgeons by comanagement and sharing of resources, so that they are more available to see outpatients and serve as consultants. Hospitalists allow the department's ambulatory care faculty to remain focused in the outpatient setting and not feel compelled to leave to manage inpatients. The quality and quantity of medical student and house staff educational experiences may be enhanced. Finally, the presence of a hospitalist group may serve as a recruitment tool, encouraging local practitioners to refer their patients.

The Value-Added Issue

Hospitals frequently are asked to contribute to pediatric hospitalist revenue. The most common argument is that hospitalists contribute value to the mission of the hospital and deserve to be paid for this additional time. This includes hours spent toward streamlining discharge processes, improving communication with primary care pediatricians, facilitating interactions with nursing and ancillary staff, and participating on hospital-wide performance and safety committees. This also includes hours spent on low-revenue overnight shifts and care provided to self-pay uninsured patients, which may be vital to the hospital's service to the community.

Regardless of the group structure (academic vs nonacademic), it is in the hospitalist's best interest to track and provide regular updates about administrative work that is undertaken and attempt to define the value to the hospital.

Quantitative data are most readily reported as financial data, but meaningful quantitative metrics can also be developed. These may include increased patient and staff satisfaction scores, tracked interactions with students and/or residents, and improved on-site availability for emergencies (such as overnight shifts). Participation in outcome management and performance improvement initiatives, which is always a priority to hospital administrators, will further confirm the nonclinical value added by a hospitalist group and strengthen the hospitalist's position in financial negotiations.

The Question of Costs

An argument supporting the value added by hospitalists is the presumption that they will contribute to a decrease in the cost of care, and thus an increase in hospital revenue. This is often measured by metrics such as a decreased length of stay and less resource (laboratory, radiology, etc) utilization, translating into hospital savings. The validity of this concept is often determined locally or regionally, depending on the types of contracts that hospitals have with payers. Other potential sources of savings include less unreimbursed care, fewer insurance denials, fewer readmissions, and improved quality of care (fewer central line and nosocomial infections, etc).

In Medicare-driven adult medicine, the Inpatient Prospective Payment System shifts the financial risk of patient care from the payers to the providers. Specifically, patients are grouped into diagnosis-related groups (DRGs), and a single payment is provided without any consideration of resource utilization. It is understood that some patients will cost more, some less, and the DRG system tries to target the average and incentivize the provider to decrease expenditures. This DRG model has only recently entered pediatric medicine, where there are state-based public financing Medicaid models, as opposed to the federal Medicare program. As a result, there is no uniform model on implementing Medicaid payment because each program is different and managed at the state level. So, for states and hospitals with significant DRG contracts, there may be validity to the idea that shortening stays or ordering less magnetic resonance imaging is beneficial to the hospital's bottom line. In contrast, if a pediatric hospitalist program takes care of inpatients reimbursed on a per-diem basis, the hospital can potentially lose revenue if length of stay is shortened, since both revenue and costs are decreased.

In contrast, DRGs are uniformly employed by adult hospitalists working under Medicare reimbursement. Hospitals clearly save costs, which directly contributes to the profitability of adult hospitalist groups. This is a fundamental difference between adult and pediatric hospital medicine programs that group leaders and chief medical officers must consider when evaluating different contract and reimbursement paradigms for pediatric versus adult programs.

Other common payment models may not fall under the same hospitalist cost logic. The details within percentage fee-for-service and per-diem contracts may make a case against the typical metrics of a hospitalist's value. In the former, hospitals are paid a percentage of charges. There is essentially no incentive to decrease charges, especially if the negotiated payment percentage is highly profitable to the hospital. In the per-diem model, the most expensive days, with the most studies, often are early in the stay, so there is actually an incentive for patients to stay longer for less expensive days when the hospital still gets paid the same daily rate.

It is therefore critical for a hospitalist to understand the hospital's types of contracts. DRG-based hospitals may be vested in length-of-stay metrics, while per-diem–based hospitals may be similarly interested in this metric but for the exact opposite reason.

Charges Versus Costs

Hospital charges are often used as a surrogate marker for the cost of a patient encounter, although the amount the hospital truly spends to provide the care is highly variable and often difficult to determine. It is important to understand the difference between fixed costs and variable costs. To account for expenses, hospitals often use a percentage model, whereby service lines (radiology, pharmacy, supplies, etc) are assigned a percentage-of-charges value, which is then used to estimate the direct-plus-variable cost of a stay. So a $9,000 hospital stay, by charges, may be estimated at $4,500 cost if the average of the percentages for the various services provided equal 50%. However, hospital charges, and the associated cost estimates, vary so widely by region that they can be almost incomparable. There have been efforts to establish correction coefficients, but this represents assumptions atop assumptions. As a result, determining the true cost of care is an elusive goal, which makes it difficult to determine how hospitalist interventions actually contribute.

Conclusion

In almost every scenario, hospitalist groups and hospitals must develop a partnership, both in clinical pursuits and financial discussions. In the scope of their everyday practice, pediatric hospitalists clearly have an opportunity to improve the hospital's bottom line. By limiting charges and providing more efficient care, hospitalists may also help the insurer's bottom line. Since a healthy hospital can provide robust services to a community and a healthy insurance company may be able to provide more affordable, broad coverage to more families, this further strengthens the argument for the existence and support of pediatric hospitalist programs. As the specialty continues to mature and hospitalists enter into leadership roles, they may have increased influence over the national debate and contribute more directly to the efforts to limit the growth of health care costs at the national and state levels.

Bibliography

Frank E, Paul DP, Nersesian R. Hospitalists at an academic medical center, part 1: impact of a voluntary pilot hospitalist program. *Hosp Top.* 2011;89:75–81

Greeno R. Funding a hospitalist program: which approach will you take? *Healthc Financ Manage.* 2010;64:76–80

Lundberg S, Balingit P, Wali S, Cope D. Cost-effectiveness of a hospitalist service in a public teaching hospital. *Acad Med.* 2010;85:1312–1315

Mitchell DM. The critical role of hospitalists in controlling healthcare costs. *J Hosp Med.* 2010;5:127–132

Sprague L. The hospitalist: better value in inpatient care? *Issue Brief Natl Health Policy Forum.* 2011 Mar 30;1–17

CHAPTER 52

Family-Centered Rounds

Introduction

Family-centered rounds (FCR) is defined as "interdisciplinary work rounds *at the bedside* in which the patient and family *share in the control* of both the management plan and the evaluation of the process itself." The essential component of FCR is the equal relationship between the family and medical staff, which usually includes the bedside nurse and the physician team. Rounding at the bedside allows the team to disperse the same information about the patient to everyone. FCR offers an ideal setting to role-model professional skills to trainees and to conduct case-specific teaching. Medical staff benefits include the opportunity to learn from families, as well as improved communication, coordination of care, and resource utilization. For patients and families, FCR is empowering, as it facilitates participation in rounds and leads to a better understanding of medical issues and the plan of care. FCR improves patient, family, and staff satisfaction. Potential drawbacks to FCR include an increase in rounding time, as well as initial team discomfort with presenting to families, soliciting family participation in case presentations, and crowding in the patient's room. However, with thorough preparation the benefits outweigh these drawbacks.

How It Works

Who

The medical team consists of the family and medical staff. The family includes the patient, parent/legal guardian, and other family members, while the physician team, nurses, care coordinators, and other health care providers comprise the medical staff. The physician component is composed of medical students, interns, residents, mid-level providers, fellows, and attending physicians.

Where

FCR occurs at the bedside, the patient's room door, or the nursing station *with the family*.

Getting Started

Begin by explaining the benefits of FCR with all participants.

Preparing Families

Introduce the family to FCR on admission, either verbally or via brochures or videos. Critical elements are the definition, purpose, and process of FCR, and the time at which the family can expect the medical team for rounds. Ask the family if they want to participate in FCR and whom to include, and then confirm before starting the rounds. If they agree, before the rounds begin, ask the family to write down their questions or any observations they want to share. When the case is being presented, have the family correct errors in the history and encourage them to question any unclear medical terminology. Tell the family whether an attending physician will perform a focused physical examination during FCR.

Solicit an adolescent's preferences regarding participating in FCR and determine who should be present. Note that for some topics, like reproductive health, mental health, and substance abuse, adolescent confidentiality laws mandate that the decision regarding parental presence is left to the discretion of the patient. However, be aware of your state's adolescent age definitions and protected health topics, as they can vary considerably. For other health topics, such as asthma and diabetes, the parents have a right to be present. If the teenager does not want a parent present for FCR, then efforts must be made to ensure good rapport with both the patient and family.

Preparing the Patient

Help the patient to understand FCR and participate in the process, although this will depend on the child's age, alertness, and developmental level. Explain that a group of people will be in the room to discuss his or her care. Encourage the patient to record and ask questions during FCR. Child life specialists are a very useful resource for facilitating the preparation of the patient for FCR and managing follow-up questions that may arise.

Preparing the Nurse and Other Clinicians

The bedside nurse has the most interaction with the family and patient and therefore is an invaluable resource on FCR. The nurse is uniquely positioned to support the family's participation, assist them in formulating questions for the physician team, and share information about the patient's progress. Other clinicians can also advocate for the family in the same way on FCR.

The Physician Team

Clearly define how the physicians will educate the patient and family about FCR. Meet with the nurse and other team members before entering the room, and assign roles and tasks to keep individuals engaged.

- **Introduction:** The team member assigned to the patient introduces the other team members to the patient and family.
- **Presentation:** Sit at the family's level, use lay terminology, and speak in a conversational manner. Talk to the family during the history, and speak to the family and team during the assessment and plan. Elicit and allow time for questions and observations by the patient, family, nurse, etc. Clarify the discharge goals.
- **Orders:** Have a physician who is not presenting write/enter any orders and repeat them verbally.
- **Discharge facilitation:** Begin, update, or complete any discharge paperwork, if appropriate for a non-presenter to do so.
- **Resident:** Guide the junior team members in developing their assessments and plans. Ask pertinent questions and introduce the on-call resident to the family, if applicable. Also function as a role model, troubleshooter, and time-keeper (the goal is <10 minutes per patient). Call consults after exiting the room.
- **Fellow/attending physician:** Be a role model by guiding learners as needed. Take advantage of the opportunity to teach about physical findings as the family and patient permit. Ensure privacy if a focused physical examination is performed. Confirm whom the primary care provider is to facilitate comanagement or transition of care at discharge.

Other Medical Staff

Include other staff, such as the care manager/discharge planner, physical and/or occupational therapist, child life specialist, respiratory and/or speech therapist, dietitian, and pharmacist, if their input is important.

Indications for Consultation

- **Child life specialist:** To help prepare children for rounds or procedures
- **Family advocacy:** To bridge communication gaps when the attending physician or charge nurse has been unable to resolve a conflict; for families to make formal statements about their experience in the hospital; to educate families and staff on patient's rights and responsibilities
- **Social work:** For resources, including social support

Follow-up

- Timely communication with the primary caregiver about the discharge plan

Pearls and Pitfalls

- Preparation for FCR includes adapting it to your hospital.
- See Table 52-1 for troubleshooting tips.
- Treat the family as equals on the team. They are the experts on their child.
- In general, families focus on the condition of their child while medical personnel focus on the plan. Spend time explaining the diagnosis and condition during the assessment.
- Every medical team has different dynamics. If problems arise, address them quickly and implement change.
- A useful form of communication is a dry-erase board inside the room that includes pertinent information.

Table 52-1. Troubleshooting

Potential Solutions: Before Rounds	Potential Solutions: During Rounds
Lack of Buy-in	
Staff: Provide a literature review documenting benefits of FCR. Family: Clarify expectations for rounds. Presenter: Introduce yourself to the family.	Decrease the number of staff in the room. Identify one person as the team spokesperson. Encourage questions and observations from the family.
Time Constraints	
Review roles of each individual. Have the presenter practice and review the plan. During pre-rounding, help the family formulate questions and answer the straightforward ones.	Start on time Be aware of time limitations (<10 minutes per patient). Politely tell the family that a team member will return later to discuss the less critical issues and set a time to return.
Family Is Absent	
Obtain the family's questions and observations, and arrange for a different time to talk.	Use a speakerphone to call the family (ie, the mother is at work).
Use of Medical Jargon	
Anticipate unavoidable medical terminology and review the definitions with the family.	Give definitions during the presentation. Encourage the family to ask questions. Give feedback to the presenter after rounds.
Lack of Consensus	
Have a "quarterback huddle" before starting to quickly review the proposed plan and options.	Ask the family about their major concerns and/or their goals for the hospitalization.
Non-English Speakers	
Arrange for a translator (not a family member).	Use an offsite translator via speakerphone or video.
Suspected Child Abuse	
Clarify with the social worker what information the parents/legal guardians can receive and who makes medical decisions. Practice how to review management decisions in a non-accusatory way.	Focus on the medical management, safety, and well-being of the patient. Inform the family that the medical staff's role is limited to medical management.

Coding

CPT

- Prolonged service, 30 to 74 minutes **99356**
- Each additional 30 minutes **99354**

Bibliography

Children's Hospital of Philadelphia. *Patient and Family Tips for Participation on Rounds* http://www.chop.edu/export/download/pdfs/articles/family-centered-care/rounds-tips-families.pdf. Accessed April 20, 2012

Cincinnati Children's Hospital. *Family-Centered Rounds.* http://www.cincinnatichildrens.org/professional/referrals/patient-family-rounds/default/. Accessed April 20, 2012

Committee of Hospital Care and Institute for Patient- and Family-Centered Care: Family-centered care and the pediatrician's role. *Pediatrics.* 2012;129:394–404

Rosen P, Stenger E, Bochkoris M, Hannon MJ, Kwoh CK. Family-centered multidisciplinary rounds enhance the team approach in pediatrics. *Pediatrics.* 2009;123:e603–e608

Sisterhen LL, Blaszak RT, Woods MB, Smith CE. Defining family-centered rounds. *Teach Learn Med.* 2007;19:319–22

Videos Explaining FCR for Families

Cincinnati Childrens Hospital. *Family-Centered Rounds at Cincinnati Children's Medical Center.* http://www.youtube.com/watch?v=XZQ7Yy3gxZU and http://www.cincinnatichildrens.org/professional/referrals/patient-family-rounds/videos/

Texas Children's Hospital. *Family-Centered Care in Pediatric Hospital Medicine.* http://www.youtube.com/watch?v=TdgU0VZNfSg

CHAPTER 53

Hospitalist Comanagement

The Society of Hospital Medicine defines comanagement as the "shared responsibility, authority, and accountability for the care of a hospitalized patient." This term was created to describe the increasing prevalence of diverse medical teams working together to care for complex patients. In pediatrics, this primarily involves children with surgical conditions or complex medical diseases being managed by subspecialists.

Comanagement of children requires a unique perspective. The impact of family involvement and, more specifically, the importance of patient family-centered care (PFCC) affect the success of any comanagement collaboration. The principles of PFCC must therefore be incorporated into every comanagement arrangement. Also, the multidisciplinary team must include the patient's medical home and primary care physician, while at hospital discharge home health care professionals may also be incorporated.

Models of Comanagement

Models of comanagement vary, but all place the primary responsibility for patient care on one team. Secondary members of the comanagement group assume a consulting role in care, as in the case of a hospitalist involved with a surgical patient. In the role of consultant, the hospitalist may need to review guidelines and "etiquette" in providing pediatric expertise while maintaining boundaries and modeling medical professionalism. An excellent template for this service comes from Goldman's "Ten Commandments for Effective Consultation": (1) clarify the question, (2) determine the urgency, (3) gather data independently, (4) be brief and avoid recapitulation, (5) be specific in all recommendations, (6) anticipate potential problems and provide therapeutic options, (7) honor the roles of the caregivers, (8) teach with tact, (9) maintain direct contact with the referring physician, and (10) follow up with notes and recommendations.

In an alternative model of comanagement of the surgical patient, the hospitalist team assumes the role of primary physician while the surgical team is the consultant. The hospitalist may also serve as the gatekeeper for the surgeons by providing preoperative evaluations on complex patients with multiple medical comorbidities. By using hospitalists, surgeons can identify which patients may have unexpected complications and assist in preparing the medically fragile patient when surgery cannot be postponed. Regardless of which model is employed, the importance of a single primary team cannot be overemphasized when caring for complicated patients.

Benefits of Comanagement

As the field of hospital medicine has evolved, pediatric subspecialists and surgeons have discovered the benefits of using the expertise of hospitalists, including reduced length of stay, fewer medical complications, and improved patient and ancillary staff satisfaction. In addition, hospitalists have intimate experience with the specific hospital policies and procedures, so patients and their families can rely on them to coordinate care through the increasingly confusing hospital system. Finally, in teaching hospitals, new guidelines from the Accreditation Council for Graduate Medical Education continue to limit the hours of resident physicians. In-house hospitalist coverage can offset some of the effects of these restrictions.

Another benefit of early and well-defined comanagement arrangements is to decrease the use of laboratory testing and radiologic procedures. Hospitalist services improve surgical patient outcomes by giving expert advice to consultants on medications and medical disease states, while early intervention for medical complications can prevent unforeseen outcomes. Hospitalist groups are encouraged to meet with their comanagement partners regularly to come to consensus on how particular medical conditions will be treated prior to and after surgery.

The creation of comanagement arrangements can broaden the exposure of hospitalists in an institution and support their need to hospital administration. In addition to interactions with surgical teams, hospitalists may also strengthen associations with anesthesiologists and subspecialists. Comanagement can also create a means to introduce quality assurance initiatives to a broader physician base in the hospital.

Potential Pitfalls of Comanagement

Use of comanagement can create obstacles for the hospitalist group if certain guidelines are not followed. Groups working together must clearly define the roles of both the surgical teams and the hospitalist groups, and patients and staff must have a clear understanding as to who the attending and consulting teams are at admission. Issues can arise if roles are not defined, and medical mistakes occur when there is no clear assignment of duties. This is especially important when laboratory and radiology overview is needed.

Comanagement can lead to mistakes if nursing and ancillary staff do not understand the relationship or if there are conflicting orders. Communication, in the form of daily rounds between the hospitalist group and a member of the surgical team, is imperative. It is incumbent on all members of a comanagement team to update one another directly when unexpected changes in patient status occur and not presume that written notes suffice for ample communication to others on the comanagement team.

Finally, hospitalist groups should be mindful of "mission creep" when establishing a comanagement model. This term applies to a situation in which a project expands into areas where it was not initially intended. The use of hospitalists on all surgical patients in a given specialty may be unnecessary, while expansion of hospitalist workload in a short amount of time can lead to decreases in job performance and dissatisfaction. Comanagement is not effective for the hospitalist team if they do not feel valued or have autonomy to select which patients are most benefited from their consultative roles.

Billing and Coding

When participating in a comanagement model, hospitalists must be familiar with the correct billing codes required for their services. Under most comanagement models, the hospitalists will not bill for the initial admission history. The exception is a situation in which the hospitalist directly admits a patient requiring surgery from the emergency department. The patient may be admitted to the surgery team but a hospitalist provides the service of overnight admission history and physical examination. In some comanagement models the hospitalists evaluate surgical patients preoperatively and would use outpatient consultant codes **99241–99245.** (See example of protocol.)

Changes continue to occur in reimbursement from Medicare and private insurance companies. These changes are expected to follow with Medicaid and will affect pediatric hospitalists. In January 2010, Medicare eliminated the use of inpatient consultation codes for most patients. As a result, hospitalists now bill an initial hospital visit under the codes **99221–99223.** These codes are used for the first encounter and examination by a hospitalist. After the primary assessment, subsequent hospitalist team members use the care codes **99231–99233.** These codes cover general medical care of the patient after surgery. Rare exceptions may exist in which the hospitalist is asked to address a specific medical issue, such as hyponatremia, and in this situation the pediatric hospitalist may bill under the **99251–99254** codes for medical consultation. All hospitalist groups should review coding with a hospital billing specialist on a regular basis.

An important point to remember when billing is to follow the requirements for complete and accurate documentation. This includes listing the name of the referring, or comanaging physician, and completing a written note that includes the key components needed for a selected billing designation.

Hospitalist groups may encounter denials from insurance companies when initiating comanagement agreements if staff is not educated on billing practices. Experts also recommend that denials be followed up with appeal letters to ensure payment, and most claims will be paid after physician documentation is reviewed.

Comanagement Implementation Guidelines

When embarking on a comanagement agreement, hospitalist groups have access to guidelines from the Society of Hospital Medicine. Position papers from the Co-Management Advisory Council provide a good resource to institutions. The following is a checklist for implementation of comanagement:

1. Identify a comanagement champion on both the hospitalist and surgical teams. These individuals will initiate dialogue and meet regularly to start the process. Each champion will represent their specialty to negotiate, educate, and update other staff members.
2. Identify comanagement stakeholders. Hospital support should be sought at this point to identify who in the hospital administration can facilitate the comanagement. Include in the initial meetings ancillary staff such as nursing, pharmacy, emergency department physicians, and case managers.
3. Hold a consensus meeting. Early in the development of the project bring together the comanagement project champions and the stakeholders. Issues to be discussed are related to how the comanagement model will improve patient care and staff satisfaction, as well as promote quality improvement within the institution. Introduce a general framework for the project and prepare a value proposal for the stakeholders on how the program might benefit the hospital.
4. Determine stakeholders' goals. Solicit input from people who will be directly impacted by the creation of a comanagement project. This increases chances of success by allowing these personnel to assist in identifying potential institutional or work-flow issues. Allow each stakeholder to give input on how a comanagement project might affect their given area of interest.
5. Develop a service agreement. This document is needed to define the roles, responsibilities, and expectations of the comanagement project. Use it to delineate specifics on the comanagement project, including admission and discharge procedures and attending and consulting team responsibilities. Also include a consensus on communication protocols, patient selection, and financial and billing arrangements. Use this agreement to resolve issues that arise, and revise it frequently as the team gains experience.

6. Define key program metrics. The comanagement program must have a process to identify outcome measures so that quality assurance can be documented. A list of must-have measures can be found in the consensus panel's report. These measures include both financial and patient outcome data, although each institution may vary in the accessibility of certain data. Discuss and determine who will be responsible for collection and assimilation of the data.
7. Address financial considerations. It is important to decide financial compensation prior to institution of the comanagement project. Issues to be determined are who will bill for what services and which providers will be involved. All physicians involved in the comanagement agreement must be trained in correct billing practices and be accountable for timely submission.
8. Select patients appropriate for comanagement. Be proactive at this process to ensure that they will benefit from the comanagement project. Develop inclusion and exclusion criteria that include patient factors such as age and comorbidity status. Also include criteria for selection of the phase of the surgical process (presurgical, perioperative, and postoperative) in which the hospitalists will be involved in comanagement. Other important issues to consider are the hospital admission rate for surgical patients, the size and expertise of the hospitalist service, and the capability of adding surgical patients to the hospitalist workload.
9. Establish a staffing model and communication plan. Address staffing issues prior to institution of the comanagement agreement, including assessment of current staffing in nursing and ancillary staff and whether new hires will be needed. Also decide whether nurse practitioners and residents will be included in the model. Within the communication plan, determine who will be included in daily rounds and how often comanagement team meetings will be held.
10. Develop program support materials. The success of the comanagement project is improved when teams collaborate on clinical guidelines, order sets, and other important policies and procedures prior to launching the program. Early in the process, implement agreed-on standards of care to help decrease errors and miscommunication.
11. Pilot the comanagement program. Start the comanagement program with a small, preselected group of patients. This decreases initial errors in the system, allows timely evaluation of early obstacles and flaws in the program, and facilitates making adjustments in the model.

Summary

The definition of comanagement remains vague and differs substantially from one institution to another. Multiple models for combined care exist, and the guidelines for best practices in comanagement continue to evolve. Task forces have been established to assist with improving this growing trend and ensuring that hospitalist groups enter into comanagement arrangements in a way that benefits their practice and patient outcomes. More information and time are needed to assess what impact comanagement will have on the field of pediatric hospital medicine. The incorporation and success of comanagement in the field of pediatrics will need to focus on the family as a part of the medical team and the critical importance of impeccable communication that serves as a cornerstone to safe and effective pediatric patient care.

Bibliography

Hinami K, Whelan CT, Konetzka RT, Meltzer DO. Provider expectations and experiences of comanagement. *J Hosp Med.* 2011;6:401–404

Rappaport DI, Pressel DM. Pediatric hospitalist comanagement of surgical patients: challenges and opportunities. *Clin Pediatr (Phila).* 2008;47:114–121

Simon TD, Eilert R, Dickinson LM, et al. Pediatric hospitalist comanagement of spinal fusion surgery patients. *J Hosp Med.* 2007;2:23–30

Stille CJ. Communication, comanagement, and collaborative care for children and youth with special healthcare needs. *Pediatr Ann.* 2009;38:498–504

Whinney C, Michota F. Surgical comanagement: a natural evolution of hospitalist practice. *J Hosp Med.* 2008;3:394–397

CHAPTER 54

Leading a Team

Introduction

A pediatric hospitalist team leader must be able to balance the needs of the patient and family (diagnosis, treatment, comfort) with those of the hospital (efficiency, cost awareness). A physician may lead many different types of teams, such as the rounding team, a quality committee, a code team, or a community response to a disease. However, all have the same ultimate goal: to provide high-quality, family-centered care that emphasizes efficiency and safety.

Key Elements for a Pediatric Hospital Medicine Team Leader

Knowledge of Disease States and Procedures

This is a career-long, ongoing process. The best leaders know when to admit they do not know an answer and how to find assistance.

Knowledge of Team Members and Skill Sets

The ward team may include some combination of trainees, nurses, respiratory therapists, case managers, and social workers, among others. The patient care team will also include the patient and family. It is critical to understand the strengths and weaknesses of each member, yourself included, in order to provide or seek mentorship. This creates a better group and helps improve patient outcome. A leader will set a direction for this team with interdisciplinary input and ensure (without micromanaging) that the team optimizes its performance. This may need to be done at a systems level (ie, changing the admission process) or at the patient level. The leader will not simply give orders and leave, but direct this collaboration on patient care needs and delivery.

Knowledge of Health Care and Related Systems

In order to provide better care to patients in the hospital, a leader must explore the following:

- Community needs and strengths, including those of referring physicians or unaffiliated organizations, in order to ensure safe transfers of care
- Hospital needs and strengths, including bed numbers, growth strategies, budgets, etc
- Hospital-based support systems (These range from quality teams and resource utilization committees to reporting systems for adverse events to social supports for families.)

When issues arise, an effective leader can work with others to design a systems-based approach or change.

Understanding the Importance of Communication

Communication is a key element to successful care and partnership with the patient, family, team members, and primary care provider. While systems for communication may exist, ultimately communication is a personal experience that relies on the expressive and receptive skills of all involved parties. A leader must be aware of how information is both given and then received by the recipients. A leader must also model respect for the wishes of the patient and family. Finally, documentation of communication is an equally important part of a leader's oversight responsibilities.

Key Attributes of a Leader

- Sets an example to others in terms of dedication to patients and team performance
- Invests the time to develop leadership skills outside of medical training (This will include coursework and reading as well as a process of active feedback on skills sets.)
- Always seeks personal mentors while learning how to provide mentorship to others
- Understands how to alter the style of communication and negotiation based on the personal style of any given team member, patient, family member, or primary care provider
- Effectively manages conflict
- Uses time management skills
- Understands the importance of documentation, billing, and coding in the success of the team, program, and hospital
- Evaluates all processes to ensure family-centered care

Bibliography

Black J. *The Toyota Way to Healthcare Excellence: Increase Efficiency and Improve Quality with Lean.* Chicago, IL: Health Administration Press; 2008

Burkhardt U, Erbsen A, Rüdiger-Stürchler M. The hospitalist as coordinator: an observational case study. *J Health Organ Manag.* 2010;24:22–44

Fisher R, Ury W, Patton B. *Getting to Yes: Negotiating Agreement without Giving In.* 2nd ed. New York, NY: Penguin Books; 1991

The Myers-Briggs Foundation. http://www.myersbriggs.org/

O'Leary KJ, Williams MV. The evolution and future of hospital medicine. *Mt Sinai J Med.* 2008;75:418–423

CHAPTER 55

Patient Safety

Introduction

Hospitalists are expected to integrate quality improvement and patient safety as core practices and expected competencies. This requires a combination of reactive (ad hoc for acute event occurrence), responsive (Joint Commission continual readiness), and proactive (trigger tools) programs.

Developing systems to prevent or respond to a medical error or patient harm always requires personal accountability. However, the single greatest impediment to error prevention is that often the institution punishes people for making mistakes, rather than embracing a "culture of safety." This culture supports learning and focuses on proactive management of system design and behavior choices. The culture of safety distinguishes reckless human actions from those caused by an unintended failure or a lack of training or education. Each occurrence is treated as unique and addressed in a thoughtful, collegial manner.

The most frequently reported errors involve medications. However errors in communication, patient identification, diagnosis, left/right confusion, and others are common, but suffer from limited reporting.

Basic Terms

Adverse Event: Any medical error, regardless of severity or cause.

At-risk Behavior: A behavior choice that increases risk, such as not consistently using 2 patient identifiers when indicated. Either the risk is not recognized or it is mistakenly believed to be justified.

Culture of Safety: A commitment to safety at all levels in the organization that acknowledges the high-risk, error-prone nature of an organization's activities. This is a blame-free environment with an expectation of collaboration across ranks and a willingness to direct resources to address safety concerns.

Error: An inadvertent action; a slip, lapse, or mistake. Mistakes are errors due to failure to choose correctly, while slips are lapses in concentration.

Hard Stop: A step in a process that must be completed in order to continue, such as scanning a patient ID bar code in order for a medication to be dispensed.

Harm: An unintended injury resulting from, or exacerbated by, medical care. This then requires additional monitoring, treatment, or hospitalization, or results in death.

High Reliability Organization (HRO): Any organization operating under hazardous conditions yet having few adverse events. HROs are preoccupied with failure, resilient when failure occurs, and sensitive (attentive) to operations, while maintaining a culture of safety.

Sentinel Event: An unexpected occurrence involving death or serious physical or psychological injury or risk thereof. Requires immediate investigation and response.

Basic Tools, Resources, and Committees

Ad hoc Committee: A committee formed to address a specific patient safety issue, separate from standing patient safety meetings or committees.

Clinical Nurse Leader: A staff member who focuses on patient safety, evidence-based practice, care coordination, and risk assessment. The role and certification have been developed by the American Association of Colleges and Nursing.

Failure Mode and Effect Analysis (FMEA): Error analysis done either retrospectively (as in a root cause analysis) or prospectively to determine failures and the relative impact of each failure. Allows for prioritization of targets for improvement based on a number (criticality index).

Patient Safety Officer: The designated safety officer has primary oversight for the facility-wide patient safety program and directs process improvements to reduce medical errors (and other factors) that contribute to unintended adverse patient outcomes.

Root Cause Analysis (RCA): Problem-solving methods used to identify and evaluate contributing or causal factors associated with adverse events or near misses. Includes implementation of solutions and monitoring of the effect of those solutions.

Trigger Tool: The use of "triggers," or clues, to identify adverse events. This is an effective method for measuring the overall level of harm from medical care in a health care organization.

Selected Best Practices

Antimicrobial Stewardship: A program to optimize antimicrobial therapy (choice, dose, timing, duration) based on individual patient data, local resistance patterns, cost, ease of use, and other criteria.

Disclosure Team: Members may include a quality/safety officer, attending physician, and a treating nurse who presents information to a patient and/

or family, in a way they can clearly understand, about an adverse event or serious error.

Fatigue Recognition Training/Abatement: This provides ongoing education on the effects of fatigue on cognition and motor performance and is usually paired with sleep education. The training encourages self-awareness and includes prevention tips.

Peer Review: A clinical review of a case with unintended or complicated outcome and/or unexpected variability in care among similar cases. The review addresses best practices, diagnostic errors, and systems failures (communication, products, environment, etc); classifies the error; and lists actions to be taken to address these failures.

Safety Walk Rounds: Perform on all units, 1 to 2 times per week. Include senior leadership (chairman, board member, patient safety officer, chief nursing officer, etc) so that they can connect with front-line staff. Ask the staff, "What is the next thing to harm your patient today?" or "Is there anything that might be causing your patient to feel in harm's way?" Then focus on immediately remediable safety issues.

SBAR: SBAR is a communication tool that describes the situation, background, assessment, and recommendation related to an acute event or patient care handoff.

Stop the Line: This is a policy and procedure that gives all staff, parents, trainees, and visitors the responsibility and authority to immediately intervene to protect the safety of a patient. All staff are expected to immediately stop and respond to the request by reassessing the patient's safety.

Team Building: A system, such as Team STEPPS (Department of Defense and Agency for Healthcare Research and Quality), to improve communication and teamwork skills, including conflict resolution and defining team roles and responsibilities.

How to Be Involved

Advocate: Encourage the development and use of health information systems that address pediatric-specific needs, offer data element tracking, and allow for modifications such as hard stops for error prevention.

Engage: Contribute to patient safety teams, national patient safety goal initiatives, and hospital safety committees. Include patients and families in patient safety endeavors wherever possible.

Lead: Be involved in safety walk rounds or a local initiative (eg, procedure documentation).

Participate: Be part of ad hoc reviews of and action plans developed from critical events.

Report: Undergo training on the use of safety reporting systems and report near misses.

Support: Support a culture of safety and HRO attributes.

Teach: Integrate safety practices into clinical rounds, conferences, and journal clubs.

Coding and External Reporting

Insurers and Medicare may not pay for care that is necessary because of preventable errors. Many of these are termed "never events" and currently include things such as hospital-acquired skin breakdown/decubitus ulcers and nasal cannula nares erosion. Payment may also be affected by proof of adherence to best practices and documenting better outcome. Pay for performance is the act of paying a provider for performing at or above a certain standard of quality for the given indicator.

Some examples of external reporting include sentinel events (state), asthma measures (The Joint Commission), infections (state public health), and negligent care delivery (state medical board). Each can result in mandatory action plans, on-site audits, fines, or other disciplinary or legal actions.

Pearls and Pitfalls

- Put one safety measure into every quality project.
- Use hard stops whenever possible.
- Seek patient and family input to prevent and address errors. Anticipate problems by assessing how processes will be completed by patients and families.
- Integrate safety role modeling on clinical rounds.
- Work with interdisciplinary teams in a family-centered manner. Engage trainees on hospital committees (chief residents are particularly well suited for this role).
- Arrange a test run to assess the potential impact of a change prior to implementation.
- Do not use just education and reminders to address a problem. These are the least effective methods of error avoidance.
- Perform a thorough RCA when investigating errors. Situational, behavioral, and patient-specific issues are often lost if an RCA is not complete.

Information and Training

Agency for Healthcare Research and Quality Patient Safety Tools: http://www.ahrq.gov/qual/pips/

American Academy of Pediatrics Safer Health Care for Kids Culture of Safety: www.aap.org/saferhealthcare/resources_04.html

Institute for Healthcare Improvement: www.ihi.org

The Joint Commission: http://www.jointcommission.org/topics/patient_safety.aspx and http://www.jcrinc.com

Bibliography

Billman G, Kimmons H. Pediatric hospital medicine core competencies: patient safety. *J Hosp Med.* 2010;5(S2):104–105

Ranji SR, Shojania KG. Implementing patient safety interventions in your hospital: what to try and what to avoid. *Med Clin North Am.* 2008;92:275–293

Takata GS, Mason W, Taketomo C, et al. Development, testing, and findings of a pediatric-focused trigger tool to identify medication-related harm in US children's hospitals. *Pediatrics.* 2008;121:e927–e935

CHAPTER 56

Pediatric Hospitalists in Transport

Hospitalist involvement in pediatric inter-facility transport is an evolving role. Pediatric hospitalists find themselves on both ends of the transport spectrum—either as the referring physician looking for a higher level of care or as the accepting physician at the higher-level institution. The first priority for the hospitalist is proper communication so that the correct site/unit, team, and vehicle are available for the patient.

Communication

Transport programs differ in the method of access for referring physicians. Some have communication centers with specialized staff trained in answering calls, alerting the appropriate team members, and arranging the transport. Others have registered nurses (RNs) or physicians who answer the calls and organize all aspects of the transport. Either way, having one telephone number that referring sites can call is the safest and most efficient means to conduct transports. Incorporate a time-out to focus on the exchange of demographic information. In addition, request that the referring physician remain in contact with the receiving center in case there are additional questions or problems. Therefore, all systems require 24-hour coverage. Finally, log and save all communications for later review.

The information that must be obtained and then become part of the medical record is outlined in the sample intake and accepting forms (Figures 56-1 and 56-2). Triage decisions will depend on the patient's diagnosis and whether the potential receiving hospital has the capabilities to manage that illness or injury. For instance, is it necessary for the receiving institution to be a trauma or burn center or have an intensive care unit bed or a specific subspecialist available? It is critical that the personnel answering the telephone know to whom to triage the call (ward, emergency department [ED], or pediatric intensive care unit [PICU] attending) and where to refer the intake call if services are not available at that center. See the American Academy of Pediatrics (AAP) "Guidelines for Developing Admission and Discharge Policies for the Pediatric Intensive Care Unit" and "Guidelines for Intermediate Care" for decisions regarding when to refer a child to a PICU or an intermediate level of care.

Figure 56-1. Hospitalist Transport Activation—Guidance Card (Referring)

1. Discuss patient with accepting physician
2. Location recommendation: ED, ward, PICU, NICU?
3. Time-out: provide information

   Today's date and time ______________________

   Referring physician ______________________

   Referring hospital ______________________

   Hospital address (if needed) ______________________

   Referring hospital phone number ______________________

   Where is patient located in hospital? ______________________

   Patient name ______________________

   Patient date of birth ______________________

   Patient telephone ______________________

   Chief concern ______________________

   Medical history ______________________

   Vital signs ______________________

   Pertinent labs and x-rays ______________________

   Get medical advice until transport arrives ______________________
4. Ask for anticipated arrival time
5. Ask for call-back number in case patient status changes

Team Composition

Transport team composition varies among institutions with several different possible combinations: physician, nurse practitioner (NP), RN, respiratory therapist, emergency medical technician (EMT), and paramedic. It is the role of the medical control physician (MCP) to assess the needs of the patient and determine the team composition based on the scope of practice of the available personnel. Flexibility in a program ensures assembling the appropriate team for a specific patient.

Choosing the level of transport therefore coincides with deciding on the team composition. There are 3 levels of transport: basic life support (BLS), advanced life support (ALS), and critical care transport. Each state has pediatric guidelines for emergency medical services (EMS), some more stringent than others. BLS transports involve only EMTs, usually no medications or intravenous (IV) fluids, and minimal oxygen administration. EMTs are trained

Figure 56-2. Hospitalist Transport Activation—Guidance Card (Accepting)

1. Discuss patient with referring physician—assess
2. Consider bed situation?
3. Time-out: collect information

   Today's date and time ______________________

   Referring physician ______________________

   Referring hospital ______________________

   Hospital address (if needed) ______________________

   Referring hospital telephone number ______________________

   Where is patient located in hospital? ______________________

   Patient name ______________________

   Patient date of birth ______________________

   Patient telephone ______________________

   Chief concern ______________________

   Medical history ______________________

   Vital signs ______________________

   Pertinent labs/x-ray ______________________

   Give medical advice until transport arrives
4. Give referring site anticipated arrival time
5. Activate transport: xxx-xxx-xxxx
6. Call admitting resident
7. Await notification of transport arrival at referral site

in basic CPR and just a small percentage of their training and encounters involve children. ALS transports use paramedics and/or RNs and can administer various medications, infuse IV fluids, provide oxygen, and maintain temperature control. Critical care transport teams include specialized RNs, NPs, and/or physicians and provide higher-level, critical care needs, often for patients with one or more failing organ systems.

There are pros and cons to the different team compositions and levels of transport. If a patient is seriously ill and unstable, a critical care team is essential because of the need for specialty monitoring, equipment, and medication. However, if response time is crucial (ie, the patient urgently requires a critical procedure that can only be performed at the accepting institution), then it may be more beneficial to send a BLS team, which can be mobilized in much less time than a critical care team. In addition, sending a critical care team for a stable patient that BLS providers could have transported is an inappropriate utilization of resources that may be needed elsewhere during the same period. It is often helpful to speak with the referring physicians and understand their preferences. The MCP must then weigh all of these factors when making a decision.

When accepting a patient from a private practitioner's office or clinic, ensure that the child will not be exposed to a lower level of care during transit to the hospital (eg, the parents' car) compared with the higher level of care in the office (eg, supplemental oxygen). Also, since these are prehospital locations, the MCP may decide that the safer approach would be using local EMS services to transport the patient to a nearby ED.

Referral hospitals must abide by the federal Emergency Medical Treatment and Active Labor Act, which requires the hospital to evaluate all patients who arrive with emergent conditions and to stabilize them before transfer. The MCP must review the case with the referring physician when deciding about the proper composition of the transport team, personnel, and mode. Medicolegally, responsibility is shared once a receiving hospital accepts a patient. Therefore, the MCP must work in conjunction with the referring physician to help make these decisions.

Role of the MCP

As discussed above, the MCP determines team composition and the level of transport. This process occurs after discussion with a referring physician, once the necessary clinical information is obtained (see Figure 56-2). The MCP starts caring for the patient at that moment and provides advice to the referring physician about the continuing evaluation and management of the child. At this point, the MCP may also need to consult with various subspecialists for further information and guidance. Once the transport team assumes care of the patient, they may use direct communication (online) and/or written protocols (offline) to care for the patient. It is important for the MCP to have easy, online communication with the team (via radio, cell phone) if difficult decisions arise. Therefore, the MCP should have knowledge of the transport environment and equipment. The MCP and/or transport team also need to communicate with the receiving unit so preparations can be made for the patient.

Of note, state regulations may dictate who can act in the role of an MCP. In many cases, it can be any pediatrician, but in some states, it needs to be a critical care or ED physician. The role of an MCP is evolving, though, and with the increased presence of pediatric hospitalists who are familiar with transport program protocols and the transport environment, a program can rely on the hospitalist to act as the primary MCP.

Equipment

Do not assume that the referring hospital can provide all of the equipment that is required for transport. Rather, develop and maintain a supply of dedicated specialized storage packs, designed to cover pediatric critical care needs for all age and weight ranges. See appendices C1 and C2 of the AAP *Guidelines for Air and Ground Transport of Neonatal and Pediatric Patients* for sample supplies. The packs must be able to withstand the stress of the transport environment and, for air medical transport, may need to meet guidelines for space and weight capacity. Check the equipment daily to ensure that oxygen and battery supplies are sufficient for the expected duration of any potential transport.

Vehicle Selection

The 3 different types of vehicles are ambulance, fixed-wing plane, and helicopter. The MCP makes the decision about which vehicle to use in coordination with the referring hospital. Selection criteria include severity of the illness or injury, distance to the referring hospital, travel time required, weather conditions, vehicle availability, equipment needs, and expense. When considering distance, typically a ground ambulance is preferred when the transport is less than 100 miles. At more than 100 miles, air transport may be preferable. Factors to keep in mind are that fixed-wing planes require several ambulance transfers, flying at certain altitudes can affect partial pressure in body cavities and increase the volume of entrapped air (worsening a pneumothorax), and space is a constraint in air transport so equipment and personnel may be limited.

Safety

Safety is a priority with each transport. Air transport may be faster but carries inherent risks, including weather, mechanical failure, and collisions. Weather can also play a significant role in ground ambulance transport. The Commission on Accreditation of Medical Transport Systems offers guidelines for minimal safe weather conditions. If a transport is delayed because of weather, the MCP must continue to guide the management of the patient until a transport can take place. In addition, advise ambulances to never go "code 3" or use "lights and sirens" as the data indicate this has no positive effect on patient outcome.

Bibliography

American Academy of Pediatrics Section on Transport Medicine. *Guidelines for Air and Ground Transport of Neonatal and Pediatric Patients.* 3rd ed. Elk Grove Village, IL: American Academy of Pediatrics; 2006

Frankel LR. Interfacility transfer of the critically ill infant and child. In: Kliegman RM, Behrman RE, Jenson HB, Stanton BF, eds. *Nelson Textbook of Pediatrics.* 18th ed. Philadelphia, PA: Saunders; 2007:380–382

MacGilvray S. Stabilization of the newborn for transport. In: Perkin RM, Swift JD, Newton DA, Anas NG, eds. *Pediatric Hospital Medicine: Textbook of Inpatient Management.* 2nd ed. Philadelphia, PA: Lippincott, Williams & Wilkins; 2008:637–642

Orr RA, Han YY, Roth K. Pediatric transport: shifting the paradigm to improve patient outcome. In: Fuhrman BP, Zimmerman JJ, eds. *Pediatric Critical Care.* 3rd ed. Philadelphia, PA: Mosby; 2006:141–150

CHAPTER 57

Pediatric Palliative Care

Introduction

Pediatric palliative care (PPC) offers physical, psychological, social, and spiritual support to children with life-threatening or life-shortening conditions and their families. PPC places emphasis on comfort, quality of life, and goal-directed decision-making, with the objective of preventing and relieving suffering through interdisciplinary collaboration. Ideally, PPC supportive interventions should be initiated at the time of diagnosis, introduced as a routine part of therapy, and continued during all subsequent phases of therapy.

PPC is provided by an interdisciplinary team consisting of physicians, nurse practitioners, nurses, social workers, case managers, psychologists, physical and occupational therapists, speech pathologists, child life specialists, music/art therapists, and chaplains. Regardless of whether an institution has a dedicated PPC program, health care providers should still strive to adhere to the goals and principles of PPC in order to provide comprehensive and compassionate care to patients and their families.

Indications for PPC

Refer a patient and family for a PPC consultation if there are life-threatening or life-shortening conditions, including (but not limited to) the following:

- Cancer; heart failure; cystic fibrosis and other pulmonary diseases; renal failure; cerebral palsy; progressive or severe genetic, neurologic, metabolic, or immunologic disorders; or advanced HIV/AIDS
- Uncertain prognosis and accompanying symptom burden
- Dependence on feeding tube, tracheostomy, or ventilatory support for a condition that is not expected to resolve and may preclude a full, long life
- Disabling or uncontrolled symptoms, such as pain, fatigue, insomnia, depression, anxiety, agitation, spasms, nausea, vomiting, diarrhea, constipation, or dyspnea
- Facilitation of patient-centered and family-centered communication and decision-making, both at initial diagnosis and when the goals of care are changing
- Need for psychological, social, or spiritual support, whether for the patient, family, or siblings
- Multiple admissions for the same diagnosis with undefined goals of care
- Admissions of increasing frequency or severity for the same underlying condition or its complications

- Reliance on full-time medical daycare
- Need for coordination of care across settings (hospital, home, skilled nursing facility, hospice)
- Care and support at the end of life and during bereavement
- Prenatal consultation for a fetus with a life-limiting condition

Statements by Patients and Families That Can Trigger Consultation

- I don't know how much longer we can do this.
- It hurts me to see my child in pain like this.
- We feel like the doctors have given up on us.
- I am so confused. Every new provider tells me something different.
- My child seems to be getting worse no matter what they are doing.
- My child is so tired of being in the hospital.
- I just want my child to get to be a kid and play.
- We just want to go home.
- There are so many people involved and no one is really listening.
- I am so worried about my other kids and whether I'll still have my job.

How to Introduce PPC to Patients and Families

The introduction of PPC may be challenging if the family has a preexisting negative perception about PPC. For example, they may equate PPC with hospice or view PPC as a signal that the medical team is "giving up" on their child. If either of these difficulties arises, consider introducing PPC as an extra layer of support for the family, one that emphasizes "doing everything possible to improve the quality of life for the child and family." Also, reassure the family that PPC emphasizes "goal-directed care," which will be integrated with curative care. Emphasize that the medical services in your institution often consult the PPC team when the care plan is complex or the outcome is uncertain.

PPC Introduction Example

"To best meet the goals of care for your child, we believe it would be helpful to have the PPC service visit with you. The PPC team works with both families and other health care providers. They specialize in improving your child's quality of life by helping to manage symptoms such as pain, nausea, and fatigue, as well as providing support to your child and family. They can also help you clarify your goals of care, and help us think through any decisions as they might arise. Our goal is for all of the teams to work together to provide your child with the best care possible."

Goals of Care

The goals of care are different for every patient and family. To determine an individual's goals, ask the following key questions:

- What is your understanding of your child's condition?
- What do you expect in the future?
- What are the most important things that you desire for your child right now?
- What are you hoping for?
- What are your child's greatest needs right now?
- What are you most worried about, or what keeps you awake at night?

Spiritual Assessment

A spiritual assessment may also be helpful to gain a better understanding of the family's goals. Use the acronym HOPE for assessing the patient's and family's spiritual status and needs.

- Sources of **H**ope: What are your sources of hope, strength, comfort, and peace? What do you hold on to during difficult times? What or who sustains you and keeps you going?
- **O**rganized Religion: Are you a part of a religious community? How is this helpful to you?
- **P**ersonal Spirituality and **P**ractices: Do you have other personal spiritual beliefs that are helpful to you? What aspects of your spirituality are most helpful (eg, prayer, meditation, music, nature)?
- **E**ffects on Medical Care and **E**nd-of-Life Issues: Has your child's health condition affected your spiritual practices? Are there conflicts between your beliefs and medical situation? Would it be helpful to speak to a chaplain or other spiritual leader?

Continuity of Care

PPC emphasizes interdisciplinary collaboration among the patient's primary medical team, consult services, the family, and community-based care providers with the intention of enhancing communication and improving continuity of care. The process of PPC also includes supporting the family in making difficult decisions. In addition, continuity of care also encompasses end-of-life care, whether in hospital or at home, as well as the provision of bereavement resources for long-term support to the family.

Language Selection

Communication is a key component to successful PPC. Language choices have a meaningful impact on both patients and families, and it is important to choose words carefully (Table 57-1).

Opioids for Pain Management

- Say "opioid," not "narcotic."
- Titrate opioids based on clinical response.
- The "right dose" is the dose that best controls pain with the fewest side effects.
- Base dose increases on percentage of current dose: 30% increase for mild pain, 50% increase for moderate pain, 100% increase for severe pain.
- When using opioids, always start a bowel regimen that consists of more than just a stool softener (osmotic agent, with or without a stimulant laxative).
- Encourage dosing by schedule, typically every 4 hours (unless the drug is delayed release or is methadone), to avoid the pain roller coaster that can occur with PRN dosing.

Non-Pharmacologic Symptom Management

- Limit painful procedures.
- Address coincident depression and anxiety through counseling and the use of psychopharmacologic agents as needed.
- Use alternative therapies such as relaxation, meditation, breathing exercises, hypnosis, guided imagery, Reiki, biofeedback, yoga, massage, acupuncture/acupressure, or art/pet/play/music therapy.

Table 57-1. Appropriate Language Selection

Language to Avoid	Therapeutic Language
The sickler	The child with sickle cell disease
Your child failed therapy.	Our treatments were not successful in curing your child.
I know how you feel, I know how difficult this situation is for you.	I cannot imagine how difficult this situation is for you.
Do you want us to do everything to keep your child alive?	What is your understanding of the decision to attempt life-sustaining interventions?
Are you ready to sign the "do not resuscitate" orders?	Do you agree with the medical recommendation for "do not attempt resuscitation"?
We are going to withdraw support now. We will be pulling the ventilator at this time.	We will stop mechanical ventilation as it is no longer clinically indicated, but we will continue to provide maximal supportive care.

- Fatigue: Consider contributing factors (anemia, depression, medication side effects), sleep hygiene, gentle exercise.
- Dyspnea: Try suctioning, repositioning, loose clothing, fans, minimize hydration, relaxation exercises, opioids.
- Nausea: Try dietary modifications (bland/soft, timing/volume), aromatherapy (peppermint, lavender), ginger, acupuncture/acupressure.

Support for Families

- Provide respite care when feasible, such that families may have some time without the burden of caring for the affected child.
- Child life specialists and volunteers can also provide support for siblings.

Provider Fatigue

Providing PPC to children and families is most often a highly rewarding personal undertaking, but in some instances it can be an overwhelming experience, leading to frustration, stress, hopelessness, or burnout. In order to avoid or ameliorate these adverse emotional responses, it is critical to maintain open channels of communication with professional colleagues and other health care providers. Establish consistent forums for self-reflection and discussion, in order to provide a safe place for providers to share and reflect on their experiences.

Disposition and Follow-up

Hospice

The transition into a hospice program can be complex. Prior to hospital discharge, it is important to clarify and clearly document the goals of care. If the child is being enrolled into hospice, have a representative meet the child, family, and primary care team, ideally prior to discharge, to communicate the management plan for symptom control and end-of-life care. Optimize all medications to enhance quality of life. In addition, be aware that hospice does not necessarily require discontinuation of active therapy. For example, a cancer patient may continue to receive chemotherapy while under the care of a hospice.

Home Care

The philosophy of PPC may be successfully implemented in the home, provided the focus remains on quality of life, physical and psychological comfort, and the prevention or alleviation of suffering. A PPC provider may be on call to provide support in the home and can serve as a link among the hospital, specialists, and community caregivers. This provider can help to prevent or facilitate hospital admissions, as well as organize and supervise the provision of respite care and increased home services as needed. The family can benefit from knowing how to obtain help quickly when the clinical condition changes (eg, pain flares, behavioral changes, breathing difficulties, color changes).

If the patient is being discharged to home with goals of care such that resuscitative measures should be limited, then complete an out-of-hospital "do not attempt resuscitation" form. These forms are state-specific, and may be found online through the individual state's Department of Public Health. The form protects a patient from aggressive interventions, such as CPR and intubation, in the event that emergency medical services are called. Even if the family has signed the form, they still may choose full resuscitative measures at any time.

Pearls and Pitfalls

- If your hospital does not have a dedicated interdisciplinary PPC team, advocate for the creation of one.
- In the absence of a dedicated PPC team, palliative care may still be provided by using the basic skills and competencies required of all physicians and health care professionals.
- The role of the hospitalist may be challenging when PPC concepts have not been addressed with a patient prior to hospital admission at the end of life. However, all hospitalists can readily learn the basic skills and competencies of PPC in order to provide compassionate care to patients and families at the end of life.

Coding

ICD-9

- Long-term (current) use of opiate analgesic **V58.69**
- Encounter for palliative care **V66.7**
  - List underlying condition first

Bibliography

Anandarajah G, Hight E. Spirituality and medical practice: using the HOPE questions as a practical tool for spiritual assessment. *Am Fam Physician.* 2001;63:81–89

Children's Project on Palliative/Hospice Services (ChiPPS). www.nhpco.org/pediatrics

End of Life/Palliative Care Education Resource Center (EPERC). http://www.eperc.mcw.edu/

Klick JC, Hauer J. Pediatric palliative care. *Curr Probl Pediatr Adolesc Health Care.* 2010;40:120–151

Liben S, Papadatou D, Wolfe J. Paediatric palliative care: challenges and emerging ideas. *Lancet.* 2008;371:852–864

Weissman DE, Meier DE. Identifying patients in need of a palliative care assessment in the hospital setting: a consensus report from the center to advance palliative care. *J Palliat Med.* 2011;14:17–23

Wolfe J, Hinds P, Sourkes B. *The Textbook of Interdisciplinary Pediatric Palliative Care.* Philadelphia, PA: Elsevier; 2011

CHAPTER 58

Quality Improvement

Introduction

The Institute of Medicine (IOM) has defined quality as the degree to which health care systems, services, and supplies for individuals and populations increase the likelihood for positive health outcomes and are consistent with current professional knowledge. The IOM has proposed 6 specific aims for improvement. Quality health is

- Safe: Avoid injury from care that is intended to help.
- Effective: Avoid underuse or overuse of services.
- Patient-centered: Provide respectful, responsive, individualized care.
- Timely: Reduce waits and harmful delays in care.
- Efficient: Avoid waste of equipment, supplies, ideas, and energy.
- Equitable: Provide equal care regardless of personal characteristics, gender, ethnicity, geographic location, and socioeconomic status.

The goal of quality improvement in health care is to provide the right care for every patient, every time.

Right Care: Practice evidence-based medicine with judgment, experience, and adaptation to the patient's needs. However, the IOM reported that it may take an average of 17 years for new knowledge generated by randomized, controlled trials to be incorporated into practice, so that knowing what is right care is not enough. The goal is to translate evidence-based medicine into clinical judgment and patient-centered care.

Every Patient: Many reports have demonstrated how care varies for even the most common inpatient pediatric diagnoses, such as gastroenteritis and bronchiolitis. Quality improvement methodology is focused on reducing inappropriate variation and improving the delivery of value-based outcomes.

Every Time: Most physicians are familiar with the most recent and relevant clinical research (evidence-based medicine) and work to incorporate this knowledge into our daily practice. Unfortunately, it is difficult to do this on a consistent basis.

Pediatric hospitalists must be leaders in working toward optimal quality improvement. This requires the knowledge, skills, and attitudes to be successful in leading a system that provides the right care for every patient, every time. The following 5 concepts are critical for hospitalists to recognize as they develop into leaders of quality improvement in their organizations.

System Improvement

Quality improvement is not accomplished by forcing people to work harder/faster/safer, reusing traditional quality assurance or peer-review methodologies, or creating order sets or protocols without monitoring their use or effects. To generate meaningful positive outcomes the hospitalist must focus on the processes of care, reduce variations in care by shifting entire practices, and change the design of care. Traditional quality assurance focuses on outliers, without changing the process or reducing inappropriate variation, whereas quality improvement focuses on process improvements leading to more reliable outcomes.

Understand How to Measure Quality

Measurement of quality is critical to the quality improvement process. Although measurement systems are inherently imperfect, create local assessment tools to use within the hospital organization. These metrics may further evolve during multiple improvement cycles, allowing individual units (eg, hospital floors or physicians) ready access to transparent data that will be meaningful to individuals and motivate change. Measure relevant information in small samples, over time, and use it for providing feedback to the clinical staff, who can then affect the specific indicators. Provide feedback in a collaborative and nonpunitive manner, so as to build trust, which is essential for further change.

The dashboard of quality contains 2 types of indicators: the process indicator, which is analogous to speed measured by a speedometer, and the outcome indicator, which is similar to miles travelled on the odometer. Process indicators measure the completion of steps in the process, such as "X% of patients with asthma receiving an asthma action plan." Outcome indicators measure the result of the process, such as mortality, length of stay, and complications. Current research documents that improvement in the process indicators almost always leads to positive changes in the outcome indicators. However, it may take multiple rapid improvement cycles to show measurable change in outcomes.

It is important to recognize that government agencies or payers do not initiate the development of quality indicators. Rather, they often result from the recommendations of professional societies and research studies. Therefore, hospitalists must become involved with national professional bodies and participate in the decision-making process of what are meaningful process and outcome measures.

Build Teams

Traditional medical school education focused on training physicians to be autonomous and individualistic, but this model is no longer viable for hospitalists. Today, a quality physician works as part of an effective team, with members representing 3 different components within an organization: system leadership (hospital administrator), technical leadership (physician), and day-to-day leadership (nurses, clerks, housekeepers, respiratory therapists etc). Also, the principles of family-centered care also apply to quality improvement. Involvement of patients and their families within quality improvement teams is also critical to help break traditional silos.

Implement the PDSA Model for Improvement

The model for improvement using PDSA (Plan-Do-Study-Act) is a powerful and proven tool for accelerating improvement. It provides structure to the improvement process just as a history and physical examination provides structure to a patient encounter.

- Set aims: "What are we trying to accomplish?" Define an aim that is time-specific and measurable, and define the population that will be affected.
- Establish measures: "How will we know that a change is an improvement?" Measures help the team determine if a change leads to quantitative improvement.
- Select changes: "What changes can we make that will result in improvement?" Improvement requires change, but not all change leads to improvement. It is the test of change by using rapid cycle methodology that will allow quality improvement teams to determine whether meaningful improvement can be measured.
- Test change: "How can we make changes in the real world setting?" Rapidly initiate a PDSA cycle, with a narrow focus, using smaller "tests of change," before disseminating across a larger population.
  - Plan: Answer the questions in the first 3 steps above by setting aims, establishing measures, and selecting changes.
  - Do: Implement the changes. This may range from a "baby step," one small change for a small number of patients to the widespread use of "bundles," which are packages of evidence-based interventions that help provide consistency of care.
  - Study: Evaluate the pilot change to see if the desired effect occurred and identify any unintended consequences.
  - Act: Adopt, reject, or modify the change plan, so that the next cycle can begin.

Sustain the Changes

"We know this works, what do we do now?" After several successful PDSA cycles, create a "control" plan to ensure that the "new change" is integrated into a system of care. Quality improvement must be sustainable over time, leading to the delivery of reliable outcomes regardless of changes in team composition.

Spread the Changes

"How can we help others bring about change?" After the hospital or unit has benefitted from the improvement, share the process with other organizations in order to spread best practices. This will also serve as an educational opportunity for the team.

These simple steps have brought profound changes within health care organizations. By developing a system-level approach to improve measurement, building teams, and employing the PDSA model of improvement, pediatric hospitalists can be leaders in transforming the culture of an organization, one that is focused on quality improvement. In this way, all members of an organization, from the boardroom members to the ward clerks, work together to provide the *right care for every patient, every time.*

Bibliography

Berwick DM. The science of improvement. *JAMA.* 2008;299:1182–1184

Harrison JP, Curran L. The hospitalist model: does it enhance health care quality? *J Health Care Finance.* 2009;35:22–34

Kohn LT, Corrigan JM, Donaldson MS, eds. *To Err Is Human: Building a Safer Health System.* Washington, DC: National Academies Press; 1999

Lloyd R. Tapping the knowledge that hides in data. In: Lloyd R, ed. *Quality Health Care: A Guide to Developing and Using Indicators.* Sudbury, MA: Jones and Bartlett Publishers; 2004:151–172

Sachdeva RC, Jain S. Making the case to improve quality and reduce costs in pediatric health care. *Pediatr Clin North Am.* 2009;56:731–743

Speroff T, O'Connor GT. Study designs for PDSA quality improvement research. *Qual Manag Health Care.* 2004;13:17–32

Nephrology

CHAPTER 59

Acute Glomerulonephritis

Introduction

The term acute glomerulonephritis (AGN) encompasses the spectrum of diseases leading to variable degrees of inflammation in the glomeruli. AGN can be an isolated, self-limited illness or the first presentation of chronic glomerulonephritis (GN). Clinical manifestations vary from asymptomatic microscopic hematuria to acute nephritic syndrome, characterized by abrupt onset of gross hematuria, proteinuria, and edema, often with hypertension and some degree of renal insufficiency.

Postinfectious AGN is the classic example of AGN and the most frequent cause in children. It most commonly occurs after a pharyngitis or skin infection with group A streptococcus, although it can be seen with many other bacterial, mycobacterial, viral, fungal, or parasitic infections. Postinfectious GN classically presents 7 to 14 days after pharyngitis or up to 3 to 12 weeks following pyoderma. It typically occurs in school-aged children and is rare before 2 years of age. The gross hematuria and edema of postinfectious GN usually resolve within 3 to 7 days, with gradual normalization of urine output and blood pressure over the following 2 to 4 weeks.

Berger disease, or immunoglobulin (Ig) A nephropathy, is the most common GN worldwide. It occurs most often in patients older than 10 years and can frequently present as recurrent episodes of gross hematuria in childhood.

Other causes of pediatric AGN include membranoproliferative GN and vascultic diseases, including Henoch-Schönlein purpura (HSP).

Clinical Presentation

History

Painless gross hematuria and edema are the most common presenting symptoms. The patient may report the abrupt development of puffy eyes or facial edema accompanied by foamy cola-colored urine and decreased urine volume. A patient with postinfectious GN will often develop hypertension, but a hypertensive emergency with hypertensive encephalopathy is uncommon. This presents with headaches, seizures, altered mental status, and visual disturbances. Other rare complaints include dyspnea, orthopnea, or cough as a result of pulmonary edema.

Ask about recent or concurrent infections to determine the etiology of the AGN. Exacerbations of IgA nephropathy often occur concurrently with mild infections. Note any other preceding infections, particularly endocarditis, deep-seated visceral abscess, osteomyelitis, and shunt infection.

Ask about prior history of microscopic or gross hematuria. Since a patient with Alport syndrome may occasionally develop AGN, determine whether there is a family history of hematuria, sensorineural hearing loss, or chronic kidney disease. While fever and systemic symptoms are typically absent in postinfectious AGN, a history of fever, malaise, abdominal pain, arthralgia, arthritis, or rash may be present in a patient with a systemic vasculitis, such as systemic lupus erythematosus or HSP.

Physical Examination

With the possible exception of an elevated systolic and/or diastolic blood pressure, the physical examination may be normal, although pallor, edema (localized or generalized), and/or pulmonary rales may be appreciated. A patient with postinfectious AGN may have evidence of a resolving skin infection, but is otherwise usually well-appearing. A patient with hypertensive encephalopathy may exhibit seizures or altered mental status. There may also be physical findings (eg, hair loss, epistaxis, joint swelling, and rash) specific to the systemic etiology. Also, carefully assess growth parameters since chronic kidney disease may initially manifest as AGN.

Laboratory

Hematuria is the hallmark of AGN and is defined by the presence of 5 or more red blood cells (RBCs) per high-power field. For any patient presenting with dark urine, obtain a complete urinalysis with urine microscopy to distinguish among various causes of red urine, including RBCs, hemoglobinuria, myoglobinuria, and discoloration from drugs or foods. Gross hematuria is turbid, while urine containing myoglobin or hemoglobin is dark, but clear. To further differentiate the latter 2, examine centrifuged serum, which will be clear in myoglobinuria, but have a pink tinge with hemoglobinuria.

Once the presence of RBCs is confirmed, obtain a urine culture, complete blood cell count, basic chemistry panel, and C3 and C4. To screen for postinfectious AGN, check the anti-streptolysin O (ASO) and anti-DNAse titers. A positive ASO does not confirm the diagnosis of AGN, but only establishes that either colonization or infection (old or new) with streptococcus has occurred. Moreover, AGN that is unrelated to streptococcal infection will feature negative results for both ASO and anti-DNase antibody responses. Obtain a renal/bladder ultrasound if the patient presents with bright red blood (to rule out a mass) or has recurrent hematuria or a systemic disease.

In postinfectious AGN, the urine will be reddish-brown or cola-colored, with dysmorphic RBCs, RBC casts, and often white blood cells. Non-nephrotic range proteinuria is commonly present. Anemia is usually hemodilutional, but postinfectious AGN has been associated with autoimmune hemolytic anemia. Depending on the degree of renal dysfunction, the blood urea nitrogen (BUN) and creatinine may be elevated. The C3 is depressed in 90% of patients, while the C4 is typically normal. In general, the ASO is elevated in a patient with pharyngitis, and poststreptococcal AGN, while the anti-DNAse titer is high if there is a streptococcal pyoderma, AGN, and streptococcal infection.

If the AGN does not seem to be postinfectious and/or the patient has acute and severe deterioration in renal function (ie, rapidly progressive GN), obtain antibodies to the glomerular basement membrane (anti-glomerular basement membrane; Goodpasture syndrome) or those associated with other forms of vasculitis (anti-neutrophil cytoplasmic antibodies).

Differential Diagnosis

The differential diagnosis of hematuria is extensive, but painless gross hematuria suggests a glomerular etiology. Potential causes can be further classified according to complement levels. GN associated with normal complement levels include IgA nephropathy, Alport syndrome, and HSP, while low complement levels occur in poststreptococcal AGN, membranoproliferative GN, shunt nephritis, and systemic lupus erythematosus. Additional details for each of these conditions are summarized in Table 59-1.

Treatment

Treatment is largely supportive and focuses on control of hypertension and fluid overload. Since these are primarily caused by enhanced salt and water retention, fluid and salt restriction is the first-line treatment. Limit sodium to 1 to 2 mEq/kg/day. Fluid restriction varies based on the degree of edema and circulating volume, but may be as strict as 1 to 2 times the amount needed to replace insensible losses (400–800 mL/m^2/day).

If further treatment is needed to control volume overload and/or mild to moderate hypertension, give a loop diuretic (furosemide 0.5–1 mg/kg intravenous [IV] every 8 hours). If the hypertension persists, provide a calcium-channel blocker such as nifedipine (0.25–0.5 mg/kg oral, every 4–6 hours, 10 mg maximum) or amlodipine (0.05–0.4 mg/kg oral every day). Consult with a nephrologist before ordering an angiotensin-converting enzyme inhibitor as there is a risk of decreasing the glomerular filtration rate and causing hyperkalemia.

Table 59-1. Differential Diagnosis of Painless Gross Hematuria	
Diagnosis	**Clinical Features**
Alport syndrome	X-linked dominant Sensorineural hearing loss Ocular disease: retinopathy, cataracts, lenticonus
Berger disease/IgA nephropathy	>10 years of age Macroscopic hematuria concurrent with infections ↑ IgA in 50%; normal complement
Henoch-Schönlein purpura	Purpuric rash, arthritis, abdominal pain Normal complement
Lupus nephritis	Photosensitive malar rash, arthralgia, serositis ↓ C3 and C4 (+) ANA, anti-dsDNA
Membranoproliferative glomerulonephritis	Similar to PSAGN Persistent ↓ C3, +/- ↓ C4
PSAGN	2–12 years of age Pharyngitis or skin infection 1–12 weeks prior ↓ C3, normal C4, (+)ASO/anti-DNAse
Shunt nephritis	History of shunt Arthralgias, lymphadenopathy, hepatosplenomegaly ↓ C3

Abbreviations: ANA, antinuclear antibody; ASO, anti-streptolysin O; IgA, immunoglobulin A; PSAGN, poststreptococcal glomulernephritis.

Initial IV treatment options for a hypertensive emergency include hydralazine (start at 0.1 mg/kg/dose, titrate to desired blood pressure with 0.2–0.4 mg/kg/dose, maximum 20 mg) or labetalol (0.2–1 mg/kg/dose, maximum 40 mg, avoid use with significant acute respiratory disease or asthma). If these measures do not provide adequate control of blood pressure, options include nicardipine (0.5–4 mcg/kg/minute, start at 0.1–0.2 mcg/kg/minute), nitroprusside (0.3–0.5 mcg/kg/minute, maximum 10 mcg/kg/minute), or labetalol (0.25–3 mg/kg/hour). If the patient has hypertension and volume overload, give furosemide (1 mg/kg/dose; maximum 6 mg/kg/day). For any patient treated with IV antihypertensive medications, check the blood pressure at least every 5 to 15 minutes and titrate the infusion to reach the target blood pressure. There are a number of specific guidelines for safe blood pressure reduction. One approach is to target a normal blood pressure in a stepwise fashion by reducing the blood pressure by 25% over the first 8 hours, followed by another 25% over the next 8 to 12 hours, and the remaining 50% over the next 24 hours.

Indications for Consultation

- **Nephrology:** Blood pressure difficult to control, renal insufficiency, need for biopsy, concern for a systemic disease

Disposition

- **Intensive care unit transfer:** Hypertensive emergency, need for dialysis or hemofiltration, need for ventilator support
- **Discharge criteria:** Blood pressure controlled, renal impairment improving

Follow-up

- **Primary care:** 1 week for blood pressure check, BUN/creatinine, and urinalysis
- **Nephrology:** 4 weeks to check C3 (if it was low)

Pearls and Pitfalls

- Poststreptococcal AGN runs a typical course. Evaluate for other etiologies of AGN if the presentation is unusual in terms of clinical and/or laboratory features.
- Up to 50% of patients with AGN and an abnormal urinalysis are asymptomatic.
- A patient with hypertensive encephalopathy or acute renal failure may have a marginally abnormal urinalysis.

Coding

ICD-9

- AGN, unspecified **580.9**
- Acute renal failure, unspecified **584.9**
- Chronic GN, unspecified **582.9**
- Edema **782.3**
- Hypertensive chronic kidney disease, unspecified **403.90**
  — Use additional code to identify the stage of chronic kidney disease **(585.x)**

Bibliography

Ahn S, Ingulli E. Acute poststreptococcal glomerulonephritis: an update. *Curr Opin Pediatr.* 2008;20:157–162

Chadban SJ, Atkins RC. Glomerulonephritis. *Lancet.* 2005;365:1797–1806

Chan JCM, Williams DM, Roth KS. Kidney failure in infants and children. *Pediatr Rev.* 2002;23:47–60

Eison TM, Ault BH, Jones DP, Chesney RW, Wyatt RJ. Post-streptococcal acute glomerulonephritis in children: clinical features and pathogenesis. *Pediatr Nephrol.* 2011;26(2):165–180

Flynn JT, Tullus Kjell. Severe hypertension in children and adolescents: pathophysiology and treatment. *Pediatr Nephrol.* 2009;24:1101–1112

Srivastava RN. Acute glomerulonephritis. *Indian J Pediatr.* 1999;66:199–205

Vinen CS, Oliveira DBG. Acute glomerulonephritis. *Postgrad Med J.* 2003;79:206–213

Zaffanello M, Cataldi L, Franchini M, Fanos V. Evidence-based treatment limitations prevent any therapeutic recommendation for acute poststreptococcal glomerulonephritis in children. *Med Sci Monit.* 2010;16(4):RA79–RA84

Hemolytic Uremic Syndrome

Introduction

Hemolytic uremic syndrome (HUS) is a disorder characterized by the triad of microangiopathic hemolytic anemia, thrombocytopenia, and acute renal injury that classically follows the prodrome of a diarrheal illness. While most (60%) patients will have a complete recovery, 3% to 5% will progress to renal failure, so that HUS is the most common cause of renal failure in children.

Classic HUS is associated with a diarrheal illness prodrome (D+HUS), most often caused by Shiga toxin-producing *Escherichia coli* O157:H7. Other Shiga-toxin producing agents include non-O157 strains of *E coli*, *Shigella*, and *Salmonella dysenteriae*. HUS affects boys and girls equally and is more common during the first decade of life and during the summer and fall.

Atypical HUS (D-HUS) is usually not associated with a diarrheal prodrome and can be caused by non-Shiga toxin–associated bacterial infections (particularly *Streptococcus pneumoniae*), viral infections, drugs, or malignancies. D-HUS can also be due to inherited deficiencies in the complement system. D-HUS is less common, but more severe than D+HUS, with higher rates of both relapse and end-stage renal disease. This chapter will focus on classic HUS.

Clinical Presentation

History

Classic HUS is preceded by a nonspecific diarrheal illness (often bloody) that presents with nausea, vomiting, abdominal pain, tenderness, and low-grade fever. A patient with HUS will then develop the sudden onset of pallor, irritability, weakness, and oliguria or anuria. These symptoms occur several days (often 5–7) after the onset of the diarrheal illness, typically when the colitis is improving. Approximately one-third of patients may have neurologic changes at the onset of symptoms ranging from mild irritability and lethargy to seizures, stroke, or coma.

Physical Examination

Perform a thorough physical examination, as abnormal findings reflect the severity of the cascade of hematologic and renal dysfunction. The patient is often ill-appearing, with significant pallor and possibly mild jaundice. Hypertension and tachycardia are common. There may be petechiae, but purpura is rare. Generalized edema is often present and is more prominent in dependent areas. Nonspecific neurologic findings are often present and include irritability and generalized weakness or fatigue. However, more severe neurologic changes such as seizures, encephalopathy, coma, or focal neurologic deficits consistent with stroke may be seen secondary to metabolic derangements or thrombotic events.

Generalized abdominal pain and tenderness are common and are typically related to the inciting infectious colitis. More focal abdominal pain and tenderness can be seen with complications such as hepatitis (right upper quadrant tenderness, hepatomegaly), pancreatitis (epigastric pain and tenderness radiating to the back, severe emesis), obstruction, intussusception, or perforation (distension, severe emesis, decreased bowel sounds). Cardiovascular complications include severe tachycardia, hypertension, or signs of heart failure (dyspnea, tachypnea, rales, hepatomegaly, cool extremities, delayed capillary refill). These physical findings are secondary to severe anemia, fluid overload, electrolyte abnormalities, and acute renal insufficiency. Myocarditis is a rare complication.

Laboratory

Follow the complete blood cell count every 6 to 8 hours, as HUS produces a microangiopathic hemolytic anemia. The hemoglobin is typically less than 8 g/dL and may fall rapidly as a result of ongoing intense hemolysis. The cells are normochromic and normocytic with schistocytes/helmet cells seen on peripheral smear. Assess for other markers of nonimmune-mediated hemolysis, including increased reticulocyte count, indirect bilirubin, and lactate dehydrogenase with decreased haptoglobin and a negative Coombs test. The patient may have thrombocytopenia with a platelet count less than 60,000/mm^3 and megakaryocytes on peripheral smear, but the coagulation factors (prothrombin/partial thromboplastin time, D-dimer, fibrinogen) are all normal. Mild leukocytosis is seen, but it is rarely greater than 20,000/mm^3. A low C3 complement raises the possibility of atypical HUS.

During the acute phase, monitor the electrolytes every 6 to 8 hours, looking for hyperkalemia, hyper- or hyponatremia, metabolic acidosis, hyperphosphatemia, and hypocalcemia. The blood urea nitrogen and creatinine might be markedly elevated, although there is no correlation between the degree of anemia and the severity of the renal disease. Obtain a urinalysis to assess for hematuria, proteinuria, and possible red blood cell casts. The patient may also have elevated liver transaminases and hypoalbuminemia from enteric losses. If the pancreas is involved, amylase and lipase will be elevated, and the patient may be hyperglycemic.

Send a stool Shiga-toxin assay as well as a stool culture for enterohemorrhagic *E coli*. Stool cultures obtained more than 6 days into the diarrheal illness may have a low yield, and blood cultures are typically negative.

Radiology

While imaging is not routinely indicated, obtain abdominal imaging (anteroposterior abdominal x-ray [commonly referred to as KUB], computed tomography [CT] scan, ultrasound) if there is a concern for obstruction, perforation, or intussusception. Renal ultrasound can exclude renal vein thrombosis and assess for cortical necrosis. Obtain magnetic resonance imaging or a non-contrast head CT scan if there are seizures, coma, or signs of a stroke. Order an electrocardiogram if the patient has severe hyperkalemia and an echocardiogram if there are signs of congestive heart failure, pericardial effusion, or myocarditis.

Differential Diagnosis

The differential diagnosis is summarized in Table 60-1.

Treatment

The management of HUS is mostly supportive and includes meticulous attention to fluid and electrolyte balance. For an anuric patient, restrict fluids to provide only insensible losses (400–600 mL/m^2 body surface area) and replace output (emesis, diarrhea, urine) with isotonic fluid. Correct electrolyte abnormalities and follow daily weights. Give furosemide (1 mg/kg/dose every 6–24 hours) to help maintain some urine output and prevent progression from oliguria to anuria. Antimotility agents and antibiotics are contraindicated and may worsen the course. Optimization of nutritional support is essential, preferably by the enteral route, if the clinical status permits.

Despite rigorous management of fluid and electrolyte status, dialysis may eventually be required. Indications for dialysis include refractory hyperkalemia (>6.0–6.5 mEq/L), severe metabolic acidosis, symptomatic uremia, calcium/phosphate imbalance, or volume overload with persistent anuria that is not responsive to diuretic therapy. In addition, management of nutritional support and transfusions for severe anemia may require administration of large volumes of fluid, necessitating dialysis.

Emergent antihypertensive treatment may be required. Give a bolus of hydralazine (0.2–0.6 mg/kg, 20 mg/dose maximum) or labetalol (0.2–1 mg/kg, 40 mg/dose maximum) intravenous, followed by continuous infusions of either nicardipine (start with 0.5–1 g/kg/minute and titrate to a maximum of

Table 60-1. Differential Diagnosis of Hemolytic Uremic Syndrome

Diagnosis	Clinical Features
Gastrointestinal: Microangiopathic hemolytic anemia and thrombocytopenia not seen	
Appendicitis	Acute onset of periumbilical pain ⟶ right lower quadrant Diarrhea uncommon Normal blood urea nitrogen/creatinine and liver function tests
Infectious colitis	Fever, severe abdominal pain, tenesmus (+) Fecal leukocytes
Inflammatory bowel disease	Diarrhea or constipation Weight loss and/or growth failure Oral ulcers and perianal skin tags/fissures
Henoch-Schönlein purpura	Arthralgia/arthritis Palpable purpura of extensor surfaces of lower extremities Heme (+) stools
Hematologic	
Bilateral renal vein thrombosis	Flank pain No gastrointestinal symptoms
Disseminated intravascular coagulation	Prolonged prothrombin time/partial thromboplastin time ↓ Fibrinogen
Sepsis	Absence of microangiopathic hemolytic anemia Signs/symptoms of infection/systemic inflammatory response system
Thrombotic thrombocytopenia	Usually occurs in adults More central nervous system involvement
Renal	
Acute glomerulonephritis	Absence of hemolysis No gastrointestinal symptoms
Severe dehydration	Return of renal function with fluid resuscitation No hematologic findings
Vasculitis	Rash, arthralgia/arthritis No gastrointestinal symptoms Persistent systemic symptoms

4–5 g/kg/minute) or labetalol (0.25–3 mg/kg/hour). In the setting of hypertensive urgency in a patient who can tolerate oral medications, give isradipine (0.05–0.1 mg/kg, 5 mg/dose maximum) or clonidine in an older child or adolescent (0.05–0.1 mg/dose every 1 hour, 0.8 mg total dose maximum). In the acute phase of renal injury, avoid nephrotoxic drugs, such as angiotensin-converting enzyme inhibitors and nonsteroidal anti-inflammatory medications, as they alter glomerular perfusion.

Transfuse packed red blood cells (5–10 mL/kg) if the hemoglobin is less than 6 to 7 g/dL or there are signs of cardiovascular compromise. Transfuse slowly and monitor the patient closely for signs of fluid overload. A diuretic (furosemide 1 mg/kg/dose) may be required before and/or during the transfusion to prevent overload. Avoid a platelet transfusion unless there is a significant hemorrhage or an invasive procedure is necessary. A patient with atypical HUS or thrombic thrombocytopenic purpura may require plasmapheresis.

Indications for Consultation

- **Cardiology:** Carditis or heart failure
- **Gastroenterology/surgery:** Complications from colitis or acute abdomen
- **Hematology:** Complications from anemia or thrombocytopenia
- **Nephrology:** All patients
- **Neurology:** Coma, stroke, or seizure

Disposition

- **Intensive care unit transfer:** Severe electrolyte abnormalities, refractory hypertension requiring antihypertensive infusions, status epilepticus, coma, stroke, or heart failure
- **Discharge criteria:** Improving renal function, anemia, and thrombocytopenia, with stable electrolytes; adequate oral intake and nutrition; hypertension resolved or stable with oral medication

Follow-up

- **Primary care:** 2 to 3 days
- **Nephrologist:** 1 week; however, long-term follow-up needed for persistent or recurrent hypertension and proteinuria

Pearls and Pitfalls

- Maintain a high index of suspicion for a patient with a recent diarrheal illness and abrupt onset of pallor or change in urine output or activity.
- Avoid using antibiotics or anti-motility agents in a patient with a diarrheal illness.
- Consider obtaining central access early to facilitate management and monitoring of fluid and electrolyte status, nutritional support, hematologic derangements, transfusions, and possible dialysis.
- There is no correlation between the severity of the hematologic findings and the renal disease.
- Avoid platelet transfusions.

Coding

ICD-9

Hemolytic uremic syndrome **283.11**

Bibliography

Amirlak I, Amirlak B. Haemolytic uraemic syndrome: an overview. *Nephrology (Carlton)*. 2006;11:213–218

Bitzan M, Schaefer F, Reymond D. Treatment of typical (enteropathic) hemolytic uremic syndrome. *Semin Thromb Hemost*. 2010;36:594–610

Razzaq S. Hemolytic uremic syndrome: an emerging health risk. *Am Fam Physician*. 2006;74:991–996

Scheiring J, Andreoli SP, Zimmerhackl LB. Treatment and outcome of Shiga-toxin-associated hemolytic uremic syndrome (HUS). *Pediatr Nephrol*. 2008;23:1749–1760

Scheiring J, Rosales A, Zimmerhackl LB. Clinical practice. Today's understanding of the haemolytic uraemic syndrome. *Eur J Pediatr*. 2010;169:7–13

CHAPTER 61

Henoch-Schönlein Purpura

Introduction

Henoch-Schönlein purpura (HSP), also known as anaphylactoid purpura, is a systemic vasculitis characterized by some combination of non-thrombocytopenic palpable purpura, abdominal pain, arthritis/arthralgia, and/or renal manifestations. HSP is the most common vasculitis of childhood, with 75% of the cases occurring between 2 to 11 years of age and a peak incidence at 5 years of age. Males are affected twice as often as females, and there is a seasonal predilection in the spring and fall. Although the precise etiology is unknown, most cases are preceded by upper respiratory tract infections caused by organisms such as group A streptococcus, Epstein-Barr virus, *Mycoplasma,* and parvovirus B19.

Generally HSP is a benign illness, but if the patient develops any renal manifestations, the risk for end-stage renal disease is about 2%.

Clinical Presentation

History

As noted above, there is usually a history of a preceding upper respiratory tract infection, often associated with malaise and low-grade fever. The classic symptoms then begin to appear simultaneously or sequentially over a period of days to weeks. About three-quarters of patients complain of colicky, episodic, abdominal pain that is rarely associated with vomiting, hematemesis, and/or gross blood in the stools. About two-thirds of the time the patient complains of pain and swelling of the large joints, such as knees and ankles. Rarely, gross hematuria is noted. In as many as 50% of cases the classic purpuric rash is not evident at presentation, although eventually all patients or parents report an erythematous rash on the buttocks and lower extremities (which can also be seen on face and scalp in children <2 years old).

Physical Examination

The typical finding is an erythematous, blanching, lacy, macular rash that quickly evolves into palpable purpura on the buttocks and lower extremities. Lesions may also be on the face and scalp of a patient younger than 2 years, who may also have edema (acute hemorrhagic edema of infancy). The patient may also have a toxic appearance. There may be abdominal tenderness, and if intussusception (page 208) is present, rebound and guarding. The patient can also present with warmth, tenderness, and swelling, without erythema, of the knees and ankles. Hypertension may be noted, but it is more common in patients with renal involvement.

Laboratory

There are no definitive or diagnostic tests for HSP. The workup depends on the presentation, but obtain blood and urine cultures if there is any concern for bacterial sepsis or a tick-borne disease. The remainder of the laboratory evaluation depends on the differential diagnosis.

Afebrile Patient With the Classic Rash and No Signs of Sepsis

Obtain a complete blood cell count (platelet count is normal), stool guaiac, and urinalysis, but coagulation studies are unnecessary. While approximately 50% of patients develop microscopic hematuria, a minority have gross blood, white blood cells, and protein in the urine. If proteinuria is found, obtain electrolytes, blood urea nitrogen, creatinine, and albumin. To quantify the degree of proteinuria (if present), calculate the spot urine protein/creatinine ratio to determine whether the patient has nephrotic range proteinuria (>2).

Ill-Appearing Patient With the Classic Rash

In addition to the tests mentioned above, obtain blood and urine culture. If the patient has meningeal signs or an altered mental status, perform a lumbar puncture.

Arthritis Without the Classic Rash

Send an erythrocyte sedimentation rate and/or C-reactive protein, as well as a rheumatologic workup, including rheumatoid factor, antinuclear antibodies, and complement levels.

Possible Intussusception (Crampy Abdominal Pain, Drawing Up the Legs)

Obtain an abdominal ultrasound or computed tomography, as well as testing for occult blood, which is positive in 30% to 50% of cases (page 208). A contrast enema is neither diagnostic nor therapeutic for the small bowel intussusception that occurs in HSP.

Scrotal Pain and Swelling

Order a Doppler ultrasound of the scrotum to evaluate for testicular torsion.

Differential Diagnosis

See Table 61-1 for the differential diagnosis of purpura. If diagnostic uncertainty persists, consult with dermatology to arrange a skin biopsy. In both HSP and acute hemorrhagic edema of infancy, a leukocytoclastic vasculitis will be found.

Treatment

If the patient has palpable purpura (especially widespread or involving all 4 extremities), along with fever and a toxic appearance, immediately obtain a blood culture and treat with intravenous (IV) antibiotics, either ceftriaxone (100 mg/kg/day divided every 12 hours) or cefotaxime (200 mg/kg/day divided every 12 hours, 6 g/day maximum). Add doxycycline (2 mg/kg, then 1 mg/kg every 12 hours, 200 mg/day maximum) if Rocky Mountain spotted fever is suspected.

There is no specific treatment for HSP. In most cases the illness is benign and self-limiting, and symptoms usually resolve in 4 weeks. If the patient has joint swelling and pain, give a nonsteroidal anti-inflammatory drug (NSAID) such as naproxen (10–20 mg/kg/day divided every 12 hours; 1,000 mg/day maximum) or ibuprofen (10 mg/kg/dose every 6 hours; 40 mg/kg/day maximum), although NSAIDs may be contraindicated with renal impairment.

Treat a patient with severe abdominal pain and a normal ultrasound and/or radiologic studies with methylprednisolone (1 mg/kg/day for 2 weeks, 80 mg/day maximum) and slowly wean over 1 to 2 weeks, or longer depending on the response. Use the IV route to start as oral absorption is poor secondary to the gastrointestinal vasculitis. Also place the patient on bowel rest for 48 hours.

Table 61-1. Differential Diagnosis of Purpura

Diagnosis	Clinical Features
Septicemia (bacterial, Rocky Mountain spotted fever)	Fever, toxicity Purpura not limited to lower extremities
Idiopathic thrombocytopenic purpura	Petechiae without purpura Mucosal bleeding Thrombocytopenia
Coagulopathy	Ecchymoses Abnormal prothrombin time and/or partial thromboplastin time
Subacute bacterial endocarditis	Heart murmur or history of heart disease Osler nodes, Janeway lesions, splinter hemorrhages
Drug reaction	History of taking offending agent (penicillin, sulfonamide, oral contraceptives)

Indication for Consultation

- **Nephrology:** Hypertension, decreased renal function, nephrotic syndrome, or proteinuria for more than 1 week
- **Surgery:** Intussusception, intestinal hemorrhage, obstruction, or perforation
- **Urology:** Testicular torsion

Disposition

- **Intensive care unit transfer:** Severe hypertension
- **Discharge criteria:** Symptoms (abdominal pain, arthritis) are no longer incapacitating and renal function is normal or improving

Follow-up

- **Primary care:** Blood pressure check and urinalysis in 1 week for an uncomplicated case (normal urinalysis and renal function). Continue weekly for 3 weeks, then monthly until 6 months after presentation
- **Nephrology:** 1 week if the patient has proteinuria for more than 1 week; immediate consultation if the patient has renal failure or nephrotic syndrome

Pearls and Pitfalls

- In as many as 30% to 50% of patients the classic rash will develop up to 2 weeks after other clinical manifestations.
- Renal disease can develop over the subsequent 6 months, despite a normal initial urinalysis.
- Intussusception in HSP is usually ileoileal and may resolve spontaneously. Otherwise, an air enema is not effective and surgery will be required.

Coding

ICD-9

- Allergic purpura **287.0**
- Vascular disorders of skin **709.1**

Bibliography

Bogdanović R. Henoch-Schönlein purpura nephritis in children: risk factors, prevention and treatment. *Acta Paediatr.* 2009;98:1882–1889

Gedalia A, Cuchacovich R. Systemic vasculitis in childhood. *Curr Rheumatol Rep.* 2009;11:402–409

González LM, Janniger CK, Schwartz RA. Pediatric Henoch-Schönlein purpura. *Int J Dermatol.* 2009;48:1157–1165

McCarthy HJ, Tizard EJ. Clinical practice: diagnosis and management of Henoch-Schönlein purpura. *Eur J Pediatr.* 2010;169:643–650

Saulsbury FT. Henoch-Schönlein purpura. *Curr Opin Rheumatol.* 2010;22:598–602

CHAPTER 62

Nephrolithiasis

Introduction

Nephrolithiasis is a relatively uncommon diagnosis in the pediatric population, accounting for about 1 in 1,000 pediatric admissions in the United States. Consequences of untreated nephrolithiasis include severe pain, increased risk for infection and, rarely, kidney injury.

Physiological risk factors for nephrolithiasis include low urine volume, low urine pH, bacterial urinary tract infection, and increased urinary concentrations of stone-forming metabolites. Clinically, these risks manifest in the setting of metabolic derangements, anatomical abnormality of the urinary tract, and infection. Metabolic factors are found to cause more than 50% of pediatric renal calculi, with hypercalciuria and hypocitraturia being the most common. Hyperoxaluria, hyperuricosuria, and cystinuria are also well-known causes of renal stones.

Repeated infection, with or without anatomical abnormality, can lead to nephrolithiasis in children. Urease-producing bacteria, such as *Proteus*, *Providencia*, *Klebsiella*, *Pseudomonas*, and enterococci, promote renal stone formation by lowering urinary pH, leading to struvite precipitation and the "staghorn" type of renal stone. A history of surgical correction of genitourinary abnormalities further increases the risk of nephrolithiasis. In addition, prolonged immobilization can also lead to kidney stones.

Clinical Presentation

History

Nephrolithiasis presents with some combination of abdominal pain, flank pain, back pain, vomiting without diarrhea, and gross hematuria. In the first few months of life, the presentation may seem consistent with infantile colic. Ask about a history of renal disease, urinary tract infections, calcium intake, and other chronic medical conditions. Determine if the patient is taking any medications, such as calcium supplements, loop diuretics, acetazolamide, prednisone, and adrenocorticotropic hormone, which can predispose to renal stones. A first-degree relative affected by nephrolithiasis suggests a genetic etiology.

Physical Examination

Examination findings are inconsistent and nonspecific. Abdominal pain with palpation and costovertebral angle tenderness may be present. Usually there is no guarding or rebound tenderness.

Laboratory

Obtain a urinalysis and urine culture to evaluate for hematuria, oxalate crystals, and markers of infection such as pyuria, leukocyte esterase, nitrites, and bacteria. However, as many as one-third of pediatric patients with nephrolithiasis do not present with hematuria.

An anterioposterior abdominal x-ray (commonly referred to as KUB) is an appropriate initial radiographic study, although many stones may be missed if they are small in size or composed of material that is less radio-opaque, such as uric acid or cystine. Ultrasound may identify a stone or show unilateral hydronephrosis, which may be indirect evidence of an obstructing calculus. However, the most useful test is a non-contrast computed tomography, which is 96% sensitive and 98% specific.

Once the presence of a stone is confirmed, it is important to identify the exact type before initiating specific treatment. Arrange for the nursing staff or patient to strain the urine and send any recovered stones for analysis. A 24-hour urine collection is the best way to identify any abnormal metabolites, although this may be difficult to perform in a younger patient. Therefore, send a random urine sample for calcium, citrate, cystine, oxalate, and uric acid and calculate the metabolite:creatinine (Cr) ratio for each and compare to standard values. For example, divide the spot calcium level in milligrams by the spot Cr level in milligrams to determine the urinary calcium:Cr ratio. (See Table 62-1 for reference values.)

Order further laboratory tests based on the stone composition and urine metabolite evaluation. For example, in a patient with a calcium stone or high calcium:Cr, consider a broad differential for hypercalciuria, including abnormal gastrointestinal absorption of calcium, renal tubular dysfunction, endocrine derangements, and metabolic disorders.

Differential Diagnosis

The differential diagnosis for renal colic is extensive and includes most of the common causes of significant abdominal pain (Table 62-2).

Table 62-1. Normal Values for Urine Metabolite:Creatinine (Cr) Ratios (mg/mg)		
Metabolite Ratio	**Age**	**Normal Range**
Calcium:Cr	0–6 months of age 6–12 months of age 2–18 years of age	<0.8 <0.6 <0.2
Oxalate:Cr	0–6 months of age 6 months–4 years of age >4 years of age–adult	<0.3 <0.15 <0.1
Cystine:Cr	All ages	<0.02
Citrate:Cr	All ages	<0.51

Table 62-2. Differential Diagnosis of Nephrolithiasis	
Diagnosis	**Clinical Features**
Appendicitis	Fever, vomiting Periumbilical → right lower quadrant pain Guarding and rebound tenderness
Cholelithiasis	Risk factors: hemolysis, postpartum, rapid weight loss Right upper quadrant pain, hyperbilirubinemia Positive abdominal ultrasound
Glomerulonephritis	No colic Hypertension Tea-colored urine with red blood cell casts
Intussusception	Intermittent abdominal pain, drawing legs up No hematuria Guaiac positive → currant jelly stools
Malrotation	Vomiting, abdominal distension, no colic No hematuria
Ovarian/testicular torsion	Intermittent lower abdominal pain No hematuria Positive ultrasound
Pancreatitis	Epigastric or left upper quadrant pain relieved by leaning forward ↑ Amylase and lipase
Pyelonephritis	Fever, toxicity, Costovertebral angle tenderness but no colic ↑ White blood cells Pyuria, bacteriuria, (+) nitrites and leukocyte esterase

Treatment

The treatment of nephrolithiasis varies based on the underlying cause of stone formation. However, the mainstays of therapy are aggressive intravenous hydration and adequate analgesia. Give D5 ½ normal saline + 20 mEq/L potassium chloride at 1.5 to 2 times maintenance, provided there is no evidence of urinary obstruction and urine output is adequate. This will dilute the stone components and encourage excretion of excess metabolites. In addition, prescribe morphine (0.1–0.2 mg/kg every 2–4 hours, maximum 2 mg infant, 4–8 mg child, 15 mg adolescent), although nonsteroidal anti-inflammatory drugs such as ibuprofen (10 mg/kg every 6 hours, 800 mg maximum) or ketorolac (0.5 mg/kg every 6 hours, 120 mg/day maximum) may suffice if there is no evidence of acute kidney injury or history of chronic kidney disease. If infection is suspected, start empiric antibiotic treatment with ceftriaxone (50 mg/kg/day divided every 12 hours, 4 g/day maximum), then tailor the antibiotics to the culture results.

A urology consult is indicated for significant hydronephrosis causing obstruction, a stone larger than 5 mm, or recurrent pain. Among the treatment options are extracorporeal shock wave lithotripsy or surgical stone excision.

Once the underlying cause for nephrolithiasis is found, specific long-term pharmacologic treatments may be implemented in conjunction with a consulting nephrologist. For example, thiazide diuretics reduce calcium excretion and slow the formation of calcium stones.

Indications for Consultation

- **Metabolism/genetics:** Abnormal urine metabolic profile, recurrent stones
- **Nephrology:** Abnormal urine metabolic profile, recurrent stones
- **Urology:** Hydronephrosis or other stone-related obstruction, recurrent stones

Disposition

- **Discharge criteria:** Adequate oral intake of both fluids and pain medication with normal urine output

Follow-up

- **Primary care:** 1 to 2 weeks
- **Urology and/or nephrology:** 1 week

Pearls and Pitfalls

- An infant with nephrolithiasis may have a colic-like presentation.
- The absence of hematuria does not rule out nephrolithiasis.
- There may be an iatrogenic cause for nephrolithiasis, such as medications and prolonged immobilization.

Coding

ICD-9

• Calculus of the kidney	**592.0**
• Renal colic	**788.0**

Bibliography

Alon US. Medical treatment of pediatric urolithiasis. *Pediatr Nephrol.* 2009;24:2129–2135

Hoppe B, Kemper MJ. Diagnostic examination of the child with urolithiasis or nephrocalcinosis. *Pediatr Nephrol.* 2010;25:403–413

Spivacow FR, Negri AL, del Valle EE, et al. Metabolic risk factors in children with kidney stone disease. *Pediatr Nephrol.* 2008;23:1129–1133

Straub M, Gschwend J, Zorn C. Pediatric urolithiasis: the current surgical management. *Pediatr Nephrol.* 2010;25:1239–1244

Nephrotic Syndrome

Introduction

Nephrotic syndrome (NS) is a consequence of increased glomerular filtration of macromolecules with resultant heavy proteinuria. This causes hypoalbuminemia, hyperlipidemia, hypercoagulability, and an increased susceptibility to bacterial infections, especially due to encapsulated organisms (*Streptococcus pneumoniae*). When fluid retention exceeds 3% to 5% of body weight, edema appears, secondary to low plasma oncotic pressure and sodium retention. In chronic NS, renal losses of thyroxin-binding proteins predispose to the development of hypothyroidism.

Minimal change NS (MCNS) accounts for most primary cases, occurring most commonly in children younger than 6 years. Other primary diseases are focal segmental glomerulosclerosis (FSGS), membranoproliferative glomerulonephritis (MPGN), diffuse mesangial sclerosis (DMS), and membranous nephropathy.

Secondary causes include infections (HIV, hepatitis C, hepatitis B), drugs (nonsteroidal anti-inflammatory drugs, penicillamine), and malignancies (lymphoma). Most cases of congenital NS present in the first 3 months of life and are due to mutations in genes affecting podocyte structure or function. Other causes of congenital NS include syphilis, toxoplasmosis, cytomegalovirus, measles, and HIV. A patient younger than 1 year at presentation has a high likelihood of congenital NS while a child older than 10 years at presentation has an increased risk of another underlying disease.

Clinical Presentation

History

The illness begins with nonspecific symptoms such as anorexia, irritability, and malaise. There may also be gastrointestinal complaints such as abdominal discomfort and diarrhea. However, the chief complaint is usually edema, most often periorbital, but also pedal, pretibial, or labial/scrotal. Occasionally the patient complains of decreased urine output.

Urinary loss of anticoagulant proteins can predispose the patient to venous thromboembolism, which can manifest as a deep venous thrombosis (page 25) with calf pain and Homans sign (calf pain on forceful foot dorsiflexion), or a pulmonary embolism with chest pain and dyspnea.

Physical Examination

The hallmark of NS is edema, which appears in areas of low tissue resistance. These include the periorbital, pedal, pretibial, scrotal, and labial regions, as well as the abdominal cavity (ascites). The edema is characteristically dependent, so that in the morning it is periorbital and later in the day localizes primarily to the lower extremities. It can generalize and evolve into anasarca.

As a consequence of the low oncotic plasma, the patient may have intravascular volume depletion manifested by tachycardia and signs of peripheral vasoconstriction. More severe hypoalbuminemia may lead to pleural effusions and dyspnea, as well as ascites, with resultant abdominal pain, umbilical or inguinal hernias, and peritonitis.

Laboratory

If NS is suspected, obtain a urinalysis and spot urine for protein:creatinine ratio (normal <0.2, non-nephrotic range proteinuria 0.2–2, nephrotic range proteinuria >2). If the ratio is greater than 2, consider ordering a 24-hour urine collection. Nephrotic range proteinuria in a child is defined as greater than 50 mg/kg/24 hours, greater than 40 mg/m^2/hour, or greater than 1 g/m^2/24 hours. For an adult it is greater than 3 g/24 hours.

Although gross hematuria is rare in NS, microscopic hematuria occurs in up to 20% of patients. Gross hematuria is most often seen in MPGN or acute glomerulonephritis.

Other laboratory tests to obtain include

- Complete blood cell count: There may be hemoconcentration and/or thrombocytosis, which can contribute to thrombotic complications.
- Serum electrolytes, including calcium, phosphorous, and magnesium: Hyponatremia is common secondary to antidiuretic hormone secretion and there may be apparent hypocalcemia (normal ionized) secondary to a low albumin.
- Blood urea nitrogen (BUN)/creatinine: There may be prerenal azotemia secondary to intravascular volume depletion.
- Total protein and albumin: Hypoalbuminemia less than 2.5 g/dL is typical, with a low total protein.
- Lipid profile: Hyperlipidemia is typical, with both elevated total serum cholesterol and triglycerides levels.

Additional laboratory testing, to be obtained on an individualized basis, includes

- Complement levels: These are normal in MCNS and DMS, while a low C3 is associated with glomerulonephritis.
- Viral serologies to look for an etiology: HIV antibody, hepatitis B surface antigen, hepatitis C antibody.
- Venereal Disease Research Laboratory and antinuclear antibodies, especially in a patient older than 10 years.

In addition, obtain a renal ultrasound to ensure the presence of normal kidneys and rule out congenital malformations as well as renal masses.

Differential Diagnosis

NS is the most common cause of edema in childhood, and the only diagnosis associated with significant proteinuria (Table 63-1). A patient with MCNS usually has a normal blood pressure, renal function, and complement levels (Table 63-2).

Treatment

Initial Presentation

As the most likely cause of NS is MCNS, initially treat all patients with steroids (after a purified protein derivative is placed). Use prednisone 60 mg/m^2/day (divided every day or twice a day; 80 mg/day maximum). Proteinuria may

Table 63-1. Differential Diagnosis of Nephrotic Syndrome

Diagnosis	Clinical Features
Edema	
Cirrhosis/liver disease	Abnormal liver function tests Signs of portal hypertension
Congestive heart failure	Heart murmur, S3 gallop Pulmonary edema and/or hepatomegaly Abnormal electrocardiogram
Protein losing enteropathy	Diarrhea Failure to thrive Elevated stool α-1-antitrypsin
Dark-Colored Urine	
Acute glomerulonephritis	Gross hematuria Hypertension more likely Evidence of recent strep infection Decreased C3, normal C4

Table 63-2. Differential Diagnosis of Primary Etiologies of the Nephrotic Syndrome	
Diagnosis	**Clinical Features**
Minimal change nephrotic syndrome	Age 2–6 years Microscopic hematuria (20%) Response to steroids (>80%)
Focal segmental glomerulosclerosis	Hematuria (60%–80%) Hypertension (20%) Response to steroids (15%–20%)
Membranous nephropathy	Age >18 years Hematuria (60%) Venous thromboembolism
Membranoproliferative glomerulonephritis	Hematuria (80%) Hypertension (35%) Low C3

persist for 7 to 10 days after initiation of steroids, so being proteinuria-free is not a discharge criterion. For most patients with MCNS, the proteinuria will clear by the third week of oral prednisone treatment.

Manage edema with dietary sodium restriction (<2 g/day or 1–2 mEq/kg/day [1 mEq = 23 mg sodium]). If the patient has severe edema or complications such as pulmonary edema, administer a single dose of intravenous (IV) furosemide (1 mg/kg) and monitor response. If the patient does not respond, administer low sodium 25% albumin (0.5–1 g/kg IV over 4 hours) concomitantly with the furosemide to enhance the intravascular oncotic pressure, as well as delivery of furosemide to the nephron. Repeat this regimen as frequently as every 8 hours. An alternative regimen in a patient who is refractory to furosemide is to use the same dose of albumin along with a continuous furosemide infusion (0.3 mg/kg/hour for 24 hours). However, do not use a diuretic if the patient has signs of significant intravascular volume depletion.

Closely monitor the patient's intravascular volume status and obtain daily electrolytes and BUN/creatinine. Monitor daily weights and urine output per shift to ensure response to treatment.

Continue the daily steroids for 4 to 8 weeks, followed by alternate day therapy for 4 to 8 weeks, and then a gradual taper until treatment is discontinued. If the patient does not respond and has persistent edema and proteinuria after 4 weeks of treatment with prednisone, consult a nephrologist to consider initiating other treatments such as angiotensin-converting enzyme inhibitor or angiotensin II receptor blockers.

A renal biopsy is indicated if there is no response to treatment within 4 to 6 weeks. Other indications include steroid-responsive NS with more than

2 relapses in a 6-month period or more than 4 relapses in any 12-month period, low serum complement C3 level at the time of initial presentation of the NS (not related to acute poststreptococcal glomerulonephritis), hypertension at presentation (higher likelihood of FSGS), renal failure with elevated BUN/creatinine, and age younger than 1 year.

Relapses

The baseline risk of relapse after 3 months of initial treatment with steroids is 60%. Consult a nephrologist and resume the same steroid regimen as above. Continue until the urine is protein-free for 3 consecutive days, and then taper the dose in the same fashion as described in the initial treatment.

Complications

A patient with NS is at increased risk of infections as a result of decreased concentration of immunoglobulins, decreased complement levels, and the immunosuppressive therapy. Up to 15% of patients with ascites may develop bacterial peritonitis, usually caused by *S pneumoniae* and *Escherichia coli*. Suspect peritonitis if the patient has ascites and fever, abdominal pain, and/or vomiting, although the presentation may be subtle. Promptly arrange for an abdominal paracentesis to obtain the fluid for cell count, Gram stain, and culture. Infected fluid usually has more than 250 white blood cells/mm^3. Give IV ceftriaxone (50 mg/kg every day, 4 g/day maximum) or cefotaxime (150 mg/kg/day divided every 8 hours, 8 g/day maximum), for 10 days. Ascites fluid cultures may be negative in up to 50% of cases of primary peritonitis. Therefore, complete the course of antibiotics if the clinical presentation and ascites fluid cell count are consistent with peritonitis, regardless of a negative culture.

Indications for Consultation

- **Genetics:** Congenital or infantile NS (<1 year old), if there is no clear etiology
- **Hematology:** Hypercoagulable event
- **Nephrology:** All patients

Disposition

- **Intensive care unit transfer:** Severe anasarca, acute pulmonary edema, hypercoagulable syndrome
- **Discharge criteria:** No anasarca or respiratory distress and family education complete

Follow-up

- **Primary provider:** Outpatient dipstick monitoring of proteinuria once weekly, either in the office or by family at home
- **Nephrology:** 2 to 4 weeks

Pearls and Pitfalls

- The patient may not initially present with edema.
- NS is a risk factor for a hypercoagulable state.
- Most cases are caused by steroid-responsive MCNS, while most patients refractory to steroids will have FSGS.

Coding

ICD-9

• Edema	**782.3**
• Hyperlipidemia	**272.4**
• Hypoalbuminemia	**273.8**
• NS	**581.9**
• NS with focal glomerulosclerosis	**581.1**
• NS, minimal change	**581.3**
• Proteinuria	**791.0**

Bibliography

Gipson DS, Massengill SF, Yao L, et al. Management of childhood onset nephrotic syndrome. *Pediatrics.* 2009;124:747–757

Gordillo R, Spitzer A. The nephrotic syndrome. *Pediatr Rev.* 2009;30;94–105

Hodson EM, Willis NS, Craig JC. Corticosteroid therapy for nephrotic syndrome in children. *Cochrane Database Syst Rev.* 2007;(4):CD001533

Hodson EM, Willis NS, Craig JC. Interventions for idiopathic steroid-resistant nephrotic syndrome in children. *Cochrane Database Syst Rev.* 2010; 11:CD003594

Urinary Tract Infection

Introduction

Urinary tract infection (UTI) is the most common serious bacterial infection of childhood and is a frequent admitting diagnosis. About 5% of febrile infants younger than 12 months have a UTI, although most can be treated as an outpatient. Indications for inpatient treatment include age younger than 1 to 2 months, dehydration, inability to tolerate oral antibiotics, and concern for a serious complication (renal abscess, obstructive uropathy, urosepsis). The most common pathogen isolated is *Escherichia coli*, which is responsible for 80% of infections. Girls younger than 3 years are twice as likely as boys to have UTIs, although uncircumcised boys are at least 4 times more likely than circumcised boys to have a UTI.

Clinical Presentation

History

Typically, the patient presents with fever and some combination of dysuria, urgency, frequency, incontinence, and malodorous urine. However, the fever may be accompanied only by nonspecific complaints, such as irritability (infants), nausea, vomiting, diarrhea, abdominal pain, and flank pain. Ask about risk factors, including a history of previous UTIs, sexual activity (for an adolescent), underlying urinary tract anomaly, chronic constipation, diseases of the central or peripheral nervous system, and family history of renal anomalies.

Physical Examination

The patient is typically febrile and may have a toxic appearance, but hypertension is unusual in the absence of chronic renal disease. Perform a thorough examination to determine if there may be other causes of the fever. Check for abdominal tenderness, distension, or mass, as well as suprapubic and costovertebral angle tenderness. Examine the external genitalia for abnormalities and signs of irritation or local infection and note the circumcision status. Poor growth may be seen in a patient with recurrent UTIs.

Laboratory

The diagnosis of a UTI requires both inflammation on urinalysis (UA) and growth of a single pathogen from a urine culture. Confirmation of a UTI in a patient 2 to 24 months of age now entails a positive culture of a single uropathogen (colony count >50,000 cfu/mL) along with an abnormal UA. Use a minimum of more than 100,000 cfu/mL for a clean-catch specimen in an older child. After the first few months of life, a positive UA is extremely sensitive (about 99%), but not specific for the diagnosis of UTI. However, the single most sensitive (91%) and specific (96%) test is the urine Gram stain. Obtain a urine culture prior to administration of antibiotics. If the patient is too young to effectively perform a clean catch, obtain the urine culture via straight catheterization (page 175) or suprapubic aspiration (page 167). Suprapubic aspiration may result in less contamination but has a lower success rate than urethral catheterization, unless aided by direct visualization of a full bladder by ultrasonography. Do not rely on a bag specimen for culture, which is frequently contaminated, although a negative is likely a true negative. Bag specimens are useful for UA.

As many as 10% of infants younger than 2 months with a UTI will have a concomitant bacteremia. Therefore, perform a complete sepsis evaluation (blood, urine, and cerebrospinal fluid cultures) for a febrile infant younger than 2 months (page 291), Also obtain a blood culture for a toxic-appearing patient of any age.

Differential Diagnosis

The signs and symptoms of UTI in a young child are relatively nonspecific. Given the frequency of UTI, maintain a low threshold for obtaining a urine culture. Consider pyelonephritis in any patient, especially girls up to 2 years of age, with high fever (>103°F; 39.4°C) without a source. Other common causes of dysuria, frequency, and/or pyuria include viral cystitis, vaginitis, urethritis, and dysfunctional voiding.

Treatment

Antibiotics

Choose the initial treatment based on local antibiograms. Ultimately, use the urine culture identification and sensitivity to guide therapy. The dosing for some antibiotics may require adjusting if the patient has renal insufficiency.

Younger Than 2 Months

Initially treat intravenously with ampicillin 200 (mg/kg/day divided every 6 hours) *and* either gentamicin (3.5–5 mg/kg every day) *or* ceftriaxone (100 mg/kg/day divided every 12 hours) or cefotaxime for infants younger than 4 weeks (when still at risk for hyperbilirubinemia), at least until bacteremia and/or meningitis is excluded. Treat intravenously until the patient is afebrile for 24 hours and the blood culture (if obtained) is negative, then complete a 10-day course with oral antibiotics.

2 Months or Older

If the patient fits the criteria for inpatient treatment of a UTI, initiate treatment with intravenous (IV) antibiotics. Since most *E coli* are resistant to ampicillin, use ceftriaxone (50 mg/kg every day) or cefotaxime (150 mg/kg/day divided every 8 hours). If the patient is at increased risk for *Pseudomonas* (prior history of *Pseudomonas* UTI, chronic indwelling catheter, neurogenic bladder), give ciprofloxacin 20 to 30 mg/kg/day IV or oral divided every 12 hours (>12 months of age). If there is a risk factor for *Enterococcus*, such as genitourinary instrumentation or renal anomaly, or if gram-positive rods are noted on Gram stain, add ampicillin (100 mg/kg/day divided every 6 hours) empirically. If *Staphylococcus aureus* grows from the urine culture, consider hematogenous spread. Confirm a negative blood culture, and perform a thorough physical examination looking for signs of soft tissue, joint, pulmonary, or cardiac involvement.

Treat urosepsis (or concomitant bacteremia) and complicated pyelonephritis, such as with a renal abscess or in a pregnant adolescent, with a 10- to 14-day course of therapy, based on bacterial identification and sensitivities.

Transition to oral antibiotics after the child no longer meets criteria for inpatient treatment. Depending on the sensitivities of the identified organism (if available), use cephalexin 50 mg/kg/day divided every 8 hours), cefixime (8 mg/kg every day), amoxicillin/clavulanate (40 mg/kg/day divided every 12 hours), or sulfamethoxazole-trimethoprim (trimethoprim 10 mg/kg/day divided every 12 hours).

Treat for a total of 7 to 14 days, although a 2- to 4-day course may suffice for a patient older than 3 months with a presumed only lower tract UTI.

Antibiotic Prophylaxis

Do not give antibiotic prophylaxis after a first UTI. While prophylaxis may result in a small reduction in recurrent UTIs, there is no proven difference in future renal scarring. In addition, there is a risk of increased antibiotic resistance with subsequent UTIs. However, a child with Grade IV or V vesicoureteral reflux (VUR) or a preadolescent with more than 1 UTI may benefit. Use either sulfamethoxazole-trimethoprim (2 mg/kg every day if >2 months of age, 160 mg/day maximum) or nitrofurantoin (2 mg/kg every day if >1 month, 100 mg/day maximum). Prescribe an initial 3- to 6-month course, since most UTIs recur within 6 months.

Radiology

As per the 2011 American Academy of Pediatrics guidelines, after a first febrile UTI, screen all patients 2 to 24 months of age with a renal bladder ultrasound (RUS). Obtain a follow-up voiding cystourethrogram (VCUG) if the RUS is abnormal. This approach will facilitate the identification of a patient who is most likely to have high-grade VUR. Also order a VCUG if posterior urethral valves are suspected in a male infant (palpable bladder distension).

A technetium-99m dimercaptosuccinic acid scan is indicated only if recommended by a consulting nephrologist or urologist.

For a patient who has not had any imaging, but presents with a second or third febrile UTI, obtain a follow-up RUS and VCUG.

Indications for Consultation

- **Nephrology:** Renal insufficiency
- **Urology:** Renal abscess, urinary obstruction, obstructive uropathy, neurogenic bladder, Grade III–V VUR

Disposition

- **Intensive care unit transfer:** Septic shock, multisystem organ failure, renal failure
- **Discharge criteria:** Afebrile for more than 24 hours, adequate oral intake including antibiotics, radiologic workup arranged (if indicated)

Follow-up

- **Primary care:** Within 1 week to assess completion of antibiotic course and assess the need for prophylaxis or radiologic studies
- **Urology:** 1 to 2 weeks if there is a known genitourinary abnormality
- **Nephrology (if the patient has renal insufficiency):** 1 to 2 weeks

Pearls and Pitfalls

- Instruct the family to seek medical care promptly for a UTI evaluation if there is a new febrile illness or a change in urine odor. This is more important than any follow-up imaging study.
- Test of cure is not necessary if the patient has a prompt clinical response to the antibiotics. Lack of response suggests bacterial resistance or another cause, such as a renal abscess or ureterocele.
- Reproductive health counseling is indicated for adolescents with new-onset recurrent UTIs.

Coding

ICD

• Acute pyelonephritis	**590.1**
• Renal abscess	**590.2**
• UTI of newborn	**771.82**
• UTI, site not specified	**599.0**

CPT

• Insert bladder catheter	**51701**
• Aspiration of bladder by needle	**51100**

Bibliography

American Academy of Pediatrics Subcommittee on Urinary Tract Infection; Steering Committee on Quality Improvement and Management. Urinary tract infection: clinical practice guideline for the diagnosis and management of the initial UTI in febrile infants and children 2 to 24 months. *Pediatrics.* 2011;128:595–609

Brady PW, Conway PH, Goudie A. Length of intravenous antibiotic therapy and treatment failure in infants with urinary tract infections. *Pediatrics.* 2010;26:196–203

Herz D, Merguerian P, McQuiston L, et al. 5-year prospective results of dimercapto-succinic acid imaging in children with febrile urinary tract infection: proof that the top-down approach works. *J Urol.* 2010;184:1703–1709

Hodson EM, Willis NS, Craig JC. Antibiotics for acute pyelonephritis in children. *Cochrane Database Syst Rev.* 2007;(4):CD003772

Round J, Fitzgerald AC, Hulme C, Lakhanpaul M, Tullus K. Urinary tract infections in children and the risk of ESRF. *Acta Paediatrica.* 2012;101:278–282

Williams G, Craig JC. Long-term antibiotics for preventing recurrent urinary tract infection in children. *Cochrane Database Syst Rev.* 2011;3:CD001534

Neurology

Acute Ataxia

Introduction

Ataxia is the inability to coordinate or modulate movements. It can be caused by a disorder anywhere in the nervous system, but is commonly attributed to dysfunction of the cerebellum or posterior columns of the spinal cord. Acute ataxia implies that the symptoms evolved in less than 72 hours in a previously well child, differentiating it from chronic and episodic progressive ataxias, which are rare in children and are usually caused by genetic or metabolic disorders.

The etiologies of most cases of acute ataxia in childhood can be divided into the following categories: infectious or immune-mediated, drug or toxin exposure, mass lesions, trauma, and paraneoplastic syndromes. The most common diagnoses are acute cerebellar ataxia (ACA), toxic exposure, and Guillain-Barré syndrome (GBS). ACA is a postinfectious, autoimmune phenomenon that leads to cerebellar demyelination. Common preceding infections include varicella, coxsackievirus, and echovirus. Toxic exposure may be accidental (organic chemicals, heavy metals) or recreational (alcohols), as well as from prescribed medications (antiepileptic drugs, benzodiazepines, antihistamines, and alcohols).

In GBS, the associated ataxia may be caused by ascending muscle weakness or sensory derangement, as seen in the Miller Fisher variant.

Clinical Presentation

History

Symptoms of ataxia may be subtle or profound, limited to extremity disability or compromising coordination of all movements. The patient usually presents shortly after the onset of symptoms, which may include slurred speech; clumsiness of extremity movements; refusal to walk; and wide-based, "drunken" gait. The goal of the initial history is to quickly rule out a life-threatening condition, such as a mass lesion, central nervous system (CNS) infection, or hydrocephalus. Ask about progression, duration, and frequency of the ataxia, as well as accompanying symptoms, including recent or current infection, fever, recent immunizations, recurrent or persistent headache, diplopia, change in mental status, exposure to toxins, and recent history of trauma.

ACA occurs primarily in children younger than 6 years. It presents days to weeks following a viral illness and is characterized by the sudden onset of ataxia. Vomiting, visual disturbances, and slurred speech may also be seen, but fever, stiff neck, and abnormal behavior are absent.

Physical Examination

Perform a thorough physical examination, including a fundoscopic examination, as well as a detailed neurologic evaluation. Ataxia may present with abnormalities of gait, trunk, extremity control, and/or speech. An ataxic patient may compensate for imbalance by widening the base of support while standing or walking. Evaluate variations of gait (walking on heels or toes) and balance on one leg to uncover subtle degrees of ataxia. Ataxia caused by weakness can be determined by a thorough manual muscle test targeting the muscle groups exhibiting the instability. Muscle tone and reflexes are usually preserved in cerebellar disorders, whereas GBS often presents with ascending weakness and diminished reflexes. Specific signs consistent with ACA include wide-based gait, dysarthria, dysmetria, and nystagmus.

Dyssynergia (the loss of smoothness of execution of a motor activity), dysmetria (overshooting or undershooting while attempting to reach a target), dysdiadochokinesia (the inability to perform rapid alternating movements), and dysarthria may accompany ataxia and are specific to a cerebellar etiology. Evaluate dyssynergia and dysmetria with finger-to-nose or heel-to-shin testing. Test for dysdiadochokinesia by having the patient repeatedly tap a foot or pat the examiner's hand. Use the Rhomberg test (proprioception) to determine whether the cause of ataxia is sensory in nature. The test is positive when the patient is able to stand with feet together and eyes open without losing balance, but is unable to remain steady when the eyes are closed. This occurs because the patient is using visual cues to compensate for a lack of sensory feedback from the lower extremities. In the toddler or young child, assess coordination by having the patient reach for and use toys.

Fever usually accompanies an infectious etiology of ataxia. Mental status integrity helps differentiate ACA from more serious conditions, such as toxic exposure, acute disseminated encephalomyelitis, mass lesions, and encephalitis. An ophthalmologic examination may identify papilledema, which is indicative of an intracranial lesion or hydrocephalus. Cushing triad, bulging of the fontanelle, and cranial nerve palsies are other hallmarks of an emergent intracranial process.

A fixed and dilated pupil may occur when a rapidly expanding intracranial mass, such as blood from a hemorrhage, causes compression of cranial nerve III. It may also herald impending herniation. Certain drugs, such as alcohol and opioids, cause constriction of the pupils; others, including anticholinergics and sympathomimetics, may cause pupillary dilation.

Laboratory

If there is no obvious etiology for the acute onset of ataxia, obtain urine and serum drug screens to rule out a toxic exposure. As drug screens detect a limited number of substances, testing for specific agents may be necessary. In addition, in most cases a complete blood cell count, C-reactive protein and/or erythrocyte sedimentation rate, glucose, electrolytes, and liver function tests will help screen for an infectious or inflammatory etiology.

Ataxia associated with trauma is an indication for an emergent computed tomography (CT) of the head, neck, and/or spine. Emergent neuroimaging is also indicated when there is evidence of increased intracranial pressure, focal neurologic findings, or altered mental status. Magnetic resonance imaging (MRI) is superior to CT for identifying posterior fossa disease, demyelinating disease, and intracranial tumors. However, CT is generally more readily available and can usually detect conditions requiring urgent intervention, such as hydrocephalus, traumatic injury, evolving hematoma, and many mass lesions.

Perform a lumbar puncture with opening pressure if a CNS infection or inflammatory disorder cannot be ruled out. Marked pleocytosis and a highly elevated protein are indicative of an active infectious process, such as meningitis or encephalitis. In GBS, the cerebrospinal fluid will often have an elevated protein without significant pleocytosis, while in ACA, the white blood cell count and protein will be normal to mildly elevated.

Nerve conduction studies can help to confirm the diagnosis of GBS (slowed nerve velocity). ACA is generally a diagnosis of exclusion based on clinical findings, although MRI may reveal bilateral diffuse abnormalities of the cerebellar hemispheres. Obtain urine and serum catecholamine levels for a patient presenting with ataxia accompanied by opsoclonus or myoclonus. This constellation of symptoms may be due to a paraneoplastic syndrome secondary to neuroblastoma.

Order a simple electroencephalogram (EEG) if the patient has an altered consciousness, a history consistent with seizure, or fluctuating clinical signs. Long-term (24-hour) EEG monitoring may be indicated if symptoms persist and the simple EEG is non-diagnostic.

Differential Diagnosis

The differentiation of ataxia from vertigo can be difficult, especially in a nonverbal patient. Nausea and nystagmus often accompany vertigo and may be elicited or worsened by sudden changes in the patient's head position. The differential diagnosis is summarized in Table 65-1.

Table 65-1. Differential Diagnosis of Ataxia	
Diagnosis	**Clinical Features**
Acute cerebellar ataxia	Symptoms evolve over days Afebrile, normal mental status Nystagmus, slurred speech
Acute disseminated encephalomyelitis	Altered mental status, seizures Multifocal neurologic dysfunction Magnetic resonance imaging: multifocal white matter demyelination
Bacterial meningitis	Fever, meningismus, ill-appearance Cerebrospinal fluid (CSF): pleocytosis, ↑ protein, ↓ glucose
Encephalitis	Fever, altered mental status Cranial nerve abnormalities (ocular palsies, facial weakness) Reflexes preserved CSF: pleocytosis
Guillain-Barré syndrome (GBS)	Afebrile, normal mental status Paresthesias common Ascending weakness with areflexia CSF: mild initial pleocytosis, moderate ↑ protein
Intracranial hemorrhage	May have had preceding head or neck trauma Afebrile, mental status usually altered Focal neurologic deficits Hemorrhage on computed tomography scan
Labyrinthitis	Fever variable, normal mental status Otitis media, hearing loss, vomiting Intense vertigo
Miller Fischer variant of GBS	Ataxia, areflexia Ophthalmoplegia
Post-concussive syndrome	Afebrile, mental status normal, vertigo, unsteady gait Onset often acute Prior mild traumatic brain injury Duration: 1–6 months
Posterior fossa tumor	Afebrile, altered personality, mental status variable Headache, vomiting, head tilt, nuchal rigidity Papilledema, diplopia
Toxic ingestion	Afebrile, altered mental status Acute onset Duration: hours to days

Treatment

The priority is the treatment of life-threatening symptoms, such as respiratory failure (pages 614–617) in GBS, and increased intracranial pressure (pages 441–442) in a patient with an intracranial hemorrhage, mass, or stroke. Consult with the appropriate subspecialist (infectious disease, neurology, neurosurgery, oncology) to manage an intracranial infection, tumor, or hemorrhage. Obtain the necessary imaging and diagnostic tests while awaiting emergent consultation.

The treatment for ACA is supportive, including physical and occupational therapy and emotional support. Monitor and support nutrition and hydration as needed. Up to 90% of patients will recover fully, with improvement starting within a week.

The treatment of toxic exposure may require consultation with the local poison control center and depends on the specific agent and quantity of the exposure.

A patient with GBS requires close observation until the evolution of symptoms has stopped. In particular, monitor respiratory and bulbar function closely, as progressive dysfunction can be life-threatening. Monitor the negative inspiratory force (NIF), also known as maximum inspiratory force, and perform early intubation if the NIF is greater than -25 cm H_2O, the symptoms are progressing rapidly, or there is severe autonomic instability. Treating progressive GBS with intravenous immunoglobulin (2 g/kg as a single dose; or 1 g/kg/day for 2 days; or 0.4 g/kg/day for 5 days) or plasmapheresis may truncate the progression and hasten recovery.

Institute a bowel program to ensure daily stooling by providing a stool softener (docusate) combined with a bowel stimulant suppository (bisacodyl) each evening, if the patient has not defecated in the prior 24 hours. Monitor urinary void volumes and the abdominal examination to evaluate for evidence of retention. If the bladder is enlarged or void volumes are high, obtain a bladder scan to estimate the bladder volume. Elevated post-void volumes suggest retention secondary to incomplete bladder evacuation and dysfunctional voiding. Initiate a program of intermittent catheterization every 4 to 6 hours as needed to avoid an excessive bladder volume ([normal bladder volume in ounces] = [patient's age in years] + 2).

Indications for Consultation

- **Neurology:** Unclear etiology, primary neurologic disorder such as GBS
- **Physical medicine and rehabilitation:** Persistent, significant functional deficit
- **Neurosurgery, infectious disease, oncology:** Depending on the etiology

Disposition

- **Intensive care unit transfer:** Compromised neurologic state affecting brain stem function, declining mental status, hemodynamic instability, respiratory insufficiency
- **Discharge criteria:** Stabilization and/or improvement of the ataxia, adequate oral intake

Follow-up

- **Primary care:** 2 to 3 days, with close follow-up until the ataxia resolves
- **Physical therapy and occupational therapy, physical medicine and rehabilitation if functional deficit persists:** 1 week
- **Pediatric neurology:** 1 to 2 weeks

Pearls and Pitfalls

- Relapse can occur in up to 10% of children with ACA.
- Antiepileptic medications, such as phenytoin, are common causes of acute ataxia.

Coding

ICD-9

• Ataxia	**781.3**
• Cerebellar ataxia	**334.3**
• GBS	**357.0**
• Poisoning by unspecified drug or medicinal substance	**977.9**

Bibliography

Menkes JH, Moser FG. Neurologic examination of the child and infant. In: Menkes JH, Sarnat HB, Maria BL, eds. *Child Neurology.* 7th ed. Philadelphia, PA: Lippincott, Williams & Wilkins; 2006:1–27

Ryan MM, Engle EC. Acute ataxia in childhood. *J Child Neurol.* 2003;18:309–316

Salas AA, Nava A. Acute cerebellar ataxia in childhood: initial approach in the emergency department. *Emerg Med J.* 2010;27:956–957

Weinberg GA, Moran MM. Neurologic symptom complexes. In: Long SS, Pickering LK, Prober CG, eds. *Principles and Practice of Pediatric Infectious Diseases.* 3rd ed. New York, NY: Churchill Livingstone Elsevier; 2008:187–188

Willoughby RE. Cerebellar ataxia, transverse myelitis and myelopathy, Guillain-Barré syndrome, neuritis, and neuropathy. In: Long SS, Pickering LK, Prober CG, eds. *Principles and Practice of Pediatric Infectious Diseases.* 3rd ed. New York, NY: Churchill Livingstone Elsevier; 2008:317–319

CHAPTER 66

Acute Hemiparesis

Introduction

Acute hemiparesis typically implicates the contralateral corticospinal tract, which travels from the cortex, through the internal capsule, to the medulla. In the medulla it decussates to the contralateral side, and descends in the lateral spinal cord. It then synapses on the anterior horn cells, which give rise to the peripheral nerves. Because unilateral spinal cord injury is rare, especially acutely, cerebral pathology is the most common cause for acute hemiparesis.

Clinical Presentation

History

The most likely causes of any acute neurologic symptoms fall into the categories of seizure, stroke, and migraine. Therefore, priorities in the history include evidence for prior seizures (with subsequent Todd paralysis) or infection (meningitis, cerebral abscess), risk factors for stroke (especially trauma for arterial dissection and family history of hypercoagulability), and gradual progression of weakness over 1 hour in the setting of headache (suggestive of hemiplegic migraine). Ask about recent illness or immunization followed by abrupt neurologic symptoms (including hemiparesis), which raises the concern of a demyelinating process (acute disseminated encephalomyelitis [ADEM]).

Physical Examination

The presence of fever suggests an infectious or inflammatory process. Hypertension is typical for stroke (ischemic or hemorrhagic). However, a normal blood pressure does not exclude stroke, but makes it less likely. With rare exception, involvement of the corticospinal tract results in weakness in contiguous limbs or face. That is, there will be weakness in the face/arm, or arm/leg, or face/arm/leg. Although a monoplegia implies a peripheral nervous system insult, an exception is an anterior cerebral artery infarct causing unilateral leg weakness.

A patient younger than 12 months has immature myelination of the corticospinal tract and may present with subtle signs of weakness. Careful observation at the bedside is typically more revealing than overzealous examination.

Laboratory

Laboratory testing includes screening tests as well as more directed evaluations once a diagnosis is established. Obtain a complete blood cell count and complete metabolic panel, including liver function tests, which may be elevated with certain viral infections (herpes). Also obtain urine toxicology if the clinical presentation suggests a stroke or new onset seizures. If infectious etiologies are being considered perform a lumbar puncture (LP), either before or after the head computed tomography (CT), unless the patient has a platelet count lower than 20,000/mm^3. If an intracranial hemorrhage (ICH) is suspected or confirmed, order a prothrombin time/partial thromboplastin time and bleeding studies. Also consider evaluation for systemic lupus erythematosus, vasculitis, or sickle cell disease.

While the hematologic studies for ischemic stroke are not standardized, in the absence of a clear vascular or cardiac etiology a reasonable evaluation includes obtaining homocysteine, antiphospholipid antibodies, protein C and S, activated protein C resistance, lipoprotein a, and ferritin. If these are unremarkable, genetic studies, including Factor V Leiden, PT G20201A, and methylenetetrahydrofolate reductase, can be helpful. A tiered approach to diagnosis potentially limits unnecessary and expensive studies, and it is reasonable to defer genetic testing to the outpatient setting unless the results will change management acutely (unlikely).

Radiology

The evaluation for an acute ischemic stroke includes looking for cardiac, vascular, infectious, immune-mediated, or hematologic causes. After 3 to 6 hours ischemic stroke may be visible on CT. However, magnetic resonance imaging (MRI) can identify an ischemic stroke within minutes of symptom onset, and is therefore the preferred modality, if immediately available. In addition to the head imaging, also obtain an electrocardiogram and transthoracic echocardiogram.

Arrange a head CT if there is a concern for an ICH, which will be immediately evident on CT.

A magnetic resonance angiography neck with fat suppression images can identify arterial dissections in the setting of trauma. Also order a brain MRI with contrast (if immediately available) when a tumor or abscess is being considered.

Differential Diagnosis

The initial priority is the diagnosis of an acute ischemic stroke or intracerebral hemorrhage (Table 66-1).

The key to diagnosing a cerebral abscess is the identification of risk factors in a patient with new focal weakness, seizures, or change in level of alertness with or without fever. In a child, the infection is typically due to contiguous spread of sinusitis, mastoiditis, or a dental abscess. Other potential sources of bacteremia include cellulitis, a pulmonary infection, and endocarditis.

Hemiplegic migraine is a diagnosis of exclusion, after alternative diagnoses such as strokes and seizures have been ruled out. The typical history involves the gradual spread of neurologic symptoms over 20 to 30 minutes, followed by headache. The development of symptoms, visual loss, numbness, and weakness correlates with the progression of cortical depression.

ADEM is a multifocal, monophasic, demyelinating illness that develops over hours to days. It is typically postinfectious or parainfectious, with multiple potential infectious causes (most often viral). The patient presents with the new onset of multifocal neurologic disease consisting variously of change in mental status, visual loss, ataxia, limb weakness, and sometimes seizures.

Treatment

Stroke and Increased Intracranial Pressure

Obtain a non-contrast head CT. Transfer the patient to the intensive care unit (ICU), and then (if necessary) to a center with immediately available pediatric neurosurgery, as well as the capability to perform diagnostic imaging (MRI) and monitoring of intracranial pressure (ICP) (pediatric ICU). Consult with a neurologist to determine whether to give intravenous (IV) tissue plasminogen activator (tPA), which has limited use in children because of the risk of an ICH with its use. The adult neurology stroke service may be helpful in evaluation and treatment decision-making.

Obtain urgent neurosurgical consultation if the patient has a posterior fossa ICH, or an ICH with mass effect (displacement or compression of adjacent structures). Elevate the head of the bed to 30 degrees, but defer intubation if the patient is alert in order to avoid sedation and its subsequent effects on the neurologic examination. There is no standardized goal blood pressure. Permissive hypertension is the rule-in order to maintain an adequate cerebral perfusion pressure, but discuss these parameters with a neurology or neurosurgery consult. Monitor closely for signs of deterioration, such as a change in mental status (becoming more difficult to arouse), anisocoria, or worsening limb

Table 66-1. Differential Diagnosis of Acute Weakness

Diagnosis	Clinical Features
Acute ischemic stroke Intracerebral hemorrhage	Face and/or arm and/or leg weakness Hypertension
Acute disseminated encephalomyelitis	Abrupt onset of weakness Encephalopathy associated with a febrile illness
Brain tumor (complicated by intracranial hemorrhage or seizure)	Prior subtle signs of weakness and headache
Cerebral abscess	Headache Penetrating trauma Contiguous infection Cyanotic congenital heart disease
Complex migraine	May have a personal/family history of migraines Gradually migrating cortical depression over 30–60 min: followed by headache
Encephalitis (especially herpes)	Lateralizing weakness Fever, confusion +/- seizures Electroencephalogram: paroxysmal lateralizing epileptiform discharges
Hypoglycemia	Focal weakness History of diabetes
Mitochondrial myopathy, encephalopathy, lactic acidosis, and stroke	Unexplained lateralizing weakness Magnetic resonance imaging signal changes do not follow vascular distribution Headache and/or confusion Can present with seizures
Seizure/Todd paralysis	Acute history of paroxysmal movements Weakness or somnolence
Viral meningitis (especially West Nile virus)	Fever, headache, vomiting Meningismus

weakness. An acute alteration in the neurologic examination warrants a repeat head CT. If the patient had been receiving chronic anticoagulation, consult with a hematologist to initiate reversal.

The evaluation for an acute ischemic stroke includes looking for cardiac, vascular, infectious, immune-mediated, or hematologic causes. Obtain the laboratory tests and imaging studies mentioned above. Consider viral etiologies, especially varicella, which is a treatable cause of viral vasculopathy and strokes in children. Discuss antiplatelet agents or anticoagulation with a neurologist. However, neurosurgical involvement is not usually necessary in the early management of ischemic stroke.

Seizures

The evaluation and treatment of seizures is detailed elsewhere (page 475). In general, give prophylactic antiepileptic drug therapy (fosphenytoin 5 mg/kg/day divided twice a day or leviteracetam 20–30 mg/kg/day divided twice a day) for 7 days to a patient with moderate or severe ICH. Except as noted above, most first-time seizures do not require short- or long-term antiepileptogenic treatment.

Encephalitis

If there is any concern about herpes simplex virus (HSV) encephalitis, initiate acyclovir immediately (>28 days–12 years: 20 mg/kg every 8 hours for 21 days; >12 years: 10 mg/kg every 8 hours for 21 days). Note that while the sensitivity of HSV cerebrospinal fluid (CSF) polymerase chain reaction (PCR) is high, it is not 100%, so that a patient with herpes encephalitis can have a negative PCR. Therefore, rely on both clinical suspicion and the HSV PCR results to determine whether to initiate and continue acyclovir. Also, the PCR can remain positive for days after treatment has begun, so a lumbar puncture performed after the initiation of acyclovir is still useful. The response to acyclovir is not immediate, so that a patient who is back to baseline mental status within less than 24 hours of the initiation of treatment is unlikely to have HSV encephalitis. In contrast, the combination of a normal CSF, the absence of periodic lateralized epileptiform discharges on electroencephalogram, and a normal brain MRI essentially excludes HSV encephalitis.

Hemiplegic Migraine

This is a diagnosis of exclusion, after diagnoses such as strokes and seizures have been ruled out. Treat with ketorolac (15 mg IV every 6 hours) and metoclopramide (0.1 mg/kg slow IV push, 10 mg maximum). Do not use sumatriptan, which causes vasoconstriction and might worsen the hemiplegic migraine.

Cerebral Abscess

Obtain an MRI of the brain with and without contrast. Obtain an infectious disease consult and treat empirically with IV antibiotics for 6 to 8 weeks. The choice of antibiotic therapy is based on the presumed source of infection (oral flora, hematogenous spread, post-neurosurgical procedure), but in some cases a brain biopsy is necessary for identification of pathogens. In the setting of significant mass effect, manage increased ICP as above for ICH and consult neurosurgery. A focal neurologic examination is a contraindication to LP.

ADEM

An MRI of the brain or spinal cord is diagnostic, with evidence for demyelination on T2-weighted imaging. Perform an LP and send CSF for cell count, glucose, protein, oligoclonal bands, myelin basic protein, and immunoglobulin (Ig) G index (requires simultaneous serum IgG). Typical findings are an elevated cell count (>6 white blood cell count/mm^3) and elevated protein (>25 mg/dL in a patient <18 years of age). IV steroid treatment is controversial, as it does not clearly affect outcome in mild to moderate cases, but may speed the recovery. Consult with a neurologist to determine whether to treat with methylprednisolone (15–30 mg/kg every day IV for 15 days, 1 g/day maximum), IVIG, or plasmapheresis.

Indications for Consultation

- **Hematology:** Stroke patient receiving anticoagulation
- **Neurology:** All cases of acute hemiparesis
- **Neurosurgery:** Hemorrhagic stroke, brain tumor, cerebral abscess
- **Oncology:** Brain tumor

Disposition

- **Intensive care unit transfer:** Acute hemiparesis associated with acute encephalopathy (delirium), airway concerns, stroke, status epilepticus, or rapidly evolving neurologic changes
- **Discharge criteria:** Stable, non-evolving condition, action plan in place for recurrent events (eg, seizures, migraines), adequate plan for administrating and monitoring of therapy and rehabilitation (if needed)

Follow-up

- **Primary care:** 1 to 2 weeks
- **Neurology:** 1 to 2 weeks

Pearls and Pitfalls

- If the patient has a history of recent trauma, consider embolic stroke due to arterial dissection.
- New hypertension in the setting of hemiparesis is suggestive of stroke.
- Todd paralysis following a seizure implies a focal seizure, and is often associated with a structural lesion such as remote stroke, cortical dysplasia, or in older patients a brain tumor.

- Obtain a CT scan early if a stroke is suspected to identify a patient for whom tPA is a potential option (within 4.5 hours of symptom onset).
- For questions about thrombolysis therapy, consult 800/NO-CLOTS, a pediatric thromboembolic hotline staffed by Toronto Sick Kids.

Coding

ICD-9

- Cerebral embolism, with cerebral infarction **434.11**
- Cerebral embolism, without cerebral infarction **434.10**
- Cerebral thrombosis, with cerebral infarction **434.01**
- Cerebral thrombosis, without cerebral infarction **434.00**
- Flaccid hemiparesis unspecified side **342.00**
- Hemiplegic migraine, without mention of intractable migraine without mention of status migrainous **346.30**
- Intracranial abscess **324.0**
- ICH **431**
- Metabolic encephalopathy **348.31**
- Viral encephalitis(list first underlying viral condition) **323.01**

Bibliography

Black DF. Sporadic and familial hemiplegic migraine: diagnosis and treatment. *Semin Neurol.* 2006;26:208–216

Frazier JL, Ahn ES, Jallo GI. Management of brain abscesses in children. *Neurosurg Focus.* 2008;24:E8

Goodman S, Pavlakis S. Pediatric and newborn stroke. *Curr Treat Options Neurol.* 2008;10:431–439

Lopez-Vicente M, Ortega-Gutierrez S, Amlie-Lefond C, Torbey MT. Diagnosis and management of pediatric arterial ischemic stroke. *J Stroke Cerebrovasc Dis.* 2010;19:175–183

Lynch JK, Pavlakis S, Deveber G. Treatment and prevention of cerebrovascular disorders in children. *Curr Treat Options Neurol.* 2005;7:469–480

Pohl D. Epidemiology, immunopathogenesis and management of pediatric central nervous system inflammatory demyelinating conditions. *Curr Opin Neurol.* 2008;21:366–372

CHAPTER 67

Acute Weakness

Introduction

Acute muscle weakness is the decreased ability to move muscles against resistance. It can be the result of pathology anywhere in the neuromuscular system and may occur abruptly or evolve over the course of hours to days. Acute weakness can be life-threatening if it advances to include the respiratory muscles or is secondary to an intracranial process.

The most common cause of acute weakness in children is Guillain-Barré syndrome (GBS), also known as acute inflammatory demyelinating polyneuropathy. Other common etiologies of acute weakness include viral myositis, intracranial tumor, seizure, medication side effect, toxin exposure, and conversion disorder. Diseases that cause chronic weakness may present acutely and therefore require consideration in the differential diagnosis.

Clinical Presentation

History

Ask about the timing and severity of the weakness and whether there is any associated fever, rash, headache, double vision, altered mental status, changes in sensation, or bowel or bladder dysfunction. Other pertinent points include a history of trauma, seizure, preceding viral or bacterial illness, possible medication or toxin exposure, and a family history of childhood weakness.

Physical Examination

The first priorities are airway, breathing, and circulation. After the patient has been stabilized, perform a thorough neuromuscular examination, attempting to localize the affected portion of the neuromuscular system. Grade the muscle strength (grade 5: normal; grade 4: active movement against gravity and resistance; grade 3: active movement against gravity; grade 2: active movement with gravity eliminated; grade 1: flicker or trace of contraction; grade 0: no contraction), note the distribution of weakness and any sensory loss, and assess the muscle tone.

Upper motor neuron lesions are caused by pathology of the cerebral cortex and spinal cord. These lesions typically present with acute onset of weakness, either unilateral or bilateral. Other symptoms include spasticity, hypertonicity, hyperreflexia, and encephalopathy. However, in the early phase, the patient may have decreased muscle tone prior to the development of spasticity.

Lower motor neuron lesions include disorders of the anterior horn cell, neuromuscular junction, and peripheral nerve. Symptoms include absent or diminished reflexes, decreased muscle tone, muscle atrophy, and fasciculations. Primary disorders of the muscle typically present with a subacute or an indolent course of muscle weakness, associated with muscle pain, swelling, or tenderness. Muscle atrophy may be a late finding.

Mental status changes are indicative of an intracranial process, while nuchal rigidity is caused by meningitis or an epidural abscess. Focal tenderness along the back is suggestive of spinal cord lesion, focal inflammation, or infection. Evaluate the skin, looking for the heliotrope rash of dermatomyositis, tick bite marks, or signs of trauma.

Laboratory

Obtain a complete blood cell count, C-reactive protein, and/or erythrocyte sedimentation rate if there is concern for an infectious or inflammatory disease. Check a basic metabolic panel, including electrolytes, calcium, and creatinine, as electrolyte abnormalities can cause acute weakness. If there is proximal muscle weakness; muscle tenderness; or a history of dark, tea-colored urine, obtain a creatinine kinase (CK) and urinalysis (dipstick and microscopic). Perform a lumbar puncture if meningitis, encephalitis, GBS, or multiple sclerosis (MS) is suspected. Send the cerebrospinal fluid for cell count and differential, total protein and glucose, culture and, if MS is a concern, oligoclonal bands.

Radiology

An emergent computed tomography of the head is indicated for abrupt onset of weakness with deterioration of mental status, focal neurologic deficits, or preceding trauma. Obtain magnetic resonance imaging (MRI) of the brain in a clinically stable patient with symptoms of intracranial pathology. If spinal cord pathology is suspected, perform an emergent MRI to evaluate for trauma, infection, transverse myelitis, or tumor. Order an electroencephalogram if seizure is suggested by the history or physical examination.

Differential Diagnosis

Upper Motor Neuron Disorders

Pathology located in the cerebral cortex presents with acute onset of unilateral weakness, headache, vomiting, seizure, and/or mental status changes. The persistence of neurologic deficits is an indication for an urgent evaluation to rule out an evolving process, such as stroke, intracranial abscess, and epidural hematoma. Spinal cord injury, spinal epidural hematoma, and other causes of spinal cord compression may predominantly affect the upper motor neurons. The symptoms associated with this mixed injury include unilateral or bilateral weakness, altered sensation below the level of the lesion, and bowel and/or bladder dysfunction. Focal back pain at the level of the lesion may be present, while reflexes below the level of the lesion are absent.

Lower Motor Neuron Disorders

With disorders of the anterior horn cell, the patient will have normal or decreased reflexes, muscle atrophy, and fasciculations. Diseases of the peripheral nerves cause diminished reflexes (bilateral or unilateral), paresthesias, and dysesthesias. The most common etiology is GBS, which is a group of diseases that result in an acute inflammatory demyelinating polyneuropathy. The classic presentation occurs 2 to 4 weeks following a benign febrile respiratory or gastrointestinal illness. Symptoms start with paresthesias of the distal extremities, followed by ascending symmetrical paralysis. Pain and dysesthesias may be absent or pronounced. There can also be associated autonomic dysfunction with changes in blood pressure, cardiac arrhythmias, or bowel and bladder dysfunction. In up to 25% of patients, paralysis will ascend to include the respiratory muscles, necessitating observation in a unit capable of providing assistance with ventilation.

Disorders of the neuromuscular junction cause generalized weakness and hypotonia. These include botulism, tick paralysis, myasthenia gravis, and organophosphate toxicity.

Primary Muscle Disorders

Disorders of the muscle are often associated with a slower onset of weakness and an elevated CK.

Other

Suspect a conversion disorder when the physical examination is not consistent with an organic lesion. Often the patient has an inconsistent neuroanatomical constellation of symptoms, as well as a negative medical workup.

The differential diagnosis of acute weakness is summarized in Table 67-1.

Treatment

General management of all patients with acute weakness includes close observation of respiratory status, nutrition, feeding, and functional abilities. Closely follow bulbar function by assessing the strength of the gag reflex and monitoring for the onset of drooling, dysarthria, and/or decrease in oral motor integrity.

Table 67-1. Differential Diagnosis of Acute Weakness	
Diagnosis	**Clinical Features**
Disorders of the Cerebral Cortex	
Acute disseminated encephalomyelitis (ADEM)	Acute encephalopathy Seizures, headache, vomiting May have ataxia
Acute intracranial hemorrhage Cerebrovascular accident	Abrupt onset Altered mental status Headache, vomiting, seizure
Encephalitis Meningitis	Fever Altered mental status Weakness may be global
Alternating hemiplegia of childhood Hemiplegic migraine	Acute onset of hemiplegia and headache Family history of migraines
Multiple sclerosis	Presentation similar to ADEM Oligoclonal bands present in cerebrospinal fluid (CSF) Frequent relapses following remission
Todd paralysis	Unilateral weakness following seizure
Transient ischemic attack	Unilateral weakness Duration <24 hours
Tumor	Headache, clumsiness, behavior changes Vomiting (especially in the morning)
Disorders of the Spinal Cord	
Anatomical abnormalities: atlantoaxial instability, Chiari, tethered cord	History of chronic weakness Progressive worsening of symptoms
Discitis Epidural abscess	Fever Back pain
Spinal cord concussion	History of trauma Symptoms resolve within a few hours
Transverse myelitis	Progressive symptoms Paresthesias Typically unilateral limb weakness Neck or back pain
Traumatic injury: epidural hematoma, vertebral body compression fracture, dislocation, transection	History of trauma Abrupt onset of symptoms Paresthesias, bowel and bladder dysfunction
Tumor	Focal back pain Weight loss
Disorders of the Anterior Horn Cell	
Paralytic poliovirus	Preceded by fever, malaise, sore throat Typically unilateral weakness Extremely rare in the United States
Spinal muscle atrophy	Tongue fasciculations in an infant Motor delay

Table 67-1. Differential Diagnosis of Acute Weakness, continued	
Disorders of the Peripheral Nerves	
Acute intermittent porphyria	Abdominal pain, sensory changes Family history of porphyria
Guillain-Barré syndrome (GBS)	Ascending weakness (usually symmetrical) Elevated CSF protein (> twice normal) May have mild CSF pleocytosis
Toxins: heavy metals	History of exposure Weakness typically distal
Disorders of the Neuromuscular Junction	
Botulism	*<6–12 months* Honey exposure Poor feeding, constipation, lethargy *>6–12 months* Direct ingestion of toxin Dry mouth, blurred vision, nausea, vomiting Symptoms can rapidly progress to weakness of the bulbar and skeletal muscles.
Myasthenia gravis	Ptosis, diplopia Extraocular muscle weakness Weakness worsens with activity
Organophosphate toxicity	Diarrhea, emesis Miosis, bradycardia
Tick paralysis	GBS-like ascending weakness and paresthesias Tick usually found on scalp
Primary Muscle Disorders	
Inflammatory myopathies: dermatomyositis, polymyositis	Fever, heliotrope rash in dermatomyositis Proximal muscle weakness Elevated creatinine kinase (CK)
Congenital myopathies Metabolic myopathies Mitochondrial disease Muscular dystrophies	Slowly progressive weakness Muscle tenderness and wasting May have hypertrophy in advanced stages Elevated CK
Periodic paralysis	Episodic weakness Associated with potassium abnormalities May also occur with sodium abnormalities
Pyomyositis	Multifocal muscle abscesses Typically immunocompromised patient
Rhabdomyolysis	Myalgias Dark urine (hemoglobin/myoglobin positive) Markedly elevated CK
Viral myositis	Preceding viral illness Myalgias

Table 67-1. Differential Diagnosis of Acute Weakness, continued	
Other Conditions	
Conversion disorder	Inconsistent neurologic examination Medical workup negative
Toxic exposure: antineoplastics, ciguatoxin, isoniazid, nitrofurantoin, paralytic shellfish toxin, zidovudine	Paresthesias History of possible exposure

Screen respiratory integrity via assessment of oxygen saturations or consult with respiratory therapy to assess forced vital capacity and negative inspiratory forces (NIFs). These measures provide an early warning of impending respiratory compromise. If respiratory compromise is suspected, obtain a blood gas (see respiratory failure, page 613).

If MS, myasthenia gravis, botulism, muscular dystrophy, peripheral neuropathy, or a disorder of the neuromuscular junction is suspected consult a neurologist, who may recommend nerve conduction velocities, electromyography or, rarely, a muscle biopsy. If myasthenia gravis is suspected, arrange for a Tensilon test, which involves administering a short-acting acetylcholinesterase inhibitor. The diagnosis is confirmed if the symptoms resolve.

Early in the hospitalization, institute a bowel regimen of stool softeners daily and suppositories as needed. Monitor pre- and post-void bladder volumes for evidence of urinary retention. If volumes are consistently greater than predicted for age, initiate a catheterization program and consult with urology. (See Acute Ataxia on page 433.)

Immediate neurosurgery consultation is imperative in the case of acute intracranial or spinal cord mass, abscess, or hemorrhage. An epidural abscess will require decompression and culture from the wound, followed by broad-spectrum intravenous (IV) antibiotics, including coverage for methicillin-resistant *Staphylococcus aureus*. Acute intracranial hemorrhage may require immediate evacuation. If an intracranial tumor is suspected, consult with pediatric oncology.

A patient with GBS requires close inpatient observation until the nadir of the illness has been reached, typically within 4 weeks of the onset of symptoms. Follow the respiratory status closely with oxygen saturations, forced vital capacity, and negative inspiratory forces. Transfer to a pediatric intensive care unit (ICU) is indicated if the weakness is rapidly progressing, NIFs are less than 30 cm H_2O, oxygen saturations are consistently less than 90%, vital capacity is declining, or if there is advancing bulbar muscle weakness. If the onset of symptoms occurred within 2 weeks of diagnosis, first-line treatment is IV immune globulin (0.4 mg/kg daily for 5 days).

Treat tick paralysis with immediate removal of the tick. Symptoms will typically resolve within several days. Treat transverse myelitis with high-dose pulse methylprednisolone (0.5–1 mg/kg/day IV, 1,000 mg/day maximum, for 3–5 days). Treat viral myositis with rest, analgesia, and hydration. However, if there is rhabdomyolysis, give IV hydration and perform serial assessments of renal function and output.

If conversion disorder is suspected, limit the medical workup. Assess the psychological status of the patient and consult with psychiatry and/or psychology.

Indications for Consultation

- **Neurology:** All patients with acute weakness
- **Neurosurgery:** Tumor, abscess, or hemorrhage of the brain or spinal cord
- **Physical, occupational, and/or speech and swallow therapy:** Significant functional impairment

Discharge Criteria

- **Discharge:** Depending on the primary process, the weakness has improved or stabilized, and an adequate plan is in place to meet functional needs
- **ICU transfer:** Rapid escalation of weakness, respiratory compromise, signs of increased intracranial pressure

Follow-up

- **Primary care:** 1 to 2 weeks
- **Neurology:** 1 to 2 weeks

Pearls and Pitfalls

- Ongoing observation and evaluation are essential to monitor respiratory integrity.
- A thorough history and physical examination are key to determining the location of the pathology along the neuromuscular pathway.
- GBS is the most common cause of acute weakness in children.

Coding

ICD-9

• Acute disseminated encephalomyelitis	**323.61**
• Botulism, infant	**040.41**
• Dermatomyositis	**710.3**
• GBS	**357.0**
• Muscle weakness (generalized)	**728.87**
• Myasthenia gravis, with (acute) exacerbation	**358.01**
• Transverse myelitis, acute, unspecified	**341.20**

Bibliography

El-Bohy AA, Wong BL. The diagnosis of muscular dystrophy. *Pediatr Ann.* 2005;34:525–530

Harris MK, Maghzi AH, Etemadifar M, et al. Acute demyelinating disorders of the central nervous system. *Curr Treat Options Neurol.* 2009;11:55–63

Hughes RA, Swan AV, van Doorn PA. Intravenous immunoglobulin for Guillain-Barré syndrome. *Cochrane Database Syst Rev.* 2010;(6):CD002063

Hughes RA, Wijdicks EF, Benson E, et al. Supportive care for patients with Guillain-Barré syndrome. *Arch Neurol.* 2005;62:1194–1198

Krupp LB, Banwell B, Tenembaum S; International Pediatric MS Study Group. Consensus definitions proposed for pediatric multiple sclerosis and related disorders. *Neurology.* 2007;68(16 suppl 2):S7–S12

Tsarouhas N, Decker JM. Weakness. In: Fleisher G, Ludwig S, eds. *Textbook of Pediatric Emergency Medicine.* 6th ed. Philadelphia, PA: Lippincott, Williams & Wilkins; 2010:626–634

Altered Mental Status

Introduction

Altered mental status (AMS) is a derangement in consciousness, which is defined as arousal and awareness of one's self and environment. Awareness is determined by the cerebral hemispheres, whereas arousal is controlled by the ascending reticular activating system (ARAS). Although derangements in either one or both systems may alter mental status, there is a spectrum of decreasing states of consciousness, ranging from confusion (loss of clear thinking) to coma (no response to stimuli, including pain, and the eyes remain closed).

The etiology of AMS can be either structural (mass, hemorrhage) or medical (infection, ingestion, intoxication, inborn error of metabolism, diabetic ketoacidosis [DKA]). Structural causes are associated with focal neurologic deficits due to the proximity of the ARAS to brain stem reflex pathways, whereas medical etiologies lead to cerebral dysfunction and generally do not cause focal neurologic deficits.

While there are numerous possible etiologies for AMS, a rapid thorough assessment of the patient's history and a physical examination are crucial for determining the appropriate initial interventions targeting the underlying cause.

Clinical Presentation

History

Ask about the onset of the change in consciousness (acute versus subacute), along with a history of recent illnesses, behavioral changes, and specific associated symptoms (ie, focality). For an infant, determine whether there are symptoms suggestive of an inborn error of metabolism, such as poor feeding, lethargy, failure to thrive, and seizures. In an older child, a careful review of the patient's medical history may yield clues, such as diabetes (DKA) and kidney (uremia) or liver disease (encephalopathy). Inquire about sick contacts, recent travel, immunization status, and any potential immunodeficiency. Key information to collect for both suspected accidental ingestion in toddlers and intentional overdose in adolescents includes a current medication list and the availability of medications in the home or environment. Also inquire about any recent history of trauma, particularly head trauma.

A patient with sickle cell anemia or congenital heart disease may develop AMS due to a thrombotic or ischemic stroke. A patient with a seizure disorder can be postictal or having nonconvulsive status epilepticus (subclinical seizures) and present with AMS. A patient with ventriculoperitoneal shunt (VPS) malfunction will complain of acute headache and/or vomiting, while a patient with a brain tumor may present with headaches and vomiting over weeks to months. Such tumors can cause mass effect leading to focal neurologic deficits (such as eye deviation, papillary changes, and motor weakness) or hydrocephalus with increased intracranial pressure (ICP).

Physical Examination

Immediately assess the vital signs and airway, breathing, and circulation (ABCs) and evaluate the patient for signs of trauma (ecchymoses, hematomas). Priorities on a focused physical examination include features that can help differentiate between structural and medical etiologies. Perform a thorough neurologic examination evaluating the pupillary response, fundi, cranial nerves, reflexes, upper and lower motor neuron functions, and sensory responses. Specific findings associated with structural lesions include abnormal pupillary light reflexes (either asymmetrical or dilated pupils), abnormalities in extraocular movements, asymmetry of motor response, and decorticate or decerebrate posturing.

As a result of the relatively fixed volume within the skull, insults causing a mass effect can increase ICP, which is characterized by irritability, headache, vomiting, and a unilaterally dilated pupil suggesting uncal herniation. In addition, downward eye deviation ("setting sun"), papilledema, and cranial nerve palsies (particularly III, IV, and VI) may be seen. Cushing triad (hypertension, bradycardia, and irregular respirations) are late signs of increased ICP and signify impending herniation.

If the neurologic examination is non-focal and structural lesions are not suspected, a more thorough physical examination may elucidate which of the medical etiologies may be responsible. Classic signs of infection include fever, nuchal rigidity, lymphadenopathy, and rash. For metabolic derangements, the focused physical examination varies with the specific organ system that is responsible. Liver disease may present with hepatomegaly, ascites, and jaundice. DKA may present with signs of dehydration, Kussmaul breathing, and fruity breath odor.

A patient with an ingestion or intoxication can present with varied symptoms and altered vital signs, thus knowledge of common toxidromes (page 321) is essential for identification, intervention, and treatment.

Laboratory

Initial laboratory tests to obtain include an immediate bedside serum glucose determination, complete blood cell count, serum electrolytes and calcium, liver function studies, ammonia, and a coagulation profile, as well as an arterial blood gas if the patient is breathing abnormally or a toxic ingestion is suggested. If the patient is comatose order a head computed tomography (CT) (without contrast) to immediately rule out a central nervous system bleed, mass lesion, or hydrocephalus. Also obtain a CT if there are signs or symptoms of elevated ICP, particularly if the patient requires a lumbar puncture. If an intracranial infection is suspected in a patient with signs of elevated ICP, treat with appropriate antibiotics (page 466) and defer the lumbar puncture until the patient is clinically stable. Culture additional sites as indicated. Obtain serum and urine toxicology to guide management if an ingestion or intoxication is suspected. A stool guaiac may be positive in cases of intussusception.

Differential Diagnosis

While there are many causes of AMS (Table 68-1), a focused history, physical examination, laboratory tests, and imaging will help narrow the differential diagnosis. Structural causes of AMS are often associated with focal neurologic findings, such as abnormal pupils, extraocular movements, focal weakness, asymmetrical reflexes, and posturing. Medical etiologies cause global cerebral dysfunction and generally do not produce focal neurologic deficits. In addition, a gradual change in mental status is more suggestive of a medical etiology while an abrupt onset may indicate a structural lesion.

AMS accompanied by fever, photophobia, headache, and vomiting suggests an infectious etiology. Intoxications and ingestions may present with similar symptoms, such as temperature derangements and vomiting. Maintain a high level of clinical suspicion, as often there is no reported history of ingestion. In addition to exogenous toxins, there are numerous metabolic derangements that can result in AMS, including electrolyte imbalance, hypoxia, thyroid and adrenal disease, acid-base disturbance, and extremes of temperature.

Consider non-convulsive status epilepticus, in which there are electrographic seizures without motor movements, in a patient who remains with AMS for more than 60 to 90 minutes after a seizure.

Any mechanism of injury that is inconsistent with the clinical findings or is unlikely, given the patient's developmental capability, raises the concern for non-accidental trauma (pages 587–589).

Intussusception (page 208) is an unusual cause of AMS in a young infant who may also present with vomiting and guaiac-positive stools.

Table 68-1. Differential Diagnosis of AMS

Diagnosis	Clinical Features
Brain tumor/ICP	Headache, vomiting Cushing triad: bradycardia, hypertension, Cheyne-Stokes Asymmetrical pupils, VIth nerve palsy
CNS infection	Fever, photophobia, headache, vomiting Nuchal rigidity
Concussion/head trauma	(+) History Confusion, headache, memory loss Scalp/skull hematoma or ecchymoses
Confusional migraine	History of migraines Headache, confusion, aphasia
Diabetic ketoacidosis	Abdominal pain, vomiting, polyuria Fruity breath odor Kussmaul breathing Hyperglycemia and ketonuria
Hemorrhagic stroke	Headache, vomiting Signs of ICP Focal neurologic deficits
Hypertension	Headache
Hypoglycemia	Dizziness, tremor, diaphoresis ↓ Glucose
Hypotension	Dizziness Poor perfusion
Inborn errors of metabolism	Lethargy, poor feeding Seizures Hypoglycemia
Ingestion/intoxication	Confusion, slurred speech, hallucinations Hyperthermia, respiratory depression Seizures
Intussusception	Episodic abdominal pain, currant jelly stools
Ischemic stroke	Headache, vomiting, focal neurologic deficits Signs of ↑ ICP
Liver failure	Jaundice Easy bleeding Ascites
Non-accidental trauma	Story inconsistent with injuries Fracture in nonmobile infant Retinal hemorrhages
Psychiatric conditions	Catatonia (can maintain posture) Echolalia Resists eye opening
Seizure	Shaking, twitching, eye rolling Incontinence
Sepsis	Fever, poor perfusion, widened pulse pressure Source of infection

Diagnosis	Clinical Features
Subarachnoid hemorrhage	Headache, photophobia, irritability Meningismus
Uremia	Anorexia, lethargy, fatigue
Venous thrombosis	Headache, seizures Signs of ↑ ICP
VPS malfunction	History of hydrocephalus and shunt Headache, vomiting Signs of ↑ ICP

Table 68-1. Differential Diagnosis of AMS, continued

Abbreviations: AMS, altered mental status; CNS, central nervous system; ICP, intracranial pressure; VPS, ventriculoperitoneal shunt.

Treatment

Initial management of AMS involves addressing the ABCs and restoring and ensuring stable respiratory and hemodynamic status. Continuously monitor the vital signs and provide oxygen by facemask or non-rebreather mask until normal oxygenation is documented. A patient with a Glasgow Coma Scale (GCS) score below 8 may require intubation. Secure large-bore intravenous (IV) access for the administration of medications and isotonic fluids. Correct hypoglycemia (<40 mg/dL) with 5 mL/kg of D10 (0.5 mg/kg). Administer a 20 mL/kg bolus of isotonic fluid (0.9% sodium chloride or lactated Ringer solution) for hypotension, poor perfusion, or signs of dehydration. Monitor the clinical response and repeat as necessary. Identify and treat abnormalities in temperature, blood pressure, and electrolytes.

In a case of known or suspected trauma, stabilization of the C-spine is essential until a fracture can be ruled out. Assess the patient for other signs of injury and obtain imaging as indicated. Obtain an emergent head CT and consult neurosurgery for any intracranial hemorrhage as surgical intervention may be necessary.

Electively intubate a patient with increased ICP to protect the airway and allow hyperventilation to a $PaCO_2$ of 35 to 40 mm Hg. Also elevate the head of the bed to 45 degrees with the head maintained midline. Give mannitol (0.5–1 g/kg) or hypertonic (3%) saline (3–5 mL/kg) for treatment of suspected cerebral edema and consult with a neurosurgeon.

See page 475 for the management of seizures.

There are specific antidotes (page 323) for some ingestions or intoxications. Treat a suspected opiate intoxication with IV naloxone (0.1 mg/kg IV, 2 g maximum) and repeat every 2 to 3 minutes as needed. Note that the opiate antagonist has a shorter half-life than the opiate, so multiple doses or a continuous infusion of naloxone may be required.

The radiologist will attempt to reduce the intussusception with an air or barium enema. If this is unsuccessful, surgical intervention will be required.

Indications for Consultation

- **Neurology:** New-onset seizures, focal seizures
- **Neurosurgery:** Head trauma, increased ICP, VPS malfunction, brain tumor, intracranial hemorrhage
- **Poison control:** Ingestion or overdose
- **Surgery:** Intussusception

Disposition

- **Intensive care unit transfer:** AMS, unstable airway, GCS of 8 or less, intracranial bleed
- **Discharge criteria:** The patient's mental status is at or near baseline and the underlying cause has been addressed.

Follow-up

- **Primary care:** 1 to 2 weeks
- **Neurology:** 1 week

Pearls and Pitfalls

- Lethargy may be the only presenting symptom in a child with intussusception.
- Consider child abuse in an infant with AMS, regardless of the presence of bruising.
- Kernig and Brudzinski signs may be absent in a comatose patient with meningitis.
- Structural lesions such as hydrocephalus or bilateral subdural hematomas may cause a non-focal examination.

Coding

ICD-9

- Altered mental status **780.97**
- Coma **780.01**
- Persistent vegetative state **780.03**
- Semicoma, stupor **780.09**
- Transient alteration of awareness **780.02**

Bibliography

Avner JR. Altered states of consciousness. *Pediatr Rev.* 2006;27:331–338

Conway EE. Altered states of consciousness. In: Fisher MM, Alderman EA, Kreipe RE, Rosenfeld WD, eds. *Textbook of Adolescent Health Care.* Elk Grove Village, IL: American Academy of Pediatrics; 2011:1321–1332

Kochanek PM, Carney N, Adelson PD, et al. Guidelines for the acute medical management of severe traumatic brain injury in infants, children, and adolescents—second edition. *Pediatr Crit Care Med.* 2012;13(suppl 1)1:S1–S82

Lehman RK, Mink J. Altered mental status. *Clin Pediatr Emerg Med.* 2008;9:68–75

Sharma S, Kochar GS, Sankhyan N, Gulati S. Approach to the child with coma. *Indian J Pediatr.* 2010;77:1279–1287

Cerebrospinal Fluid Shunt Complications

Introduction

Cerebrospinal fluid (CSF) shunts are named for the positions of the proximal and distal catheters. Proximal catheters are in the lateral, third, or fourth ventricles or in an intracranial cyst, and exit the skull via a burr hole. Distal catheters are tunneled under the skin to their final location, which can be in the peritoneal space, right atrium, and pleural space, among others. Most commonly, ventriculoperitoneal shunts are placed.

Between the proximal and distal catheters is a one-way valve system that allows drainage of CSF at a predetermined pressure differential. This valve system may be separate or integrated into distal catheter and is located exterior to the skull. It may be programmable and therefore must be reset following any magnetic resonance imaging. Other components may include on-off valves, which permit intermittent shunting and assessment of shunt function; anti-siphon devices, which prevent overdrainage of CSF; and reservoirs (single or double chamber), which allow withdrawal of CSF or infusion of medications. The latter are located on the exterior of the skull, proximal to the one-way valve.

The most common acute complications of CSF shunts are shunt malfunctions and shunt infections. CSF shunt malfunction is most frequent, occurring in two-thirds of patients within 2 years of placement, secondary to debris, fibrosis, choroid plexus, or parenchymal occlusion of the proximal catheter. Delayed malfunctions (>2 years after insertion) are frequently caused by obstruction, breaking of the catheter, migration of the distal catheter and, rarely, kinking or knotting. A CSF shunt infection is the second most common complication, most of which occur within 6 months of shunt surgery. The most common pathogens include *Staphylococcus epidermidis*, *Staphylococcus aureus*, and gram-negative bacilli.

A rare complication is slit-ventricle syndrome (slit-like ventricles on brain imaging with poor ventricular compliance). If CSF shunt malfunction then develops, the patient's intracranial pressure (ICP) can rise quickly and without radiologic evidence of ventricular expansion, making the diagnosis difficult. Other complications include perforation of a hollow viscus (signs of shunt infection with peritonitis, meningitis, ventriculitis), migration of the distal catheter tip, intussusception, volvulus around the catheter, and omental cyst torsion.

Less acute complications of CSF shunts include an abdominal pseudocyst, which is a loculated fluid mass within the peritoneum around the catheter tip. It can present with signs of shunt malfunction along with decreased appetite, abdominal pain, tenderness, distention, mass, guarding, an inguinal hernia, and intractable hiccups.

CSF overdrainage can also occur, generally within 1 month after either shunt insertion or revision. Symptoms include positional headaches and vomiting, which is worse when upright and improved when recumbent.

Clinical Presentation

History

With a CSF shunt malfunction the symptoms are highly variable and nonspecific, including, but not limited to, lethargy, irritability, headache, increased seizures, nausea, vomiting, feeding problems, neck pain, back pain, blurred vision, "not acting right," and parental suspicion. The nonspecific presentation of a CSF shunt infection is similar to a shunt malfunction, with or without infectious symptoms such as fever, wound erythema or exudate, abdominal pain, and peritonitis.

Physical Examination

A patient with a CSF shunt malfunction may have altered mental status, irritability, non-erythematous swelling around the shunt tract, a bulging or full fontanel, increased head circumference, VIth nerve palsy, papilledema, and ataxia. Reservoirs (which abut the valves) that remain depressed or fail to depress are suspicious but nonspecific findings. Rarely, a patient will present with signs of severe increased ICP, including sun-setting eyes, hypertension, bradycardia, and irregular respirations. If the shunt is infected, there may be the nonspecific signs of a shunt malfunction (see above), fever, a cellulitis or signs of a wound infection around the shunt tract, and signs of peritonitis.

Laboratory and Radiology

Shunt Malfunction

If a patient presents with signs and symptoms consistent with shunt malfunction, immediately obtain a shunt series and either a flash/fast magnetic resonance imaging (MRI) or computed tomography (CT) of the brain. A shunt series includes plain radiographs of skull, neck, chest, and abdomen, and will detect disconnections, kinks, and migration of catheters. While proximal and distal catheters are radio-opaque, reservoirs and connectors can be radiolucent, therefore the films must be reviewed very carefully. A CT or MRI of the brain will determine the location of the proximal catheter tip and size of the ventricles. Comparison to a prior study is critical, but if these are unavailable, evidence of transependymal flow and sulcal effacement are suggestive of malfunction. Order an abdominal ultrasound if an abdominal pseudocyst is suspected.

Less commonly, immediate cranial ultrasound can be used, but only for a patient with an open anterior fontanelle. If the presentation is subacute, the diagnosis may be confirmed with a radionucleotide scan, in which the isotope is injected into the shunt reservoir and observed as it flows proximally and distally.

Shunt Infection

If a patient presents with signs or symptoms of a shunt infection, immediately arrange a shunt series, CT/fast MRI of the brain, or cranial ultrasound to rule out coincident malfunction. Also obtain a complete blood cell count, C-reactive protein and/or erythrocyte sedimentation rate, and blood and urine cultures to rule out other infectious etiologies. If this workup is negative and the patient is within 6 months of a previous shunt operation, or a shunt infection is highly suspected, consult with a neurosurgeon to arrange a shunt tap. Send the CSF for Gram stain, culture, cell count, glucose, and protein, and measure the opening pressure, if possible.

Differential Diagnosis

The differential diagnosis of shunt complications is summarized in Table 69-1.

Treatment

Shunt Malfunction

For the rare patient presenting with signs of severe increased ICP, start emergent treatment, including elevating the bed to 30 degrees, intubating and hyperventilating to a pCO_2 of 28 to 33 mm Hg, and giving a bolus of either intravenous (IV) mannitol (0.5–1.0 g/kg) or 3% saline (5 mg/kg). If the patient is moribund, consult with neurosurgery to arrange an emergency shunt tap or ventricular tap through the burr hole or open fontanelle, prior to urgent definitive shunt revision. For most other patients, who are ambulatory with headaches and vomiting over several days, urgent neurosurgery consultation is indicated to plan a shunt revision within 24 hours.

Table 69-1. Differential Diagnosis of CSF Shunt Complications	
Diagnosis	**Clinical Features**
CSF shunt infection	Shunt operation within the last 6 months Purulent wound Erythema along shunt tract
CSF shunt malfunction	Non-erythematous swelling around shunt tract Disconnection on shunt series Increase in ventricle size on CT/MRI
Gastroenteritis	Sick contacts May have diarrhea
Meningitis	Meningismus, fever, decreased level of consciousness No change in ventricle size on CT/MRI
Urinary tract infection	No shunt operation within the last 6 months Dysuria Positive urinalysis
Viral syndrome	Sick contacts May have rhinorrhea, cough, conjunctivitis, pharyngitis

Abbreviations: CSF, cerebrospinal fluid; CT, computed tomography; MRI, magnetic resonance imaging.

Shunt Infection

Urgent neurosurgery consultation is necessary. Surgical approaches to hardware removal vary among neurosurgeons, but most will completely remove the shunt and place an external ventricular drain (EVD). However, with small ventricles or medically complex patients, the distal end of the existing shunt may instead be externalized at the level of the clavicle or abdomen. Treat with IV vancomycin (20 mg/kg every 8 hour, 1 g maximum) and IV ceftriaxone (50 mg/kg every 12 hours, 2 g maximum). Tailor the antibiotic coverage once the culture and sensitivity results are available. Generally, the course of antibiotics is 7 to 21 days, with 14 days being typical. Alternatively, discontinue antibiotics once there have been 3 consecutive negative CSF cultures, each separated by 2 days. At that point, arrange for the shunt to be replaced.

Indications for Consultation

- **Infectious disease:** CSF shunt infection
- **Neurosurgery:** Any suspicion for a CSF shunt malfunction or infection

Disposition

- **Intensive care unit transfer:** Severely increased ICP, meningitis, and/or sepsis; depending on the institution, externalized shunts and EVDs
- **Discharge criteria:** No further symptoms/signs of the acute complication and recovery from surgical treatment of the hydrocephalus (eg, repaired CSF shunt after malfunction, re-internalized CSF shunt after infection)

Follow-up

- **Primary care:** 1 to 2 weeks
- **Neurosurgery:** 2 to 4 weeks

Pearls and Pitfalls

- In general, CSF shunt malfunctions present in a consistent fashion for a given patient. Ask the family how the child's shunt failure usually presents.
- The most predictive symptoms of CSF shunt malfunction are vomiting, lack of fever, parental suspicion, and headache in a verbal child.
- Shunt infection is very unlikely if the patient has not had a shunt operation within the last 6 months and/or is presenting with diarrhea. Neurosurgery services are therefore quite reluctant to tap the shunt in these circumstances for fear of introducing infection during the procedure.
- If a shunt complication is highly suspected, arrange for rapid transfer to a pediatric neurosurgical center, if services are not available locally.

Coding

ICD-9

• CSF shunt infection	**996.63**
• CSF shunt malfunction	**996.2**

Bibliography

Browd SR, Gottfried ON, Ragel BT, Kestle JR. Failure of cerebrospinal fluid shunts: part II: overdrainage, loculation, and abdominal complications. *Pediatr Neurol.* 2006; 34:171–176

Browd SR, Ragel BT, Gottfried ON, Kestle JR. Failure of cerebrospinal fluid shunts: part I: obstruction and mechanical failure. *Pediatr Neurol.* 2006;34:83–92

Duhaime AC. Evaluation and management of shunt infections in children with hydrocephalus. *Clin Pediatr (Phila).* 2006t45:705–713

Khan AA, Jabbar A, Banerjee A, Hinchley G. Cerebrospinal shunt malfunction: recognition and emergency management. *Br J Hosp Med (Lond).* 2007;68:651–655

Prusseit J, Simon M, von der Brelie C, et al. Epidemiology, prevention and management of ventriculoperitoneal shunt infections in children. *Pediatr Neurosurg.* 2009;45:325–336

Rekate HL. The slit ventricle syndrome: advances based on technology and understanding. *Pediatr Neurosurg.* 2004;40:259–263

Headache

Introduction

Although headache is a common presenting complaint in pediatrics, it rarely requires admission for workup and management. However, a patient may be admitted when a headache is associated with altered mental status, seizures, or an abnormal neurologic examination. Examples include primary headaches, such as severe migraine or migraine variants, and secondary conditions, such as intracranial infection (encephalitis, meningitis), and increased intracranial pressure (ICP) secondary to mass effect, trauma, or thrombosis.

Clinical Presentation

History

Ask about the onset of the headache (including any aura) and its intensity; frequency; and associated symptoms, such as fever, vomiting, visual changes, photophobia, seizures, and neck stiffness. Inquire about medication use, possible toxin exposure, and significant medical problems (ventriculoperitoneal shunt, immunodeficiency or suppression, coagulopathy). Finally, perform a thorough psychosocial assessment, including substance abuse history.

Physical Examination

Priorities on the physical examination include vital signs (looking for hypertension alone or as part of Cushing triad), growth parameters, and neurocutaneous findings such as hamartomas, neurofibromas, café au lait macules, or hemangiomas. Perform a comprehensive neurologic examination to investigate for signs of increased ICP, focal neurologic findings, and meningismus. If none of these signs are present, the likelihood of a secondary headache related to significant central nervous system (CNS) pathology is quite low.

Laboratory

If the clinical presentation is suspicious for a primary CNS condition, obtain a complete blood cell count, erythrocyte sedimentation rate, and/or C-reactive protein to screen for an infection and/or inflammatory process. If meningitis is a concern, also obtain electrolytes, a blood culture, and cerebrospinal fluid for Gram stain and culture, cell count, and protein and glucose. Always measure the opening pressure when lumbar puncture is performed. In general, if signs of increased ICP are absent, a head computed tomography (CT) is not necessary prior to lumbar puncture. If increased ICP is suspected, delay the lumbar puncture, regardless of the CT results.

If the history and physical examination are consistent with a toxidrome (page 321), perform toxicology screening and contact local poison control.

If a focal neurologic deficit exists, neuroimaging is usually indicated to rule out secondary intracranial causes of headache. Since there is no consensus of opinion over the routine use of CT and/or magnetic resonance imaging (MRI) for headache, undertake a careful analysis of the benefits and probable yield prior to exposing patients to the risks associated with each (radiation, contrast, sedation, anesthesia). A CT is indicated if acute bleeding or thrombosis is suspected, but obtain an MRI if there is concern about an intracranial mass or inflammatory condition.

Differential Diagnosis

The priority is to rule out an intracranial mass lesion, hemorrhage, thrombosis, and meningitis/encephalitis (Table 70-1).

A positive family history in a first- or second-degree relative is suggestive of a primary headache, while recurrent, chronic, severe, progressive, or unconventional headaches are more likely with a secondary headache. Headaches that raise a concern for primary CNS pathology include those that waken a child from sleep, are worse in the morning or improve over the course of the day, or are worse when recumbent or with a Valsalva maneuver. Sudden onset of severe headache, the so-called thunder clap headache, demands urgent evaluation to rule out subarachnoid hemorrhage or venous sinus thrombosis.

Treatment

Treat a migraine with a full dose of ibuprofen (10 mg/kg) at the first symptom of onset. Have the patient rest in a quiet, dark room when possible. Give sumatriptan (5 mg intranasally, 25 mg orally, or 0.1 mg/kg/dose intradermally) and repeat in 2 hours, if necessary. Consult a pediatric neurologist for status migrainosus or migraine variants.

Treat the underlying cause of a secondary headache. For a headache associated with a systemic infection or inflammatory condition, give acetaminophen (10–15 mg/kg/dose every 4–6 hour) or ibuprofen (5–10 mg/kg every 6 hour). See page 466 for the treatment of suspected meningitis.

Venous sinus thrombosis often requires anticoagulation (pages 28–30) with low molecular weight heparin, such as enoxaparin (1 mg/kg every 12 hours) unless significant bleeding has occurred, as well as treatment of the cause of the thrombosis. Obtain emergent consultation with a pediatric

Table 70-1. Differential Diagnosis of Headaches

Diagnosis	Clinical Features
Central nervous system infection (bacterial meningitis)	Fever, altered mental status Nuchal rigidity, photophobia Positive Kernig and/or Brudzinski signs
Idiopathic intracranial hypertension	Overweight/obese Visual disturbances Papilledema
Inflammatory conditions	Fever, malaise, myalgias, fatigue, weight loss Rash/skin changes Arthralgias/arthritis
Intracranial mass	Headache awakens patient at night, also worse in the morning Abnormal neurologic examination Signs of increased intracranial pressure
Migraine	Positive family history Multiple previous episodes Nausea and/or vomiting Phono-, photophobia
Non–central nervous system infection	May have a upper respiratory infection, pharyngitis, or facial pain Fatigue, myalgias, abdominal pain
Posttraumatic	Antecedent history of trauma (acute or chronic)
Vascular	Abnormal headache character Focal neurologic findings, especially cranial nerve deficits
Viral meningitis	Fever Headache +/- photophobia May not have meningeal signs

neurosurgeon for intracranial bleeding and treat with platelets, fresh frozen plasma, cryoprecipitate, and/or other clotting factors as indicated for any underlying coagulopathy.

Diagnostic and therapeutic lumbar puncture is often adequate in the acute setting of idiopathic intracranial hypertension, but long-term treatment requires identification of the underlying cause. In addition, a headache secondary to summertime enteroviral meningitis is also often relieved by the lumbar puncture.

Indications for Consultation

- **Infectious diseases:** Unusual organism causing a systemic or CNS infection
- **Neurology:** Status migrainosus, migraine variants, seizure

- **Neurosurgery:** Intracranial hemorrhage, intracranial mass, increased ICP
- **Ophthalmology:** Possible papilledema or to assess for eye involvement in systemic illness, especially inflammatory conditions
- **Rheumatology:** Systemic inflammatory conditions affecting the CNS

Disposition

- **Intensive care unit transfer:** Signs of impending herniation/increased ICP, hemodynamic instability associated with systemic illness/infection
- **Discharge criteria:** Baseline mental status and neurologic examination

Follow-up

- **Primary care:** 4 to 7 days
- **Subspecialists involved in care during the hospitalization:** 1 week

Pearls and Pitfalls

- Risk factors for a serious cause of a headache include a new headache in a preschool-aged patient, occipital headache, inability to characterize the quality of headache, atypical headache pattern, and abnormal neurologic findings.

Coding

ICD-9

• Headache	**784.0**
• Benign (idiopathic) intracranial hypertension	**348.2**
• Migraine, unspecified, without mention of intractable migraine without mention of status migrainosus	**346.90**
• Shunt malfunction	**996.2**
• Venous sinus thrombosis	**325**

Bibliography

Abend NS, Younkin D, Lewis DW. Secondary headaches in children and adolescents. *Semin Pediatr Neurol.* 2010;17:123–133

Alehan FK. Value of neuroimaging in the evaluation of neurologically normal children with recurrent headache. *J Child Neurol.* 2002;17:807–809

Conicella E, Raucci U, Vanacore N, et al. The child with headache in a pediatric emergency department. *Headache.* 2008;48:1005–1011

Detsky ME, McDonald DR, Baerlocher MO, et al. Does this patient with headache have a migraine or need neuroimaging? *JAMA.* 2006;296:1274–1283

Lateef TM, Grewal M, McClintock W, et al. Headache in young children in the emergency department: use of computed tomography. *Pediatrics.* 2009;124:e12–e17

Lewis DW. New practice parameters: what does the evidence say? *Curr Pain Headache Rep.* 2005;9:351–357

CHAPTER 71

Seizures

Introduction

About 5% of children will have a seizure and 1% will have recurrent seizures. Provoked seizures occur in the context of fever, infection, trauma, or metabolic abnormality, while those without an identifiable cause are defined as idiopathic. Status epilepticus is a seizure lasting more than 30 minutes or recurring seizure events without a return to a normal level of consciousness between episodes. Brief idiopathic seizures are typically not associated with significant morbidity, while status epilepticus may result in long-term neurologic sequelae.

Seizures are further classified by the patient's level of consciousness. Generalized seizures imply impaired consciousness, while a patient with partial seizures has a normal level of consciousness. Partial seizures often involve abnormal motor activity and can progress to be generalized.

Febrile seizures occur in children 6 months to 6 years of age, who have a temperature higher than 38°C (100.4°F) within 24 hours of the seizure. A simple febrile seizure is a generalized tonic-clonic episode, with no focality, lasting less than 15 minutes, and occurring only once in 24 hours. A febrile seizure is classified as complex if it has one of the following features: it is partial, has focality, persists more than 15 minutes, or more than one seizure occurs within a 24-hour period. In the absence of prior neurologic abnormality, febrile seizures carry a favorable prognosis but can recur in up to 30% of children.

Infantile spasms are a subset of epilepsy that occur in children younger than 24 months. The seizures are repetitive jerking motions, often with flexion of the neck and adduction of the extremities. The electroencephalogram (EEG) shows a characteristic hypsarrhythmia pattern, and the patient often has cognitive and functional deterioration associated with the seizures.

A patient with a known seizure disorder may have breakthrough seizures, which occur while on a medication regimen for seizure control. If a patient has been stabilized and seizure-free while on antiepileptogenic medication, any subsequent seizure is a potential treatment failure, or breakthrough. However, breakthrough seizures most often occur in the context of illness, change in sleep/eating patterns, or subtherapeutic medication levels secondary to missed doses or outgrowing previous dosing.

Clinical Presentation

History

Determine the details of the seizure activity, including behavior prior to onset, how the episode started (body site first noted to have seizure-like activity), length of episode, movement of extremities, presence of/and direction of eye deviation, cyanosis, incontinence, and interventions performed to halt the seizure. Ask about a history of prior seizures, as well as recent head trauma, illnesses, current home medications, or possible toxic ingestion. A history of premature birth, known intracranial anomaly, developmental delay, or other neurologic abnormalities may suggest a possible cause of the seizure. Since many seizure disorders are genetic, inquire about a family history of seizures or neurologic diseases.

Physical Examination

As with all initial assessments, focus on airway, breathing, and circulation when stabilizing a patient with a seizure. During seizure activity or in the postictal period, a patient may have hypoxia, respiratory distress, hypoventilation, and difficulty tolerating secretions.

After the brief initial assessment, perform an evaluation for seizure activity. Frequently, seizure activity involves both a tonic phase and clonic movements. However, seizure activity can be less obvious, without extremity involvement, especially in an infant. Eye deviation, repetitive eye movements, increased jaw tone, tachycardia, and lack of response to external stimuli can be subtle signs of seizure activity. After resolution of the seizure activity, perform a thorough neurologic examination looking for localizing abnormalities that may suggest a mass effect, such as limited extraocular movements, asymmetrical pupillary response, facial droop, altered speech, or asymmetrical movement and tone in the extremities. Also include an assessment for signs of increased intracranial pressure, such as Cushing triad (bradycardia, hypertension, irregular respirations-Cheyne-stokes breathing), asymmetrical pupillary response, papilledema, or obtundation. Always check for the presence of meningeal signs, such as meningismus and Brudzinski and Kernig signs.

A patient with partial seizures can develop a Todd paralysis, which is a transient postictal paralysis of muscles, most often of the extremities. It generally lasts a few hours. However, persistence more than 24 hours raises the concern of a stroke.

Signs of non-accidental trauma, such as bruising and extremity swelling, raise the concern for intracranial injury as a cause of the seizure. Dermatologic abnormalities may be suggestive of a neurocutaneous disorder predisposing the patient to seizure. These include a port-wine stain indicative of Sturge-Weber, café au lait spots seen in neurofibromatosis, and ash leaf spots or shagreen patches associated with tuberous sclerosis.

Laboratory

Febrile Seizures

A patient with a simple febrile seizure and a normal non-focal neurologic examination requires only an age-appropriate fever evaluation, without a routine lumbar puncture. The same is true for a child with a complex febrile seizure, but maintain a low threshold to pursue an infectious etiology if there is a concerning history or abnormal neurologic examination. A complete evaluation for bacterial infection, including lumbar puncture, is indicated for a patient with febrile status epilepticus.

Afebrile Seizures

Direct the initial evaluation at identifying a potential correctable cause of the seizure, such as hypoglycemia or other electrolyte abnormalities. Hyponatremia can occur with syndrome of inappropriate antidiuretic hormone, inappropriate water intake, or iatrogenic administration of hypotonic fluids. Hypocalcemia can be seen in a premature neonate, an infant of a diabetic mother, and in DiGeorge syndrome, in which seizures can be the primary presentation. In an infant younger than 3 months, the absence of fever does not necessarily preclude the need for a lumbar puncture, and one is indicated if the patient has abnormal laboratory results or an abnormal neurologic examination. Also consider an inborn error of metabolism in a young infant with altered mental status or acidosis.

In an older infant and child, the history and physical examination guide the choices for laboratory testing, especially if there is a prior illness, concern about an ingestion, or dehydration.

For a patient with a known seizure disorder, check the serum level(s) of antiepileptic medications, as subtherapeutic regimens frequently lead to breakthrough seizures. Although levels may not be available acutely, they can guide subsequent outpatient management.

An EEG is indicated to rule out subclinical status epilepticus if the patient has persistent alteration in mental status after the seizure activity has ceased. Obtain an urgent EEG if infantile spasms are a concern. While brief afebrile seizures are an indication for a follow-up outpatient EEG, do not order one for a patient with a simple febrile seizure.

Radiology

Afebrile seizure

Emergent head imaging is necessary for an afebrile infant younger than 6 months with definitive seizure activity and an abnormal neurologic examination, such as altered mental status, abnormal tone, focal weakness, or abnormal pupillary response or reflexes. Up to 10% of such patients will have a finding that will alter the acute medical management. While magnetic resonance imaging (MRI) is the preferred modality, obtain a non-contrast computed tomography if the MRI is not available emergently or the patient is not clinically stable to allow for sedation for the study. The indications for neuroimaging of a patient with afebrile seizures are summarized in Table 71-1.

Febrile Seizure

- Any age, abnormal neurologic examination: Emergent imaging
- Younger than 6 months, normal neurologic examination: Urgent or delayed imaging

A patient older than 6 months with a simple febrile seizure does not require imaging or follow-up with a neurologist. However, imaging is indicated if the patient has a developmental delay or focal seizures. For a patient with complex febrile seizures, EEG and neuroimaging are recommended, although the timing can be based on the child's clinical status.

Differential Diagnosis

Differentiation of a seizure from non-epileptiform events can be very difficult in a young child. The history often provides adequate details to detect characteristics of the non-epileptiform events described in Table 71-2. Otherwise, direct observation of the events or video recording allows the most accurate assessment. Episodes that can be extinguished with a change in position or immobilization of extremities are unlikely to be epileptiform. Atypical movements during sleep in infants are most often benign myoclonus.

Table 71-1. Indications for Neuroimaging After an Afebrile Seizure

	Normal Neurologic Exam		Abnormal Neurologic Exam
Age	**Generalized**	**Focal**	**Generalized or Focal**
<6 months	Emergent imaging for inflicted trauma	Emergent imaging	Emergent imaging
>6 months	None	Consider delayed imaging	Emergent imaging

Table 71-2. Differential Diagnosis of Seizures	
Diagnosis	**Clinical Features**
Benign myoclonus	Symmetrical repetitive jerks during sleep Extinguished when aroused
Breath-holding spell	Occurs when child is upset or after occipital head trauma 2 types: pallid or cyanotic
Migraine	May have an aura Associated with headache, nausea, photophobia
Reflux (Sandifer syndrome)	History of spitting up Generalized stiffening and opisthotonic posturing Occurs within 30 minutes of a feed
Syncope	Episodes occur when standing or overheated Preceded by nausea and/or dizziness Patient remembers "fainting"

Treatment

First Time Seizure

The goal is the emergent cessation of all seizure activity. Since all of these drugs can cause respiratory depression, always be prepared to secure the airway and ventilate the patient. Give the medications in rapid succession, as cessation of seizure is essential for neuroprotection. Fosphenytoin can cause hypotension, vasodilatation, tachycardia, and bradycardia.

If the seizure activity lasts more than 5 minutes or the patient has respiratory depression, give lorazepam (0.01 mg/kg/dose intravenous [IV] once over 2–4 minutes, 2 mg maximum). Use diazepam (0.5 mg/kg/dose rectal once, 10 mg maximum) if the patient does not have IV access. If the seizure activity persists for another 5 minutes, repeat the lorazepam and give a loading dose of fosphenytoin (20 mg/kg of phenytoin equivalents IV, 1,000 mg phenytoin equivalents maximum) over 7 minutes. If the seizure activity lasts more than 15 minutes and does not respond to lorazepam and fosphenytoin, add phenobarbital (20 mg/kg/dose IV over 20 minutes).

Institute treatment of metabolic derangements that may be the primary cause of seizure. For a patient at risk for hypoglycemia, give IV dextrose (0.5–1 g/kg = 1–2 mL/kg of $D5_0$). For a patient with known hyponatremia, give 3% hypertonic normal saline 2 mL/kg IV over 1 hour, but discontinue the infusion once the seizure activity ceases. Treat hypocalcemia with 10% calcium gluconate (100 mg/kg = 1 mL/kg IV over 5–10 minutes).

Defer treatment of infantile spasms to a neurologist once the diagnosis has been confirmed.

Treat seizures secondary to an intracranial infection with broad-spectrum antibiotics (see meningitis, page 466). Do not delay treatment if a lumbar puncture cannot be performed in a timely manner. See page 443 for the treatment of possible herpes encephalitis.

Recurrent Seizures

Treat breakthrough seizures in a patient who has a seizure disorder and is receiving maintenance medication(s) with a bolus of the maintenance medication(s), after consultation with the primary neurologist. However, lorazepam (as above) remains the first-line agent for seizure treatment.

Indications for Consultation

- **Neurology:** Focal neurologic findings, persistent altered mental status, continued seizure activity despite treatment, new seizure in an infant younger than 6 months, afebrile seizure in a patient younger than 24 months, concern for infantile spasms
- **Neurosurgery:** Signs of increased intracranial pressure or abnormal head imaging

Disposition

- **Intensive care unit transfer:** Status epilepticus, respiratory depression second to antiepileptics, persistent altered mental status
- **Discharge criteria:** Baseline neurologic examination

Follow-up

- **Neurology:** 1 to 2 weeks

Pearls and Pitfalls

- Rapidly consider all of the possible treatable causes of seizure.
- Perform a very limited workup of a child with simple febrile seizure.

Coding

ICD-9

• Grand mal status	**345.3**
• Petit mal status	**345.2**
• Generalized non-convulsive epilepsy	**345.0x**
• Generalized convulsive epilepsy	**345.1x**

- Partial (focal) epilepsy with complex partial seizures **345.4x**
- Partial (focal) epilepsy with simple partial seizures **345.5x**
- Infantile spasms **345.6x**
- Other forms of epilepsy and recurrent seizures **345.8x**
- Epilepsy, unspecified **345.9x**
  - Use one of these digits for the fifth digit (x) to identify
    0 without mention of intractable epilepsy
    1 with intractable epilepsy
    - pharmacologically resistant
    - poorly controlled
    - treatment resistant
    - refractory (medically)
- Convulsions in newborn **779.0**
- Febrile convulsions, simple or unspecified **780.31**
- Complex febrile convulsions **780.32**
- Posttraumatic seizures **780.33**
- Seizure not otherwise specified **780.39**

Bibliography

Abend NS, Gutierrez-Colina AM, Dlugos DJ. Medical treatment of pediatric status epilepticus. *Semin Pediatr Neurol.* 2010;17:169–175

American Academy of Pediatrics Subcommittee on Febrile Seizures. Neurodiagnostic evaluation of the child with a simple febrile seizure. *Pediatrics.* 2011;127:389–394

Gaillard WD, Chiron C, Cross JH, et al. Guidelines for imaging infants and children with recent-onset epilepsy. *Epilepsia.* 2009;50:2147–2153

Harden CL, Huff JS, Schwartz TH, et al. Reassessment: neuroimaging in the emergency patient presenting with seizure (an evidence-based review): report of the Therapeutics and Technology Assessment Subcommittee of the American Academy of Neurology. *Neurology.* 2007;69:1772–1780

Hsieh DT, Chang T, Tsuchida TN, et al. New-onset afebrile seizures in infants: role of neuroimaging. *Neurology.* 2010;74:150–156

Kimia AA, Capraro AJ, Hummel D, Johnston P, Harper MB. Utility of lumbar puncture for first simple febrile seizure among children 6 to 18 months of age. *Pediatrics.* 2009;123:6–12

Nutrition

CHAPTER 72

Failure to Thrive

Introduction

Failure to thrive (FTT) is generally defined as a weight lower than the third or fifth percentile on a growth chart or a change in weight that has crossed down 2 major percentile lines over 3 to 6 months.

FTT is due to inadequate calorie intake, excessive calorie losses, or increased calorie requirements. The most common cause, found in 85% of cases in the United States, is inadequate calorie intake, which may be associated with significant psychosocial issues. However, this approach is too rigid, as often inadequate nutrition reflects a complex interaction among a child's medical, nutritional, and social issues. Therefore, a thorough psychosocial evaluation is an important part of patient assessment.

Indications for hospitalization include failure of outpatient therapies, severe FTT or malnutrition, serious infections, neglect or a concern for the patient's safety, or the need for a multidisciplinary team approach and/or services for parental education and coordination of care that are best performed in the inpatient setting.

Clinical Presentation

History

A detailed history is critical to making the diagnosis. Take a thorough dietary history, including foods and formula (preparation, frequency), feeding/breastfeeding patterns, juice/water intake, and behaviors at mealtime. Quantify the daily caloric intake. It is best to do a 24-hour diet recall or to have the family keep a 3-day diet log. Inquire about gastrointestinal (GI) symptoms (vomiting or spitting up, difficulty swallowing or eating), stooling (pattern, frequency, consistency, diarrhea, bloody, mucoid), respiratory issues (difficulty breathing, chronic cough, snoring), and recurrent infections. Pregnancy and birth history, including birth weight, as well as a complete medical history and review of symptoms are essential. Document the developmental milestones in infants, and confirm the newborn screen results.

As noted above, there is often a psychosocial component to FTT. A complete assessment of the family and social situation is important, including who is caring for the child during the day. Ask about the parents' income and other economic issues; mental health and intellectual capacity; family dysfunction; parent-child interaction; child maltreatment, including Munchausen by proxy;

and other stressors in the home. Obtain a complete family history, focusing on systemic disease (inflammatory bowel disease, asthma, cystic fibrosis, renal tubular acidosis), FTT, and short stature (note the height and weight of both parents).

Review the growth chart trends. Inadequate nutrition leads to poor weight gain, which will be followed, over time, by decreased height velocity. Head circumference is typically spared unless the problem is severe.

Physical Examination

The vital signs and general appearance (dysmorphic features, cachexia, general activity) are priorities. Examine the oropharynx for a cleft palate, poor suck or swallow, dental caries, and enlarged tonsils. Assess the work of breathing, auscultate for a murmur, and palpate the abdomen for hepatomegaly. Note any loose skin, edema, poor hygiene, rash, or bruises or evidence of trauma. Perform a neurologic examination for tone, reflexes, social interaction, and developmental milestones. One final, important part of the physical examination is an observation of the parent/child interaction and feeding routine.

Laboratory

Limit the use of laboratory tests and evaluations to those suggested by the history and physical examination, as without specific evidence for organic disease, laboratory testing is rarely helpful in determining the etiology of FTT. When indicated, screening tests may include a complete blood cell count; comprehensive chemistry (including electrolytes, blood urea nitrogen/creatinine, calcium, phosphorus, magnesium, and albumin); liver function tests; erythrocyte sedimentation rate; urinalysis; and stool samples for occult blood, pH, and reducing substances (Table 72-1). Other tests to consider, if indicated by the findings on history and physical examination, are thyroid function tests, ammonia, lactate, HIV, purified protein derivative, and bone age, only if indicated by the findings.

Differential Diagnosis

The diagnosis of FTT is primarily a clinical endeavor. Perform a comprehensive review of the growth chart trends and identify chronic illnesses and syndromes that alter growth. In comparison to a patient with an endocrinologic disorder, a child with FTT will "fall off" the weight curve before "falling off" the height/length curve, with the weight being lower down on the curve than the height/length.

Base the differential diagnosis on caloric intake (Table 72-1). The etiology may be secondary to inadequate caloric intake, inadequate caloric absorption/

Table 72-1. Differential Diagnosis of Failure to Thrive

Diagnosis	Clinical Features	Initial Laboratory Tests and Evaluations
Inadequate Caloric Intake		
Cleft palate	Milk regurgitated through nose HEENT examination	Speech/swallow consult
Excess juice consumption	Dietary history	None
Incorrect formula preparation	Dietary history History of economic pressures	CBC, electrolytes
Oromotor dysfunction	Observation of feeding	Speech/swallow consult
Poor feeding technique	Observation of feeding	Observe patient feeding
Psychosocial—insufficient food	Stressors in the home	CBC, electrolytes Social work consult
Inadequate Caloric Absorption/Utilization		
Celiac disease	Family history Diarrhea	CBC, albumin Anti-tissue transglutaminase (anti-tTG) Stool pH, reducing substances, fecal fats
Cystic fibrosis	Family history Abnormal newborn screen Respiratory symptoms Diarrhea	Review newborn screen Sweat test Stool pH, reducing substances, and fecal fats
Gastroesophageal reflux	Vomiting history	Response to treatment +/- swallowing study or pH probe
Increased intracranial pressure	Vomiting history Cushing triad Abnormal neurologic exam	Head CT Neurology consult
Inflammatory bowel disease	Family history Diarrhea, bloody stools	CBC, ESR/CRP, albumin Stool occult blood
Liver disease	Jaundice Diarrhea	Liver function tests Hepatitis serologies
Milk protein allergy	Family history Vomiting history Diarrhea, bloody stools Eczema	Stool occult blood GI consult Possible endoscopy
Increased Caloric Requirements		
Adrenal diseases	Vomiting, diarrhea Hyperpigmentation Hypotension	Chemistry Glucose
Blood disorders	Fatigue Pallor	CBC
Cardiopulmonary diseases	Fatigue, especially with feeds Respiratory illnesses	Chest x-ray EKG and echocardiogram
Diabetes mellitus	Polydipsia, polyuria, polyphagia	Chemistry, fasting glucose Urinalysis

Table 72-1. Differential Diagnosis of Failure to Thrive, continued		
Diagnosis	**Clinical Features**	**Initial Laboratory Tests and Evaluations**
Genetic diseases	Family history Dysmorphic features	Specific for suspected diseases
Hyperthyroidism	Fatigue, increased sweating, polyphagia Nervousness, sleep disturbance Diarrhea Tachycardia, exophthalmos	Thyroid studies
Renal tubular acidosis	Normal anion gap metabolic acidosis	Venous blood gas and urinalysis (compare serum and urine pH)

Abbreviations: CBC, complete blood cell count; CRP, C-reactive protein; CT, computed tomography; EKG, electrocardiogram; ESR, erythrocyte sedimentation rate; GI, gastrointestinal; HEENT, head, eyes, ears, nose, and throat; tTG, tissue transglutaminase.

utilization, or increased caloric requirements (excess metabolic demand as occurs in chronic diseases). Inadequate caloric intake is by far the most common cause of FTT. However, some diseases, such as congenital heart disease or bronchopulmonary dysplasia, present with a mixed picture of inadequate intake and a hypermetabolic condition.

Physiological causes of decreased growth that are not considered to be FTT include a history of prematurity or small for gestational age, familial short stature, and constitutional growth delay.

Treatment

The treatment is to provide adequate nutrition for catch-up growth (Box 72-1). Therefore, the patient will require 150% or more of the usual maintenance calories to transition from negative to positive nitrogen balance.

Once adequate nutrition is delivered, typical rates of weight gain are 0 to 4 months: 23 to 34 g/day, 4 to 8 months: 10 to 16 g/day, 8 to 12 months: 6 to 11 g/day, and 12 to 24 months: 4 to 9 g/day. However, there may be a lag of several days before weight gain finally begins. Close, continued outpatient follow-up is essential.

When a patient does not gain weight on a regular formula (20 cal/oz), first change to a hypercaloric one (24–30 cal/oz). For exclusively breastfed infants, use expressed breast milk with fortification. As a general estimate, adding a teaspoon of a powdered formula (Similac NeoSure Advance, Enfamil EnfaCare Lipil Powder, Nestle Good Start Gentle Plus, etc) to 100 mL of breast milk will increase the caloric density to about 23 calories/ounce. If a formula concentration greater than 24 cal/oz is needed, request a nutrition consult.

For a patient older than 1 year, consult with a nutritionist and use behavioral modification and high-calorie foods. The rule of 3s is helpful (3 meals,

Box 72-1. Nutrition for Catch-up Growth

$$\text{kcal/kg required} = \frac{[\text{IBW in kg (50th percentile wt/ht)}] \times [\text{kcal/kg/day (DRI for age)}]}{[\text{actual weight (kg)}]}$$

Abbreviations: DRI, Dietary Reference Intake (available at http://fnic.nal.usda.gov/interactiveDRI/); IBW, ideal body weight.

3 snacks, and 3 choices), as is the use of high-calorie liquids (fortified whole milk or commercial formulas containing >20 cal/oz). Hypercaloric feedings are usually, but not always, hyperosmolar, which may cause side effects such as osmotic diarrhea if the feeds are advanced too quickly.

Reintroduce nutrition slowly to avoid refeeding syndrome, which occurs when a malnourished patient begins to receive adequate nutrition too quickly. This triggers insulin release, thereby causing intracellular shifts of phosphate, potassium, and magnesium. Although refeeding syndrome is rare except in severe malnutrition, marasmus, or kwashiorkor, manifestations may include hypophosphatemia (most common), hypokalemia, and hypomagnesemia. Insulin secretion can also cause renal sodium resorption, leading to edema and volume overload. To prevent refeeding syndrome in a patient at risk, consult a nutritionist and begin feeding slowly, starting with 50% of the caloric needs, then increase the intake by 25% of the daily calories every 3 to 4 days. Closely monitor the vital signs, daily weights, and physical examination (for edema). Check the electrolytes (comprehensive chemistry with magnesium and phosphorus) daily at first, but if refeeding syndrome is suspected, obtain electrolytes 2 to 3 times a day and correct any abnormalities. If there are serious derangements, transfer the patient to an intensive care unit (ICU) for closer monitoring.

Assess growth with calorie counts and daily weights. Nasogastric or transpyloric feeds are indicated when a patient cannot manage adequate oral intake due to increased energy needs and/or physiological impairment but the GI tract is fully or partially functioning. Trans- or pyloric (nasoduodenal or nasojejunal) feeding is useful when a nasogastric feed is not indicated, such as when there are congenital upper GI anomalies, inadequate gastric motility, high aspiration risk, severe gastroesophageal reflux, or upper GI obstruction.

See Table 72-2 for the details on starting continuous tube feeding. The overall rate is determined by the kilocalories per day necessary, based on the catch-up growth formula described in Box 72-1. Transition to bolus nasogastric feeds (Table 72-3) once continuous maintenance intake is tolerated, but do not use bolus feeding with a nasoduodenal or nasojejunal tube. Make one change, either volume or concentration, at a time when adjusting enteral feeds and monitor for tolerance. If the patient does not tolerate a full-strength formula,

Table 72-2. Continuous Feeding Guidelines[a]			
Age	How to Start	How to Advance	Tolerance Volume
0–12 months	1–2 mL/kg/h	1–2 mL/kg every 2–8 h	6 mL/kg/h
1–6 years	1 mL/kg/h	1 mL/kg every 2–8 h	1–5 mL/kg/h
>7 years	25 mL/h	25 mL every 2–8 h	100–150 mL/h

[a]Adapted with permission from Courtney E, Grunko A, McCarthy T. Enteral nutrition. In Hendricks KM, Duggan C, eds. *Manual of Pediatric Nutrition*. 4th ed. Hamilton, Ontario: BC Decker; 2005.

Table 72-3: Bolus Feeding Guidelines[a]			
Age	How to Start	How to Advance	Tolerance Volume
0–2 months	10–15 mL/kg every 2–3 h	10–30 mL per feed	20–30 mL/kg every 4–5 h
1–6 years	5–10 mL/kg every 2–3 h	30–45 mL per feed	15–20 mL/kg every 4–5 h
>7 years	90–120 mL every 3–4 h	60–90 mL per feed	330–480 mL every 4–5 h

[a]Adapted with permission from Courtney E, Grunko A, McCarthy T. Enteral nutrition. In: Hendricks KM, Duggan C, eds. *Manual of Pediatric Nutrition*. 4th ed. Hamilton, Ontario: BC Decker; 2005.

decrease the volume and slowly increase as tolerated. If the patient will be on a combination bolus and continuous schedule (day/nocturnal feedings), wait 2 hours from the end of the continuous schedule to initiate the bolus schedule.

Indications for Consultation

- **Gastroenterology:** Severe gastroesophageal reflux or milk protein allergy, irritable bowel disease, cystic fibrosis, celiac disease, concern about hepatitis
- **Neurology:** Increased intracranial pressure
- **Nutritionist:** All patients admitted for FTT
- **Speech therapy:** Cleft palate, oromotor dysfunction
- **Social work:** To assess the family dynamics and ability to adhere to outpatient plan

Disposition

- **Intensive care unit transfer:** Critical malnutrition (bradycardia, hypothermia, severe dehydration, altered mental status), severe electrolyte disturbances (hypophosphatemia, hypokalemia, hypomagnesemia, hypocalcemia) secondary to refeeding syndrome
- **Discharge criteria:** Adequate, consistent weight gain demonstrated for 2 to 3 consecutive days; any underlying disease identified and treated; the feeding regimen with adequate calories is established; the family demonstrates understanding of nutrition recommendations, proper feeding techniques, and growth expectations; relevant social issues resolved

Follow-up

- **Primary care:** Weekly to monitor long-term weight gain and development

Pearls and Pitfalls

- The response to hospitalization does not necessarily contribute to identifying the cause of FTT.
- FTT is a multifactorial illness requiring a multidisciplinary approach.
- Most cases of FTT are failure to (adequately) feed, so a detailed feeding history is critical.
- Laboratory testing is usually not helpful in determining an etiology.
- Careful and thorough documentation is especially important in a suspected case of child neglect or abuse.
- Suggested management algorithms may lead to quicker diagnosis, improvement in nutrition, and shorter lengths of stay.
- Use a disease-specific growth curve to plot a child with a genetic or chromosomal disease.

Coding

ICD-9

- FTT **783.41**
- FTT in newborn **779.34**
- Feeding difficulties and mismanagement **783.3**
- Feeding problems in newborn **779.31**
- Loss of weight **783.21**
- Malnutrition of moderate degree **263.0**
- Malnutrition, unspecified **263.9**
- Underweight **783.22**

Bibliography

American Academy of Pediatrics Committee on Nutrition. Failure to thrive. In: Kleinman RE, ed. *Pediatric Nutrition Handbook*. 6th ed. Elk Grove Village, IL: American Academy of Pediatrics; 2009:601–636

Gahagan S. Failure to thrive: a consequence of undernutrition. *Pediatr Rev*. 2006;27:e1–e11

Jaffe AC. Failure to thrive: current clinical concepts. *Pediatr Rev*. 2011;32:100–107

Jolley CD. Failure to thrive. *Curr Probl Pediatr Adolesc Health Care*. 2003;33:183–206

Shah MD. Failure to thrive in children. *J Clin Gastroenterol*. 2002;35:371–374

Stephens MB, Gentry BC, Michener MD, Kendall SK, Gauer R. Clinical inquiries. What is the clinical workup for failure to thrive? *J Fam Pract*. 2008;57:264–266

CHAPTER 73

Feeding Tubes and Enteral Nutrition

Introduction

Feeding tubes are commonly used to provide supplemental nutrition, hydration, and/or medication. Although feeding tubes are also used in the setting of acute self-limiting illnesses (gastroenteritis, bronchiolitis, administration of unpalatable medications), the focus here is on the patient with a chronic feeding problem. The proper use and management of feeding tubes in such a patient requires the involvement of a multidisciplinary team of specialists, nurses, dietitians, therapists, and equipment suppliers.

Types of Feeding Tubes

There are 2 general types of feeding tubes (Figure 73-1). Enterostomy tubes are inserted percutaneously. Examples include gastrostomy (G) tubes, gastrojejunal (GJ) tubes, or jejunal tubes. These are indicated for long-term use (>8–12 weeks). Tubes inserted via the oronasal passage include nasogastric (NG), orogastric, and nasojejunal tubes. These are generally reserved for short-term use due to the increased risk of dislodgment and migration.

There are several types of enterostomy tubes available, all of which have 3 components

- An internal portion (balloon, mushroom, bulb, pigtail) within the stomach that prevents the tube from being accidentally withdrawn
- The visible portion on or outside the skin (low profile or traditional tube that projects out of the skin)
- The feeding port for connection

Some tubes have an external bar or disc to provide additional security. Typically, non–low-profile tubes are placed initially, and then replaced with a low-profile device after 6 to 12 weeks. However, the timing is dependent on local practice. When evaluating a patient, always document the type and size of the tube. Note that a Foley catheter can be used as a temporary catheter.

Indications for Percutaneous Feeding Tubes

- Oral-motor feeding problem resulting in an inability to maintain hydration by oral intake; prolonged feeding times; actual or potential risk of pulmonary aspiration
- Failure to thrive as a result of inadequate caloric intake secondary to a specific disease process (cystic fibrosis, congenital heart disease, chronic renal failure, malignancy)

Figure 73-1. Types of Enterostomy Tubes

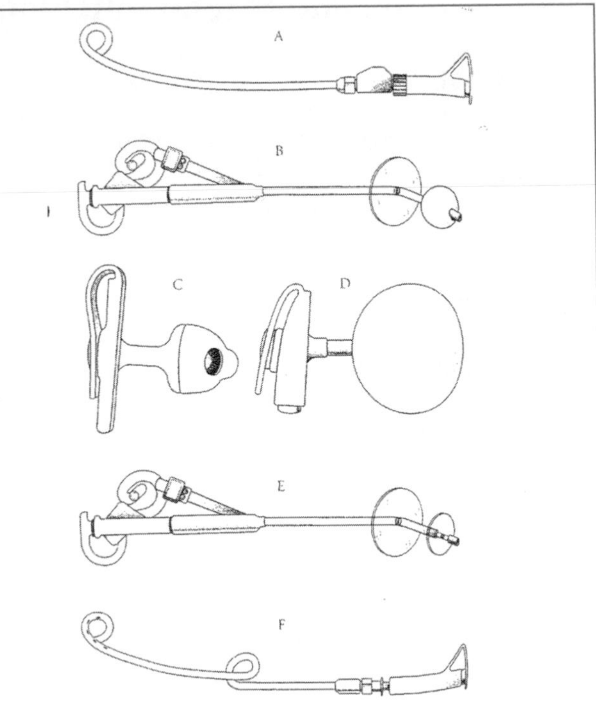

Low Profile (button tubes): Device is flush to the skin.

C: Bard button tube has a mushroom-shaped dome tip.

D: MIC-KEY device has a silicone balloon tip inflatable with saline.

Non–Low Profile: Device has long external portion

A: Mac-Loc (Dawson-Mueller catheter) is most often used by radiologists and consists of an internal pigtail loop and an external locking device.

B: Balloon style gastrostomy tube (eg, MIC gastrostomy) has an internal balloon tip and an external port for inflating/deflating the balloon.

E: Mushroom/bulb tip gastrostomy tube (eg, Malecot, de Pezzer) has a mushroom or wing tip to secure the tube to the stomach.

F: Mac-Loc gastrojejunal tube has a gastric loop and a distal loop that sits in the jejunum.

- Delivery of an elemental diet for the treatment of a disease process (inflammatory bowel disease, metabolic disease)
- Gastric venting, in conjunction with GJ-tube feeding, in a patient with severe dysmotility; gastroesophageal reflux (GER) that has not been adequately controlled medically and/or surgically
- Administration of unpalatable medications (antiretrovirals)

Indications for Jejunal Feeds (GJ-Tubes)

Use GJ-tubes very selectively, as they are associated with higher mechanical problems and greater inconvenience for families.

- Treatment of severe GER that has not been controlled medically and/or surgically, especially in a patient who is at risk for aspiration while receiving gastrostomy feeds and is already receiving maximal treatment for GER
- Gastrointestinal anomalies (superior mesenteric artery syndrome)

Techniques of G-Tube Placement

Techniques for G-tube placement vary among institutions and include surgical, laparoscopic, percutaneous endoscopic gastrostomy (PEG), and image-guided/radiologic. The PEG technique is the most commonly used method, although image-guided/radiologic gastrostomy is becoming more popular.

Complications Associated With G- and GJ-Tubes

Complications related to enteral tubes can be divided into early (within 30 days of the procedure) and late, as well as major and minor. Complication rates depend on the technique of placement. Late, minor complications are common with all techniques.

Early (Procedure-Related)

- Bleeding, infection (peristomal or systemic), puncture of other intra-abdominal organs (colon), misplacement of tube (into small or large bowel), peritonitis (about 2%), esophageal tear (PEG), aspiration, anesthetic-related, and death (rare)

Late

- Tube problem (blockage, dislodgment, breakage), peristomal wound infections, stomal enlargement with leakage around the tube, buried bumper syndrome (PEG), peritonitis caused by replacement of the tube into the peritoneum (rare), and intussusception around distal portion of tube (GJ-tube)

Management of Specific Common and/or Serious Complications

Peritonitis Following G-/GJ-Tube Placement

This usually occurs within 48 hours after insertion or during the first weeks after tube insertion when the new tract between the stomach wall and skin is not yet formed. Causes include gastric leakage of contents into the peritoneal space, dislodgment of the tube into the peritoneum, and perforation of other organs or vessels during the procedure. The patient presents similarly to other causes of peritonitis with fever, irritability, vomiting, and peritoneal signs.

Management involves general measures, including discontinuing feeds, placing an NG-tube for gastric drainage, giving broad-spectrum antibiotics (see Acute Abdomen, page 681), as well as aggressive fluid management. In addition, obtain an x-ray or fluoroscopic study with contrast (tube check) to confirm placement of the tube and the presence of pneumoperitoneum. If there is a concern about intra-abdominal collections (fever, no response to antibiotics) or bleeding, obtain an ultrasound or a cross-sectional computed tomography. Urgently consult with the radiologist, endoscopist, or surgeon. In some cases an emergent laparotomy will be necessary to investigate and manage a possible perforation.

Intussusception Around G-Tube

This has been commonly reported with the use of Mac-Loc (pigtail) catheters, as the pigtail distal portion of the tube acts as a lead point for a small bowel intussusception. The highest risk is in an infant younger than 1 year who usually presents with bilious vomiting and irritability. Obtain an abdominal ultrasound, which is diagnostic. Management includes removing the tube and placing a temporary Foley catheter into the stomach to provide acute relief. Recurrences may be prevented by cutting the distal pigtail and thus shortening the tube. However, recurrences are an indication for discontinuing the GJ feeds and trying other options, such as fundoplication and continuous gastric feeds.

Vomiting With an Enteral Tube in Place

Always consider non–tube-related causes, including GER, which may worsen after the placement of an enterostomy tube. G-tubes, particularly those with a long internal portion or without a securing mechanism (Mac-Loc, Foley catheter), can migrate into the duodenum or esophagus. Obtain a contrast study (G-tube check). GJ-tubes can also migrate, become malpositioned, or promote reflux (duodenal-gastric). In addition, a common complication in these tubes is intussusception (as above).

Blocked G-/GJ-Tube

Obstruction or clogging of an enteral tube is usually caused by a medication (Box 73-1), thickened feeds, or the failure to flush the tube after feeds. A tube with a thinner outside diameter is also more prone to blockage. To relieve the obstruction, gently flush with warm water using a 1- to 3-mL syringe. If this is ineffective, repeat with a carbonated beverage or cranberry juice. However, in some cases, as a last resort, the tube may have to be removed.

Dislodged Tube

If tube dislodgment is suspected shortly after insertion, assess the position by a contrast check before feeds are started, as there is an increased risk of peritoneal placement of the tube and subsequent peritonitis when the tract is not completely formed. The period during which a contrast check is needed is about 8 weeks, although this varies among surgeons and radiologists. During this period, do not inflate the balloon of a G-/GJ-tube (Figure 73-1B or 73-1D). Confirm the correct position by withdrawing gastric contents with a syringe. Once the tube position is confirmed, it may be used for feeds until a new tube is placed, if the G-/GJ-tube is more than 8 weeks old. For a patient with GJ-tube dislodgment, initiate temporary gastric feeds only if it is medically safe (patient is not at a high risk for aspiration).

If the tube is completely out, replace with a Foley catheter of the same size, or one size smaller, and secure with tape.

G-Tube Site Infection

Several steps in the care of G-tube sites can help prevent site infections, including cleaning the stoma daily with soap and water, keeping the stoma dry, and avoiding covering the stoma site with dressings. An infection presents with redness around the site and/or pus. Consider other causes of redness around the G-tube site, which may be confused for infection (Table 73-1).

Box 73-1. Medications and Substances That Commonly Block Enterostomy Tubes	
Cholestyramine resin Ciprofloxacin Clarithromycin Corn starch Cotazym Iron (liquid)	Kayexalate Lactulose Magnesium oxide Nelfinavir mesylate Pyridoxine (vitamin B)

Table 73-1. Differential Diagnosis of Peristomal Erythema

Diagnosis	Presentation	Management
Bacterial infection	Rarely complicated by abscess formation	Topical polysporin Oral antibiotics (cephalexin)
Fungal infection	Erythema with satellite lesions May have coexisting oral thrush or diaper candidiasis	Topical antifungal cream Oral nystatin for coexistent oral candidiasis
Granulation tissue	Pinkish-red, moist tissue May bleed May be painful	Warm saline compresses No dressings or creams Silver nitrate cautery
Irritation secondary to leakage of gastric contents	Erythema, breakdown, or ulceration	Keep area dry Barrier cream (zinc oxide) Proton pump inhibitor (omeprazole 0.2–3.5 mg/kg/day; titrate the dose to maintain gastric pH >5)
Skin sensitivity/contact dermatitis	Red, scaly, dry skin	Remove all dressings Change the adhesive tape

Feeding Via an Enteral Tube

Decisions regarding the type and route of feeds are often made in consultation with a nutritionist. Basic considerations include the following.

Bolus Versus Continuous Feeds

Generally speaking, bolus feeds are safe, as they represent physiological stomach function, although there is controversy as to whether continuous feeds are safer. A very general recommendation is to calculate the daily caloric requirement and give one-eighth of the total every 3 hours, with each feed over 1 hour. Adjustments can be made accordingly. However, if the patient is receiving trans-pyloric feeds, do not use boluses as the small intestine (unlike the stomach) is not capable of receiving fluids in this manner.

Caloric and Fluid Needs

Calories and fluids will vary widely depending on the patient and the indication(s) for tube. For example, a neurologically devastated patient with a decreased metabolic rate will have a lower caloric need than an otherwise active patient with cystic fibrosis. As a general rule, calculate a fluid/calorie estimate, then track the patient over a period of 3 to 5 days to ensure adequate tube function, adequate weight gain, and appropriate hydration.

Types of Formula

There is nothing particularly unique about a tube-fed patient in terms of choice of formula. While this may depend on the reason(s) why the tube was placed, allow the gut physiology to drive the formula choice. As an example, initially order Enfamil (infant) or Pediasure (toddler) if there is no underlying condition suggesting otherwise.

Discharge Planning

This is an area where pediatric hospitalists will need some expertise and experience to anticipate the patient's needs. In most situations, a case manager will assist in the transition of the patient and family from the inpatient to the outpatient setting in terms of medical equipment and formula delivery. One useful common strategy for facilitating the transition to the home environment is to implement daytime bolus feeds (allowing the patient time off the feeding pump) and overnight continuous feeds, then monitor for a day or two.

Pearls and Pitfalls

- The delivered tube feed volume is often less than what was ordered because the feeds are frequently stopped, delayed, or withheld for multiple reasons. Base calorie counts on volume delivered, not ordered.

Bibliography

Burd A, Burd RS. The who, what, why, and how-to guide for gastrostomy tube placement in infants. *Adv Neonatal Care.* 2003;3:197–205

Davis AM, Bruce A, Cocjin J, Mousa H, Hyman P. Empirically supported treatments for feeding difficulties in young children. *Curr Gastroenterol Rep.* 2010;12:189–194

Friedman JN. Enterostomy tube feeding: the ins and outs. *Paediatr Child Health.* 2004;9:695–699

Nijs EL, Cahill AM. Pediatric enteric feeding techniques: insertion, maintenance, and management of problems. *Cardiovasc Intervent Radiol.* 2010;33:1101–1110

Sullivan PB. *Feeding and Nutrition in Children with Neurodevelopmental Disability.* Hoboken, NJ: Wiley; 2009

CHAPTER 74

Fluids and Electrolytes

Introduction

Volume depletion (dehydration) and electrolyte disturbances are common in hospitalized children. While most instances are relatively mild, in severe cases they can result in shock, seizures, coma, and death. Hypovolemia can occur with an elevated, normal, or decreased serum sodium (hypertonic, isotonic, or hypotonic hypovolemia), and abnormalities in serum sodium can be seen in patients without hypovolemia (eg, syndrome of inappropriate antidiuretic hormone secretion [SIADH]).

Clinical Presentation

History

Usually there is a history of emesis, diarrhea, decreased oral intake and urinary output, malaise, and central nervous system (CNS) depression. High fever, high-pitched cry, and irritability can occur with hypernatremic dehydration. Markedly decreased urinary output implies greater than 10% dehydration. Assess the patient's input (volume and specific fluid) as well as the losses (vomitus, stool, urine).

Physical Examination

Evaluate the child's general appearance and look for signs of mild, moderate, and severe dehydration (Table 74-1), corresponding to approximately 5%, 10%, and 15% volume depletion, respectively. Tachycardia (pulse >95th percentile for age) is typically the earliest symptom of hypovolemia. However, fever can be a confounder, as it increases the heart rate by about 10 beats/minute per each degree above 37°C (98.6°F). Overt hypotension is a late finding in hypovolemic shock in children, and its absence does not preclude the

Table 74-1. Dehydration Score

Clinical Signs	0: Mild	1: Moderate	2: Severe
General appearance	Normal	Restless or lethargic Remains responsive	Drowsy, limp, cold Comatose
Eyes	Normal	Slightly sunken	Very sunken
Mucous membranes (tongue)	Moist	"Sticky"	Dry
Tears	Normal	Decreased	Absent

diagnosis of significant hypovolemia. Check the capillary refill by raising the extremity to be tested slightly above the heart and briefly press the nail bed on a finger or toe to compress the underlying capillaries (blanching). Observe as the skin returns to a normal color when the pressure is released. Dehydration and most types of shock cause a sluggish or prolonged capillary refill time greater than 2 seconds, although this can also occur as a consequence of simple exposure to a cold external environment. Also assess skin turgor by gently pinching a fold of the patient's abdominal skin then releasing it. The longer the skin remains tented after it is released, the more severe the degree of dehydration.

Laboratory

Obtain a complete blood cell count, electrolytes, and urinalysis. The serum sodium is not a reflection of volume status and must be interpreted in the context of whether the patient is hypovolemic, euvolemic, or hypervolemic. Investigate causes of abnormal glucose level, acidosis, and elevated anion gap (normal <12 mEq/L). Assess for ketone bodies in the urine, as products of fatty acid oxidation, during fasting or hypoglycemia.

$$\text{Anion Gap} = [\text{Sodium} - (\text{Chloride} + \text{bicarbonate})]$$

Suspect acute kidney injury (AKI) if the patient is frankly anuric, polyuric despite clinical signs of dehydration, or has a blood urea nitrogen and creatinine that are disproportionately high or continue to rise despite proper management. Suspect SIADH (postoperative; acute gastrointestinal, pulmonary or CNS illness) if the patient presents with hyponatremia and increased urine osmolality, without clinical signs of dehydration. If AKI or SIADH are suspected, calculate the serum/urine ratios and the fractional excretion of sodium (FENa), which generally will be less than 1% in a patient with normal renal function, greater than 1% in renal disease, and less than 1% to 2% in SIADH, depending on sodium intake (Table 74-2):

$$\text{FENa} = (\text{plasma Cr} \times \text{urine Na})/(\text{plasma Na} \times \text{urine Cr}) \times 100$$

When the plasma osmolality is low suggesting SIADH, use the "urine/serum osmolality ratios" as shown in Table 74-2. Repeat the electrolytes 4 to 6 hours later if the patient is not improving, has significant abnormalities in serum sodium or potassium, severe acidosis, or signs of possible renal dysfunction. If the child has persistent ongoing losses and is primarily, or exclusively, receiving intravenous (IV) fluids, check the electrolytes daily for the first 2 to 3 days and as per clinical condition afterward.

Table 74-2. Laboratory Values in Oliguria

	Prerenal	Renal	SIADH
Urine			
Sodium (mEq/L)	<20	>40	>40
Specific gravity	>1.020	~1.010	>1.020
Osmolality (mOsm/L)	>500	<350	>500
U/S Ratios			
U/S Osm	>1.3	<1.3	>2
U/S urea	>20	<10	>15
U/S creatinine	>40	<20	>30
FENa (%)	<1	>2	<1–2

Abbreviations: FENa, fractional excretion of sodium; SIADH, syndrome of inappropriate antidiuretic hormone secretion; U/S, urine/sodium.

Differential Diagnosis

Table 74-3. Causes of Sodium and Potassium Abnormalities

Diagnosis	Causes
Hyponatremia	
Pseudo	Hyperlipidemia, hyperproteinemia
Factitious	Hyperglycemia (diabetic ketoacidosis) (Na^+ ↓ 1.6 mEq/L for each ↑ 100 mg/dL of glucose)
Euvolemic	Syndrome of inappropriate antidiuretic hormone secretion (central nervous system, medications, postoperative, pulmonary)
Hypovolemic	Burns, dietary, cerebral salt wasting, gastrointestinal losses, iatrogenic
Hypervolemic	Cardiac, edema: renal (nephrotic syndrome), iatrogenic, liver failure
Hypernatremia	
With ↓ total body Na^+	Diarrhea, renal disease, sweat
With normal total body Na^+	Diabetes insipidus (central, nephrogenic), heat
With ↑ total body Na^+	Hyperaldosteronism, iatrogenic, renal disease
Hypokalemia	
	Dietary (chronically ill), gastrointestinal losses, medications (β-agonists, diuretics) renal disease
Hyperkalemia	
	Acidosis, Addison disease, congenital adrenal hyperplasia, hemolysis, iatrogenic, medications, renal disease, rhabdomyolysis

Treatment

Calculate a patient's fluid and electrolyte requirements management based on the clinical presentation and underlying diagnosis. Take into consideration the severity of illness, as well as the basal metabolic needs, initial hydration and electrolyte status (deficits), and ongoing losses. Acute changes in body weight reflect fluid losses. For example, a 20-kg patient who is 10% dehydrated has lost 2 kg, equal to 2 L of fluid.

Fluid and Electrolyte Maintenance Therapy

Maintenance therapy is required to preserve intravascular volume in a euvolemic, otherwise healthy patient who does not have any abnormal deficits or ongoing losses, such as an infant who is pre- or postoperative. Add glucose, sodium, and potassium (only if the patient is voiding, without hyperkalemia) requirements to prevent iatrogenic hypoglycemia, hyponatremia, and/or hypokalemia. Overnight maintenance IV fluid is typically not needed in a euvolemic older child without ongoing losses who is NPO for next-day surgery. However, avoid prolonged fasting prior to surgery.

Maintenance Fluid

Use the Holliday-Segar method (Table 74-4) for a patient weighing more than 3.5 kg. If the child is obese, use the ideal body weight or 50th percentile weight for height. These calculations are for an otherwise healthy child. For a patient who is ill or dehydrated, adjust the fluids to take into account the volume deficit, maintenance requirements, and clinical course (changes in oral intake, urine output, ongoing losses, etc). Use 5% dextrose to minimize catabolism, as this will provide 2 to 4 mg/kg/minute of glucose, equivalent to the liver glucose production rate.

For example, for a 30-kg patient

Fluid

$$= (100\text{ mL} \times 10\text{ kg}) + (50\text{ mL} \times 10\text{ kg}) + (20\text{ mL} \times 10\text{ kg})$$

$$= 1{,}000 + 500 + 200 = 1700\text{ mL/24 hours} \rightarrow \text{Infusion rate} = 70\text{ mL/hour}$$

Table 74-4. Holliday-Segar Method

Body Weight	Water (mL/kg/24 hours)
First 10 kg of body weight	100
Second 10 kg of body weight	50
Each additional kg (>20 kg)	20

Maintenance Electrolytes

Replace the Na^+ and K^+ losses that occur daily in the sweat, urine, and stool. Give 2 to 3 mEq/kg/day of Na^+ and 1 to 2 mEq/kg/day of K^+. Defer giving potassium if the patient has hyperkalemia, marked oliguria/anuria, or suspected renal insufficiency.

Fluid and Electrolyte Imbalance

Volume Depletion

Deficit and maintenance calculation

Example: 9-kg patient with several days of diarrhea is clinically estimated to be 10% dehydrated, with Na^+ 130 mEq/L, K^+ 2 mEq/L, and pH: 7.3.

Well weight = Current weight × 100/(100−%dehydration) = 9 × 100/90 = 10 kg

Fluid deficit = Well weight−current weight = 10 kg−9 kg = 1 kg → 1 L

Total fluid/24 hours = Fluid deficit (1 L) + daily maintenance (1 L) = 2 L/24 hours

Ongoing losses

Always consider ongoing losses of both volume and sodium (emesis Na^+: 60–155 mEq/L; diarrhea: Na^+ 40–120 mEq/L; third spacing Na^+: 140 mEq/L). Measure volume losses and assess replacement needs every 4 hours.

Example: Postoperative patient with nasogastric aspirate of 100 mL/hour: measure and replace 400 mL normal saline (NS) after 4 hours

Hyponatremia (sodium <135 mEq/L)

Na^+ deficit (mEq) = (Fluid deficit × 140 mEq/L) + [(Na^+desired−Na^+plasma)] × weight × 0.6 L/kg*]

*0.6 L/kg = Na^+ correction factor

Example: 9 kg patient with several days of diarrhea is clinically estimated to be 10% dehydrated (ie, well weight = 10 kg), with Na^+ 130 mEq/L, K^+ 2 mEq/L, and pH: 7.3

Na^+ deficit mEq = (1 L × 140 mEq/L) + [(135–130 mEq/L) × 10 kg × 0.6 L/kg] = 170 mEq

Total Na^+/24 hours = Na^+ deficit + Na^+ maintenance/24 hours

= 170 mEq + (2 mEq/kg × 10 kg) = 170 + 20 = 190 mEq

= 190 mEq/2 L/24 hours = 85 mEq/L (approximately ½ NS)

Increase the serum sodium by no more than 0.5 mEq/L/hour, unless the patient is actively seizing from severe hyponatremia (see below), to prevent central pontine myelinosis.

Severe hyponatremia with seizures (sodium <120 mEq/L)

Use 3% NaCl (513 mEq/L) through a central venous line until the seizures stop (1.2 mL/kg will raise serum Na^+ about 1 mEq/L). Administer very slowly if only a peripheral IV is available.

Hypernatremia (sodium >145 mEq/L)

Free water deficit = 4 mL/kg × weight × ($Na^+_{plasma} - Na^+_{desired}$)

Example: 10-kg patient with Na^+ 155 mEq/L:

Free water deficit = (4 mL/kg × 10 kg) × (155–145 mEq/L) = 400 mL

Decrease the serum Na^+ by no more than 0.5 mEq/L/hour to prevent cerebral edema.

Hypokalemia (potassium <3 mEq/L)

To properly interpret the serum K^+, consider the effect of blood pH on the intracellular-extracellular movement of K^+. A 0.1 decrease in blood pH increases the serum K^+ by approximately 1 mEq/L, while a 0.1 increase in blood pH decreases the serum K^+ by approximately 1 mEq/L. In addition, take into account that only 2% of the total body K^+ (TBK) is found in plasma. Each 1 mEq/L decrease in serum K^+ represents a fall in TBK of approximately 12%. Therefore, in general, hypokalemia implies marked TBK depletion.

Symptoms of mild hypokalemia include muscular weakness, myalgia, muscle cramps, and constipation. Severe hypokalemia leads to depressed muscle function, flaccid paralysis, diminished reflexes, respiratory depression, and potentially rhabdomyolysis. Severe hyperkalemia is characterized by electrocardiogram (ECG) abnormalities, such as prominent U wave after the T wave, ST-segment depression, and atrioventricular conduction abnormalities.

Whenever possible, correct a potassium deficiency enterally, as this is a much safer form of administration. Mild hypokalemia will usually resolve with just oral repletion. Severe symptomatic hypokalemia requires IV potassium correction of 1 mEq/kg, although a rapid infusion of K^+ is rarely needed. Correct a significant the K^+ deficit slowly over 3 to 5 days with an IV solution containing 30 to 40 mEq/L of KCl or K- acetate (if the patient is acidotic). Do not exceed an infusion rate of 0.5 mEq/kg/hour or 4 to 5 mEq/kg/day and do not use a K^+ concentration greater than 40 mEq/L through a peripheral IV, as it can cause acute phlebitis.

A simplified formula to calculate the potassium deficit is (10-kg patient with 10% dehydration):

K^+ deficit (mEq) = (Fluid deficit × 0.4[1]) × 150[2] mEq/L

= (0.9L X 0.4) × 150 mEq/L = 54 mEq

[1]0.4 L/kg = k^+ correction factor

[2]Intracellular K^+ concentration

Hyperkalemia (potassium >6 mEq/L)

Recheck the electrolytes to confirm the K^+ level, obtain an ECG looking for peaked T waves (T wave >one-half the R or S wave). Check the bicarbonate level to assess for acidosis, which causes a K^+ shift into the extracellular fluid and look for hemolysis of the sample (spurious hyperkalemia). If the ECG is abnormal (arrhythmia or peaked T waves) or the K^+ is confirmed to be higher than 7 mEq/L, discontinue the administration of exogenous potassium and use therapeutic agents that can transiently redistribute potassium: 25% dextrose (2 mL/kg over 30 minutes and repeat every 30 minutes) along with regular insulin (1 unit/kg/hour); nebulized albuterol. Also give 10% calcium gluconate (1 mL/kg = 100 mg/kg/dose every 3 to 5 minutes) to protect the myocardium. To enhance potassium excretion, use a loop diuretic (furosemide 1–2 mg/kg IV every 6 hours) and polystyrene sulfonate (1 g/kg). Dialysis is indicated for life-threatening hyperkalemia.

Summary example

For a 9-kg patient who is 10% dehydrated (10 kg when well) with Na^+ 130 mEq/L, K^+ 3 mEq/L, and pH 7.3

	D5W	Na^+	K^+
Maintenance/24 hours	1,000 mL	20 mEq	10 mEq
Deficit	1,000 mL	170 mEq	54 mEq
Total/24 hours	2,000 mL	190 mEq	64 mEq

Therefore, order D5 ½ NS, with 30 to 35 mEq/L of KCL at 83 mL/hour. Note: 0.9% NS = 154 mEq/L; 0.45% NS = ½ NS = 77 mEq/L

Ongoing Losses

Gastrointestinal (emesis, diarrhea, ileus, third spacing), renal, and insensible water losses affect fluid maintenance requirements. Assess ongoing losses frequently, as they may change rapidly (Table 74-5).

Table 74-5. Changes in Maintenance Fluid Requirements

	Increase	Decrease
Activity (eg, seizures)	30%	N/A
Anuria	N/A	50%
Diabetes insipidus	200%–400%	N/A
Diarrhea	10%–50%	
Humidified oxygen	N/A	25%–40%
Hyperventilation	50%–65%	N/A
Polyuria (eg, diabetic ketoacidosis)	100%	N/A
Sweat	5%–50%	
Temperature	12% per degree C >37°C	12% per degree C <37°C

Example: 25-kg (well weight) patient who is 10% dehydrated, tachypneic, with persistent fever (39°C; 102.2°F), and requiring humidified oxygen:

Maintenance Fluids (1000 + 500 + 100)	Deficit (10% body weight)	Ongoing losses (about 40% of maintenance)[a]	Total/ 24 hours
1,600 mL	2,500 mL	640 mL	4740 mL

[a]40% accounts for: fever (+24%), tachypnea (+50%), and humidified oxygen (-35%).

Resuscitation Fluids Practical Guidelines

What follows is a safe, simplified method to minimize common iatrogenic fluid and electrolyte disturbances. Compare the calculated rehydration plan to MedCalc, which provides in-depth electronic fluid and electrolyte calculations (www.medcalc.com/pedifen.html). However, this plan is not a substitute for clinical judgment and assessing and reassessing the status of the patient.

Start Fluid Resuscitation With an Isotonic Solution (NS or Lactated Ringer)

1. Give 20 mL/kg IV boluses over 5 to 10 minutes.
2. Reassess and repeat boluses as needed, up to 60 mL/kg in 60 minutes. Always consider possible life-threatening conditions requiring a different approach, such as sepsis (fever and hypotension), congestive heart failure (CHF) or myocarditis (respiratory distress, gallop rhythm, hepatomegaly), increased intracranial pressure (history of hydrocephalus, bradycardia, altered mental status), and adrenal crisis (unresponsive shock). When CHF or myocarditis is a consideration, give multiple smaller boluses of 10 mL/kg. Monitor the changes in pulse, blood pressure, and urine output.
3. If the patient is in shock, rapidly secure intraosseous access if IV access appears suboptimal.

Subsequent Fluid and Electrolyte Therapy

1. Calculate the maintenance (Holliday-Segar method) and deficit fluid volumes (as above), while monitoring ongoing losses.
   a. Isonatremic/hyponatremic dehydration: Use D5 ½ NS with 20 mEq/L KCl. This will provide additional NaCl to slowly compensate the deficit, as well as the K^+ and glucose requirements (2–4 mg/kg/minute).
   b. Hypernatremic dehydration: Use D5 ¼ NS with 20 mEq/L KCl, over *48 hours.*
   c. Make sure the patient has voided before adding potassium to the IV fluids
   d. Resume oral feeding as early as possible.
   e. Monitor the pulse, blood pressure, and urine output.
2. If the patient child is stable and well hydrated (post-rehydration, NPO)
   a. Weight <10 kg: D5 ¼ NS with 20 mEq/L KCl
   b. Weight >10 kg: D5 ½ NS with 20 mEq/L KCl

Indications for Consultation

- **Endocrinology:** Hypernatremia and increased urine output greater than 5 mL/kg/hour (diabetes insipidus)
- **Metabolism:** Laboratory suggestive of a metabolic disorder (severe acidosis, unexplained elevated anion gap and/or hypoketotic hypoglycemia)
- **Nephrology:** Anuria or signs of renal disease (elevated creatinine), severe hypo- or hypernatremia or hypo- or hyperkalemia

Disposition

- **Intensive care unit transfer:** Shock not responding to resuscitation fluids, acute kidney injury, hyperkalemia requiring IV medications, severe hypokalemia, severe hypo- or hypernatremia
- **Discharge criteria:** Back to premorbid weight, tolerating maintenance oral fluids, with adequate urine output (≥1 mL/kg/hour)

Follow-up

- **Primary care:** 1 to 3 days

Pearls and Pitfalls

- To avoid fluid overload, use ideal body weight or 50th percentile weight for height for an obese patient.
- Assume greater than 10% dehydration if the patient is anuric/oliguric or has hypernatremic dehydration.

- As a result of reperfusion, severe metabolic acidosis can worsen immediately after rehydration.
- In the context of oliguria, FENa less than 1% suggests prerenal azotemia, rather than intrarenal injury/acute tubular necrosis.
- Proteinuria and glucosuria can falsely elevate the urine specific gravity and thereby mask renal insufficiency.
- Always consider the possibility of acute adrenal insufficiency in a hypotensive, unresponsive patient with hyponatremia and/or hyperkalemia.

Coding

ICD-9

- Dehydration **276.51**
- Electrolyte and fluid disorders not otherwise specified **276.9**
- Hyperkalemia **276.7**
- Hyperosmolality and/or hypernatremia **276.0**
- Hypokalemia **276.8**
- Hyposmolality and/or hyponatremia **276.1**
- Shock unspecified **785.50**

Bibliography

Favia I, Garisto C, Rossi E, Picardo S, Ricci Z. Fluid management in pediatric intensive care. *Contrib Nephrol.* 2010;164:217–226

Friedman A. Fluid and electrolyte therapy: a primer. *Pediatr Nephrol.* 2010;25:843–846

Friedman, JN, Goldman RD, Srivastava R, Parkin P. Development of a clinical dehydration scale for use in children between 1 and 36 months of age. *J Pediatr.* 2004;145:201–207

Goff DA, Higinio V. Hypernatremia. *Pediatr Rev.* 2009;30:412–413

Hanna M, Saberi MS. Incidence of hyponatremia in children with gastroenteritis treated with hypotonic intravenous fluids. *Pediatr Nephrol.* 2010;25:1471–1475

Peruzzo M, Milani GP, Garzoni L, et al. Body fluids and salt metabolism—part II. *Ital J Pediatr.* 2010;36:78

Obesity

Introduction

Since 1980 the prevalence of obesity has nearly tripled among American school-aged children and adolescents. This epidemic has led to an increasing number of patients with associated comorbidities, which can have significant implications when caring for inpatients.

There are also some rare but important causes of obesity in children that are not related to diet or exercise. These include Prader-Willi syndrome, Bardet-Biedl syndrome, and Albright syndrome, as well as the use of various psychotropic medications, such as risperidone (Risperdal) or quetiapine (Seroquel). Consider syndromic obesity if the patient has short stature, hypogonadism, developmental delay, or dysmorphic features. Similarly, most primary endocrinologic causes of obesity (hypothyroidism, Cushing syndrome) will have other symptoms at time of presentation. Otherwise, most obese children will not have a specific genetic or metabolic etiology identified.

Definition

For a patient 2 years of age or older, the definition of obesity relies on the calculation of the body mass index (BMI): BMI = (mass in kg)/(height in m)^2. A patient with a BMI greater than the 95th percentile is classified as obese, while a child with a BMI greater than the 85th percentile is classified as overweight. For a patient younger than 2 years, use a weight-for-length percentile greater than the 95th percentile as a screen for overweight.

Clinical Presentation

History

Ask about diet history, physical activity, and menstrual history, as well as a family history of type II diabetes, thromboembolic events, hypertension, and dyslipidemias. Assess for any psychological comorbidities (depression, bullying, anxiety, disordered eating).

Physical Examination

Priorities on physical examination are BMI, blood pressure, and skin inspection for acanthosis nigricans, abdominal striae, skin breakdown, and intertrigo, as well as hirsutism and acne, which may suggest polycystic ovary syndrome (PCOS). Also assess the patient for limp and hip or knee pain and pes planus.

Comorbidities

As with adults, there are significant comorbidities associated with childhood obesity that may affect inpatient management.

Endocrine

Metabolic Syndrome

Metabolic syndrome, a group of risk factors for cardiovascular disease and type 2 diabetes, is well defined in the adult population. However, the definition is less exact for children. Adult criteria include a fasting plasma glucose of 110 mg/dL or higher, abdominal obesity (waist circumference >40 inches male; >35 inches female), hypertriglyceridemia 150 mg/dL or higher, decreased high-density lipoprotein (HDL) (<40 mg/dL male; <50 mg/dL female), and blood pressure 130/85 mm Hg or higher.

Type 2 Diabetes

Type 2 diabetes is now the most common form of diabetes in children, as hyperinsulinemia and abnormal glucose tolerance are common consequences of obesity. Screen for type 2 diabetes in any overweight patient with 2 or more of the following criteria: (1) family history (first- or second-degree relative) of type 2 diabetes, (2) African-American, Latino, American Indian, or Asian-Pacific Islander ethnicity, and (3) physical findings or signs of insulin resistance (hypertension, dysplipidemia, PCOS, acanthosis nigricans). Screen at 10 years of age or at the onset of puberty, whichever comes first, preferably with a fasting plasma glucose (≥110 mg/dL). An elevated hemoglobin A1C (>6.0%) is not as sensitive, but may be useful when confirming that a patient's elevated glucose level is secondary to intravenous fluids, stress, or corticosteroid use.

While most endocrinopathies will not primarily present with obesity, PCOS is frequently a comorbid condition in obese adolescent girls. Clinical history and findings include menstrual irregularity, hirsutism, acne, and elevated insulin levels. Screening for PCOS may include obtaining free testosterone level as well as luteinizing and follicle-stimulating hormones.

Cardiovascular

Hypertension

An obese child has more than 4-fold greater risk of elevated systolic pressure and a 2-fold greater risk for elevated diastolic pressure. Persistent elevated blood pressure may also warrant further testing and assessment of renal and cardiac function.

Dyslipidemia

An obese patient is more likely to have elevated total cholesterol, triglycerides, and low-density lipoprotein cholesterol and reduced levels of HDL cholesterol. Obtain a fasting lipid profile in any child who has a BMI above the 85th percentile.

Respiratory

Up to 50% of obese children develop obstructive sleep apnea (OSA), which may also contribute to insulin resistance independent of BMI. Nocturnal polysomnography is the gold standard for diagnosis of OSA. In addition, obesity hypoventilation syndrome may occur in an extremely obese patient when the weight of the fat on the chest and abdomen disrupt ventilation. This can occur while asleep or awake.

Neurologic

An obese child is at risk for developing idiopathic increased intracranial pressure and pseudotumor cerebri. This may present with papilledema and severe headache, but otherwise normal cerebrospinal fluid parameters.

Gastrointestinal

Non-Alcoholic Fatty Liver Disease (NAFLD)

Although there are other disorders of liver dysfunction that can cause elevated transaminases, up to 10% of overweight children may have histologic evidence of hepatosteatosis and elevated transaminases, as well as alkaline phosphatase and γ-glutamyltransferase. If NAFLD is suspected, obtain an ultrasound of the liver and consult with a pediatric gastroenterologist.

Gallstones

Up to 2% of obese adolescents may develop gallstones. The risk is greatest among older, female, and severely obese patients.

Musculoskeletal

Blount Disease

Blount disease is characterized by abnormal growth of the proximal tibial physis. It is more common among African Americans and males, and occurs in up to 2.5% of obese preadolescent boys. Blount disease presents with progressive bowing (genu varum), gait disturbance, and arthritis.

Slipped Capital Femoral Epiphysis (SCFE)

An obese child is at increased risk for SCFE. The incidence appears to be increasing, with some cases occurring in prepubertal males. The patient presents with a limp associated with hip or referred knee pain.

Pharmacologic

Most pediatric medications are dosed based on body weight, so that some obese children may require more than an adult dose of a particular drug. In addition, there may be significant variations in drug distribution and metabolism. In such cases, consultation with a clinical pharmacologist may be helpful.

Complications of Obesity Specific to the Inpatient Setting

An obese patient is at increased risk for complications during hospitalization, including an increased length of stay following surgery. Factors involved may include longer times to full diet and ambulation, prolonged wound healing, and postoperative airway issues.

Airway

An obese patient is at increased risk anatomically for airway obstruction following general anesthesia. Previously undetected obstructive sleep apnea and hypopnea may be discovered, while incomplete ventilation during or following anesthesia may lead to ventilation/perfusion mismatch, hypoxemia, and hypercapnia. Although continuous pulse oximetry may be very helpful, it does not substitute for formal nocturnal polysomnography, if indicated, along with consultation with a pulmonologist and/or otolaryngologist.

An extremely obese patient is also at risk for obesity-hypoventilation syndrome (Pickwick syndrome). The normal central response to hypercapnia may be blunted, significantly increasing post-anesthetic complications.

Infection

An obese child may be at increased risk for postinfectious complications. The mechanism is likely multifactorial, including metabolic derangement and the relatively avascular condition of adipose tissue. Give careful attention to hygiene and candidal infection (intertrigo).

Venous Thromboembolism (VTE)

VTE appears to be increasing among pediatric patients, although there is currently no universally accepted screening tool for children. Risk factors to consider include BMI greater than 30; surgery or trauma; smoking; prolonged immobility or length of stay (≥3 days); malignancy; respiratory disease; inflammatory bowel disease; hypercoagulable states (adolescent taking oral contraceptives); presence or history of an indwelling central venous catheter; history of thrombotic events; family history of hypercoagulability or thrombosis; and musculoskeletal sepsis, osteomyelitis, or staphylococcal infections.

VTE prophylaxis with low-molecular-weight heparin (such as enoxaprin), regular heparin, and warfarin have all demonstrated efficacy (see pages 28–29), although safety profiles may vary. If it is not clear whether the patient requires anticoagulation, consult with a thrombosis specialist or hematologist. Sequential compression devices have also been shown to be effective for prevention, particularly for non-ambulatory patients.

Ergonomics

Standard-sized hospital equipment (blood pressure cuffs, wheelchairs, scales, etc) may not be sufficient to meet the needs of an extremely obese adolescent. Such a patient may not be able to undergo such routine hospital procedures as magnetic resonance imaging (due to weight limits and/or size limits of the machine) or an echocardiogram (due to thoracic diameter), so that transesophageal echocardiogram or other modalities may be needed.

Approach to the Hospitalized Overweight or Obese Child

Management of an acute illness usually takes priority over the treatment of obesity. However, always consider the comorbidities and potential complications associated with obesity. Hospitalization for an acute illness may provide a "teachable moment" or motivation for a patient and family to consider lifestyle modification, especially if encountering an obesity-related complication for the first time.

Since obesity is often emotionally charged, approach the overweight or obese patient in a nonjudgmental and empathetic manner. Simply asking for the family's permission ("Would it be all right if we discuss your child's weight?") can often initiate a constructive discussion. Involve other staff members, such as a registered dietitian, who can assist with nutritional counseling, and a physical therapist, who can assess physical activity and develop an exercise plan. Referral to an outpatient center that specializes in pediatric weight management may be helpful. Identification of eating disorders, emotional eating, other mental health conditions, and behavioral therapy may be useful adjuncts.

Hospitalization may also provide an opportunity for an evaluation by a physical therapist or exercise physiologist if available, with assessment of flexibility, strength training, and conditioning. An overweight child may have patellar maltracking, foot overpronation, and low back pain, all of which may benefit from an individualized exercise plan.

Finally, there is ample evidence that many health care professionals may be biased (even unconsciously) against overweight patients. Obese individuals frequently feel stigmatized in health care settings, which can amplify vulnerability to depression, low self-esteem, and motivation to change. Unkind or insensitive comments by hospital staff, the hospital environment, and procedures can all affect the quality of an obese individual's experience in the hospital setting. Having correct instruments and equipment (eg, blood pressure cuffs, wheelchairs, beds) is vital. Focusing on the patient, rather than the obesity, will provide a more positive experience. Resources for preventing weight bias among health professionals are currently available online from the Yale Rudd Center for Food Policy and Obesity.

Options for the Morbidly Obese Patient

Modalities available for this population include very low calorie diets, typically administered in liquid form, and bariatric interventions (such as gastric bypass and laparoscopic banding). Refer the patient to an obesity center.

Indications for Consultation

- **Cardiology:** Severe hypertension
- **Endocrinology:** PCOS, diabetes
- **Gastroenterology/liver:** Dyslipidemia, NAFLD
- **Neurology:** Increased intracranial pressure
- **Orthopaedics:** Blount disease, SCFE
- **Psychiatry:** Disordered eating, depression, suicide
- **Pulmonology:** Obstructive sleep apnea, obesity hypoventilation syndrome
- **Surgery:** Gallstones

Pearls and Pitfalls

- Do not visually categorize a patient as overweight or obese without calculating the BMI.
- Do not overlook the opportunity to address lifestyle changes while the patient is admitted.

Coding

ICD-9

• Acanthosis nigricans	**701.2**
• Blount disease	**732.4**
• Dyslipidemia	**272.4**
• Hypertension, unspecified	**401.9**
• Metabolic syndrome X	**277.7**
• NAFLD	**571.8**
• Obesity hypoventilation syndrome	**278.03**
• Obesity, unspecified	**278.00**
• Overweight	**278.02**
• OSA	**327.23**
• Polycystic ovaries	**256.4**
• SCFE	**732.2**
• BMI, pediatric, 95th percentile or greater for age	**V85.54**

Bibliography

Cole CH. Primary prophylaxis of venous thromboembolism in children. *J Paediatr Child Health.* 2010;46:288–290

Doyle SL, Lysaght J, Reynolds JV. Obesity and post-operative complications in patients undergoing non-bariatric surgery. *Obes Rev.* 2010;11:875–886

Fennoy I. Metabolic and respiratory comorbidities of childhood obesity. *Pediatr Ann.* 2010;39:140–146

King DR, Velmahos GC. Difficulties in managing the surgical patient who is morbidly obese. *Crit Care Med.* 2010;38:S478–S482

Yale Rudd Center for Food Policy and Obesity. Weight bias & stigma. http://yaleruddcenter.org/what_we_do.aspx?id=10. Accessed May 15, 2012

Young KL, Demeule M, Stuhlsatz K, et al. Identification and treatment of obesity as a standard of care for all patients in children's hospitals. *Pediatrics.* 2011;128:S47–S50

Parenteral Nutrition

Introduction

Parenteral nutrition (PN) is a form of complete intravenous (IV) nutrition that bypasses the gastrointestinal tract. It is indicated for a patient who is unable to receive or tolerate adequate nutrition through an oral or enteral route, such as a child with bowel surgery, prematurity, short gut syndrome, severe pancreatitis, Stevens-Johnson syndrome, burns, and trauma. Nutrition is then provided in an IV solution containing dextrose, protein, lipids, electrolytes, vitamins, and trace elements.

In comparison to an adult, a child has fewer energy and protein stores and can develop nutritional deficiencies more rapidly. In addition, the calorie and protein requirements for growth can significantly increase the nutrient demands, so that the need for PN often arises sooner in a child. If a patient will be NPO for more than 3 days, some sort of nutritional support is indicated (enteral or parenteral). In a patient with no other comorbidities, PN is necessary when there has been inadequate caloric intake for 3 days, but resume enteral feedings as soon as the patient is able to tolerate adequate oral caloric intake.

Access

Ideally, achieve IV access selection well in advance of PN order writing. The delivery route will depend on the duration of PN therapy, calorie needs, and the nutritional goals. Peripheral generally means that the catheter tip is in a vein other than the superior or inferior vena cava. Peripheral and midlines are not appropriate for vesicant chemotherapy, central PN solutions, and/or medications with pH less than 5 or greater than 9, and solutions/medications with an osmolarity greater than 900 mOsm/L. Most institutions have policies and procedures regarding the osmolarity of a solution that may be delivered via peripheral vein. In general, peripheral PN solutions range from 10% to 12.5% dextrose and 2% to 2.5% amino acids. Electrolytes and minerals contribute to the final osmolarity of the solution as well. Consult with a clinical pharmacist if there are any questions regarding the suitability of a solution for a peripheral line.

A central venous catheter is for long-term use in a patient who requires a PN solution with an osmolality greater than 900 mOsm/L. In general, there are 4 types of catheters: peripherally inserted central catheter, non-tunneled, tunneled, and totally implanted venous access (ports). The tips of these catheters reside in the superior or inferior vena cava and are therefore considered central. Discuss with the surgeon or interventional radiologist the goals of PN and the other needs for the central line in order to determine if a single, double, or triple lumen line is required. Advance planning can then save a patient from needless discomfort.

Clinical Presentation

History and Physical Examination

The goals of PN, and the patient's nutritional and medical status, guide the decisions regarding the nutrient needs, mixture, and rate of delivery. First, assess whether or not the patient can tolerate enteral (oral or tube) feeds. If not, determine the patient's medical history, current nutritional status, the expected duration of being NPO, and the percentage of the total daily caloric requirement to be given parenterally. Look for oral lesions, a murmur, hepatomegaly, and old surgical scars, as these may be important clues for ongoing medical problems, liver dysfunction, or need for fluid restriction. Next, assess the overall nutritional status and determine if the patient is malnourished or overweight.

Calculating PN

Minimum amounts of glucose, fat, and protein are required to prevent hypoglycemia, essential fatty acid deficiency, and hypoproteinemia, respectively. However, feeding an excess of these nutrients can be a factor in the development of hepatic steatosis, excessive carbon dioxide production, increased infection risk, or prerenal azotemia. In general, consider protein requirements first and then energy when determining PN (Table 76-1). A patient with a significant fluid restriction, for example, may need protein intake provided at the expense of decreasing energy intake. There are larger gains in protein accretion with increases in protein intake than with increases in energy intake. Unless a patient has renal or liver impairment or disease, there is no reason to limit initial protein intakes to less than calculated needs.

There can be considerable variation in intra- and interindividual, as well as day-to-day, energy needs. Energy requirements for the hospitalized child can be difficult to define accurately. In most cases the provision of resting energy to critically ill patients is sufficient. The Dietary Reference Intake (DRI) values (Table 76-1) may overestimate the caloric requirements for a given patient. Thus an initially conservative approach to calorie delivery initially will minimize overfeeding or excessive weight gain. Use the tables as a starting point, to

Table 76-1. Estimated Energy and Protein Requirements for Infants Through Adolescents[a]

	Age	Reference Weight (kg)[b]	Reference Height (cm)[b]	BMR (kcal/kg/day)[c]	DRI: Energy Based on EER With PAL = Sedentary		DRI: Protein	
					kcal/day	kcal/kg/day		
Infants (age in months)	0–2	N/A	N/A	--	--	--	--	1.52[d]
	2–3	6	62	54	610	102	9.1	1.52[d]
	4–6	6	62	54	490	82	9.1	1.52[d]
	7–12	9	71	51	720	80	11	1.2[e]
	13–35	12	86	56	990	82	13	1.05[e]
Boys (age in years)	3	12	86	57	1019	85	13	1.05[e]
	4–5	20	115	48	1405	70	19	0.95[e]
	6–7	20	115	48	1279	64	19	0.95[e]
	8	20	115	48	1186	59	19	0.95[e]
Girls (age in years)	3	12	86	55	986	82	13	1.05[e]
	4–5	20	115	45	1291	65	19	0.95[e]
	6-7	20	115	45	1229	61	19	0.95[e]
	8	20	115	45	1183	59	19	0.95[e]
Boys (age in years)	9–11	36	144	36	1756	49	34	0.95[e]
	12–13	36	144	36	1601	45	34	0.95[e]
	14–16	61	174	29	2385	39	52	0.85[e]
	17–18	61	174	29	2230	37	52	0.85[e]
	> 18	70	177	28	2550	36	56	0.8[e]
Girls (age in years)	9–11	37	144	33	1550	42	35	0.95[e]
	12–13	37	144	32	1491	40	35	0.95[e]
	14–16	54	163	26	1760	33	46	0.85[e]
	17–18	54	163	26	1684	31	46	0.85[e]
	>18	57	163	22	1939	34	46	0.8[e]

Abbreviations: BMR, basal metabolic rate; EER, estimated energy requirement; DRI, Dietary Reference Intake; PAL, physical activity level.

[a] This table is meant to be a quick reference guideline, as calculations are based on reference heights and weights. Various sources present age groups differently. Therefore, some calculations reflect the average between genders and age groups.

[b] Reference weights and heights taken from *Dietary Reference Intakes: The Essential Guide to Nutrient Requirements Divided Into Smaller Groupings*. Based on National Center for Health Statistics/Centers for Disease Control and Prevention 2000 growth charts. Institute of Medicine, 2006.

[c] Estimates based on Schofield equations for calculating basal metabolic rate in children.

[d] Adequate intake.

[e] Recommended daily allowance.

be adjusted based on the pediatric dietitian's assessment and patient's response to treatment.

PN calculations are often complex, therefore it is important to have a consistent and reproducible system. Although each hospital uses a somewhat different system to calculate PN, there are a number of key steps for ensuring that the appropriate PN is delivered to the patient. Contact the nutrition service to get assistance with the local ordering system.

PN Order Writing

1. Assess protein and energy requirements: Estimate the energy requirements using the resting energy expenditure or DRI listed in Table 76-1. If the patient is adequately nourished, use the actual weight in kilograms. Use the ideal body weight (weight-for-length or body mass index at the 50th percentile) if the patient is malnourished and needs additional energy for catch-up growth. For an obese patient (>150% ideal body weight), use an adjusted or ideal weight to determine energy needs. The protein requirement may range from the DRI (Table 76-1) or greater, depending on the individual requirements (Table 76-2).
2. Maintenance fluid requirements: Calculate the maintenance IV fluid requirement based on the patient's weight, body surface area, and medical condition.
3. Determine contribution of energy from fat, dextrose, and amino acids: Order a solution that delivers 20% to 30% of the calories from fat and 60% to 70% from the dextrose and amino acid solution. In general, an appropriate solution has 40% to 60 % of the calories from dextrose and a glucose infusion rate (GIR) of 6 to 14 mg/kg/minute.
4. Volume of lipid: Divide the energy required from fat (in kcal/day) by 2 kcal/mL to determine the milliliters per day of lipid. Generally, a patient will tolerate 20% to 40% of total calories supplied by the fat emulsion, but avoid more than 50% to 60%, which may result in ketosis. IV fat may be administered on the same day as amino acid and dextrose initiation. Initiate fat delivery at 2 to 5 mL/kg/day and increase in a stepwise fashion to a goal of 5 to 10 mL/kg/day, or approximately 30% of the daily caloric intake. One determinant of the rate of fat clearance is the amount infused per unit time. Thus the longer the infusion time the less likely the patient will experience intolerance (hypertriglyceridemia).
5. Determine the energy density for amino acid–dextrose solution: From Table 76-3, choose the concentrations of amino acids and dextrose that are desired.

Table 76-2. Protein Needs Are Estimated Based on ASPEN Clinical Guidelines[a]	
Age (Years)	**Protein Recommendations (g/kg/day)**
0–2	2.5–3
2–13	1.5–2
13–18	1.5

Abbreviation: ASPEN, American Society of Parenteral and Enteral Nutrition.

[a]Adapted from Mehta NM, Compher C; ASPEN Board of Directors: ASPEN clinical guidelines: nutrition support of the critically ill child. *J Parenter Enteral Nutr.* 2009;33:260–276.

Table 76-3. Energy Density of Solution (kcal/mL of Total Parenteral Nutrition)[a]

		% Amino Acids								
		1	**2.2**	**2.4**	**2.8**	**3**	**3.5**	**4**	**5**	**6**
% Dextrose	**7.5**	0.30	0.34	0.36	0.37	0.38	0.40	0.42	0.46	0.50
	10	0.38	0.43	0.44	0.45	0.46	0.48	0.50	0.54	0.58
	12.5	0.47	0.51	0.51	0.54	0.55	0.57	0.59	0.63	0.67
	15	0.55	0.60	0.61	0.62	0.63	0.65	0.67	0.71	0.75
	17.5	0.64	0.68	0.69	0.71	0.72	0.74	0.76	0.80	0.84
	20	0.72	0.77	0.78	0.79	0.80	0.82	0.84	0.88	0.92
	25	0.89	0.94	0.95	0.96	0.97	0.99	1.01	1.05	1.09
	30	1.06	1.11	1.1	1.13	1.14	1.16	1.18	1.22	1.26
	35	1.23	1.28	1.29	1.30	1.31	1.33	1.35	1.39	1.43
	40	1.40	1.45	1.46	1.47	1.48	1.50	1.52	1.56	1.60

[a]Adapted from Bunting KD, Mills J, Phillips S. *Texas Children's Hospital Pediatric Nutrition Reference Guide.* 9th ed. Houston, TX: Texas Children's Hospital; 2010.

6. Volume for amino acid–dextrose solution: Divide the energy from amino acids and dextrose (from Step 3) by the energy density of the solution (Table 76-3). Compare the protein provided with estimated protein needs (grams per day).
7. Total protein (g) × 100 = % protein (mL of amino acid/% dextrose)
8. Determine electrolyte dosages: Table 76-4
9. The addition of the vitamins, minerals, and trace elements is weight-based. Most hospitals will automatically add these to PN.
10. Advancing PN: Table 76-5.

Table 76-4. Parenteral Nutrition Electrolyte Dosing Guidelines[a,b]

Electrolyte	Preterm Neonate	Infant/Child	Adolescent/Child >50 kg
Sodium	2–5 mEq/kg	2–5 mEq/kg	1–2 mEq/kg
Potassium	2–4 mEq/kg	2–4 mEq/kg	1–2 mEq/kg
Calcium	2–4 mEq/kg	0.5–4 mEq/k	10–20 mEq/day
Phosphorus	1–2 mmol/kg	0.5–2 mmol/kg	10–40 mmol/day
Magnesium	0.3–0.5 mEq/kg	0.3–0.5 mEq/kg	10–30 mEq/day
Acetate	As needed to maintain acid base-balance		
Chloride	As needed to maintain acid base-balance		

[a]Adapted from Mirtallo J, Canada T, Johnson D, et al. Safe practices for parenteral nutrition. *J Parenter Enteral Nutr.* 2004;28:S39–S70, with permission.
[b]Assumes normal organ function and losses.

Table 76-5. Recommendations for Initiation and Advancement of Parenteral Nutrition[a]

	Initiation		Advance By		Goals	
Infant (<1 year of age)						
	Preterm	Term	Preterm	Term	Preterm	Term
Protein (g/kg/day)	1.5–3	1	1	1	3–4	2–3
Carbohydrate (mg/kg/min)	5–7	6–9	1%–2.5% dextrose/day	1–2 or 2.5%–5% dextrose/day	8–12 14–18 max	12 14–18 max
Fat (g/kg/day)	1–2	1–2	0.5–1	0.5–1	3–3.5 0.17 g/kg/h max	3 0.15 g/kg/h max
Child (1–10 years of age)						
Protein (g/kg/day)	1–2		1		1.5–3	
Carbohydrate (mg/kg/min)	10% dextrose		5% dextrose/day		8–10	
Fat (g/kg/day)	1–2		0.5–1		2–3	
Adolescent						
Protein (g/kg/day)	0.8–1.5		1		0.8–2.5	
Carbohydrate (mg/kg/min)	3.5 or 10% dextrose		1–2 or 5% dextrose per day		5–6	
Fat (g/kg/day)	1		1		1–2.5	

[a]Adapted from Corkins MR, ed. *The ASPEN Pediatric Nutrition Support Core Curriculum*. Silver Spring, MD: American Society for Parenteral and Enteral Nutrition; 2010, with permission.

Complications

Complications related to PN administration can be categorized as metabolic, mechanical, and infectious. Metabolic complications include electrolyte abnormalities related to refeeding syndrome (significant decreases in potassium, phosphorous, and magnesium), drug nutrient interactions (furosemide, amphotericin), or metabolic acidosis. The exact cause of PN-related complications is unknown, but there are several factors that increase the risk: intestinal resection, recurrent episodes of infection, lack of enteral feeds, or overfeeding of carbohydrate or protein. The severity of injury varies from minimal, with transient increases in liver-related blood tests to biliary cirrhosis and, ultimately, liver failure. The younger the patient, the greater the risk of developing refeeding syndrome. Mechanical problems include line occlusions related to precipitants (calcium and phosphorus, drug or lipid), line fractures (due to excessive pressure), and kinks in the line.

Monitoring PN

Monitoring PN includes the routine assessment of metabolic factors as well as growth, developmental, and psychological parameters (Table 76-6). Initial laboratory assessment is based on the patient's nutritional status, medical condition, and medications. Subsequently, measure the serum electrolytes and blood sugar daily until full PN is achieved and the electrolytes are stable. Provide meticulous attention to blood drawing procedures. Discontinue all fluid infusions prior to phlebotomy, minimize the blood volumes withdrawn, and time these measurements with the middle or latter end of the PN infusion to minimize spurious results. In addition, limiting entry into the line will decrease the risk of developing iatrogenic blood stream infections.

An initial or baseline measurement of serum proteins, calcium, magnesium, phosphorous, and triglycerides may be helpful in some patients (eg, malnutrition, liver or renal disease, sepsis). A patient with significant malnutrition, liver or metabolic diseases, or at risk for refeeding syndrome may require more frequent monitoring of some electrolytes and minerals.

Glucose

Monitoring the urine glucose and blood glucose levels, as well as calculating the GIR (mg glucose/kg/minute) is important for minimizing the potential complications of overfeeding this nutrient. Insulin increases potassium, magnesium, and phosphorous uptake by the cells. Therefore, these minerals will also need to be monitored frequently with insulin use. Measure blood glucose in patients on cyclic (<24 hours) PN at the beginning, middle, and end of the cycle to assess tolerance.

Fat

A malnourished patient will have a decreased capillary mass and, as a result, less lipoprotein lipase, which resides there. Therefore, a malnourished patient will have a slower rate of lipid clearance. IV fat tolerance may need to be monitored more frequently than suggested in Table 76-6 in such a patient.

Table 76-6. Monitoring Parenteral Nutrition in Pediatrics[a]

Parameter	Initial	Follow-up
Growth		
Weight	Daily	Daily to monthly
Length/stature	Weekly to monthly	Monthly
Head circumference	Weekly	Weekly to monthly
Body composition	Monthly	Monthly to annually
Metabolic: Serum		
Electrolytes	Daily to weekly	Weekly to monthly
BUN/creatinine	Weekly	Weekly to monthly
Ca, PO_4, Mg	Twice weekly	Weekly to monthly
Acid/base	As indicated until stable	Weekly to monthly
Albumin/prealbumin	Weekly or every other week	2 weeks to monthly
Glucose	Daily to weekly	Weekly to monthly
Triglyceride	Daily with changes	Weekly to monthly
Liver function	At 2 weeks	Weekly to monthly
CBC	Weekly	Weekly to monthly
PT/PTT and platelets	Weekly	Weekly to monthly
Iron indices	As indicated	Every 3–4 months
Trace elements	Monthly	Every 6–12 months
Fat-soluble vitamins	As indicated	Every 6–12 months
Carnitine	As indicated	Every 6–12 months
Folate/B_{12}	As indicated	Every 6–12 months
Ammonia	As indicated	As indicated
Metabolic: Urine		
Glucose/ketones	2–6 times per day	Daily to weekly
Specific gravity Urea nitrogen	As indicated	As indicated
Other		
Bone Density	As Indicated	As indicated
Verify line placement	As indicated with growth	Every 6–12 months
Developmental	Monthly	Every 6–12 months
Occupational therapy Physical therapy	At 1 month, as indicated	Annually

Abbreviations: Ca, calcium; CBC, complete blood cell count; BUN, blood urea nitrogen; Mg, magnesium; PO_4, phosphate; PT, prothrombin time; PTT, partial thromboplastin time.

[a]Adapted from Davis AM. Initiation, monitoring, and complications of pediatric parenteral nutrition. In: Chernoff R, ed. *Pediatric Parenteral Nutrition*. New York, NY: Chapman and Hall; 1997:212–237. Reprinted with permission.

Protein

In addition to the traditional protein monitors (albumin, prealbumin, transthyretin, transferrin), a patient receiving PN may need other parameters measured as well. In liver disease, the serum ammonia may need to be followed if the patient has elevated direct bilirubin and transaminases. In a patient with short gut, malabsorption, or protein-losing enteropathy, there is an increased loss of enteric protein, so that fecal α-1-antitrypsin excretion is useful in assessing protein losses and the need for additional protein intake. The blood urea nitrogen can also be used, if renal function and hydration are normal.

Liver Function Tests

Liver injury is associated with PN therapy. Monitor liver function (aspartate transaminase, alanine transaminase, γ-glutamyltransferase, bilirubin, prothrombin time, partial thromboplastin time) if the patient receives PN for 2 weeks or longer. A patient with liver disease or no enteral intake will need more frequent assessments (weekly or greater).

Pearls and Pitfalls

Vitamin, mineral, and amino acid shortages make PN order writing a challenge. Maintain an ongoing dialogue with the nutrition support team and clinical pharmacist.

- Iron is not routinely added to parenteral nutrition solutions. A patient on long-term (>1 month) PN may need IV iron infusions if unable to tolerate oral intake.
- Sodium bicarbonate is contraindicated in PN solutions as it will change the pH of the solution and may result in calcium/phosphorous precipitation. Sodium or potassium acetate may be added, but some patients may require additional bicarbonate administration through a separate line.

Bibliography

American Academy of Pediatrics. Parenteral nutrition. In: Kleinman RE, ed. *Pediatric Nutrition Handbook*. Elk Grove Village, IL: American Academy of Pediatrics; 2009: 519–540

Bunting, D Mills J, Phillips, S, et al. *Pediatric Nutrition Reference Guide*. 9th ed. Houston, TXs: Texas Children's Hospital; 2010

Corkins MR. *The A.S.P.E.N. Pediatric Nutrition Support Core Curriculum*. Silver Spring, MD: American Society for Parenteral and Enteral Nutrition; 2010

Mehta NM, Compher C; A.S.P.E.N. Board of Directors. A.S.P.E.N. clinical guidelines: nutrition support of the critically ill child. *J Parenter Enteral Nutr.* 2009;33:260–276

Shulman RJ, Phillips P. Parenteral nutrition indications, administration, and monitoring. In: Baker S, Baker RD, Davis AM, eds. *Pediatric Nutrition Support.* Missiassauga, Ontario: Jones and Bartlett Publishers; 2007:273–286

Singla S, Olsson JM. Enteral nutrition. In: Perkin R, Swift J, Newton D, Anas N, eds. *Pediatric Hospital Medicine.* 2nd ed. Philadelphia, PA: Lippincott, Williams & Wilkins; 2008:797–808

Ophthalmology

CHAPTER 77

Acute Vision Loss in the Hospitalized Child

Introduction

Acute vision loss may be secondary to pathology in the cornea, lens, vitreous, retina, optic nerve, or the central nervous system (CNS). Vision loss in a hospitalized child can occur secondary to a serious systemic condition (malignant hypertension, meningitis).

In the context of trauma, vision loss may be related to traumatic iritis, hyphema, optic nerve avulsion, vitreous hemorrhage, retinal detachment, or a perforated globe. However, vision loss does not always present with ocular abnormalities, as it may represent a neuro-visual pathway disorder, ranging from chiasmal pathology to other CNS diseases.

Acute vision loss can often be associated with a red eye, which may or may not be painful. Uveitis is a common cause of vision loss and can be secondary to an underlying systemic illness such as juvenile idiopathic arthritis. In addition, conjunctivitis (from various etiologies), chemical injuries, microbial keratitis, acute glaucoma, and endophthalmitis can present similarly.

Clinical Presentation

History

Ask about any recent facial trauma, history of a red eye, ocular discharge, illnesses or infections, and a very detailed review of systems (including fevers, weight loss, weakness, etc). In general, very young children may have difficulty verbalizing vision loss. However, the parents may be able to detect subtle acute visual changes based on the patient's behavior.

Physical Examination

Check the visual acuity in each eye, using a near vision card. If testing is unsuccessful, check the ability to discern light or fingers at a close distance. The visual acuity may range from just slightly diminished to no light perception, in one or both eyes. In the hospital setting, check the visual acuity daily to monitor for any changes. The pupillary examination is a priority, especially in a patient with functional vision loss.

Depending on the etiology, the external examination may range from normal to evidence of facial trauma (eyelid edema, erythema, ecchymosis) or eyelid inflammation. Evaluation of the visual fields is important to rule out a homonymous defect. Examine the red reflex, which will be abnormal if there is an obstruction anterior to the retina or a central retinal artery occlusion. Perform or arrange for a slit lamp examination, to assess the clarity of the cornea, anterior chamber, lens, and vitreous, as well as a dilated fundoscopic examination to evaluate for vitreous, retinal, or optic nerve issues, such as vitreous hemorrhage, retinal detachment, vascular occlusions, optic nerve pallor, and retinal hemorrhages.

Laboratory

Order either computed tomography or magnetic resonance imaging (MRI) of the brain and orbits to evaluate for orbital trauma; orbital cellulitis; globe trauma; optic neuritis; intraocular foreign body (do not obtain an MRI if the object might be metallic); or a tumor of the orbit, optic nerve, or globe. If the ophthalmology examination reveals evidence of uveitis or a neuroretinitis, obtain a complete blood cell count, rapid plasma reagin, fluorescent treponemal antibody–absorbent, blood culture, rheumatoid factor, and antinuclear antibodies, and place a purified protein derivative. A lumbar puncture is indicated if there is a concern for neurologic issues, such as a meningitis or neuromyelitis optica.

Differential Diagnosis

It is essential to identify the potential location of the abnormality causing the acute decrease in vision. This typically is (1) an opacification of the normally transparent ocular structures (cornea, lens, anterior chamber, vitreous), (2) a retinal abnormality, or (3) an abnormality of the optic nerve or visual pathways. The external examination, pupil reactivity, slit lamp examination, and fundus examination are critical in the evaluation of the child with acute vision loss, and immediate ophthalmology consultation is warranted if a gross abnormality is noted. However, with CNS pathology the patient may not have any other abnormal neurologic or physical examination findings. The ophthalmologic causes of acute vision loss are summarized in Table 77-1.

Treatment

Treatment will generally be determined by the consulting ophthalmologist, along with neurology and/or neurosurgery consults, depending on the underlying etiology. Acute vision loss due to an intracranial mass may be life-threatening and requires an urgent neurosurgical consult and management. In contrast, retinal detachment and dense vitreous hemorrhage are not urgent causes of vision loss. Arrange for outpatient ophthalmology follow-up with surgical correction in the near future.

Table 77-1. Ophthalmologic Causes of Acute Vision Loss	
Diagnosis	**Clinical Features**
Chemical injury	Photophobia, blepharospasm Ischemia of the conjunctiva Altered pH of the ocular surface
Endophthalmitis	Painful red eye
Glaucoma	Photophobia Corneal clouding Enlarged eye
Keratitis	Painful red eye Ocular discharge Corneal opacity
Orbital cellulitis	Fever, toxicity Proptosis, chemosis Decreased extraocular motility

The treatment of a perforated globe (page 537) and orbital cellulitis (page 119) is detailed elsewhere in this text.

Indications for Consultation

- **Neurology:** Migraines, multiple sclerosis
- **Neurosurgery:** Suspected intracranial mass, subdural hematoma or abscess, hydrocephalus
- **Ophthalmology:** Acute vision loss
- **Otolaryngology:** Orbital cellulitis associated with sinusitis

Disposition

- **Intensive care unit transfer:** Subdural or intracranial hemorrhage, intracranial extension of orbital cellulitis, intracranial mass with midline shift
- **Discharge criteria:** Visual acuity stable or improving on oral (or no) medication and any concerns about inflicted trauma have been addressed

Follow-up

- **Ophthalmology:** Daily or weekly, depending on the etiology
- **Other subspecialists (otorhinolaryngology, neurosurgery, neurology):** Depending on the etiology

Pearls and Pitfalls

- Acute vision loss in a child may represent a life-threatening condition, necessitating urgent evaluation.
- Vision loss does not always present with ocular abnormalities.

Coding

ICD-9

- Acute and subacute iridocyclitis, unspecified **364.00**
- Acute endophthalmitis **360.01**
- Central opacity of cornea **371.03**
- Glaucoma associated with ocular trauma **365.65**
- Optic neuritis, unspecified **377.30**
- Orbital cellulitis **376.01**
- Primary optic atrophy **377.11**
- Retinal detachment with retinal defect unspecified **361.00**
- Unspecified visual loss **369.9**
- Vitreous hemorrhage **379.23**

Bibliography

Beran DI, Murphy-Lavoie H. Acute, painless vision loss. *J La State Med Soc.* 2009;161: 214–216, 218–223

Goold L, Durkin S, Crompton J. Sudden loss of vision—history and examination. *Aust Fam Physician.* 2009;38:764–767

Goold L, Durkin S, Crompton J. Sudden loss of vision—investigation and management. *Aust Fam Physician.* 2009;38:770–772

Vortmann M, Schneider JI. Acute monocular visual loss. *Emerg Med Clin North Am.* 2008;26:73–96

Ocular Trauma

Ocular trauma is a leading cause of vision loss in children. Traumatic injury may broadly be classified as either an open or closed globe. The defining feature of "closed globe" versus "open globe" injury is a full-thickness wound of the eye wall (either sclera or cornea). Within the closed globe category, there is contusion, lamellar laceration, or extraocular injury. Within the open globe category, there is rupture, penetrating laceration, or perforating laceration. An open globe injury may also be complicated by a retained foreign body.

Ocular trauma injuries requiring urgent care include an open globe, traumatic optic neuropathy, extraocular muscle entrapment (secondary to orbital fracture), rhegmatogenous retinal detachment, and retrobulbar hemorrhage.

Clinical Presentation

History

Obtain a detailed account of the injury, including time, location (periorbital, head), mechanism of injury (hit with what), extent (how hard and how many times), and whether there are any other associated injuries. Determine the patient's visual function prior to injury (history of amblyopia, strabismus, patching) and inquire about prior head, periorbital, or ocular trauma and surgery.

Assess the pain level and qualifiers (onset, location, duration, quality, severity, associated symptoms), changes in vision (decreased, flashes, floaters, curtain), diplopia (monocular or binocular, variation with gaze), foreign body sensation, tearing, and photophobia.

Physical Examination

Ocular trauma has a highly variable presentation and requires a comprehensive examination. However, the priorities are visual acuity, pupillary response, and pressure. *Prior to dilation,* perform a careful pupil examination looking for relative afferent pupillary defect, which may indicate significant retinal or optic nerve pathology, which then necessitates special attention paid to the visual field and color perception examinations. If the patient cannot cooperate for a comprehensive examination, arrange for an examination under anesthesia.

On external examination, note ecchymoses and edema of periorbital soft tissues, subcutaneous emphysema, palpable step-off along the orbital rim, enophthalmos/hypoglobus, proptosis, lacerations of the globe or periorbital tissues, and evidence of foreign body.

For lacerations external to the globe, assess if there is lid margin or canalicular (medial to the puncta) involvement of the laceration or violation of the septum (prolapsed orbital fat).

One of the few true ocular emergencies is an open globe. This is a potentially sight-threatening and organ-threatening injury. However, on examination a full-thickness violation of either the sclera or cornea is not always evident. Signs of a potential open globe include prolapse of uveal tissue, severe subconjunctival hemorrhage, deep or shallow anterior chamber (shine a light held at the lateral aspect of the globe, looking to see if the iris fully illuminates), hyphema, peaked or irregular pupil, laceration of the cornea or sclera, and an intraocular foreign body. If the clinical picture is suspicious for an open globe, *do not* place pressure on the globe during examination, check ocular pressure or motility, or dilate the pupil. To assess for the presence of occult leaking aqueous or exposed vitreous, an ophthalmologist may perform a Seidel test. When fluorescein is diluted (by a leak), it appears bright green instead of orange under cobalt blue light.

Motility is another critical part of the examination. The patient may present with the "white eyed" orbital blowout fracture, in which the eye is relatively well-appearing and the child may also be asymptomatic. "Greenstick" fractures are common in children and are more liable to create a "trapdoor" phenomenon of entrapping and incarcerating soft tissue. Restriction secondary to tissue entrapment is an urgent condition, as prolonged entrapment can result in ischemia and fibrosis. Entrapment may also cause decreased pulse rate via the oculocardiac reflex. The ophthalmologist may perform forced duction testing to rule out a mechanical restriction.

Arrange for a slit lamp and dilated fundus examination to assess the anterior and posterior segments. This can be essential for diagnosing a variety of the closed globe injuries, including corneal abrasion, traumatic iritis, hyphema, commotio retinae, choroidal rupture, non-accidental trauma, vitreous hemorrhage, and retinal detachment. Note that with non-accidental trauma, external eye findings are frequently absent.

Laboratory

If hyphema is observed, order a screen for sickle cell trait or disease. Sickle cell disease places the patient at greater risk of the complications of hyphema, such as increased intraocular pressure, non-clearing hyphema, and corneal blood staining.

Radiology

Imaging of choice for acute ocular trauma is a computed tomography (CT) of the face and orbits with axial and coronal views and 1- to 2-mm sections without contrast. The CT is helpful for assessing an open globe, traumatic optic neuropathy, entrapment secondary to orbital fracture, and retrobulbar hemorrhage. A CT can also demonstrate the integrity and shape of the globe and the presence and location of intraocular foreign bodies. Magnetic resonance imaging is contraindicated if a metallic retained foreign body is suspected.

Diagnosis

Generally, the definitive diagnostic workup will be dictated by the consulting ophthalmologist.

Treatment

If the clinical picture is suspicious for an open globe, place a Fox shield *(do not patch or apply pressure)* over the traumatized eye and determine the time of the patient's last meal, and make the child NPO. Order the above-mentioned CT series to rule out intraocular foreign body, update the patient's tetanus status, and administer intravenous antibiotics, antiemetics, and pain medications as necessary. Consult with ophthalmology, as urgent surgery is necessary.

Entrapment secondary to orbital fracture also requires urgent surgery within 48 hours to avoid ischemia and fibrosis. Other indications for orbital fracture repair include enophthalmos greater than 2 mm, greater than 50% floor fracture, and functional diplopia secondary to restriction with positive forced ductions. Depending on the time of the injury and macular involvement, a retinal detachment may also require urgent surgical intervention.

Retrobulbar hemorrhage may require emergent intervention if it causes changes in vision or pupils, or elevated intraocular pressure. Discuss assessing central retinal artery perfusion and performing lateral canthotomy and cantholysis with an ophthalmologist.

Consult with ophthalmology to determine whether a course of high-dose steroids is indicated in treating traumatic optic neuropathy.

Ophthalmology may manage both traumatic iritis and hyphema with cycloplegia and topical steroids. However, a hyphema will be followed closely due to the risk of secondary complications such as re-bleeding, elevated intraocular pressure, and corneal blood staining.

Remove a superficial corneal foreign body with irrigation, moistened cotton-tip swab, or a needle tip under slit lamp guidance. However, always assess for a full-thickness penetration. Also evert the eyelids and sweep the fornices for particulate matter. Treat a simple corneal abrasion with topical antibiotics, cycloplegia, and artificial tears.

A lid laceration, especially involving the lower lid canaliculus, will require surgical intervention.

Many closed globe injuries do not require acute intervention. However, close follow-up may be required to monitor for long-term sequelae (traumatic cataract, angle recession, retinal detachment, and choroidal neovascularization).

If there is suspicion for non-accidental trauma (page 587), contact child protective services, assess for other potential injuries, and admit the patient pending investigation.

Indications for Consultation

- **Child protection services:** Inflicted trauma
- **Ear, nose, throat/facial surgery team:** Orbital or facial fractures
- **Neurosurgery:** Orbital roof fracture
- **Ophthalmology:** Acute vision loss, open globe, orbital fracture with entrapment, lid laceration

Disposition

- **Interinstitutional transfer:** Ophthalmology services are not immediately available
- **Discharge criteria:** Vision stable and surgical issues resolved

Follow-up

- **Primary care:** 1 to 2 weeks
- **Ophthalmology:** Varies, depending on the nature of the injuries

Pearls and Pitfalls

- An open globe, entrapment secondary to orbital fracture, retinal detachment, and retrobulbar hemorrhage all require urgent surgical intervention.
- Note the "white-eyed" blow-out fracture and carefully assess for motility restriction, decreased pulse, and other signs of parasympathetic surge in the context of orbital fracture or eye movement.
- Investigate any abnormality of the ocular vitals: vision, pupils, and intraocular pressure.

Coding

ICD-9

- Secondary noninfectious iridocyclitis **364.04**
- Acute endophthalmitis **360.01**
- Glaucoma associated with ocular trauma **365.65**
- Orbital disorders, unspecified **376.9**
- Retinal detachment with retinal defect **361.00**
- Vitreous hemorrhage **379.23**

Bibliography

Ehlers JP, Shah CP. *The Will's Eye Manual.* 5th ed. Baltimore, MD: Lippincott, Williams & Wilkins; 2008:12–48

Garcia TA, McGetrick BA, Janik JS. Ocular injuries in children after major trauma. *J Pediatr Ophthalmol Strabismus.* 2005;42:349–354

Kanski JJ, Bowling B. *Clinical Ophthalmology: A Systematic Approach.* 7th ed. New York, NY: Elsevier Saunders; 2011:871–896

Levine LM. Pediatric ocular trauma and shaken infant syndrome. *Pediatr Clin North Am.* 2003;50:137–148

Salvin JH. Systematic approach to pediatric ocular trauma. *Curr Opin Ophthalmol.* 2007; 18:366–372

Upshaw JE, Brenkert TE, Losek JD. Ocular foreign bodies in children. *Pediatr Emerg Care.* 2008;24:409–414

Red Eye

Introduction

The pediatric "red eye" is one of the most common inpatient ophthalmologic diagnoses. It describes a large breadth of infectious or inflammatory conditions that may originate from the lids, conjunctiva, cornea, iris, sclera, or other internal ocular tissues. Serious etiologies of the red eye include infectious conjunctivitis in a newborn, keratoconjunctivitis, foreign body, orbital trauma, and systemic or autoimmune diseases.

Ophthalmia neonatorum is a bacterial conjunctivitis in an infant younger than 4 weeks and is usually caused by *Neisseria gonorrhea* and/or *Chlamydia trachomatis*. These infections are an ophthalmologic emergency.

Clinical Presentation

History

Obtain a thorough history of ocular and systemic symptoms, including the onset and duration of symptoms, visual changes, photophobia, discharge, burning, itching, and constitutional symptoms. Also ask about contact lens use, ocular medications, prior ophthalmologic surgery, and past episodes of red eye. The presence of eye pain suggests a foreign body, corneal abrasion or ulcer, herpes keratitis, trauma, or scleral or episcleral inflammation.

Physical Examination

First, observe the patient's spontaneous eye movements. Note areas of color change, edema, or discharge in the periorbital region, conjunctiva, and sclera. Use a light source to directly evaluate the pupil size and reactivity. Assess the presence, symmetry, and color of the red reflex with a direct ophthalmoscope in a dimly lit room. Assess visual acuity, if the patient is able. Perform a fluorescein stain examination to rule out a corneal abrasion/ulcer, herpes keratitis, or globe penetration. Evert the lid to look for the presence of a foreign body.

Differential Diagnosis

The priority is to expeditiously diagnose eye- or vision-threatening conditions. Warning signs include altered visual acuity, ocular pain, severe photophobia, excessive tearing, and a ciliary flush (Table 79-1).

Table 79-1. Differential Diagnosis of the Red Eye	
Diagnosis	**Clinical Features**
Allergic conjunctivitis	Itching and tearing Conjunctival bogginess and injection
Congenital glaucoma	Photophobia, blepharospasm Buphthalmos (enlargement of the eyeball) Increased intraocular pressure
Chemical conjunctivitis	Starts in the first 24 hours of life Bilateral watery discharge and bulbar injection
Corneal ulcer	Pain, tearing, blepharospasm Fluorescein (+) Decreased visual acuity
Dacryocystitis	Fever Erythema, swelling, and tenderness lateral to the medial canthus
Herpes keratoconjunctivitis	Pain, photophobia Vesicles on eyelids Fluorescein (+)
Infectious conjunctivitis	Bacterial: copious purulence at the lid margin Viral: watery discharge, upper respiratory infection prodrome
Keratitis	Pain, photophobia Conjunctival hyperemia Fluorescein (+)
Ophthalmia neonatorum (gonococcal)	2–5 days of life Hyperacute purulent discharge Chemosis, eyelid edema Gram stain: gram-negative diplococci
Ophthalmia neonatorum (chlamydial)	5–14 days of life Watery to mucopurulent discharge, (+) Direct fluorescent antibody or enzyme-linked immunosorbent assay
Scleritis	Pain, decreased vision Violet discoloration of the globe Anterior chamber inflammation
Subconjunctival hemorrhage	Confluent, bright red patch Does not extend past the limbus
Uveitis	Pain, photophobia, redness with ciliary flush Constricted and irregular pupil Decreased visual acuity

Laboratory

Routine laboratory testing is unhelpful in most cases of a red eye. If there is a purulent discharge, particularly in the first 2 weeks of life, swab for culture and Gram stain. If gonococcal ophthalmia neonatorum is suspected, perform a full sepsis workup, including a lumbar puncture. In cases of uveitis or scleritis obtain a complete blood cell count with differential, C-reactive protein or erythrocyte sedimentation rate, antinuclear antibody, rheumatoid factor, and uric acid.

If herpes infection is suspected in an infant younger than 6 weeks, obtain herpes simplex virus DNA via polymerase chain reaction from the cerebrospinal fluid. In addition, confirm the infection with swabs of the mouth, oropharynx, conjunctiva, rectum, and any surface lesions. Also obtain liver function tests and urine for herpes culture.

Treatment

Due to the highly specialized nature of treatment, consult an ophthalmologist prior to initiating therapy for glaucoma, uveitis, scleritis, or infectious/noninfectious corneal disease. If ocular herpes infection is suspected, immediately initiate intravenous (IV) acyclovir (60 mg/kg/day divided 3 times a day) for 14 days. Add a topical ophthalmic antiviral (1% trifluridine, 0.1% iododeoxyuridine, 3% vidarabine).

Neonatorum ophthalmia is an ocular emergency and warrants urgent ophthalmology consult. Treat with either ceftriaxone (25–50 mg/kg every day IV or intramuscular [IM], 125 mg maximum) or cefotaxime (50 mg/kg IV or IM every 12 hours <7 days old, every 8 hours >7 days). Order sterile saline eye irrigations every 2 hours to keep the eye surface clear of debris, discharge, and obstruction. Treat chlamydia with oral erythromycin (50 mg/kg/day divided every 6 hours) for 14 days.

Treat acute dacryocystitis with either ampicillin-sulbactam (150 mg/kg/day divided every 6 hours, 8 g/day maximum) or cefuroxime (100 mg/kg/day divided every 8 hours, 4.5 g/day maximum). If methicillin-resistant *Staphylococcal aureus* is a concern, add clindamycin (40 mg/kg/day divided every 6 hours, 4.8 g/day maximum) or vancomycin (40 mg/kg/day divided every 6 hours, 4 g/day maximum) after obtaining cultures of the discharge. Warm compresses may help with disease resolution. Immediate ophthalmology consultation is indicated.

Treat conjunctivitis with a topical antibiotic ointment (bacitracin, polymixin B, tobramycin) or solution (ciprofloxacin, ofloxacin, polymixin B, tobramycin) applied 3 times a day. Use a fluoroquinolone (ciprofloxacin, ofloxacin) when treating a pseudomonas corneal ulcer or conjunctivitis in a contact lens wearer.

Indications for Consultation

- **Ophthalmology:** Moderate or severe ocular pain, altered visual acuity, severe photophobia, excessive tearing, ciliary flush, corneal opacity, ophthalmia neonatorum, ocular herpes, and dacryocystitis

Disposition

- **Discharge criteria:** Good response to treatment, identification and sensitivity of infection (if any) known, close ophthalmology follow-up arranged

Pearls and Pitfalls

- Proceed with caution when adding steroids to the treatment regimen for infectious conjunctivitis as herpes keratitis will worsen.
- Antibiotic ointment is preferred in children due to difficulty with achieving appropriate antibiotic levels with drops.
- If drops are prescribed, apply them to the inner canthus (eye closed for best dosing).

Coding

ICD-9

- Conjunctivitis, acute unspecified **372.00**
- Corneal ulcer, unspecified **370.00**
- Dacryocystitis, unspecified **375.30**
- Glaucoma, unspecified **365.9**
- Gonococcal ophthalmia (infant) **098.40**
- Herpetic keratitis **054.43**
- Iridocyclitis, acute, unspecified **364.00**
- Keratoconjunctivitis, unspecified **370.40**
- Ophthalmia neonatorum **771.6**
- Scleritis, unspecified **379.00**

Bibliography

Cronau H, Kankanala RR, Mauger T. Diagnosis and management of red eye in primary care. *Am Fam Physician.* 2010;81:137–144

Granet D. Allergic rhinoconjunctivitis and differential diagnosis of the red eye. *Allergy Asthma Proc.* 2008;29:565–574

Prentiss KA, Dorfman DH. Pediatric ophthalmology in the emergency department. *Emerg Med Clin North Am.* 2008;26:181–198

Sethuraman U, Kamat D. The red eye: evaluation and management. *Clin Pediatr (Phila).* 2009;48:588–600

CHAPTER 80

White Eye

Introduction

The red reflex is a simple, yet imperative screening test that may alert a physician to ocular disease. A white reflex is called leukocoria and may represent significant ocular pathology, such as a retinoblastoma, cataracts, glaucoma, and infections (syphilis, toxoplasmosis, tuberculosis).

Clinical Presentation

History

Leukocoria is predominantly diagnosed by physical examination. However, the abnormal red reflex may first be noticed in a photograph of the child, when one pupil appears red while the other is darker or white. Ask about past eye trauma and a family history of ocular tumors, cataracts, or glaucoma. The parent of an infant may report that the patient is frequently poking and rubbing the eyes.

Physical Examination

Check the red reflex in a dimly lit room using the largest white light of an ophthalmoscope from a distance of 2 to 3 feet. Visualize both eyes and compare the red reflex size and color. Instead of the typical red light reflex, the center of one or both eyes will appear to have a bright white appearance.

Laboratory

No immediate laboratory tests are indicated on discovering a white reflex.

Differential Diagnosis

The most common causes of leukocoria are retinopathy of prematurity, cataracts, persistent hyperplastic primary vitreous, coloboma, and Coat disease. Neonatal infections, which can result in a white ocular reflex, include *Toxocara canis*, toxoplasmosis, and syphilis. Retinoblastoma, one of the most common ocular malignancies of childhood, also presents with leukocoria.

Treatment

Immediately consult an ophthalmologist if there is any suspicion of leukocoria.

Indications for Consultation

- **Pediatric ophthalmologist:** All patients
- **Pediatric hematologist/oncologist:** Any suspicion of retinoblastoma

Disposition

- **Discharge criteria:** Evaluation complete and appropriate treatment plan arranged

Pearls

- Failure to dim the lights in the examination room may yield false-negative red reflex results.
- Urgent ophthalmology referral is indicated for any red reflex abnormality.

Coding

ICD-9

• Cataract, unspecified	**366.9**
• Leukocoria	**360.44**
• Retinoblastoma	**190.5**
• Retinopathy of prematurity	**362.2x**

— Use one of these digits for the fifth digit (x) to identify stage
- 0 unspecified
- 2 stage 0
- 3 stage 1
- 4 stage 2
- 5 stage 3
- 6 stage 4
- 7 stage 5

Bibliography

Haider S, Qureshi W, Ali A. Leukocoria in children. *J Pediatr Ophthalmol Strabismus.* 2008;45:179–180

McLaughlin C, Levin AV. The red reflex. *Pediatr Emerg Care.* 2006;22:137–140

Simon JW, Kaw P. Commonly missed diagnoses in the childhood eye examination. *Am Fam Physician.* 2001;64:623–628

Orthopaedics

Fractures

Introduction

The 3 main causes of fractures are accidental trauma (most common), non-accidental trauma (child abuse), and abnormal bone (pathologic fractures). The most common fractures necessitating inpatient treatment involve the femur, tibia-fibula, elbow (supracondylar), and pelvis.

Fractures are categorized as displaced or non-displaced and open or closed. In a displaced fracture, the bone snaps into 2 or more parts. If the bone is in many pieces, it is called a comminuted fracture. In a non-displaced fracture, the bone either partially breaks or completely breaks, but maintains its proper alignment. An open fracture is one in which the bone breaks through the skin. A closed fracture is when the bone breaks but there is no open wound in the skin.

The most serious direct complications of a fracture are infection, neurovascular compromise (most common with supracondylar fractures), and compartment syndrome, when ischemia is caused by tissue pressure that exceeds the arteriolar and capillary pressures. The causes of compartment syndrome include hematoma and soft-tissue swelling, particularly under a newly placed cast or splint.

Clinical Presentation

History

Attempt to determine the mechanism of injury. Ask about the type and direction of the injuring force, position of the involved bone(s) at that time, and the events immediately following the incident. Other important information includes whether there was any treatment in the field, ongoing medical conditions, previous orthopaedic injuries (particularly at the same site), and chronic medication use. Also ask about any underlying disorders that could predispose to pathologic fractures, such as known bone cysts, osteogenesis imperfecta, chronic steroid use, and other causes of osteopenia.

Physical Examination

Most often the patient's status is either post some attempt at reducing the fracture or awaiting either operative reduction or resolution of the swelling to allow for optimal reduction. Whether the attempt was successful or not, there will be swelling at the fracture site, which raises the risk for compartment syndrome. Carefully examine distal to the fracture site, which in some cases may be very distal due to the presence of a cast or splint. Assess for pain, pallor, pulses, paresthesias, and capillary refill of the affected extremity. Also check active and passive ranges of movement. Note, however, that pulselessness and pallor can also be secondary to a vascular injury without compartment syndrome.

A femur fracture has the additional risk of significant loss of blood into the thigh. Measure the thigh circumference at a fixed point on the thigh on admission and then repeat every 8 hours.

If the patient's status is post–fracture reduction, address the resultant rotation, length, and angulation. Although these are usually assessed by the orthopaedic team, the post-reduction examination must evaluate for correction of any rotational displacement. Length can be assessed by x-ray, while angulation of long bones is rarely an issue, as angles less than 30 degrees will self-resolve.

Laboratory

If the patient has a femur fracture, obtain a complete blood cell count as baseline in case of continuing blood loss. The need for other laboratory testing for underlying bone abnormalities is dictated by the clinical circumstances, with the possible exception of an evaluation for inflicted trauma (page 587). Do not obtain a wound culture of an open fracture before surgical intervention.

Radiology

Although imaging is usually performed prior to admission, it is important to review the post-reduction images. In contrast to adults, overlap is necessary in long bone fractures in a young child to allow for expansion at the callous site. This is very important for the lower extremities to prevent a future leg length discrepancy. Further imaging may be necessary if there is ongoing severe pain at the fracture site, since most pain is relieved by reduction and stabilization.

A computed tomography (CT) scan may be useful in cases of displaced or angulated fractures, potentially complex intra-articular fractures, and vertebral and pelvic fractures.

Diagnosis

Consider possible inflicted injury or child abuse if the mechanism of injury does not adequately explain the type or severity of the fracture found, there was an unusual delay in seeking medical care, unexplained fractures in different stages of healing are present on the x-rays, a patient younger than 1 year has a fracture of the femur, or there is a scapular fracture without a clear history of violent trauma. Other concerns include epiphyseal and metaphyseal fractures of the long bones and corner or "chip" fractures of the metaphysis.

A non-displaced fracture may not be evident on initial plain x-ray. If there is significant suspicion for a fracture due to extreme pain or mechanism of injury, obtain a CT or magnetic resonance imaging acutely or a follow-up x-ray in 10 to 14 days to look for callous formation.

Complications

There are complications that are particularly associated with certain types of fractures. For example, nonunion of tibial fractures, thromboembolism and hemorrhagic shock with pelvic fractures, and neurovascular compromise secondary to brachial artery injury with supracondylar fractures. Persistence of intense pain after fracture reduction may be an indication of ischemia, compartment syndrome, or neurovascular compromise.

Compartment Syndrome

The signs of compartment syndrome are reduced pulses or capillary refill, paresthesias, pain out of proportion to the severity of the injury, pallor of the distal part of the affected extremity, and reduced sensation. The most reliable signs are hyperesthesia and increasing pain with passive stretching of the muscles within the compartment. Decreased pulses may not manifest until late in the process, although the absence of a pulse is not necessarily a danger sign and its presence does not guarantee that ischemia will be avoided. Maintain a high index of suspicion, as not all of these signs need to be present to diagnose compartment syndrome.

Fat Embolism

Fat embolism and respiratory distress syndrome can occur in a patient with a femur fracture. The risk increases if surgical repair is delayed more than 24 hours.

Treatment

Analgesia

For moderate to severe pain in a patient with no cardiovascular or central nervous system contraindications, give morphine (0.1 mg/kg/dose intravenous [IV] or subcutaneous every 4 hours to start, then increase the dose or frequency as needed; maximum 2 mg/dose infant, 4–8 mg/dose child, 15 mg/dose adolescent). If a patient older than 5 to 7 years requires morphine more frequently than every 2 hours, change to either patient-controlled analgesia (pages 665–666) or add ketorolac (1 mg/kg/dose IV every 6 hours, 15 mg/dose maximum, for 8 doses). Effective analgesia will not obscure physical findings and may increase cooperation during the examination.

Fever and Infection

The risk of infection increases when surgical hardware (nails and fixator pins) is placed into the area or if the patient has an open fracture. For this reason, irrigation and debridement are vitally important. Usually the orthopaedist will request skin prophylaxis (per local preference) for open reductions or hardware placement.

"Bone fever" can occur in the hours immediate post-reduction, then spontaneously resolve. High fever or subsequent spikes, increased pain and swelling, and discharge from the wound or hardware sites are signs of potential infection. Although pin sites can have some serosanguinous discharge initially, this is never purulent. Discourage the patient from using any devices to scratch under the casts, which can then create abrasions. Order an incentive spirometer to promote respiratory expansion in a postoperative or sedated patient.

Neurovascular

The key to preventing neurovascular injury is frequent neurovascular checks. Correct mild edema by maintaining the affected extremity elevated above the level of the heart, although this will not prevent true compartment syndrome. Urgent management consists of removal of any splint or cast. Continued or worsening symptoms are an emergency that requires surgical consultation and intervention.

Fat Embolism

The treatment is supportive care, possibly in an intensive care unit.

Deep Venous Thrombosis (DVT)

DVT prophylaxis remains controversial, but is indicated for at-risk patients. (See page 25.)

Pressure Ulcers and Immobilization

In general, children tolerate immobilization well, as they do not have underlying peripheral vascular disease and they continue to move as much as possible. Nevertheless, skin ulcers can occur. Pay close attention to relieving pressure spots with special mattresses and frequent turning of the nonmobile patient.

Other risks of prolonged immobilization are constipation and hypercalciuria. If a prolonged period of immobilization is expected, immediately begin a bowel regimen. In addition, ensure that the patient is receiving appropriate physical therapy. Obtain a spot calcium/creatinine ratio (page 414) weekly while immobilized to screen for hypercalciuria.

A problem unique to spica casts is hypertension, thought to be due to pressure on autonomic ganglia. Ensure that the cast is scooped off the abdomen.

Indications for Consultation

- **Child abuse team:** Suspected non-accidental trauma
- **Orthopaedics:** Urgently for any fracture at risk for or with the symptoms of neurovascular compromise
- **Pain team/anesthesiology:** Difficulty providing adequate analgesia
- **Physical therapy:** As needed, for crutch training and help with other activities of daily living that may be limited by casts or hardware
- **Vascular surgery:** Any concern about vascular compromise

Disposition

- **Intensive care unit transfer:** Compartment syndrome, respiratory distress due to fat emboli
- **Interinstitutional transfer:** Pediatric orthopaedic specialist not available locally for a patient with a complex fracture
- **Discharge criteria:** Fracture reduced, no risk for neurovascular compromise, pain controlled with oral medication

Follow-up

- **Primary care:** 1 to 2 weeks
- **Orthopaedics:** 1 to 2 weeks

Pearls and Pitfalls

- Persistence of intense pain after fracture reduction may be an indication of ischemia.
- Always obtain a repeat x-ray post-reduction.
- Properly treated physeal injuries are still at risk for longitudinal or angular abnormalities. This is particularly true for the distal femur, proximal tibia, or radial head or neck.
- In a case where non-accidental trauma is strongly suspected, a report to the state child protective services is mandatory.
- After crutch training has been performed, document that the patient has demonstrated safe crutch use.

Coding

ICD-9

• Compartment syndrome, traumatic, unspecified	**958.90**
• Fat embolism	**958.1**
• Fracture of unspecified part of femur closed	**821.00**
• Fracture of unspecified part of femur open	**821.10**
• Pathologic fracture	**733.10**
• Supracondylar fracture of humerus closed	**812.41**
• Supracondylar fracture of humerus open	**812.51**

Bibliography

Beaty JH, Kazzer JR. *Rockwood and Wilkins' Fractures in Children, Plus Integrated Content Website.* 7th ed. Philadelphia, PA: Lippincott, Williams & Wilkins; 2009

Chasm RM, Swencki SA. Pediatric orthopedic emergencies. *Emerg Med Clin North Am.* 2010;28:907–926

Laine JC, Kaiser SP, Diab M. High-risk pediatric orthopedic pitfalls. *Emerg Med Clin North Am.* 2010;28:85–102

Omid R, Choi PD, Skaggs DL. Supracondylar humeral fractures in children. *J Bone Joint Surg Am.* 2008;90:1121–1132

Pandya NK, Baldwin K, Kamath AF, Wenger DR, Hosalkar HS. Unexplained fractures: child abuse or bone disease? A systematic review. *Clin Orthop Relat Res.* 2011;469:805–812

Price CT, Flynn JM. Management of fractures. In: Morrissy RT, Weinstein SL, eds. *Lovell and Winters Pediatric Orthopedics.* 6th ed. Philadelphia, PA: Lippincott, Williams & Wilkins; 2006:1429–1526

Wall CJ, Lynch J, Harris IA, et al; Liverpool (Sydney) and Royal Melbourne Hospitals. Clinical practice guidelines for the management of acute limb compartment syndrome following trauma. *ANZ J Surg.* 2010;80:151–156

Osteomyelitis

Introduction

Osteomyelitis is most often caused by hematogenous seeding of bacteria to bone. In an older child, the thick periosteum contains the infection, creating a subperiosteal abscess. In a young infant, the periosteum is thinner so that inflammation easily spreads to deep tissues. In addition, in an infant younger than 18 months, the presence of end-loop capillaries feeding the epiphyses increases the risk of epiphyseal osteomyelitis and contiguous septic arthritis. Other mechanisms include trauma or the presence of foreign material (spinal rods).

Approximately 90% of cases occur in the metaphyses of long bones (femur, tibia, humerus), 6% to 8% in the pelvis (ischium, ilium), and 1% to 3% in the vertebrae. Chronic osteomyelitis (>3 weeks' duration) results from insufficiently treated acute osteomyelitis, with unusual pathogens or mechanisms of injury (pressure ulcers) often implicated. Complications of osteomyelitis include subperiosteal abscess, myositis, secondary bacteremia, pathologic fracture, growth disturbance, and fistula.

Staphylococcus aureus is the most common pathogen in all ages, followed by group A β-hemolytic streptococcus (*Streptococcus pyogenes*) in children and group B β-hemolytic streptococcus (*Streptococcus agalactiae*) in infants. Coagulase-negative staphylococci are associated with foreign bodies and implants.

Gram-negative and atypical pathogens are less common and are usually implicated in specific clinical situations: unvaccinated (*Haemophilus influenzae* type B), toddlers (*Kingella kingae*), cat scratch or bite (*Bartonella henselae*), reptile or fowl exposure (*Salmonella* species), sickle cell disease (*Salmonella* species), complement deficiency (*Salmonella* species), neonates or intravenous (IV) drug users (*Enterobacteriaceae*, yeast), bites (*Pasturella, Capnocytophaga, Eikenella* species), foot puncture wound (*Pseudomonas aeruginosa*), ingestion of unpasteurized dairy (*Brucella* species), epidemiologic risk factors (*Mycobacterium tuberculosis;* accounts for 5% to 10% of extrapulmonary disease), contaminated wound (atypical mycobacteria), foreign material (*Staphylococcus epidermidis*), or chronic fistula (polymicrobial).

Clinical Presentation

History

In acute long-bone osteomyelitis, the patient presents with a few days of fever and either a limp or decreased use of the limb. An infant or disabled child may present with a subtle pseudoparalysis of the affected limb. Pelvic osteomyelitis presents with buttock or deep perineal pain and refusal to bear weight or sit. Vertebral osteomyelitis presents with back or abdominal pain, decreased back flexion and extension, and decreased weight-bearing. In contrast, chronic osteomyelitis progresses over weeks, and may not significantly affect function.

Ask about exposure to *S aureus*, *S pyogenes*, unpasteurized milk, tuberculosis, and animals (kittens and puppies, reptiles, fowl), as well as a history of furuncles, trauma, bite wounds, contaminated wounds, pressure ulcers, foreign material, and asplenia. Check the vaccination and immune status.

Physical Examination

Acute osteomyelitis presents with point tenderness, erythema, warmth, and/or swelling over the bone. These classic symptoms may be subtle or absent, particularly when the affected limb is large due to muscle mass or obesity. A pelvic osteomyelitis may cause hip tenderness, in addition to localized bone pain. Vertebral osteomyelitis may present with leg pain, focal bony back tenderness, and neurologic signs of the lower extremities that may suggest spinal cord irritation. Referred pain is common in a child, so examine the joint above and below the affected area. Chronic osteomyelitis presents with point tenderness, but may lack swelling or warmth, although a draining fistula is sometimes present. Finally, carefully examine all other bony sites to exclude a multifocal infection.

Laboratory

If osteomyelitis is suspected, obtain a complete blood cell count, erythrocyte sedimentation rate (ESR) and/or C-reactive protein (CRP.), and a blood culture. Leukocytosis is present in about one-third of cases. CRP and ESR are often elevated in acute osteomyelitis, but may be normal in chronic osteomyelitis. In acute, febrile osteomyelitis, blood cultures obtained prior to antibiotics are positive in up to 50% of patients. If possible, arrange for a bone aspirate for culture (65%–70% positive) prior to antibiotics. However, a bone biopsy is indicated if there is an unusual history (penetrating trauma, foreign body, treatment failure) or unusual risk factors (gram-negative organism, tuberculosis, immunocompromised host).

Radiology

Obtain plain films to look for fracture, neoplasm, and signs of inflammation. Deep soft tissue inflammation is evident on plain films at more than 3 days, periosteal elevation at more than 10 days, and cortical changes at 14 to 21 days. Magnetic resonance imaging (MRI) is the most sensitive and specific for bone marrow changes in acute and chronic osteomyelitis (sensitivity 82%–100%, specificity 75%–96%). While a computed tomography scan is less sensitive and specific, it may be helpful in cases of chronic osteomyelitis or when MRI is not an option.

A bone scan may be helpful when an occult osteomyelitis is suspected but difficult to localize (fever of unknown origin in an infant) or when MRI is not an option. Bone scan (99m-Tc-methyldiphosphonate) reports 3 phases: (1) angiographic phase: occurs in seconds and highlights vessels, (2) blood pool phase: occurs in 5 to 10 minutes and highlights soft tissue phase, (3) delayed bone phase: occurs in 2 to 4 hours and highlights the deposition of labeled tracer into bone secondary to osteoblast activity. Focal hyperperfusion, hyperemia, and bone uptake are present in osteomyelitis. However, a bone scan is less accurate in an infant.

Ultrasound imaging may be useful for guided aspiration of a subperiosteal abscess. In addition, ultrasound is not impeded by orthopaedic implants.

Differential Diagnosis

Once osteomyelitis has been ruled out, consider other infectious and noninfectious causes (Table 82-1). Vasoocclusive crises in sickle cell disease (page 267) may be difficult to distinguish from infection, so that dual therapy may be necessary. Often the pain is at multiple or "typical" sites. Otherwise, multiple simultaneous sites of involvement suggest a common source (endocarditis) or a systemic inflammatory process (juvenile idiopathic arthritis; chronic recurrent multifocal osteomyelitis [CRMO]; synovitis, acne, pustulosis, hyperostosis, and osteitis [SAPHO]; psoriatic arthritis).

CRMO presents with recurrent episodes of focal bone pain and swelling at different sites, bone inflammation on biopsy, but negative cultures. SAPHO is an inflammatory syndrome that has recurrent bony involvement, in addition to skin findings. The typical patient is a young female who may have associated palmoplantar pustulosis, psoriasis vulgaris, or acute neutrophilic dermatosis.

Table 82-1. Differential Diagnosis of Osteomyelitis	
Diagnosis	**Clinical Features**
Infectious	
Brodie abscess or sequestrum	Chronic history Abnormal imaging
Septic arthritis	Erythema and warmth of affected joint Decreased range of motion Joint effusion
Noninfectious	
Sickle cell vasoocclusive crisis	At-risk patient May or may not be febrile Pain in "typical" location(s) Pain may be diffuse rather than point tenderness
Trauma	(+) History No fever
Other	
Bone neoplasm	Gradual onset Constitutional symptoms: weight loss, fatigue Pain may be worse at night
Chronic recurrent multifocal osteomyelitis	Recurrent episodes of focal bone pain and swelling Multiple sites Negative cultures
Juvenile idiopathic arthritis	Prolonged fevers Recurrent arthralgias/arthritis Morning stiffness
Langerhans histiocytosis	Lytic skull lesions Chronic otorrhea Chronic seborrheic-like rash
Leukemia	Abnormal complete blood cell count May have pallor or bleeding Constitutional symptoms: weight loss, fatigue
Synovitis, acne, pustulosis, hyperostosis, and osteitis	Acne and pustulosis Synovitis, hyperostosis, osteitis Negative cultures

Treatment

For uncomplicated acute hematogenous osteomyelitis, chose empiric treatment based on local bacterial resistance, especially for methicillin-resistant *Staphylococcus aureus* (MRSA). When feasible, attempt to obtain a bone culture prior to administering antibiotics, as identifying the causative pathogen will facilitate definitive treatment decisions. Initial empiric therapy of acute hematogenous osteomyelitis is IV clindamycin (40 mg/kg/day divided every 8 hours, 4.8 g/day maximum). A first-generation cephalosporin or an anti-staphylococcal penicillin are *not options* in areas where MRSA is prevalent.

Other choices based on culture results include oxacillin or nafcillin (100–200 mg/kg/day divided every 6 hours, 12 g/day maximum), cefazolin (100 mg/kg/day divided every 6 hours, 6 g/day maximum), cefotaxime (150–200 mg/kg/day divided every 6–8 hours, 12 g/day maximum), and for clindamycin-resistant MRSA, vancomycin (40–60 mg/kg/day divided every 6 hours, 4 g/day maximum, goal trough 15–20). Do not use ceftriaxone as monotherapy for *S aureus.*

Since an infant aged 2 months or younger is at risk for gram-negative organisms, initiate empiric therapy with IV cefotaxime *and* (depending on the concern for MRSA) either vancomycin *or* an anti-staphylococcal penicillin (oxacillin or nafcillin).

Reassess the patient daily, provide adequate analgesia, and monitor for improvement in clinical symptoms and resolution of inflammatory markers. Improvement typically begins within 48 hours, and is significant in 3 to 5 days. A delay in resolution of inflammatory factors is associated with a poorer prognosis and suggests an ongoing focus of infection or antibiotic failure.

Transition to oral therapy once the patient is afebrile, weight-bearing/using the affected extremity, has decreased inflammatory markers, and can tolerate oral medication. Use a dose that is 2 to 3 times higher than for minor infections to achieve adequate blood levels and bone penetration. Narrow the antibiotic choice based on culture results, when possible. Common choices include clindamycin (40 mg/kg/day divided every 8 hours, 1.8 g/day maximum), cephalexin (150 mg/kg/day divided every 6 hours, 4 g/day maximum), penicillin VK (120 mg/kg/day divided every 4–6 hours, 3 g/day maximum), amoxicillin (100–200 mg/kg/day divided every 6 hours, 3 g/day maximum). Oral options without culture guidance include a first-generation cephalosporin, clindamycin, dicloxacillin (100 mg/kg/day divided every 6 hours, 2 g/day maximum), or linezolid (<12 years of age: 10 mg/kg every every 8 hours; ≥ 12 years of age: 600 mg every 12 hours; 600 mg/dose maximum). Do not use doxycycline or trimethoprim-sulfamethoxazole for *S aureus*.

Treat acute osteomyelitis typically for 4 to 6 weeks and chronic osteomyelitis for 6 to 8 weeks or more, based on clinical improvement and resolution of laboratory abnormalities. In follow-up, confirm that the CRP and/or ESR have normalized (ESR will lag behind the CRP) prior to discontinuing treatment.

Treat a chronic osteomyelitis with oral antibiotics (clindamycin or first-generation cephalosporin). Obtain an infectious diseases consult to determine the treatment of a complicated osteomyelitis (penetrating injury, pressure ulcer, or prosthetic material).

Indications for Consultation

- **Infectious diseases:** Unusual risk factors or failure to respond to empiric therapy
- **Orthopaedics:** Suspected or confirmed osteomyelitis

Disposition

- **Intensive care unit transfer:** Possible bacterial sepsis, toxic appearance
- **Discharge criteria:** Afebrile for 24 hours or more, surgical issues resolved, return of baseline functioning of the extremity, antibiotics narrowed (if sensitivities known), home treatment arranged (if needed), and CRP/ESR is improving

Follow-up

- **Primary provider:** 1 week
- **Orthopaedics:** 1 to 2 weeks
- **Infectious diseases:** 2 to 4 weeks, if involved
- **Physical therapy/rehabilitation:** As indicated

Pearls and Pitfalls

- Whenever possible, obtain a biopsy and culture prior to treatment.
- If there are multiple sites of suspected osteomyelitis, consider a common source (endocarditis) or a noninfectious etiology (rheumatologic, CRMO, SAPHO).
- Consider *K kingae* in toddlers and preschoolers in child care.
- Arrange IV access (peripherally inserted central catheter) early in the course if the expected IV antibiotic course is more than 1 week.

Coding

ICD-9

- Osteomyelitis, acute **730.0x**
- Osteomyelitis, chronic **730.1x**

For both of the above codes, use one of these digits for the fifth digit (x) to identify the affected site

- 0 site unspecified
- 1 shoulder region
- 2 upper arm
- 3 forearm
- 4 hand

- 5 pelvic region and thigh
- 6 lower leg
- 7 ankle and foot
- 8 other specified sites
- 9 multiple sites

Bibliography

Conrad DA. Acute hematogenous osteomyelitis. *Pediatr Rev.* 2010;31:464–471

Copley LAB, Dormans JP. Musculoskeletal infection. In: Dorman JP, ed. *Pediatric Orthopaedics and Sports Medicine: The Requisites in Pediatrics.* St Louis, MO: Mosby; 2004:93–110

Harik NS, Smeltzer MS. Management of acute hematogenous osteomyelitis in children. *Expert Rev Anti Infect Ther.* 2010;8:175–181

Howard-Jones AR, Isaacs D. Systematic review of systemic antibiotic treatment for children with chronic and sub-acute pyogenic osteomyelitis. *J Paediatr Child Health.* 2010;46:736–741

Karmazyn B. Imaging approach to acute hematogenous osteomyelitis in children: an update. *Semin Ultrasound CT MR.* 2010;31:100–106

Ranson M. Imaging of pediatric musculoskeletal infection. *Semin Musculoskelet Radiol.* 2009;13:277–299

Septic Arthritis

Introduction

Septic arthritis is a bacterial infection of the joint space and synovium, usually secondary to hematogenous seeding of bacteria into the joint capsule. Other mechanisms are direct inoculation by penetrating trauma and contiguous extension from an adjacent osteomyelitis. In an infant, septic arthritis may be secondary to a contiguous epiphyseal osteomyelitis. Transepiphyseal vessels, which remain present until 18 months of age, allow extension of the infection. Overall, about one-half of patients are 2 years or younger and more than 90% of cases are monoarticular, with the knee and hip being the most common sites, followed by elbow, ankle, shoulder, wrist, and sacroiliac joints.

Staphylococcus aureus is the most common pathogen in all age groups (>50% of positive cultures). Other common organisms are age-related: neonate: group B streptococcus and *Escherichia coli;* child: group A streptococcus and *Kingella kingae;* adolescent: gonococcus and group A streptococcus. Consider other etiologies based on known or suspected risk factors: tick exposure (Lyme disease), unvaccinated (*Haemophilus influenzae* type b), exposure to reptiles or fowl (*Salmonella* species), sickle cell disease (*Salmonella* species), complement deficiency (*Neisseria meningitidis, Salmonella* species), bites (*Pasturella multocida, Pasturella canis, Capnocytophaga* species, *Fusobacterium* species, *Eikenella corrodens*), puncture wound *(Pseudomonas aeruginosa)*, joint prosthesis *(Staphylococcus epidermidis)*, reactive (*Chlamydia trachomatis, Campylobacter jejuni,* post-viral or post-streptococcal), or epidemiologic risk factors *(Mycobacterium tuberculosis)*.

Septic arthritis requires *urgent* diagnosis, arthrocentesis, and treatment to prevent permanent limitation of joint mobility. If septic arthritis is complicated by osteomyelitis of the epiphysis and growth plate, long-bone growth may also be impaired. In addition, septic arthritis of the hip and shoulder has an increased risk of avascular necrosis of the femoral or humeral head, respectively, secondary to ischemia.

Clinical Presentation

History

Septic arthritis typically presents with the acute onset of a painful joint, decreased range of motion, and inability to bear weight, often associated with fever (>38.4°C). Septic arthritis in an infant or disabled child may be subtle and present as a pseudoparalysis of the affected joint. *Neisseria gonorrhoeae* can present in a sexually active adolescent as either an arthritis-dermatitis syndrome or disseminated gonococcal infection (polyarthritis, polyarthralgia, and tenosynovitis). Arthritis is a late manifestation of disseminated Lyme disease, so that the patient often reports a preceding illness consistent with early Lyme disease, including erythema migrans.

Ask about exposures and risk factors for unusual pathogens, including vaccination status, trauma, immune status, asplenia, sickle cell disease, sexual activity, unpasteurized dairy products, tick exposure, tuberculosis risk, trauma, and recent pharyngitis or enteritis.

Physical Examination

In most cases the arthritis is readily apparent, with joint swelling, erythema, warmth, and tenderness. Range of motion is significantly decreased and minimal manipulation can cause severe pain. However, the sole abnormality with an infection of a deep joint (hip, sacroiliac) may be decreased range of motion. The patient will guard the affected joint in the position of least pain (hip flexed and externally rotated; knee and elbow held carefully in neutral position). Referred pain is common (especially knee pain with a septic hip), so examine the joint above and below the presumed focus. Examine the remaining joints and palpate the long bones for point tenderness.

Polyarticular involvement can occur with *N gonorrhoeae, N meningitides,* or *Salmonella* species. Other causes of polyarticular disease include acute rheumatic fever, Lyme arthritis, and juvenile idiopathic arthritis. A patient with Lyme arthritis may have a subacute presentation with a swollen, non-erythematous joint (most often the knee), while maintaining weight-bearing and range of motion with minimal discomfort.

Laboratory

Obtain a complete blood cell count, erythrocyte sedimentation rate (ESR) and/or C-reactive protein (CRP), and a blood culture (yield 40%). Order additional tests if a specific organism is suspected, such as Lyme enzyme-linked immunosorbent assay with reflex to Western blot, nucleic acid amplification tests from urine and cervicovaginal samples for gonococcus and *Chlamydia,* and a purified protein derivative. The white blood cell count is typically elevated with a left shift, and the ESR and CRP are elevated (ESR >30 mm/hour and CRP >3 mg/dL), although an ESR greater than 100 mm/hour suggests an autoimmune arthritis.

If septic arthritis is suspected, arrange for an *immediate* percutaneous diagnostic joint aspiration, under ultrasound guidance if the hip is involved. Send joint fluid specimens for cell count, Gram stain, and culture (Table 83-1). Immediate surgical irrigation by an orthopaedist is indicated if the preliminary results are suggestive of bacterial infection. In order to improve culture yields and detect fastidious organisms such as *K kingae,* some laboratories will inoculate the fluid into a blood culture bottle. Request special cultures for *M tuberculosis,* if suspected. Polymerase chain reaction testing is available on joint fluid for *Borrelia burgdorferi* and *N gonorrhoeae.*

Radiology

Obtain plain films to evaluate for effusion, fracture, and other noninfectious causes such as bone cyst or neoplasm. In suspected septic hip, ultrasound is rapid and diagnostic and it facilitates therapeutic drainage. Additional imaging is not necessary unless a primary contiguous osteomyelitis or complication is suspected, in which case magnetic resonance imaging is indicated. However, do not delay diagnostic arthrocentesis and empiric antimicrobial therapy while awaiting imaging.

Differential Diagnosis

First, confirm that the patient has arthritis and not merely arthralgia. An arthritic joint presents with some combination of erythema, warmth, effusion, and limited range of motion. Once septic arthritis has been ruled out, consider other infectious and noninfectious causes of arthritis (Table 83-2).

Treatment

Arrange for an *immediate* percutaneous diagnostic joint tap by an orthopaedist (or other skilled personnel). If positive, surgical irrigation is necessary. Effective treatment involves urgent surgical drainage and/or irrigation *and*

Table 83-1. Interpretation of Synovial Fluid Cell Count

WBC/mm^3	% PMNs	Interpretation
<200	<25%	Normal
200–2,000	<25%	Noninflammatory (osteoarthritis)
2,000–50,000	>50%	Inflammatory, possibly noninfectious (reactive, juvenile idiopathic arthritis, Lyme disease, gonorrhea, tuberculosis, brucellosis)
>50,000	>75%	Probably infectious (*Staphylococcus aureus,* group A streptococcus, Lyme, gram-negative rods)

Abbreviations: PMNs, polymorphonuclear neutrophils; WBC, white blood cell count.

Table 83-2. Differential Diagnosis of Septic Arthritis	
Diagnosis	**Clinical Features**
Acute rheumatic fever	Preceding group A strep pharyngitis Migratory polyarthritis Severe pain out of proportion to exam findings May have carditis
Gonorrhea	Sexually active Multiple smaller joints and knees (+) Urine/cervical nucleic acid amplification test
Henoch-Schönlein purpura	Palpable purpura of lower extremities Abdominal pain May have (+) stool guaiac and/or hematuria
Irritable bowel disease	May have poor growth or weight loss May have diarrhea, possibly guaiac (+) May have iritis
Juvenile idiopathic arthritis	Pain and stiffness worse in the morning (+) Serology
Lyme disease	May have a history of tick bite and/or erythema migrans Swollen non-erythematous knee Lyme serology (+)
Osteomyelitis	Point tenderness of long bone No joint swelling or erythema
Parvovirus	Viral prodrome: fever, fatigue, headache, pharyngitis Typical rash: slapped cheeks followed by lacy appearance on trunk and extremities
Postinfectious/vaccination	Subacute onset over 2–3 weeks May not have fever Less dramatic exam: ↓ erythema, swelling, pain
Systemic lupus erythematosus	Symmetrical arthritis of hands and feet May have other features (malar rash, proteinuria, etc) (+) Serology
Sickle cell disease vasoocclusive crisis	(+) History Previous episodes with pain in typical location(s) May be afebrile
Transient synovitis	Recent viral illness Less dramatic joint examination Responds to analgesics
Trauma	(+) History (+) Radiographs
Tuberculosis	(+) Risk factors (+) Purified protein derivative and/or interferon-γ Joint fluid: lymphocytic predominance

intravenous (IV) antimicrobial therapy (Table 83-3). Consider a bacterial infection of a hip or shoulder to be a medical/surgical emergency and include vancomycin in the initial antibiotic regimen. Otherwise, review local antibiograms for the prevalence of methicillin-resistant strains (MRSA) and obtain an infectious diseases consult for a contaminated wound (trauma), joint prosthesis, or unusual or resistant organism.

Administer the initial IV antibiotics, provide adequate analgesia, and reassess the patient daily, looking for resolution of clinical symptoms and inflammatory markers. Improvement begins within 72 hours, and is significant by 5 to 7 days. Use the clinical course and identification and sensitivity of the organism (if available) to tailor the choice of antibiotics and the timing of transition to oral therapy. However, there is no absolute minimum duration of IV antibiotic treatment. The total (IV plus oral) duration of antibiotics for uncomplicated septic arthritis (including *S aureus*) is at least 3 weeks. If there is a coexistent osteomyelitis, treat for 4 to 6 weeks.

Treat Lyme arthritis for a total of 21 days. Gonococcal arthritis warrants a thorough evaluation and treatment for other sexually transmitted infections.

Indications for Consultation

- **Infectious diseases:** Patient with unusual risk factors, organism, or failure to respond to empiric therapy
- **Orthopaedics:** All cases of suspected septic arthritis
- **Physiatry/physical therapy:** As tolerated, once surgical issues are resolved

Table 83-3. Empiric Antibiotic Treatment of Septic Arthritis

Infection	Empiric Treatment
Hip or shoulder	Vancomycin[a]: 15 mg/kg every 6 h, 1 g/dose maximum; trough goal = 10–15 mcg/mL *plus* nafcillin or oxacillin (100–200 mg/kg every 6 h, 12 g/day maximum)
Other joints	Clindamycin[a] (40 mg/kg/day divided every 8 h, 4.8 g/day maximum)
Suspect gram-negative	Add ceftriaxone (75 mg/kg/day divided every 12 h, 4 g/day maximum)
Neonate	Nafcillin *or* oxacillin (as above) *plus* gentamycin *or* cefotaxime (doses for both depend on age and weight)
Penicillin allergic	Clindamycin or vancomycin or ceftriaxone
Lyme arthritis	Ceftriaxone (50 mg/kg every 12 h, 4 g/day maximum)
Gonococcal arthritis	Ceftriaxone (75 mg/kg every 12 h, 4 g/dose maximum)

[a] For methicillin-resistant *Staphylococcus aureus* coverage.

Disposition

- **Interinstitutional transfer:** If orthopaedic management is not available, especially if there is a concern about a septic hip
- **Discharge criteria:** Afebrile more than 24 hours, surgical issues resolved, return of baseline joint function, antibiotic regimen narrowed (if sensitivities are known), and improving CRP

Follow-up

- **Primary provider:** 3 days
- **Orthopaedics:** 1 to 2 weeks
- **Infectious diseases:** 2 weeks (if involved)

Pearls and Pitfalls

- If septic arthritis is suspected, arrange for an *urgent* arthrocentesis.
- Consider adjacent osteomyelitis of the epiphysis in a young infant.
- Ensure that a blood culture is obtained prior to the first dose of antibiotics.
- Arrange IV access (peripherally inserted central catheter) early in the course if the expected IV antibiotic course is more than 1 week.

Coding

ICD-9

- Gonococcal arthritis **098.50**
- Lyme disease **088.81**
- Pyogenic arthritis **711.0x**
  - Use one of these digits for the fifth digit (x) to identify site
    - 0 site unspecified
    - 1 shoulder region
    - 2 upper arm
    - 3 forearm
    - 4 hand
    - 5 pelvic region and thigh
    - 6 lower leg
    - 7 ankle and foot
    - 8 other specified sites
    - 9 multiple sites
- Tenosynovitis **727.00**

Bibliography

Kang SN, Sanghera T, Mangwani J, Paterson JM, Ramachandran M. The management of septic arthritis in children: systematic review of the English language literature. *J Bone Joint Surg Br.* 2009;91:1127–1133

Kocher MS, Mandiga R, Zurakowski D, et al. Validation of a clinical prediction rule for the differentiation between septic arthritis and transient synovitis of the hip in children. *J Bone Joint Surg Am.* 2004;86-A:1629–1635

Mathews CJ, Coakley G. Septic arthritis: current diagnostic and therapeutic algorithm. *Curr Opin Rheumatol.* 2008;20:457–462

Rathore MH. The unique issues of outpatient parenteral antimicrobial therapy in children and adolescents. *Clin Infect Dis.* 2010;51(suppl 2):S209–S215

Shah SS. Infectious arthritis. In: Bergelson JM, Shah SS, Zaoutis TE, eds. *Pediatric Infectious Diseases: The Requisites.* Philadelphia, PA: Elsevier Mosby; 2008:231–236

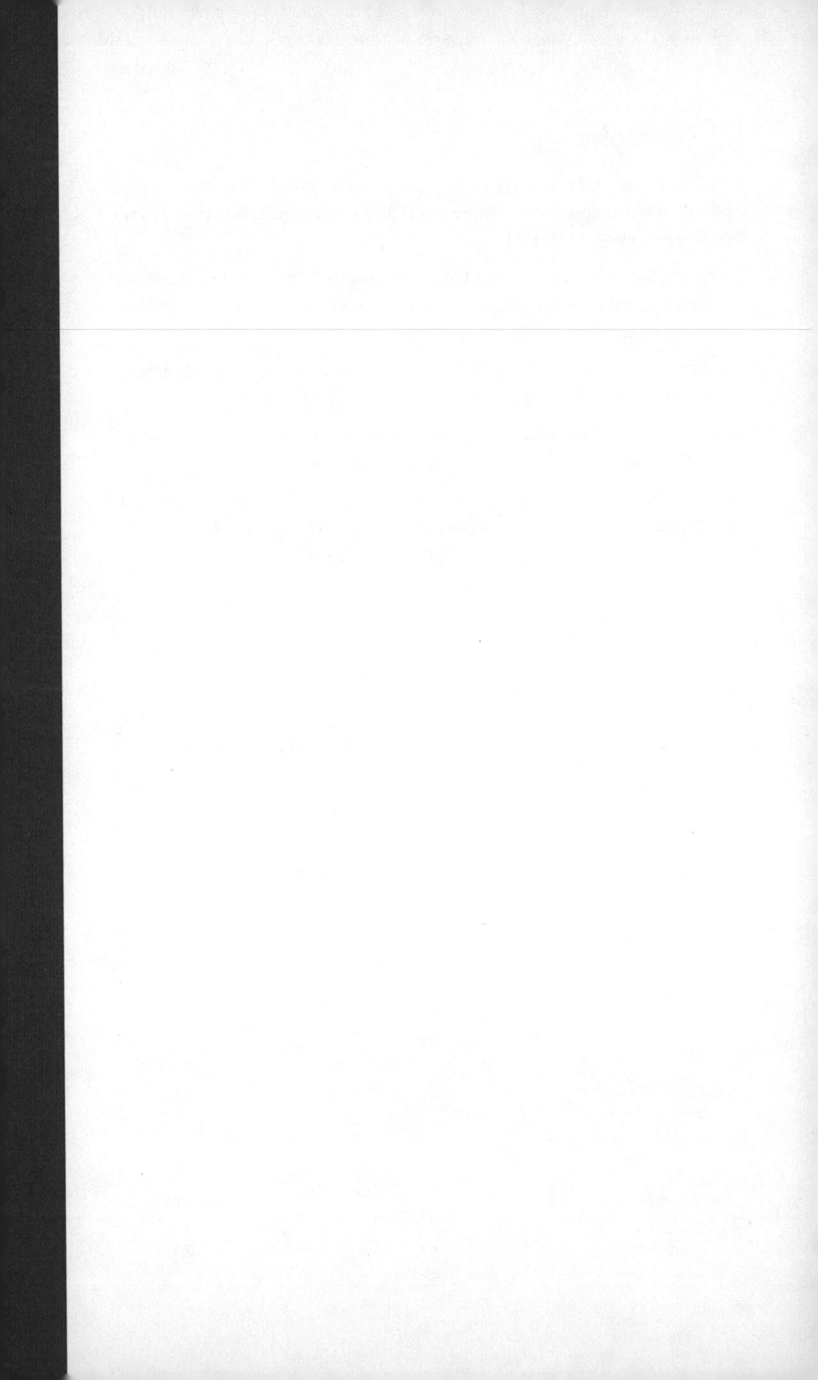

Psychiatry

CHAPTER 84

Acute Agitation

Introduction

Agitation is defined as excessive motor, verbal, and/or psychological activity. The admission to the hospital of an acutely agitated patient, or the development of agitation in an already admitted patient, can raise the anxiety level of both the patient's family and the medical team. As a result, security and safety become priorities, while the underlying etiology may be progressive and the therapies employed can themselves be toxic. In some cases the agitation may be severe enough that restraint is necessary.

The 4 etiologic categories for acute agitation are primary medical illness, trauma, underlying psychiatric or developmental illness, and intoxication/withdrawal. The most common causes of acute agitation are listed in Table 84-1.

Table 84-1. Common Causes of Acute Agitation

Drug-Induced (Iatrogenic)		Intoxication	
Antihistamines	Isoniazid	Amphetamines	Dextromethorphan
Benzodiazepines	Neuroleptic malignant syndrome	Anticholinergics (antihistamines, tricyclics)	Ketamine
Corticosteroids	Serotonin syndrome	Caffeine	MDMA (ecstasy)
		Cocaine	PCP
Drug Withdrawal		**Neurologic**	
Alcohol	Cannabinoids	CNS mass	Stroke
Baclofen	Nicotine	Confusional migraine	Traumatic brain injury
Benzodiazepines	Opiates	Pre-, postictal	
Endocrine		**Metabolic**	
Hyperthyroidism	Hyperparathyroidism	Hyper-/hypoglycemia	Hyper-/hyponatremia
Psychiatric		**Other**	
ADHD	Generalized anxiety	Acute porphyria	Hypoxia
Autism	Post-traumatic stress	Encephalitis	ICU psychosis
Bipolar disorder	Psychosis	Envenomation	SLE
Conduct disorder	Schizophrenia	Fragile X syndrome	Wilson disease
		Hypercarbia	

Abbreviations: ADHD, attention-deficit/hyperactivity disorder; CNS, central nervous system; ICU, intensive care unit; MDMA, 3,4-methylenedioxymethamphetamine; SLE, systemic lupus erythematosus.

Clinical Presentation

History

The presentation of agitation can range from simple restlessness, irritability, crying, or confusion, to loud speech, increased muscle tension, and combative behavior. Agitation is sometimes associated with elevated autonomic tone (tachycardia or diaphoresis). It is important to differentiate the chief complaint from the patient's baseline behavioral patterns by obtaining additional history from family, caregivers, outpatient providers, and other members of the patient's medical home.

Screen the patient for endogenous risk factors for agitated or violent behavior, such as a history of aggressive behavior, developmental delay, preexisting psychiatric illness, physical abuse, substance abuse at a young age, and criminal or gang behavior. Also search for risk factors for delirium, including fever, known medical illness, new or changed medications, recent hospitalizations/surgeries, and subacute trauma. Identify whether the patient suffers from seizure disorder, and inquire about relatives with sudden cardiac death or possible long QT syndrome (congenital hearing loss, seizures, syncope), which may affect the choice of a safe antipsychotic medication. Detail the patient's living situation and caregivers and whether there was a recent social stressor that may have precipitated an ingestion. Finally, identify the patient's allergies, prescribed and over-the-counter medications, and any medications in the household. Inquire about prior paradoxical reactions to antihistamines or benzodiazepines.

During the interview, speak with the patient in a consistent tone, offer frequent reassurance, employ nonthreatening body language, and monitor the patient's gestures and statements. Other strategies include avoiding prolonged eye contact, leaving the examination door open, conducting the interview while seated and with a "safety zone" between yourself and the patient, offering food or drink, and directly integrating trusted family and friends into the discussion. However, do not "negotiate" and be careful with using rewards, as the possible future perception of not following through can then precipitate further agitation.

Physical Examination

Priorities on the physical examination include the vital signs, especially fever, Cushing triad, and signs of inadequate perfusion. Perform a detailed neurologic examination and verify that the patient's "agitation" is not a misdiagnosis of a pure movement disorder, such as dystonia, akathisia, or severe tremor.

Note any gross psychiatric manifestations, such as paranoia, perseveration, psychosis, and visual/auditory/olfactory/tactile hallucinations. However, despite a history of an underlying psychiatric disorder, do not immediately ascribe the patient's entire presentation to that diagnosis.

Laboratory

If warranted by the clinical presentation and most likely diagnoses, obtain a complete blood cell count, electrolytes (including sodium, potassium, calcium, magnesium, and phosphorus), glucose, blood urea nitrogen, creatinine, and possibly a venous blood gas. Other considerations include liver function tests, ultrasensitive thyroid-stimulating hormone, and urine and serum toxicologies. An electrocardiogram is indicated if an arrhythmia is noted, a cardiotoxic ingestion is suspected, or a proarrhythmic sedative will be prescribed. Obtain an urgent noncontrast head computed tomography (CT) if the patient has had recent head trauma, partial seizure, known intracranial lesion, immunosuppression, suspected subarachnoid hemorrhage, progressive headache, papilledema, visual field deficit, or other focal neurologic findings. Perform a lumbar puncture with opening pressure with prior CT imaging if indicated; if the patient has mental status changes accompanied by fever, headache, focal neurologic deficit, or examination evidence of meningeal irritation; or if there is no reasonable alternative explanation for the agitation. Send the cerebrospinal fluid for cell count, glucose, protein, Gram stain, and culture, and save an additional tube for possible serology or polymerase chain reaction (herpes simplex virus, encephalitis panel, enterovirus, etc).

Treatment

First, determine whether the level of agitation has escalated to overt aggression or violence, which poses a risk to the patient, family, or staff. If so, alert hospital security, arrange an adequate staff-to-patient ratio, and consider physically restraining the patient. Also determine whether there is intercurrent diminished consciousness that could endanger the airway. If so, immediately assemble the appropriate equipment and staff for rapid sequence intubation and ventilatory support.

Promptly initiate treatment for the underlying cause if the patient suffers from medical delirium. While a peripheral intravenous (IV) access can facilitate medication administration, it may need to await safe physical restraint. If the patient will not accept oral or transmucosal medications, and if IV access is delayed, certain medications may be administered intramuscularly (Table 84-2).

Table 84-2. Pharmacologic Options in the Treatment of Acute Pediatric Agitation					
Medication	**Route**	**Initial Dose (mg/kg)**	**Max Dose (mg)**	**Onset (min)**	**Side Effects**
Antihistamines					
Diphenhydramine	PO	1.25	50	30	Anticholinergic CNS and/or respiratory depression Paradoxical disinhibition May worsen airway reactivity
	IM/IV	1.25	50	15	
Hydroxyzine	PO	0.6	100	30	
	IM	0.5–1	100	15	
Benzodiazepines					
Lorazepam	PO	0.02–0.1	4	60	Respiratory depression Habituation/tolerance Paradoxical disinhibition
	IV	0.02–0.1	4	20	
	IM	0.02–0.1	4	45	
Midazolam	PO	0.25–0.5	20	30	Respiratory depression Habituation/tolerance Paradoxical disinhibition
	IV	0.025–0.1	10	5	
	IM	0.05–0.15	10	30	
	IN	0.2–0.3	10	15	
Diazepam	PO	0.05–0.3	10	45	Respiratory depression Longer half-life may interfere with assessing mental status Erratic absorption after IM administration
	PR	0.5 (using the IV formulation)	20	10	
	iv	0.05–0.2	10	3	
Antipsychotics					
Haloperidol (typical antipsychotic)	PO	0.025–0.075	5	60	Dystonic reactions[a] Risk of EPS and NMS ↑ QTc Least seizure threshold reduction among typical antipsychotics IV formulation is not FDA approved
	IM/IV	0.025–0.075	5	30	
Risperidone (atypical antipsychotic)	PO	0.025–0.05	1	30	Hypotension (at ↑ doses) ↑ QTc ↓ Risk of EPS and NMS Least seizure threshold reduction among atypical antipsychotics

Table 84-2. Pharmacologic Options in the Treatment of Acute Pediatric Agitation, continued

Medication	Route	Initial Dose (mg/kg)	Max Dose (mg)	Onset (min)	Side Effects
Antipsychotics, continued					
Olanzapine (atypical antipsychotic)	PO	0.1–0.2	10	60	↑ QTc ↓ Risk of EPS and NMS Can exacerbate hypotension or bradycardia induced by concomitant agents
	IM	2.5–5	10	30	

Abbreviations: CNS, central nervous system; EPS, extrapyramidal symptoms; FDA, US Food and Drug Administration; IM, intramuscular; IN, intranasal; IV, intravenous; NMS, neuormalignant syndrome; PO, oral; PR, rectal.

[a]Treat dystonia (oculogyric crisis, torticollis, opisthotonos) with diphenhydramine (1.25 mg/kg IV/IM/PO every 30 min), with or without adjuvant benzotropine (0.02–0.05 mg/kg/ IV/IM/PO).

Restraint

Restraint is categorized into physical and chemical (or pharmacologic) methods. The goals are to reduce the patient's anxiety and discomfort; minimize the disruptive behavior and prevent further escalation; protect the patient and staff from injury; and facilitate performing physical examinations, diagnostic tests, and essential medical interventions. Consult psychiatry or the psychiatric liaison service to determine whether restraint is necessary and which option to choose. For children with baseline neurodevelopmental issues, other consult options include neurology or behavioral developmental pediatrics. Prior to initiating either method, carefully document all antecedent measures taken to calm the patient, as well as the indications for escalating to restraint, and adhere to all of the institution's restraint policies and procedures.

If chemical restraint is employed, start with the lowest dose necessary to calm the patient and titrate to the behavioral severity and urgency of the sedation. If the indications are nonsevere and nonurgent, first offer the patient an oral sedative, in tablet, suspension, or transmucosal form. This can lead to greater rapport with the patient while having a lower risk of side effects than parenteral medications. Be aware of any potential drug interactions that can cause QT prolongation or exacerbate respiratory or central nervous system (CNS) depression. Verify that the cardioactive electrolytes (corrected or ionized calcium, potassium, magnesium) are normal and provide continuous cardiorespiratory monitoring.

Therapeutic options for chemical restraint (Table 84-2) generally fall into 3 pharmacologic categories: antihistamines, benzodiazepines, and antipsychotics. However, few data exist to compare the relative efficacies for an agitated child. Atypical (second-generation) antipsychotics are gaining increasing use in the management of acute agitation, compared with typical (first-generation) neuroleptics. In the absence of evidence-based or consensus guidelines, it is best to develop a consistent and reliable approach to mild, moderate, and severe agitation. This will promote familiarity with 1 or 2 agents from each pharmacologic class, thereby ensuring proficiency with their dosing, toxicities, and contraindications.

For mild agitation, first give an antihistamine, and reserve benzodiazepines and antipsychotics for moderate agitation. Note that roughly 15% of children have an atypical "hyperactive" response to diphenhydramine. For severe agitation, intramuscular combination therapy (haloperidol + antihistamine; haloperidol + lorazepam; atypical antipsychotic + antihistamine; atypical antipsychotic + lorazepam) may be superior to monotherapy. Monitor the patient closely for CNS and respiratory depression when using any of these agents. In addition, antipsychotics carry the additional risk of cardiac toxicity and hemodynamic compromise. For severe agitation (eg, PCP ingestion), additional measures may be required to ensure safety for the patient, staff, and other pediatric patients on the ward, even to the extent of neuromuscular blockade with concomitant intubation. Pediatric wards should develop policies in advance to deal with agitated patients meeting age criteria for hospitalization on the pediatric service whose level of physical agitation presents a risk to patients, staff, families, and visitors on pediatric units.

Prevention

There are a number of basic measures that can lower the risk of new-onset agitation in an inpatient. Minimize the use and duration of indwelling catheters, implement venous thromboembolism prophylaxis in high-risk patients, reduce polypharmacy, be vigilant for drug-drug interactions, and regularly assess intensive care unit (ICU) patients to detect emergence of delirium.

Indications for Consultation

- **Child life:** Most cases of agitation (once acutely stabilized)
- **Neurology:** Stroke, neuroleptic malignant syndrome (NMS), serotonin syndrome, pre- or postictal state, confusional migraine
- **Psychiatry:** Consideration of physical restraint, moderate or severe agitation, concern for psychosis, history of psychiatric disorder, NMS, serotonin syndrome

Disposition

- **ICU transfer:** NMS, severe serotonin syndrome, moderate/severe traumatic brain injury

Coding

ICD-9

• Agitation	**307.9**
• Anxiety state, unspecified	**300.00**
• Emotional lability	**799.24**
• Irritability	**799.22**
• Nervousness	**799.21**
• Neuroleptic malignant syndrome	**333.92**
• Serotonin syndrome	**333.99**

Pearls and Pitfalls

- The goal is to achieve a cooperative state by calming, not sedating, the patient.
- Document all pre-restraint attempts at de-escalating the patient.
- Cardiorespiratory monitoring is mandatory during chemical restraint with sedatives, due to inherent risks of respiratory inhibition and cardiotoxicity.

Bibliography

Adimando AJ, Poncin YB, Baum CR. Pharmacological management of the agitated pediatric patient. *Pediatr Emerg Care.* 2010;26:856–860

Dorfman DH, Kastner B. The use of restraint for pediatric psychiatric patients in emergency departments. *Pediatr Emerg Care.* 2004;20:151–156

Hilt RJ, Woodward TA. Agitation treatment for pediatric emergency patients. *J Am Acad Child Adolesc Psychiatry.* 2008;47:132–138

Sonnier L, Barzman D. Pharmacologic management of acutely agitated pediatric patients. *Paediatr Drugs.* 2011;13:1–10

Wusthoff CJ, Shellhaas RA, Licht DJ. Management of common neurologic symptoms in pediatric palliative care: seizures, agitation, and spasticity. *Pediatr Clin North Am.* 2007;54:709–733

Depression

Introduction

Depression is a psychiatric disorder with a wide spectrum of severity that affects up to 2% of children and 8% of adolescents. In the most severe form, depression can lead to suicide, which is the third-leading cause of death among adolescents in the United States. Risk factors for depression are both genetic and environmental and include a family history of depression in a first-degree relative, personal history of anxiety disorders or attention-deficit/hyperactivity disorder, family dysfunction, low socioeconomic status, chronic illness, substance abuse, and homosexuality.

Clinical Presentation

History

A depressed patient may present with recurrent somatic complaints (abdominal pain, headaches, myalgias) for which no organic cause can be found. The patient may have recently developed a loss of interest in friends or activities once found to be enjoyable. There may be a history of oppositional behavior, aggression, running away, stealing, fire-setting, or being accident-prone. Ask about suicidal ideation and whether the patient has formulated a plan. Occasionally, the parent is concerned about a loss of appetite, poor school performance, or a change in sleep pattern. Inquire about a family history of depression or suicide.

As a part of the review of systems, perform a mental health screening for any adolescent admitted to the hospital, regardless of the admitting diagnosis. In addition, a chronically ill patient will often have a psychological overlay to their illness, even if it does not meet the *Diagnostic and Statistical Manual of Mental Disorders, Fourth Edition, Text Revision* threshold for inpatient hospitalization or medical therapy.

Physical Examination

Use the physical examination to screen for abnormalities associated with organic causes of depression. In a patient with depressive symptoms, poor hygiene and eye contact, a flattened affect, and psychomotor depression or agitation may be present. Often, abnormalities in mood, thought content, and quality of speech are significant.

Laboratory

The goal of laboratory testing is to attempt to rule out organic causes of depression. Obtain blood for a complete blood cell count, chemistries, thyroid function tests, syphilis serology, and urinary for toxicology.

Differential Diagnosis

Except for an acutely suicidal patient, the priority is to exclude medical conditions that can mimic the clinical presentation of depression. In addition, consider recent stressors (procedures, prolonged clinical course, "bad news") that may be contributing to the patient's depressive symptoms.

The definitive diagnosis of depression requires the input of psychologist or psychiatrist, based on a careful clinical history and mental status examination (Table 85-1). Screening tools, such as the Children's Depression Inventory for a prepubertal school-aged child or the Reynolds Adolescent Depression Scale for a teenager, are helpful supplements to the evaluation of depressive symptoms.

Treatment

Consult a child psychiatrist in order to develop a comprehensive treatment plan. Based on the degree of depression and underlying medical conditions, the psychiatrist may initiate a regimen of pharmacologic intervention, psychotherapy, or a combination of both. Fluoxetine is the sole US Food and Drug Administration–approved antidepressant for use in children. However, defer initiating pharmacologic treatment to the psychiatrist.

Table 85-1. Psychiatric Conditions Mimicking Depression

Diagnosis	Clinical Features
Adjustment disorder with depressed mood	Depressive symptoms start within 3 months of a significant stressor and resolve within 6 months Stressor can be chronic (ongoing abuse) leading to symptoms lasting >6 months
Bipolar disorder	Episodes of mania alternating with depression Manic episodes may present with decreased need for sleep, flight of ideas/distractibility, increased interest in pleasurable activities, or pressured speech
Medically related mood disorder	Clinical findings of a preexisting medical condition May not fulfill all *Diagnostic and Statistical Manual of Mental Disorders, Fourth Edition, Text Revision* depressive disorder criteria Higher risk of suicide with chronic or terminal illness
Post-traumatic stress disorder	Depressive symptoms follow a traumatic event Flashbacks, recurrent dreams, reliving the event

Since inpatient mental health resources for children are limited, a patient who requires inpatient psychiatric care may be admitted to a general pediatric ward until an appropriate inpatient psychiatric bed becomes available. The most frequent such indication is a suicide attempt.

Indications for Consultation

- **Psychiatry:** All patients

Disposition

- **Inpatient psychiatric service transfer:** Active suicidal ideation or attempt or the symptoms are having a severe impact on daily life
- **Discharge criteria:** Improvement in depressive symptoms, outpatient management arranged, no active suicidal or homicidal ideation

Follow-up

- **Mental health professional:** 1 week

Pearls and Pitfalls

- Depression may present with visual hallucinations, although a small number of patients can also have psychotic features, including auditory hallucinations and delusions.
- No evidence exists that "contracting for safety" is preventive for future suicide attempts.
- Discharge planning can be challenging in view of the relative paucity of inpatient and outpatient pediatric psychiatry services.

Coding

ICD-9

• Major depressive disorder single episode	**296.20**
• Major depressive disorder recurrent event	**296.30**
• Adjustment reaction, unspecified	**309.9**
• Depressive disorder not classified elsewhere	**311**

Bibliography

Garber J, Clarke GN, Weersing VR, et al. Prevention of depression in at-risk adolescents: a randomized controlled trial. *JAMA*. 2009;301:2215–2224

Gray LB, Dubin-Rhodin A, Weller RA, Weller EB. Assessment of depression in children and adolescents. *Curr Psychiatry Rep*. 2009;11:106–113

Prager LM. Depression and suicide in children and adolescents. *Pediatr Rev*. 2009; 30:199–205

Williams SB, O'Connor EA, Eder M, Whitlock EP. Screening for child and adolescent depression in primary care settings: a systematic evidence review for the US Preventive Services Task Force. *Pediatrics*. 2009;123:e716–e735

Psychosocial

CHAPTER 86

Child Abuse: Physical Abuse and Neglect

Introduction

Child maltreatment encompasses neglect, physical abuse, sexual abuse, and emotional abuse. Neglect is the most prevalent form of child maltreatment. However, by its very nature it is the presentation that is least frequently seen by health care professionals. Neglect often presents as failure to thrive (FTT), particularly in children with special health care needs. Other forms of neglect include lack of supervision, including ingestion of a toxic substance, as well as medical care neglect, which is failing to continue critical treatment or management for a child's medical condition, such as not refilling prescriptions or missing medical appointments.

Physical abuse is any punishment that is unreasonable or causes bodily injury to a child, although individual states' definitions of such may vary. Risk factors related to the parent include an adolescent mother, substance abuse, single parenthood, employment instability or overcommitment, domestic violence, maternal depression, and history of abuse of the parent. Patient risk factors include prematurity, low birth weight, special health care needs, and intellectual disability. However, child abuse is not limited to one societal group, but cuts across all cultural and socioeconomic strata.

Identification of abused children is critical because they may be repeatedly victimized. As many as 35% of the patients who are diagnosed as victims of physical abuse have evidence of old injury at the time of diagnosis, with the most likely perpetrator being a parent or someone known to the family who is trusted by them.

Clinical Presentation

History

Ask about social support at home and any family stressors. In addition, assess the parent's affective behavior toward the patient by gently, and without judgment, asking questions about how the parent responds to the patient when a need is expressed. How does the caregiver typically discipline the child or deal with difficult behaviors? Empathizing with stressors, frustration, poverty, and the medical problems that the parents may face helps to build trust and rapport.

It is critically important to carefully review the child's medical, developmental, birth, family, and social histories, including the number of previous reports to child protective services (CPS). Determine who, other than the parents, are regular caregivers, as well their relationship to the family, how long family has known them, and if other children are cared for along with the patient (other children may also be at risk).

In a case of trauma, obtain and document a step-by-step mechanism of injury from the caregiver and the child, if verbal, although the patient may be reticent to talk about the events. With physical abuse, the mechanism of injury is often inconsistent with the physical examination, so determining the exact mechanism is a priority. Important questions include: What was the patient doing just before and just after event? Who saw the patient last before the event and what was the patient's status? Who saw the patient most immediately post-event and what was the status then? Can anyone speak to if/how the patient's status changed over time after the event?

If emesis or increased sleep is reported, can they be differentiated from the patient's usual condition (eg, reflux) or an acute viral illness? Has any swelling or bruising occurred or coloration changed? If the patient has fallen, inquire about the pre-fall and post-fall position, the reported fall distance, and the type of surface that the child's body hit. If the fall occurred from the bed, note whether there is cosleeping, a "makeshift" bed or one that is an older and less safe model, or a bed that is not suited to the child's age or functional status.

Trauma may not be part of the chief complaint or history. The patient may instead present with an altered level of consciousness, new-onset afebrile seizures, vomiting, a change in the feeding pattern, or simply an unexplained or unwitnessed injury.

Accurate and detailed documentation is critical, using quotes when possible. In addition, it is essential to inquire about the child's global development, speech, temperament, sleep schedule, and behavioral issues. Can the patient tell someone, or somehow indicate, what has or has not occurred? Indicate if there is discomfort in a particular body area that a typical caregiver would have noted sooner (eg, guarding an extremity that previously was functional).

Obtaining an accurate history can be particularly challenging when the parent/caregiver has a developmental disability, communication difficulties, behavioral issues, or mental illness. In such a case, consult with a trained interviewer, such as a child abuse expert, social worker, psychologist, or psychiatrist.

Physical Examination

Measure and plot the height, weight and, if age-appropriate, the head circumference. Chronic abuse or neglect can be reflected in abnormal growth parameters, especially reduced weight (neglect) and increased head circumference (chronic subdural hematomas). The definition of FTT is a weight-for-age decreasing across 2 major percentile channels or actual weight-for-length below 80% of ideal weight. Use the Waterlow criteria for communicating the degree of malnutrition:

(Actual weight)/(predicted weight according to length *or* weight-for-length)

Most concerning is a weight that is below 70% of predicted weight-for-length. The approach to a patient with FTT is summarized on page 486. A patient with a known genetic syndrome may have persistently been below the standard curves, but has recently had a further decrease in growth velocity.

Document bruising and other skin findings with a body diagram and/or digital camera. Suspicious sites for inflicted skin injury include the scalp, ears, neck, angle of the jaw, the frenula of the lips and tongue, the inner thighs and genitals, along the spine, and soft tissue prominences such as the cheeks, abdomen, and buttocks.

After 1 to 2 days, reexamine areas that are tender but do not have visible signs of injury, as these may be sites of deep bruising. A patient with abdominal injury may have an equivocal abdominal examination, most often without visible bruising. In contrast to long bones, rib and metatarsal fractures may not present with tenderness to palpation.

Laboratory

For physical abuse, use Table 86-1 to guide the choice of laboratory and radiology examinations. See page 486 for the workup of FTT.

Obtain a complete blood cell count, looking for an acute anemia (acute trauma) or an abnormal smear to identify mimics of abuse, such as leukemia. Also obtain liver enzymes and a urinalysis to evaluate for possible occult abdominal injury. Serum amylase and lipase are less helpful. A prothrombin time and partial thromboplastin time are useful to screen for a bleeding diathesis if the patient presents with bruising or central nervous system hemorrhage, although these tests will not necessarily detect von Willebrand disease or disorders of platelet aggregation. An osteopenia workup may be indicated for an ex-premature patient to determine if the patient's osteopenia could predispose to fracture(s).

Table 86-1. Laboratory Evaluation of Suspected Abuse			
	<12 Months	12–24 Months	>2 Years
CBC with peripheral smear, AST/ALT, urinalysis	Always	Always	Per history or physical exam
CT abdomen	Per history, physical exam, and laboratory results		
Fundoscopic examination	Routine in many centers	Follow-up for intracranial bleeding or ocular injury	
Head CT (rule out intracranial bleed)	Always	With signs of inflicted trauma	
MRI of brain (first choice for infants in some centers)	Follow-up for an abnormal head CT as needed		
Skeletal survey (when stable)	Always	Always	Per history or physical exam

Abbreviations: ALT, alanine transaminase; AST, aspartate transaminase; CBC, complete blood cell count; CT, computed tomography; MRI, magnetic resonance imaging.

A head computed tomography (CT) can provide evidence of an intracranial bleed, while magnetic resonance imaging (MRI) can sometimes define the chronicity and extent of the injury. Order a skeletal survey when the patient cannot communicate pain or history of trauma because of developmental status or a disabling injury. Since this is not an urgent study, defer it until the patient is clinically stable and skilled pediatric radiology personnel are available. In many cases, a repeat skeletal survey 10 to 12 days later will show missed occult fractures that in the interim have developed callus formation.

Although up to 80% of infants with abusive head trauma have retinal hemorrhages, fundoscopy is not a useful screening study for occult head injury. Rather, arrange a dilated fundoscopic examination to evaluate for comorbid retinal hemorrhage, retinal detachment, or vitreous hemorrhage in a patient with either intracranial or external ocular injury.

Differential Diagnosis

Abuse is more likely if the caretaker's explanations are absent, vague, variable (from the same historian or between caretakers), or inconsistent with the pattern of injuries or the developmental capabilities of the patient. Consider cultural practices and healing traditions that may leave marks, burns, or bruises, such as coining, spooning, holding the child upside down to hit the feet, and treatment for sunken fontanelle. The intention of these cultural practices is to heal or treat a perceived illness rather than to inflict injury.

A child who is found unconscious without an explanation is suspicious for abuse. Consider inflicted trauma if a nonambulatory infant has any bruising. In contrast, a cruising toddler will typically have bruising on extensor surfaces (shins) or over bony prominences, such as the forehead. Recurrent injuries are suspicious for abuse if a clear and consistent explanation for each injury is absent. Injuries that are also concerning for abuse include multiple, complex, diastatic, or occipital skull fractures, as well as heterogeneous hematomas on brain imaging. Some fracture types in infants, such as posterior rib fractures or metaphyseal fractures, are highly specific for inflicted injury.

New onset seizures require neuroimaging, usually an MRI. If there is persistent altered mental status (AMS), a CT scan can confirm the diagnosis of trauma. Infections, such as meningitis or encephalitis, can cause AMS or seizures, as well as vomiting. There may be a history of fever, headache, cold symptoms, or a rash. Ingestion and purposeful administration of a toxic substance are other etiologies of AMS and seizures.

Above-average weight gain while under observed care and receiving large amounts of *ad lib* intake is suspicious for nutritional neglect. Consider food insecurity, poverty, and domestic violence, which may contribute to nutritional problems and access to appropriate foods.

See Table 86-2 for differential diagnosis of child abuse and neglect.

Table 86-2. Differential Diagnosis of Child Abuse and Neglect

Diagnosis	Clinical Features
Failure to Thrive	
Celiac disease	Presents after introduction of gluten-containing foods Can have constipation or diarrhea
Heart failure	Tires easily with feeds Hepatomegaly May have a murmur
Inadequate caloric intake	Parent errs when mixing formula or withholds food Parent is incompetent and misunderstands normal feeding Food insecurity is present in the home environment
Inflammatory bowel disease	Does not present during infancy Abdominal pain and hematochezia May have ↑ inflammatory markers (white blood cell count, C-reactive protein, erythrocyte sedimentation rate)
Severe gastroesophageal reflux	Extensive vomiting after every meal
Bleeding	
Glutaric aciduria type 1	Macrocranium Subdural hematoma, frontotemporal atrophy Sparse retinal hemorrhages
Hemophilia	Positive family history Hemarthrosis ↑ Partial thromboplastin time
Hemorrhagic disease of the newborn	History of no vitamin K prophylaxis or home birth Exclusively breastfed
Idiopathic thrombocytopenic purpura	Petechiae Thrombocytopenia

Table 86-2. Differential Diagnosis of Child Abuse and Neglect, continued

Diagnosis	Clinical Features
Cutaneous Findings	
Coining	Erythematous, linear abrasions over back/extremities
Cupping	Bruises are perfectly circular and appear in a pattern
Mongolian spots	Nontender macules No change in appearance when reexamined
Fractures	
Osteogenesis imperfecta	Numerous transverse long-bone and rib fractures Macrocephaly, blue sclerae
Rickets	History of prematurity History of poor vitamin D and/or calcium intake ↓ Calcium, ↑alkaline phosphatase Exclusively breastfed; minimal sun exposure Radiographic changes at costochondral junctions and long bones Frontal bossing (severe)
Abdominal Injury	
Volvulus with malrotation	Bilious vomiting Surgical abdomen

Treatment

Stabilization of airway, breathing, and circulation is always the priority. Ensure that the patient is hemodynamically stable before being sent for neuroimaging. If there is concern for head injury or other trauma, consult the appropriate surgical services, and for all other injuries, treat according to the standards of care. Carefully document all findings and management decisions using objective language.

Caring for a battered child is emotionally unsettling and can lead to strong protective feelings in medical staff that may compromise objectivity. The role of the medical team is to focus on the health and support of the child, not to investigate a potential crime or judge a perceived perpetrator. Consult with CPS and the appropriate hospital administration to limit family visitation if the hospital staff are threatened by a caretaker or the safety of other patients is jeopardized. However, parental visitation cannot be broadly denied unless CPS decides it is necessary for the protection of the child.

Child Safety and Protection

If there is any *reasonable suspicion* of abuse or neglect, report the case to the local CPS. It is not necessary to have a specific perpetrator or hypothesis in mind. In addition, the Health Insurance Portability and Accountability Act does not apply because communication to appropriate child protection agencies is necessary to protect children. Know your state laws, found on the US Department of Health and Human Services Web site at www.childwelfare.gov/systemwide/laws_policies/state/can/.

Indications for Consultation

- **Child protection team:** All patients
- **Dietitian:** FTT
- **Genetics:** Suspected glutaric academia type 1 or osteopenic bone disease, such as osteogenesis imperfecta
- **Hematology:** Suspected coagulopathy
- **Neurosurgery:** Intracranial injury or displaced skull fracture
- **Ophthalmology:** If a dilated fundoscopic examination is indicated
- **Orthopaedics:** Evaluation and management of fractures
- **Surgery:** Suspected intra-abdominal injury

Disposition

- **Intensive care unit transfer:** Unstable vital signs or altered mental status
- **Discharge criteria:** Injuries stable or improved; CPS identified a safe environment to which the child may be discharged; follow-up plan established

Follow-up

- **Primary care:** 2 weeks for repeat skeletal survey for a patient younger than 2 years, biopsychosocial follow-up, vaccine catch-up, etc
- **Developmental-behavioral pediatrician:** As needed for problems with regression, fears, tantrums, aggression, and sleep problems
- **Early intervention or head start:** As needed for developmental delay
- **Mental health services:** As needed for signs of depression

Pearls and Pitfalls

- A short fall (<3 feet) can result in a simple, linear skull fracture with scalp bruising and swelling, but rarely causes multiple, complex, diastatic, or occipital skull fractures or an intracranial injury.
- *Reasonable suspicion* of abuse is sufficient to report the case to the local child protection authorities. A useful strategy when a child abuse and neglect team conducts the evaluation is to make a report if just one member of the team feels it is necessary.
- Maintain a high index of suspicion, particularly with infants, as many abused children are seen for their injuries by medical professionals prior to abuse being diagnosed.

- The age of a bruise cannot be determined by physical examination or color of the bruise.
- A patient who was not involved in a motor vehicle accident, but has pancreatic or hollow viscus injuries, is more likely to be a victim of physical abuse.

Coding

ICD-9

- Child abuse, unspecified **995.50**
- Child neglect (nutritional) **995.52**
- Child physical abuse **995.54**
- Child sexual abuse **995.53**
- Other child abuse and neglect (multiple forms of abuse) **995.59**
- Shaken infant syndrome **995.55**
  - For all of the above use additional codes, such as retinal hemorrhage **(362.81),** to show any injuries and appropriate E-code to show nature of abuse **(E960–E968)** and/or perpetrator **(E967.0–E967.9).** For neglect codes also list **E904.0** (abandonment or neglect of infants and helpless persons) or **E968.4** (abandonment of child, infant, or other helpless person with intent to injure or kill), if intent is known.

Bibliography

American Academy of Pediatrics Section on Radiology. Diagnostic imaging of child abuse. *Pediatrics.* 2009;123:1430–1435

Chadwick DL, Bertocci G, Castillo E, et al. Annual risk of death resulting from short falls among young children: less than 1 in 1 million. *Pediatrics.* 2008;121:1213–1224

Cotton BA, Beckert BW, Smith MK, Burd RS. The utility of clinical and laboratory data for predicting intraabdominal injury among children. *J Trauma.* 2004;56:1068–1074

Kellogg ND; American Academy of Pediatrics Committee on Child Abuse and Neglect. Evaluation of suspected child physical abuse. *Pediatrics.* 2007;119:1232–1241

Levin AV, Christian CW; American Academy of Pediatrics Committee on Child Abuse and Neglect, Section on Ophthalmology. The eye examination in the evaluation of child abuse. *Pediatrics.* 2010;126:376–380

US Department of Health and Human Services, Administration for Children and Families, Administration on Children, Youth and Families, Children's Bureau. *Child Maltreatment 2009.* http://www.acf.hhs.gov/programs/cb/stats_research/index.htm#can

CHAPTER 87

Sexual Abuse

Introduction

Sexual abuse is defined as sexual activities that the child cannot comprehend, for which the child is developmentally unprepared and cannot give consent, and/or that violate the law or social taboos of society. Most perpetrators are male, with adolescents implicated in at least 20% of cases.

Clinical Presentation

History

Sexual abuse has a variable presentation, which ranges from parental concern alone to nonspecific physical symptoms to the demonstration of sexualized behaviors and even frank disclosure of the abuse by the child. If there are signs or symptoms concerning for abuse, interview the caregiver and the patient separately. Use open-ended questions, which will facilitate obtaining a full history and explanation. For example, ask "Has anyone ever touched you in a way you didn't like or didn't want?" rather than, "Who touched you?" Respond calmly and without strong emotions.

A thorough review of systems is necessary, including questions about abdominal pain, dysuria, enuresis, encopresis, bleeding, discharge, phobias, difficulty sleeping, and possible physical trauma. Also ask about homicidal or suicidal ideation. Specific symptoms of sexual abuse can be rectal or genital bleeding and developmentally unusual sexual behavior.

If there is enough information to raise a concern that inappropriate contact has occurred, arrange a separate, detailed interview by a trained professional. This can occur in the hospital by contacting the child protection team or social worker. Occasionally, it may be appropriate to delay the interview until the child can be seen at an advocacy center if follow-up can be arranged within a week, the patient is safe from the perpetrator after discharge, the disclosure is of remote contact, and the child has no physical complaints. Regardless, the hospital team must obtain a history pertinent to the diagnosis and treatment of the medical consequences of the sexual abuse. This includes the type of abuse, when the last incident occurred, the type of contact that happened, any signs or symptoms of sexually transmitted infections (STIs), and date of menarche in addition to the symptoms listed above. If a child protection team is available, the team's medical provider can take the expanded medical history and assist in guiding diagnosis and treatment. Do not interview a patient younger than 3 years, but document any spontaneous utterances in quotation marks, such as "You won't hurt my pee-pee like John did, will you?"

Physical Examination

If the incident(s) occurred more than 4 days ago and there are no genitourinary symptoms, the examination may be deferred until the patient can be seen at a children's advocacy center equipped with trained examiners and a colposcope. Collection of forensic evidence is warranted when the last episode of abuse occurred within 96 hours or if the child is acutely injured. Perform the examination in accordance with the protocols for sexual assault victims to properly collect the evidence. Ideally, arrange for the presence of a supportive adult who is not involved in the allegations of abuse.

Prior to starting, explain the examination to the patient. Inspect the oropharynx and skin for signs of trauma or infection. Note the child's affect and development as there is no standard victim reaction to sexual assault. The patient may be stunned and poorly interactive, weeping, or even smiling or joking with the examiner.

During the genitourinary examination note the patient's sexual maturity rating and describe each part of the genitalia, breasts, perineal region, anus, and buttocks as necessary with accompanying drawn diagrams or photographs. The best way to visualize the hymen and female genitalia is by labial traction. Place the patient in the frog-leg or lithotomy position, grasp each of the labia majora with the thumb and forefinger, and gently pull toward the examiner (as if pulling up a sock). If performed correctly, the examination is painless and the hymen will become more 3-dimensional in relation to the introitus and vaginal canal. However, the hymen can have a variety of normal configurations, which may require specialized training to recognize. Many institutions have a pediatric sexual assault nurse examiner (SANE-P) available to perform the genital and rectal examination with colposcopic viewing and photography.

It is uncommon to discover physical examination findings that are diagnostic of sexual abuse, including among victims of chronic sexual abuse. Concerning findings include abrasions or bruising of the inner thighs and labia and scarring or tears of the labia minora and fourchette. More worrisome are scarring, tears, or interruption of the posterior hymen; absent hymenal tissue; scarring of the fossa navicularis; injury to the posterior fourchette; and anal lacerations.

Laboratory

If the abuse has occurred in the last 96 hours, complete a rape kit, following the accompanying directions. To decide on testing for STIs, consider the following:

- Was there oral, genital, or rectal contact with bodily secretions? Digital fondling alone is unlikely to transmit an STI.
- How common are STIs in the community?
- Is the child symptomatic? An asymptomatic prepubertal child will almost always have negative cultures. Exceptions include a patient who shares the environment with a symptomatic, or known to be infected, child or alleged perpetrator.

Typical STI testing includes gonorrhea, chlamydia (throat swab, urine nucleic acid amplification test [NAAT] or culture), Venereal Disease Research Laboratory or rapid plasma reagin for syphilis, HIV, and a pregnancy test for a postmenarchal girl. Pregnancy or the presence of sperm or semen is diagnostic of sexual contact. A positive test for gonorrhea, chlamydia, syphilis, or HIV is diagnostic of child abuse when vertical transmission has been excluded. Since it is unusual for a prepubertal victim to present immediately after the abuse occurred, select testing on a case-by-case basis in consultation with a child abuse expert. Likewise, there are potential legal issues involved with using NAAT versus culture as evidence in prepubertal children.

Differential Diagnosis

Normal behavior surrounding genitalia is playful, driven by curiosity, and sometimes involving other children of the same age range. Sexually reactive behaviors may include a child who attempts to force another child, whether younger or an age peer, to engage in sexual behaviors or a child who performs insertive acts on herself or her toys. As with many medical conditions, a diagnosis of sexual abuse does not rely solely on the physical examination. Often a clear and consistent history is sufficient to make the diagnosis.

In the case of genital abnormalities, consult a child abuse specialist, who has the expertise to categorize abnormalities.

Reporting

A reasonable suspicion of sexual abuse is sufficient to report the case to the local child protection authorities. Health care providers are mandatory reporters for any reasonable suspicion. See Table 87-1 for guidance.

Table 87-1. Guidelines for Making the Decision to Report Sexual Abuse of Children[a]

Data Available				Response	
History	Behavioral Symptoms	Physical Examination	Diagnostic Tests	Level of Concern About Sexual Abuse	Report Decision
Clear statement	Present or absent	Normal or abnormal	Positive or negative	High	Report
None or vague	Present or absent	Normal or nonspecific	Positive[b]	High	Report
None or vague	Present or absent	Concerning or diagnostic findings	Positive or negative	High[c]	Report
Vague, or history by parent only	Present or absent	Normal or nonspecific	Negative	Indeterminate	Refer when possible
None	Present	Normal or nonspecific	Negative	Indeterminate	Possible report[d], refer or follow

[a]Adapted from Kellogg N; American Academy of Pediatrics Committee on Child Abuse and Neglect. The evaluation of sexual abuse in children. *Pediatrics.* 2005;116:506–512.
[b]Positive test for *Chlamydia trachomatis*, gonorrhea, *Trichomonas vaginalis*, HIV, syphilis, or herpes if nonsexual transmission is unlikely or excluded.
[c]Confirmed with various examination techniques and/or peer review with expert consultation.
[d]If behaviors are rare or unusual in normal children.

Treatment

Antibiotics

Treatment for STIs depends on the type of contact with the alleged perpetrator. Order prophylactic antibiotics if there was a possible exposure to bodily fluids in a pubertal (or older) patient, but prophylaxis is rarely indicated for a prepubertal victim. Give

ceftriaxone 250 mg intramuscularly once *or* cefixime 400 mg orally once

plus metronidazole 2 g orally once

plus azithromycin 1 g orally once *or* doxycycline 100 mg orally twice a day for 7 days

If the patient is not fully vaccinated for hepatitis B, start or finish the series.

HIV Prophylaxis

If there is concern for HIV, give postexposure prophylaxis with zidovudine (page 242) and contact a retrovirologist for guidance, or contact the PEPline (888/448-4911; www.nccc.ucsf.edu/about_nccc/pepline/).

Child Safety and Protection

If there is any *reasonable suspicion* of abuse or neglect, report the case to the local child protective services (CPS). It is not necessary to have a specific perpetrator or hypothesis in mind. In addition, the Health Insurance Portability and Accountability Act does not apply because communication to appropriate child protection agencies is necessary to protect children. Know your state laws, found on the United States Department of Health and Human Services Web site at www.childwelfare.gov/systemwide/laws_policies/state/can/.

There are more than 700 children's advocacy centers (CACs) in the United States. They function as centralized locations for victims of sexual abuse. They provide coordination among community agencies and professionals, including law enforcement, CPS, prosecution, medical, victim advocacy, and mental health services. To find a CAC, go to www.nationalchildrensalliance.org/ and search by zip code or state.

Indications for Consultation

- **Child protection team:** Suspected sexual abuse
- **Pediatric SANE-P, if available:** Suspected sexual abuse
- **Psychiatry:** Suicidal or homicidal ideation
- **Social work:** Suspected sexual abuse

Disposition

- **Intensive care unit transfer:** Unstable vital signs or altered mental status
- **Discharge criteria:** CPS has identified a safe environment to which the child may be discharged; a follow-up plan has been established.

Follow-up

- **Primary care:** 1 to 2 weeks
- **CAC:** 3 to 5 days, to complete information gathering, establish care with mental health services, and repeat STI screening, if indicated
- **Mental health services:** 1 to 2 weeks, if not available at the nearest CAC, or referrals not provided by CAC

Pearls and Pitfalls

- The diagnosis of sexual abuse can be made based on a clear and consistent history, such that a normal physical examination does not rule out sexual abuse.
- Genitalia, especially female, have many variations of normal. If there is uncertainty about the findings of a physical examination, consult an expert.
- Document thoroughly and clearly, using quotations when possible. Detailed notes will facilitate effective testimony in court.
- Use a colposcope or camera when conducting a physical examination for both continuity of care and collection of evidence.
- A reasonable suspicion of sexual abuse is sufficient to report the case to the local child protection authorities.
- Consult with an appropriate expert for issues concerning teen reproductive health, such as underage sexual activity and confidentiality.

Coding

ICD-9

- Child sexual abuse **995.53**
- Other child abuse and neglect **995.59**
  - For all of the above use additional codes, such as vaginal laceration **(878.6),** to show any injuries and appropriate E-code to show nature of abuse **(E960–E968)** and/or perpetrator **(E967.0–E967.9).**

Bibliography

Adams JA, Kaplan RA, Starling SP, et al. Guidelines for medical care of children who may have been sexually abused. *J Pediatr Adolesc Gynecol.* 2007;20:163–172

Asnes AG, Leventhal JM. Managing child abuse: general principles. *Pediatr Rev.* 2010;31:47–55

Bechtel K. Sexual abuse and sexually transmitted infections in children and adolescents. *Curr Opin Pediatr.* 2010;22:94–99

Kellogg ND; American Academy of Pediatrics Committee on Child Abuse and Neglect. Evaluation of suspected child physical abuse. *Pediatrics.* 2007;119:1232–1241

Kellogg ND; American Academy of Pediatrics Committee on Child Abuse and Neglect. Clinical report—the evaluation of sexual behaviors in children. *Pediatrics.* 2009;124:992–998

Watkeys JM, Price LD, Upton PM, Maddocks A. The timing of medical examination following an allegation of sexual abuse: is this an emergency? *Arch Dis Child.* 2008;93:851–856

Pulmonary

CHAPTER 88

Acute Asthma Exacerbation

Introduction

Asthma is a chronic respiratory disease characterized by airway inflammation and obstruction with a recurrent, reversible pattern of symptoms. Seven million children in the United States have a current diagnosis of asthma and acute asthma exacerbations (AAE) are among the leading causes of pediatric hospitalizations. Status asthmaticus is defined as a life-threatening asthma exacerbation with risk for respiratory failure.

Clinical Presentation

History

In a patient with a known history of asthma, focus the initial history on recent asthma symptoms, medication use, and any risk factors for death (Box 88-1). Ask about fever, upper respiratory tract symptoms, and vomiting, which can suggest a viral trigger. Once the patient has been stabilized, inquire about chronic asthma symptoms (wheezing, nighttime coughing, and limitation of activity) and prior exacerbations.

Box 88-1. Risk Factors for Death From Asthma[a]
Asthma History
Difficulty perceiving asthma symptoms or severity of exacerbations
Hospitalization or emergency department (ED) visit for asthma in the past month
Lack of a written asthma action plan or sensitivity to *Alternaria*
Previous severe exacerbation (eg, intubation or intensive care unit admission for asthma)
≥3 ED visits for asthma in the past year
≥2 asthma hospitalizations in the past year
Using >2 canisters of short-acting β_2-agonist per month
Social History
Illicit drug use
Low socioeconomic status or inner-city residence
Major psychosocial problems
Comorbidities
Cardiovascular disease
Chronic psychiatric disease
Other chronic lung disease

[a]Adapted from US Department of Health and Human Services; National Institutes of Health; National Heart, Lung, and Blood Institute; National Asthma Education and Prevention Program. *Expert Panel Report 3: Guidelines for the Diagnosis and Management of Asthma. Full Report 2007.* Bethesda, MD: National Heart, Lung, and Blood Institute; 2007:377.

Physical Examination

A patient with a moderate to severe asthma exacerbation often has decreased air movement with diffuse wheezing (classically expiratory, but may be both inspiratory and expiratory), a prolonged expiratory phase, tachypnea, dyspnea, accessory muscle use, and coughing. In status asthmaticus, the respiratory examination can be misleading, as the patient may have no wheezing because of lack of air movement ("tight" chest), so that the subsequent onset of wheezing may indicate improved air movement and a response to therapy. Tachycardia is common and can be secondary to respiratory distress, dehydration, or a side effect from the use of short-acting β_2-agonists (SABAs) (albuterol, levalbuterol). If the patient presents with or develops fever, focus the examination on an evaluation for bacterial versus viral etiologies, although musical wheezing is generally not consistent with a classical bacterial process. Unilateral wheezing may indicate a foreign body or airway mass.

Use a validated clinical scoring system, such as the PRAM (Preschool Respiratory Assessment Measurement) or PASS (Pediatric Asthma Severity Score), to facilitate reassessment among different caretakers. Most scoring systems include accessory muscle use, wheezing, air entry, and oxygen requirement.

Laboratory

To assist in the assessment of the severity of an AAE, measure the oxygen saturation via pulse oximetry and peak expiratory flow, if a child 5 years or older is able to perform the technique. Otherwise, in most cases laboratory and radiology testing are not indicated. When there is an acute deterioration or concern for impending respiratory failure, order a blood gas, electrolytes, and a chest radiograph. Evaluate a patient who has an atypical or prolonged course for potential other diagnoses (Table 88-1). When there is diagnostic uncertainty, order spirometry for a patient 5 years or older (if capable of performing the procedure), as this can be particularly useful in differentiating asthma from other respiratory diseases.

Differential Diagnosis

Asthma is a diffuse process that affects the lower airways, producing wheezing. However, consider other potential diagnoses (Table 88-1). As a result of the diffuse nature of the process, a patient with an asthma exacerbation is more likely to have hypoxia than one with a localized process (pneumonia). When the diagnosis is in doubt, give a diagnostic/therapeutic trial of a SABA. A good clinical response is consistent with asthma, but no response may reflect status asthmaticus.

Table 88-1. Differential Diagnosis of Wheezing

Diagnosis	Clinical Features
Aspergillosis	Recurrent infections not responsive to antibiotics May have chronic sputum production or hemoptysis Complete blood cell count: eosinophilia Chest x-ray: bronchiectasis
Bronchiolitis	Age <18 months Usually no prior history of wheezing Transmitted upper airway sounds and rales may accompany the wheezing Generally no response to short-acting β_2-agonist (SABA)
Bronchopulmonary dysplasia	<3 years of age History of prematurity requiring oxygen therapy >28 days Clinical examination similar to asthma exacerbation
Community-acquired pneumonia	Tachypnea not responsive to SABA Usually not hypoxic Asymmetrical breath sounds with focal rales Chest radiograph with evidence of lobar consolidation
Congestive heart disease	Dyspnea and fatigue with feeding with poor weight gain Rales and hepatosplenomegaly Chest x-ray: abnormal cardiac silhouette, ↑ pulmonary vascular markings
Foreign body aspiration	May or may not have a history of aspiration Unilateral wheezing No response to SABA Chest x-ray: asymmetrical hyperinflation
Laryngotracheomalacia	"Noisy" breather since birth Symptoms worse when agitated, lying flat, or with feeds No response to SABA
Vocal cord dysfunction	Refractory asthma symptoms with poor response to SABA Generally no nighttime symptoms Harsh stridor noted over larynx when symptomatic Spirometry: limitation of inspiratory flow

Treatment

Treat an asthma exacerbation with a SABA, supplemental oxygen as needed to maintain an oxygen saturation (O_2 sat) 92% or greater, and systemic corticosteroids (Table 88-2). Use the same initial inpatient management for a patient 6 years of age or older with first-time SABA-responsive wheezing, but always consider other etiologies (Table 88-1).

Albuterol is the preferred SABA due to its availability and cost. Levalbuterol is an alternative for a patient with unacceptable side effects from albuterol, including significant nausea, tachycardia, or agitation. Administer albuterol either via nebulizer (0.15 mg/kg/dose; 2.5 mg minimum, 10 mg maximum) or metered-dose inhaler (4–8 puffs with aerochamber and facemask/mouthpiece appropriate for age and maturity) every 1 to 4 hours. Use the patient's history

Table 88-2. Medications for the Treatment of an Asthma Exacerbation[a]

Medication	Dose	Comments
INHALED SHORT-ACTING B_2-AGONISTS		
Albuterol		
Nebulizer solution 0.63 mg/3 mL 1.25 mg/3 mL 2.5 mg/3 mL 5 mg/ mL	0.15 mg/kg (2.5 mg minimum) every 20 minutes for 3 doses, then 0.15–0.3 mg/kg (10 mg max) every 1–4 h as needed, or 0.5 mg/kg/hour by continuous nebulization	Dilute aerosols to ≥3 mL at gas flow of 6–8 L/minute. Use a large-volume nebulizer for continuous administration.
Metered-dose inhaler (MDI) 90 mcg/puff	4–8 puffs every 20 minutes for 3 doses, then every 1–4 hours inhalation maneuver as needed. Use a valved holding chamber (VHC); add mask for a patient <6 years of age.	In mild-to-moderate exacerbations, MDI plus VHC is as effective as nebulized therapy with appropriate administration technique and coaching by trained personnel.
Levalbuterol		
Nebulizer solution 0.63 mg/3 mL 1.25 mg/0.5 mL 1.25 mg/3 mL MDI 45 mcg/puff	0.075 mg/kg (1.25 mg minimum) every 20 minutes for 3 doses, then 0.075–0.15 mg/kg (5 mg max) every 1–4 hours as needed See albuterol MDI dose.	Levalbuterol administered in one-half the mg dose of albuterol provides comparable efficacy and safety. Levalbuterol by continuous nebulization has not been evaluated.
SYSTEMIC CORTICOSTEROIDS		
Methylprednisolone, Prednisolone, Prednisone		
Prednisolone (15 mg/5mL) Prednisone (2.5, 5, 10, 20, 50 mg tabs)	1–2 mg/kg divided twice a day (60 mg/day max)	No proven benefit of methylprednisolone over oral medications. At discharge, give 1–2 mg/kg/day (60 mg max) to complete 3- to 10-day course, but an extended course may be necessary. Taper over several days if the patient receives steroids for >7–10 days.
Dexamethasone		
1 mg/mL	0.6 mg/kg intramuscular, intravenous, or oral once (16 mg max)	No proven benefit over methylprednisolone, prednisolone, or prednisone.
ADJUNCTIVE THERAPIES FOR STATUS ASTHMATICUS		
Magnesium Sulfate		
1 g magnesium sulfate = 98.6 mg of *elemental* magnesium = 8.12 mEq magnesium	50 mg/kg as intravenous solution (25–75 mg/kg, 2 g max)	Dilute to a concentration of 0.5 mEq/mL (60 mg/mL of *magnesium sulfate*). Infuse over 2–4 hours. Do not exceed 125 mg/kg/hour of magnesium sulfate.

Table 88-2. Medications for the Treatment of an Asthma Exacerbation[a], continued

Medication	Dose	Comments
ANTICHOLINERGICS IN COMBINATION WITH SHORT-ACTING B_2-AGONISTS		
Ipratropium Bromide		
Nebulizer solution 0.25 mg/mL	0.25–0.5 mg every 20 minutes for 3 doses, then as needed	May mix in same nebulizer with albuterol for a severe exacerbation, although its addition has not been shown to provide further benefit once a patient is hospitalized. Do not use as first-line therapy.
MDI 18 mcg/puff	0.5 mg every 20 minutes for 3 doses, then as needed	Use with VHC and face mask for a patient <6 years of age.
SYSTEMIC (INJECTED) B_2-AGONISTS		
Epinephrine		
1:1,000 (1 mg/mL)	0.01 mg/kg up to 0.3–0.5 mg every 20 minutes for 3 doses subcutaneous	No proven advantage of systemic therapy over aerosol
Terbutaline		
(1 mg/mL)	0.01 mg/kg every 20 minutes for 3 doses then every 2–6 hour as needed subcutaneous	No proven advantage of systemic therapy over aerosol

[a]Adapted from US Department of Health and Human Services; National Institutes of Health; National Heart, Lung, and Blood Institute; National Asthma Education and Prevention Program. *Expert Panel Report 3: Guidelines for the Diagnosis and Management of Asthma. Full Report 2007*. Bethesda, MD: National Heart, Lung, and Blood Institute; 2007:405.

and prehospital management, emergency department management, and physical examination to determine the initial scheduling of albuterol. Start with aggressive treatment, then wean as tolerated. The greater the intensity of the prehospital and acute management and the more severe the physical examination, the more frequent the albuterol scheduling.

Reassess the patient frequently, initially with each inhalation, then at least with every other inhalation. Check for improvement to wean frequency of treatments or worsening that would necessitate intensifying the therapy. Assessments can also be performed by skilled members of the health care team, including respiratory therapy or nursing. A clinical scoring system (PRAM, PASS) improves communication between the health care team and helps to standardize and facilitate the weaning process. Peak expiratory flows can also be useful to assess changes in a patient who is 5 years or older and experienced in using a peak flow meter.

Provide supplemental oxygen to correct hypoxemia (defined as O_2 sat <92%), or if the patient has an acute deterioration with worsening respiratory rate, accessory muscle use, and air movement, despite an O_2 sat 92% or greater. As the patient improves, wean the supplemental oxygen, but keep the O_2 sat 92% or greater.

Administer systemic corticosteroids, such as prednisone, prednisolone, methylprednisolone (1–2 mg/kg/day given every day or divided twice a day, 60 mg/day maximum) or dexamethasone (1 dose of 0.6 mg/kg intramuscular [IM], intravenous [IV], or oral, 16 mg maximum) to any patient with an AAE. Systemic corticosteroids decrease airway inflammation, but there is no advantage to using IV or IM steroids, unless the patient cannot tolerate oral medication. Prescribe treatment for 3 to 5 days, but extend the course if the patient has prolonged symptoms requiring hospitalization or recent or chronic steroid use. Taper over several days if the patient receives steroids for more than 7 to 10 days to prevent rebound of respiratory symptoms. If the patient received more than 10 to 14 days of steroids, a longer taper is necessary because of the risk of adrenocortical insufficiency.

In a patient with status asthmaticus (severe respiratory distress, respiratory rate >60/minutes, little air movement, O_2 sat <92 %) or an acute deterioration, increase the SABA to continuous therapy at 0.15 to 0.3 mg/kg/hour (10–15 mg/hour maximum). If a patient is receiving continuous SABA therapy for more than 24 hours, check the electrolytes to assess for hypokalemia. Make the patient NPO and begin maintenance IV fluids. If there is no response after 4 to 6 hours to treatment intensification, transfer the patient to an intensive care unit (ICU) where additional therapies can be safely delivered, such as IV magnesium (25–75 mg/kg/dose) or heliox (70:30 helium-oxygen mixture to deliver albuterol nebulization). Additional therapies of *unproven* benefit that may be considered prior to intubation for respiratory failure include systemic IV β_2-agonists (IV or subcutaneous [SC] terbutaline or SC epinephrine) leukotriene inhibitors (montelukast), and noninvasive ventilation.

Treatments that do *not* improve outcomes for an inpatient with uncomplicated asthma exacerbations include theophylline or aminophylline, chest physiotherapy, and antibiotic therapy without a definite bacterial source. Although nebulized ipratropium bromide has been shown to decrease hospitalization rates, there is no documented benefit for its use during hospitalization in an uncomplicated AAE.

If the patient does not respond as anticipated or worsens acutely, evaluate for complications, such as pneumothorax, pneumomediastinum, secondary bacterial pneumonia, or other bacterial infections. Perform a complete physical examination, obtain a complete blood cell count and blood gas, and order a chest radiograph.

Many institutions currently use asthma clinical pathways (ACPs) to promote best evidence-based practices. ACPs have been shown to reduce length of stay and costs, without increasing readmissions, and increase adherence to best-practice techniques. The development of ACPs requires a multidisciplinary team, including physicians from the inpatient setting, intensive care, pulmonary, and the emergency department, as well as respiratory therapists, pharmacy, social work, and nursing.

Discharge Planning

Start discharge planning at the time of admission. Once the patient is stabilized, and prior to discharge, elicit further history to determine the patient's chronic level of control and classification of asthma (www.nhlbi.nih.gov/guidelines/asthma/asthsumm.pdf, Figures 11 and 12), as well as medication compliance and typical triggers. A specific list of requirements prior to discharge for AAE is shown in Table 88-3. Many institutions incorporate components of asthma teaching on trigger avoidance, symptom recognition, medication use, peak flow use for a patient older than 5 years, and device training into an asthma education class given by a trained nonphysician. An individualized asthma action plan (or home management plan) with written instructions gives families and patients simple directions for actions based on symptoms and is required by The Joint Commission for all patients admitted with the diagnosis of AAE. Sample asthma action plans and other patient resources can be found in Section 3, Component 2: Education for a Partnership in Asthma Care (www.nhlbi.nih.gov/guidelines/asthma/05_sec3_comp2.pdf).

Although an asthma exacerbation is an acute event, this is a chronic disease with significant morbidity. A critical aspect to quality inpatient asthma care is facilitating a chronic asthma management plan and appropriate outpatient follow-up. Ongoing discussion and communication with the family and primary care provider is essential to these goals. Prior to discharge, determine the patient's chronic level of severity (as mentioned above) and place the patient on the appropriate controller medication. The first-line therapy for persistent asthma is an inhaled corticosteroid. Further information on classification and management of chronic asthma can be found at www.nhlbi.nih.gov/guidelines/asthma.

Table 88-3. Discharge Checklist[a]		
Intervention	**Dose/Timing**	**Education/Advice**
Inhaled medications (eg, metered-dose inhaler [MDI] with valved holding chamber [VHC] or spacer; nebulizer)	Select agent, dose, and frequency (eg, albuterol) Short-acting β_2-agonist: 2–6 puffs every 4–6 hours for 2 days or as needed Inhaled corticosteroids: Dosing depends on the patient's chronic level of severity (generally low to medium dose unless asthma specialist involved).	Teach purpose. Teach and check technique. For MDIs, emphasize importance of VHC or spacer.
Oral medications	Select agent, dose, and frequency (eg, prednisone 50 mg every day for 5 days)	Teach purpose. Teach side effects.
Peak flow meter (peak expiratory flow [PEF])	For selected patients ≥5 years and able: Measure PEF in AM and PM and record best of 3 tries each time.	Teach purpose. Teach technique. Distribute peak flow diary.
Follow-up visit	Make appointment for follow-up care with primary clinician or asthma specialist within 1 week.	Advise patient (or caregiver) of date, time, and location of appointment, ideally within 5 days of hospital discharge.
Action plan	Before or at discharge	Instruct patient (or caregiver) on simple plan for actions to be taken when symptoms, signs, or PEF values suggest airflow obstruction.

[a]Adapted from US Department of Health and Human Services; National Institutes of Health; National Heart, Lung, and Blood Institute; National Asthma Education and Prevention Program. *Expert Panel Report 3: Guidelines for the Diagnosis and Management of Asthma. Full Report 2007.* Bethesda, MD: National Heart, Lung, and Blood Institute; 2007:405.

Indications for Consultation

- **Pulmonologist or asthma specialist:** Poor response to therapy or a prolonged, recurrent, or atypical course
- **Social work:** Barriers to care, including financial or psychosocial stressors, documented history of noncompliance, and any concerns by the health care team, as well as if the patient has risk factors for death

Disposition

- **ICU:** No response to therapy within a 6-hour time frame or an acute deterioration
- **Discharge criteria:** No O_2 requirement, adequate oral intake, stable respiratory status on SABA inhalations no more frequent than every 4 to 6 hours, and asthma education and follow-up appointments completed

Follow-up

- **Primary care provider:** 2 to 5 days
- **Asthma specialist:** 1 to 2 weeks, if the patient has had a previous pediatric ICU admission for asthma or another asthma admission within the past 12 months, frequent emergency department visits for asthma, severe persistent asthma
- **Allergist:** Allergic triggers and/or atopy

Pearls and Pitfalls

- Administer or recommend an influenza vaccination, unless the patient has already received it or there is a contraindication.
- ACPs standardize and improve inpatient asthma care.
- Asthma education and discharge planning begin at the time of admission.

Coding

ICD-9

• Asthma, with acute exacerbation	**493.92**
• Asthma, with status asthmaticus	**493.91**
• Pneumothorax, primary spontaneous	**512.81**

Bibliography

Cincinnati Children's health policy and clinical effectiveness department evidence-based guideline of acute exacerbation of asthma in children 2010. http://www.cincinnatichildrens.org/svc/alpha/h/health-policy/guidelines.htm

Cunningham S, Logan C, Lockerbie L, et al. Effect of an integrated care pathway on acute asthma/wheeze in children attending hospital: cluster randomized trial. *J Pediatr.* 2008;152:315–320

Ducharme FM, Chalut D, Plotnick L, et al. The Pediatric Respiratory Assessment Measure: a valid clinical score for assessing acute asthma severity from toddlers to teenagers. *J Pediatr.* 2008;152:476–480

Gouin S, Robidas I, Gravel J, et al. Prospective evaluation of two clinical scores for acute asthma in children 18 months to 7 years of age. *Acad Emerg Med.* 2010;17:598–603

National Heart, Lung, and Blood Institute. *National Asthma Education and Prevention Program 2007 Expert Panel Report 3: Guidelines for the Diagnosis and Management of Asthma.* Section 5, Managing Exacerbations of Asthma 2007. www.nhlbi.nih.gov/guidelines/asthma

Acute Respiratory Failure

There are 2 types of respiratory failure (RF). In type I, or hypoxemic RF, the patient is unable to adequately oxygenate the blood and develops hypoxemia with normal or low carbon dioxide. In type 2, or hypercarbic RF, the patient is unable to clear carbon dioxide and develops hypercarbia and hypoxemia. One type may lead to the other, and frequently a patient has elements of both. RF can also be acute or chronic. Acute RF (ARF) is an emergency and occurs over minutes to hours. If the body is unable to compensate, death is likely without rapid intervention.

Infants and toddlers are particularly vulnerable to ARF due to a variety of anatomical, neuromuscular, and other considerations. Most infants are preferential nasal breathers until 2 to 6 months of age. In addition, a younger patient has a relatively large tongue, a narrow subglottic region, small and compliant airways, fewer alveoli with poor collateral ventilation, a compliant chest wall, easily fatigued respiratory musculature, and an immature respiratory center resulting in irregular respirations or possibly apnea. Finally, there is a high incidence of metabolic, genetic, and developmental disorders that lead to poor airway control, chronic aspiration, severe muscle weakness, scoliosis, and restrictive lung disease

Clinical Presentation

History

Risk factors for ARF include young age, history of prematurity, underlying disease(s), and previous respiratory problems or airway issues. The patient may initially present with fever, cough, upper respiratory infection symptoms, shock or sepsis, apnea, cyanosis, depressed mental status, or muscle weakness. Depending on the etiology, the progression can occur over hours to days.

It is critical to learn the nature of and response to the therapies and interventions implemented at home, in the emergency department, in the outpatient setting, or in the field by emergency medical services.

Physical Examination

While a thorough physical examination is necessary, treatment takes priority to ensure that the patient's condition does not deteriorate. Much useful information can be gleaned by observing the patient "from the door" and in a caregiver's arms, including the general appearance and mental status. Irritability or anxiety suggests dyspnea, hypercarbia, hypoxemia, and more severe disease. Lethargy occurs with severe hypercarbia or hypoxemia, fatigue, and impending respiratory arrest. Extreme tachypnea and work of breathing can lead to fatigue and respiratory arrest, while bradypnea, poor air movement, and grunting are ominous findings. Stridor with poor air movement is an emergency. Hepatomegaly, facial or peripheral edema, jugular venous distension, or a gallop rhythm raises the concern of possible heart failure.

Laboratory

Although a blood gas and other laboratory results can provide helpful information, a patient with ARF often cannot tolerate the stress of restraint and phlebotomy. The results rarely help determine the best initial therapy for ARF, and the patient's distress during collection can lead to deterioration. In general, defer laboratory testing until the patient has been stabilized. In contrast, blood gases may be quite helpful in a patient with chronic RF who is well compensated and whose only sign of worsening might be increased hypercarbia. Since oxygenation can be assessed with pulse oximetry, venous or capillary blood gas samples are adequate.

Radiology

Radiographic findings are important and may help suggest a specific and potentially life-saving therapy. Obtain a chest x-ray, explicitly looking for pneumonia, effusion, pneumothorax, a widened mediastinum, cardiomegaly, mass lesion, or evidence of a foreign body aspiration.

Differential Diagnosis

Although the list is extensive (Table 89-1), the cause of a patient's acute respiratory disease rarely presents a diagnostic dilemma.

Treatment

The treatment of ARF is directed at the underlying pathophysiology. For more information, refer to other specific sections of this text.

High flow nasal cannula oxygen (HFNCO_2) therapy delivers humidified, warmed oxygen at rates up to 40 L/minute. It can decrease need for intubation in ARF and requires little technical skill.

Heliox therapy at concentrations of 60% to 80% helium may provide a temporary reduction in acute symptoms of croup, bronchiolitis, and asthma. It may "buy some time" while preparing for transfer or awaiting subspecialist consultation. However, its use can be limited by patient hypoxemia, and it has

Table 89-1. Etiologies of Respiratory Failure	
Pathophysiology	**Diagnosis**
Nasal or other upper airway obstruction	Adenoidal-tonsillar hypertrophy Choanal atresia/stenosis Croup Epiglottitis Excessive or inspissated secretions Neuromuscular disease and poor airway control Retropharyngeal abscess
Lower airway obstruction	Asthma Bronchiolitis Bacterial tracheitis
Parenchymal lung disease	Acute respiratory distress syndrome Aspiration or inhalation injury Exacerbation of chronic lung disease Non-cardiogenic pulmonary edema Pneumonia Pulmonary contusion
Pulmonary edema	Heart failure
Muscle weakness or paralysis	Botulism Guillain-Barré syndrome Muscular dystrophy Spinal cord injury Spinal muscular atrophy
Thoracic mass effect	Effusion or empyema Pneumothorax Tumor

not been shown to decrease the rate of intubation or the need for intensive care unit (ICU) transfer.

Nasal and Other Upper Airway Obstruction

Treat nasal obstruction with nasal saline drops followed by suctioning and with the judicious use of a topical α-agonist nasal decongestant (phenylephrine, 4 drops of 0.125% or 0.1mL of 0.5%, in each nostril). A patient with a large tongue, adenoidal-tonsillar hypertrophy, or poor airway control may find a position of comfort. If not, place the patient in a lateral position, with or without a chin-lift/jaw-thrust. A mechanical nasal airway, such as a soft nasal trumpet or appropriately sized endotracheal tube, is usually well tolerated and can often provide significant relief. Use the largest diameter that will pass, lubricate well, and insert to a length equal to the distance measured from the patient's nostril to tragus. Other modalities include noninvasive positive pressure ventilation (NIPPV) such as continuous positive airway pressure (CPAP) or $HFNCO_2$.

For croup, allow the patient to assume a position of comfort, provide a calm environment, and minimize stimulation. The treatment of croup (page 105) also includes corticosteroids, racemic epinephrine and, in severe cases, heliox. Cool mist is *not* beneficial and may worsen patient distress. NIPPV such as CPAP and $HFNCO_2$ may also be helpful. The patient may require endotracheal intubation, but anticipate difficulty. This is best performed with subspecialist consultation (intensivist, otolaryngologist, or anesthesiologist) if possible, and usually requires an endotracheal tube that is at least one size smaller than usual for the patient.

Lower Airway Obstruction

The treatment of asthma (page 605) and bronchiolitis (page 631) is detailed elsewhere. If respiratory support is needed, use NIPPV with CPAP, bi-level positive airway pressure, or $HFNCO_2$. Heliox may be useful if hypoxemia is not limiting. Intubate the patient for refractory hypoxemia or impending respiratory arrest. Although an infant with severe bronchiolitis may need intubation, even an extreme asthma exacerbation can usually be managed without mechanical ventilation.

Parenchymal Lung Disease

The mainstays of treatment are oxygen, antibiotics, and diuretics. A patient with ARF almost uniformly needs NIPPV or intubation with mechanical ventilation. The positive pressure given with oxygen improves airway recruitment and hypoxemia and decreases the patient's work of breathing.

Heart Failure

The treatment, including oxygen, diuretics, and inotropes, is detailed on page 22. NIPPV and mechanical ventilation improve respiratory symptoms and heart function. However, the patient is extremely fragile. Obtain subspecialist consultation early, as endotracheal intubation can lead to cardiac arrest.

Muscle Weakness or Paralysis

Provide oxygen and mechanical support. The patients may also have upper airway obstruction that requires treatment (see above).

Thoracic Mass Effect

Drain or treat surgically as indicated. Obtain appropriate subspecialist consultation (intensivist, surgeon, anesthesiologist) early, especially if sedation is required.

Indications for Consultation

- **Intensivist:** Acute respiratory failure
- **Anesthesiology:** Patient with croup requiring intubation, thoracic mass effect
- **Cardiology:** ARF secondary to congestive heart failure
- **Otolaryngology:** ARF secondary to a foreign body, croup, retropharyngeal abscess, epiglottitis
- **Surgery:** Thoracic mass effect

Disposition

- **ICU transfer:** ARF
- **Discharge from ICU:** Patient maintaining oxygenation and ventilation with just the support available in the respiratory, step-down, or inpatient unit

Pearls and Pitfalls

- Do not give a muscle relaxant to a patient if the success of airway management and ventilation is uncertain.
- The judicious use of sedation for a patient with extreme respiratory distress can be beneficial. However, anticipate the possibility of deterioration and the need for airway intervention and mechanical ventilation.
- Do not underestimate the importance of unobstructed nasal passages to adequate breathing in an infant and other patients with poor airway control.
- Lateral positioning, with or without chin-lift/jaw-thrust, helps alleviate airway occlusion and may decrease sympathetic activity.
- Hypoxemia in a patient with isolated upper airway disease (croup) is ominous and indicative of extreme hypoventilation and impending respiratory arrest.
- Heart failure is a cause of ARF that is often overlooked.

Coding

ICD-9

- Acute and chronic respiratory failure **518.84**
- ARF **518.81**
- Chronic respiratory failure **518.83**
- Hypoxemia **799.02**

Bibliography

Bingham RM, Proctor LT. Airway management. *Pediatr Clin North Am.* 2008;55: 873–886

Deis JN, Abramo TJ, Crawley L. Noninvasive respiratory support. *Pediatr Emerg Care.* 2008;24:331–338

Lakhanpaul M, MacFaul R, Werneke U, et al. An evidence-based guideline for children presenting with acute breathing difficulty. *Emerg Med J.* 2009;26:850–853

Litman RS, Wake N, Chan LM, et al. Effect of lateral positioning on upper airway size and morphology in sedated children. *Anesthesiology.* 2005;103:484–488

Thill PJ, McGuire JK, Baden HP, Green TP, Checchia PA. Noninvasive positive-pressure ventilation in children with lower airway obstruction. *Pediatr Crit Care Med.* 2004;5:337–342

CHAPTER 90

Apparent Life-Threatening Events

Introduction

An apparent life-threatening event (ALTE) is an episode in an infant that involves some combination of apnea, color change, alteration in muscle tone, choking, or gagging. Most are benign, nonrecurring, and caused by a normal physiological phenomenon, such as gastroesophageal reflux (GER). Some, however, are the manifestation of a serious, undiagnosed problem, including child maltreatment (Table 90-1). Caregivers often fear that the patient nearly

Table 90-1. Differential Diagnosis of Apparent Life-Threatening Events

Diagnosis	Clinical Features
Arrhythmia	Family history: unexplained death, arrhythmia, congenital heart disease Pathological murmur
Benign process: periodic breathing, startle reflex, perioral cyanosis, breath-holding spell	Prompt return to normal baseline without treatment Normal vital signs and physical examination May be a single episode
Child abuse	History of unexplained deaths in other children Inconsistent history or events witnessed by a single caretaker Bruising or petechiae on face, trunk, or extremities May have failure to thrive
Gastroesophageal reflux	Choking or gagging during or after feeds Vomiting and/or regurgitation May have Sandifer sign (arching of the back) Prompt return to baseline May have failure to thrive
Hypoglycemia or inborn error of metabolism	Family history of unexplained death Age <2 months May have a metabolic acidosis, failure to thrive, or seizures
Maxillofacial abnormality	Breathing difficulties since birth Abnormal facial morphology Family history of obstructive sleep apnea
Seizures	May be recurrent May be associated with focal a neurologic examination and/or developmental delay May have a positive family history
Sepsis	Fever +/- tachycardia and hypotension Toxic appearance Persistent or progressive altered mental status
Upper or lower respiratory tract infection (respiratory syncytial virus, pertussis)	Variable congestion, wheezing, coarse rales, tachypnea, especially if <2 months of age

died despite the fact that ALTEs are not related to "aborted" or "near-miss" sudden infant death syndrome (SIDS), and patients are usually asymptomatic and well-appearing on presentation. The broad differential diagnosis, potential for a rare but serious underlying etiology, and subsequent anxiety present a unique challenge.

ALTE patients will generally fall into 2 categories: those with symptoms or physical examination findings suggestive of a diagnosis and those without symptoms or an apparent cause.

Clinical Presentation

History

Complete a thorough, systematic history to fully characterize what exactly occurred during the ALTE. Attempt to distinguish concerning symptoms, such as central apnea, central cyanosis, or seizure activity, from more benign ones, like obstructive apnea, choking, pallor, "turning red," or cyanosis limited to just the perioral area or distal extremities (acrocyanosis). Understanding the temporal and contextual relationships is also important. For example, central cyanosis without a preceding event is more concerning than vomiting after a feed, followed by gagging, choking, turning red, and hypertonia.

A careful review of symptoms (upper respiratory infection symptoms, fever, growth, and development), medical history (prior ALTE, prematurity, noisy breathing), family history (cardiac disease, apnea, and unexplained sudden death), and social history (infectious exposures, caretakers, and domestic violence) can suggest comorbid conditions, genetic predispositions, medication exposures, or social concerns.

Physical Examination

Most often the patient is asymptomatic and has a negative physical examination. However, perform a thorough examination, focusing on the skin (bruising or petechiae indicating child maltreatment), head and neck (anatomical abnormalities contributing to obstructive apnea), heart (pathologic murmur), and nervous system (focality).

Laboratory

Routine laboratory testing is of minimal value, especially in an asymptomatic infant who is more than 48 weeks' corrected gestational age and with a negative history and physical examination. A complete blood cell count, sepsis evaluation, gastroesophageal reflux testing, sleep study, toxicology screen, metabolic testing, brain imaging, electroencephalogram, and electrocardiogram are all of low yield. Instead, perform targeted testing based on the findings of the history and physical examination. For example, obtain neuroimaging if there is a concern for child maltreatment (Table 90-1). In a case where more information is desired, a period of inpatient observation is often beneficial.

Treatment

Routine admission and monitoring are unnecessary and can increase parental anxiety. However, inpatient observation is beneficial for an infant who is experiencing recurrent events, had central cyanosis or central apnea, is awaiting final test results (respiratory syncytial virus [RSV] or pertussis testing, bacterial cultures), or is less than 48 weeks' corrected gestational age. This is particularly true for a newborn with a clinical picture that is not consistent with GER, as pertussis and RSV can present without viral respiratory symptoms in this age group. Inpatient observation may also be valuable in order to gather more information when there is concern for child maltreatment.

Specific treatment is not indicated unless there is a significant underlying diagnosis. If GER is likely, recommend reflux precautions (small frequent feeds, elevate head of bed, upright feeding). If feeding difficulties are suspected, arrange for an evaluation by a feeding expert. Most importantly, reassure the family that ALTEs are not related to SIDS. CPR training may offer additional reassurance for very concerned parents.

If the patient has symptoms of obstructive apnea present since birth or an anatomical maxillofacial abnormality (noisy breathing since birth or family history of obstructive sleep apnea), consult an otolaryngologist or pulmonologist and arrange a sleep study.

If an inborn error of metabolism is suspected (positive family history, increased anion gap acidosis, hypoglycemia, lactic acidosis, hyperammonemia) stabilize as necessary and give an intravenous solution that contains dextrose. Consult with a metabolic specialist to determine the necessary laboratory tests (to be obtained while the patient is *symptomatic*) and management. These generally include blood for glucose, arterial blood gas, comprehensive metabolic panel, cortisol, lactate, pyruvate, ammonia, growth hormone, amino acids, and beta-hydroxybuterate, as well as urine for ketones, pH, and organic acids.

The management of arrhythmias (page 11), bronchiolitis (page 629), child abuse (page 587), seizures (page 475), and sepsis (page 63) is detailed elsewhere.

Indications for Consultation

- **Child abuse specialist:** Any concern or risk factor for child maltreatment
- **Gastroenterology:** Recurrent ALTE with associated GER symptoms or failure to thrive
- **Metabolic diseases:** Positive metabolic screen, recurrent unexplained ALTE, or concerning family history
- **Neurology:** Concern for seizures or focal neurologic examination, although this can be deferred to the outpatient setting
- **Pulmonologist or sleep study specialist:** Recurrent ALTE or concern for central apnea
- **Feeding expert:** Concern for swallowing difficulties

Disposition

- **Intensive care unit transfer:** Recurrent, life-threatening events requiring high-intensity monitoring or medical intervention
- **Discharge criteria:** Low risk for serious underlying etiology, family reassured

Follow-up

- **Primary care:** 1 to 2 days
- **Neurology:** 1 to 2 weeks if suspected seizure disorder

Pearls and Pitfalls

- Manage patients according to risk determined from the history and physical examination features.
- Asymptomatic patient more than 48 weeks' postconceptional age (or 2 months of age if not premature) and with a negative history and physical examination is generally at low risk for a serious illness.
- Hospitalize an infant less than 48 weeks' gestation or one with recurrent ALTEs, until it is certain that the episodes are resolved or not life-threatening.

Coding

ICD-9

- ALTE **799.82**
- GER **530.81**

Bibliography

Al-Kindy HA, Gélinas JF, Hatzakis G, Côté A. Risk factors for extreme events in infants hospitalized for apparent life-threatening events. *J Pediatr.* 2009;154:332–337

Brand DA, Altman RL, Purtill K, Edwards KS. Yield of diagnostic testing in infants who have had an apparent life-threatening event. *Pediatrics.* 2005;115:885–893

Claudius I, Keens T. Do all infants with apparent life-threatening events need to be admitted? *Pediatrics.* 2007;119:679–683

Dewolfe CC. Apparent life-threatening event: a review. *Pediatr Clin North Am.* 2005;52:1127–1146

Tieder JS, Cowan CA, Garrison MM, Christakis DA. Variation in inpatient resource utilization and management of apparent life-threatening events. *J Pediatr.* 2008;152:629–635

Vellody K, Freeto JP, Gage SL, Collins N, Gershan WM. Clues that aid in the diagnosis of nonaccidental trauma presenting as an apparent life-threatening event. *Clin Pediatr (Phila).* 2008;47:912–918

Bacterial Tracheitis

Introduction

Bacterial tracheitis is a superinfection complication of viral croup, with an estimated mortality rate of 4% to 20%. The organisms most often involved are *Staphylococcus aureus* (methicillin-resistant *S aureus* [MRSA] is a concern), group A streptococcus, *Moraxella catarrhalis*, nontypable *Haemophilus influenzae*, *Klebsiella* species, and *Pseudomonas* species. Bacterial tracheitis tends to occur in the fall or winter months, mimicking the epidemiology of croup. However, while croup is most common in patients 3 months to 6 years of age, bacterial tracheitis can occur between 3 weeks and 16 years of age.

The pathophysiology involves a diffuse inflammatory process of the larynx, trachea, and bronchi with adherent or semiadherent mucopurulent membranes within the trachea. The major site of disease is at the level of the cricoid cartilage, which is the narrowest part of the trachea. Acute airway obstruction may occur secondary to subglottic edema and sloughing of epithelial lining or accumulation of the mucopurulent membrane within the trachea.

Clinical Presentation

History

The patient initially presents in a manner similar to viral croup, with fever, barking cough, and stridor. However, standard croup therapy is ineffective. Over the course of several days, when croup would typically be improving, the patient proceeds to acute respiratory decompensation.

Physical Examination

The patient is febrile and tachypneic, with a toxic appearance, stridor (can be biphasic), significant respiratory distress, retractions, dyspnea, nasal flaring, and cyanosis. Some patients will have a sore throat, odynophagia, or dysphonia. Pertinent negative findings include a lack of drooling, and the patient is able to lie supine without increased respiratory distress.

Differential Diagnosis

The differential diagnosis includes persistent croup, epiglottis, peritonsillar abscess, and retropharyngeal abscess (Table 91-1). However, a patient with bacterial tracheitis does not respond to standard croup therapy, appears toxic, and presents with an acute respiratory decompensation.

Table 91-1. Differential Diagnosis of Bacterial Tracheitis

Diagnosis	Clinical Features
Croup	Barking cough Nontoxic appearance Responds to inhaled epinephrine and steroids
Epiglottitis (rare)	Rapid onset Toxic appearance Drooling but no cough
Foreign body aspiration	No croup-like prodrome Acute onset of choking, gagging, coughing May have stridor or wheezing
Peritonsillar abscess	No croup-like prodrome Drooling No stridor or cough
Retropharyngeal abscess	Drooling Muffled stridor

Laboratory

Obtain a complete blood cell count and blood culture, as well as a bacterial culture and Gram stain of tracheal secretions.

Radiology

If bacterial tracheitis is suspected, obtain a lateral neck x-ray, which will show an irregular or "shaggy" subglottic narrowing versus the symmetrical tapering that is typical of croup.

Treatment

If bacterial tracheitis is suspected, immediately obtain an otolaryngology or pulmonology consult to arrange laryngotracheobronchoscopy or if emergent intubation is being considered. Direct visualization and culture of purulent tracheal secretions will confirm the diagnosis and may be therapeutic by allowing tracheal toilet and stripping of the purulent membranes. However, in a deteriorating patient, initiate empiric treatment and airway stabilization without waiting for the results of laboratory and/or radiologic studies.

Once the diagnosis is made, the mainstays of treatment are airway maintenance and intravenous (IV) antibiotics. Avoid agitating the patient. If the patient's respiratory status deteriorates, it is usually secondary to movement of the membrane. Attempt bag-valve-mask ventilation, but if intubation is required, use an endotracheal tube 0.5 to 1 size smaller than expected in order to minimize trauma in the inflamed subglottic area. Frequent suctioning and high air humidity are necessary to maintain endotracheal tube patency.

Treat with IV antibiotics. Use either cefotaxime (150 mg/kg/day divided every 6 hours, 8 g/day maximum) *or* ceftriaxone (100 mg/kg/day divided every 12 hours, 4 g/day maximum) *plus* MRSA coverage with either clindamycin (40 mg/kg/day IV divided every 8 hours, 4.8 g/day maximum) or vancomycin (45 mg/kg/day divided every 8 hours, 4 g/day maximum).

Consultations

- **Otolaryngology or pulmonology:** All patients (for endoscopic procedures)
- **Pediatric intensivist:** All patients

Disposition

- **Intensive care unit transfer:** All patients
- **Discharge criteria:** Afebrile, tolerating maintenance oral fluids, no respiratory distress

Pearls and Pitfalls

- Always consider bacterial tracheitis in a patient who presents with an acute life-threatening upper airway infection.
- Bacterial tracheitis is often misdiagnosed as severe or persistent croup.
- An acute deterioration in the patient's respiratory status is usually secondary to movement of the membrane.

Coding

ICD-9

Acute tracheitis	**464.1**

Bibliography

Bjornson CL, Johnson DW. Croup. *Lancet.* 2008;371:329–339

Hopkins A, Lahiri T, Salerno R, Heath B. Changing epidemiology of life-threatening upper airway infections: the reemergence of bacterial tracheitis. *Pediatrics.* 2006;118: 1418–1421

Huang YL, Peng CC, Chiu NC, et al. Bacterial tracheitis in pediatrics: 12 year experience at a medical center in Taiwan. *Pediatr Int.* 2009;51:110–113

Shah S, Sharieff GQ. Pediatric respiratory infections. *Emerg Med Clin North Am.* 2007;25:961–979

Tebruegge M, Pantazidou A, Thorburn K, et al. Bacterial tracheitis: a multi-centre perspective. *Scand J Infect Dis.* 2009;41:548–557

CHAPTER 92

Bronchiolitis

Introduction

Bronchiolitis refers to the clinical presentation of certain viral, lower respiratory tract infections in a young child, usually younger than 2 years. The typical presentation is one of obstructive lung disease due to edema and increased mucus production involving the small airways. Respiratory syncytial virus (RSV) is the classic etiologic agent accounting for most bronchiolitis. Other viruses have been implicated, including parainfluenza and human metapneumovirus, as well as coinfection with more than one respiratory virus.

In general, bronchiolitis is a self-limited disease and therapy is simply supportive. However, the risks of apnea and bacterial coinfection are areas of ongoing controversy.

Clinical Presentation

History

Obtain a timeline of the illness. Typically, a prodromal phase of rhinorrhea or nasal congestion, often accompanied with fever, is then followed by cough and tachypnea. Obtain a birth history, as prematurity may predict a more severe or prolonged hospitalization course due to the possibility of chronic lung disease. Additionally, apnea in the youngest infants may be the presenting symptom of bronchiolitis.

Inquire about a prior history of wheezing. Recurrent wheezing may indicate asthma rather than bronchiolitis. However, it is unclear whether recurrent, viral wheezing in an infant will become persistent asthma or requires anything more than supportive care.

Physical Examination

Observe the patient's general work of breathing, including respiratory rate and comfort level. The patient may have a cough and increased work of breathing characterized by retractions or visible use of accessory respiratory muscles. Periodic reexamination is helpful to assess the disease course. In a young infant who is an obligate nose breather (typically <3 months), an examination following nasal suctioning may reveal significant overall improvement.

Lung auscultation is usually remarkable for diffuse wheezing and/or rales and tachypnea. In more severe cases, decreased breath sounds and poor air entry may be more prominent than rales and wheezing. It is important to distinguish the diffuse peripheral lung findings characteristic of bronchiolitis from the localized findings or transmitted upper airway sounds, which may suggest an alternate diagnosis. To evaluate for upper airway transmitted sounds, listen over the patient's nose and mouth, then "subtract" those sounds from what is heard during lung auscultation. Hypoxia is frequently encountered and is often the sole indication for hospital admission. Less important findings include clear rhinorrhea and middle ear effusion.

Laboratory

Do not obtain routine laboratory tests or imaging for a patient presenting with clinical bronchiolitis. Do not perform specific viral testing to confirm RSV, unless cohorting in shared hospital rooms is required, as the results will not otherwise alter care. If diagnostic uncertainty exists or if the patient is not following a fairly predictable hospital course, obtain a chest x-ray to evaluate for other pathology, including the possibility of foreign body aspiration or pneumonia. However, be aware that atelectasis may be misinterpreted as pneumonia. The right upper and right middle lobes are frequently affected, and a repeat chest x-ray obtained after 24 hours usually will show complete resolution of the "infiltrate" as the affected area quickly re-expands as the patient improves.

There is considerable controversy as to the management of fever in an infant younger than 90 days who presents with a recognizable viral illness such as bronchiolitis. A blood culture and lumbar puncture are not routinely indicated in an otherwise well-appearing, febrile infant with clinical bronchiolitis. If there is diagnostic uncertainty or any concern that the patient may have a bacterial illness, obtain a urine culture (with or without a blood culture), as this will provide the highest yield. However, a fever that occurs later in the course may be caused by a secondary bacterial pneumonia or ear infection, and therefore may be an indication for further evaluation.

Differential Diagnosis

Consider a differential diagnosis to include the common symptoms of wheezing/rales, tachypnea, and fever (Table 92-1). The wheezing and/or rales characteristic of bronchiolitis involve bilateral lung fields. Unilateral or upper airway examination findings may indicate another process such as aspiration, focal pneumonia, or laryngotracheobronchitis (croup). Other causes of diffuse wheezing and rales include pulmonary edema, perinatally acquired chlamydial infection, pertussis, or para-pertussis. Distinguish between adventitial lung sounds occurring in the larger airways (rings and slings) and those occurring in the small airways (wheezing and rales). Evaluate for other systemic

Table 92-1. Differential Diagnosis of Bronchiolitis

Diagnosis	Clinical Features
Aspiration	History is more chronic Absence of fever and rhinorrhea Possible abnormal tone and/or other neurologic signs
Chlamydia	Onset <3 months of age Staccato cough Peripheral eosinophilia (>300/mm^3)
Croup	Inspiratory stridor Unusual <3 months of age Wheezing less common
External airway compression	Monophasic/monophonic wheezing Central rather than peripheral wheeze
Metabolic acidosis	Tachypnea with clear lungs ↓ Bicarbonate
Pertussis	Paroxysmal cough Wheezing is unusual Whoop may not be heard <6 months of age
Pneumonia	May have high fever Hypoxia unusual Unilateral auscultatory findings
Pulmonary edema	History of heart disease or murmur Hepatomegaly, facial or peripheral edema

processes, including acidosis or toxic ingestion, if the patient is tachypneic in the absence of abnormal airway auscultatory findings.

Treatment

The care of inpatient bronchiolitis remains controversial and widely variable. Since the primary clinical symptom is wheezing, asthma therapies (β-agonists, steroids) continue to be used, although they are generally ineffective in treating uncomplicated bronchiolitis. The American Academy of Pediatrics published a practice guideline in 2006 that allows for an objective trial of β-agonists, although this is not specifically recommended. There is no strong evidence for selecting albuterol over epinephrine (or vice versa) when ordering a bronchodilator. In addition, current data do not support the use of systemic corticosteroids in bronchiolitis.

For most inpatients, provide supportive care only, as there is no universally effective, acute medical treatment for bronchiolitis. Administer oxygen if needed to keep the saturation greater than 90%. The routine use of continuous pulse oximetry monitoring may prolong hospitalization without providing other benefits. Therefore, order spot oximetry checks only for most patients. Frequent nasal suctioning is a mainstay of therapy, particularly before feeding attempts in the obligate nose breather (<3 months). However, avoid aggressive deep suctioning, which may cause edema of the nasopharynx. Also avoid chest physiotherapy, which is ineffective and potentially detrimental in bronchiolitis.

A mainstay of inpatient bronchiolitis management is the use of a respiratory score to quantify the impact of any intervention. This strategy reduces unnecessary treatment with bronchodilators. The most widely accepted bronchiolitis score is the WARM score used at Children's Hospital and Medical Center in Cincinnati, available at www.cincinnatichildrens.org/svc/alpha/h/health-policy/bronchiolitis.htm.

Hypertonic saline (4 mL of 3% saline every 4–6 hours) is an emerging, safe therapy for bronchiolitis that may decrease length of stay.

Apnea is a common concern in the youngest infants with bronchiolitis. However, the incidence may have been overstated once patients with underlying neuromuscular disorders and prematurity are excluded. In the absence of complicating factors, apnea may still occur in an infant younger than 2 months, but it is typically the presenting complaint and occurs early in the course of illness. Therefore, do not delay discharge of a young infant because of a concern that the patient is at risk for apnea. Treat true apnea in bronchiolitis with close monitoring and stimulation, high-flow nasal cannula (HFNC) oxygen, and continuous positive airway pressure and/or mechanical ventilation, if necessary. There is some evidence that caffeine (10 mg/kg loading dose, followed by 5 mg/kg per day, intravenous or oral, inpatient use only) may be helpful in treating apnea due to bronchiolitis.

Administration of oxygen via heated, humidified HFNC devices is an increasingly popular intervention, though only weak or anecdotal evidence exists regarding its effect on overall respiratory status and/or prevention of the need for more invasive means of ventilation. Flow rates (sometimes >6–8 L/minute) and FiO_2 can be independently adjusted in this delivery model. Although young infants who are obligate nasal breathers seem to benefit most from this modality, it may be used in any patient with increasing oxygen needs, tachypnea, and/or work of breathing.

Closely monitor the safety of oral feeding in a patient with significant tachypnea (>60 breaths/minute) and respiratory distress. There is some literature to suggest that aspiration is a cause of prolonged illness in bronchiolitis. Place a nasogastric tube if a concern for aspiration exists.

Administer or ensure appropriate administration of palivizumab, a monoclonal antibody, approved for RSV prophylaxis, in high-risk infants.

Indications for Consultation

- **Pulmonologist:** Diagnosis is uncertain or the patient requires higher concentrations of oxygen for a prolonged period

Disposition

- **Intensive care unit (ICU) transfer:** Persistent hypoxia or respiratory distress despite increasing oxygen delivery; carbon dioxide retention despite tachypnea is an ominous sign, which may also prompt ICU transfer
- **Discharge criteria:** Improved respiratory status with decreased work of breathing, oxygen saturation remaining greater than 90% in room air, and adequate oral intake. There is no specific recommendation as to the amount of time that a patient must be without oxygen supplementation prior to discharge.

Follow-up

- **Primary care:** 1 to 2 days

Pearls and Pitfalls

- An infant with bronchiolitis often sounds much worse than the overall appearance ("happy wheezer").
- Elevation of the minor fissure helps distinguish a radiographic opacity as right upper lobe atelectasis and associated volume loss as opposed to right upper lobe pneumonia.
- Bronchiolitis is a prolonged disease by pediatric standards, with an average duration of symptoms ("wet" cough) for more than 2 weeks. Failure to communicate the expected course of the disease contributes to parental frustration and can result in multiple medical visits.
- In order to prevent readmissions, it may be necessary to discuss discharge criteria and the expected course with the patient's primary care provider.

Coding

ICD-9

- Acute bronchiolitis due to other infectious organisms **466.19**
- Acute bronchiolitis due to RSV **466.11**

Bibliography

American Academy of Pediatric Subcommittee on Diagnosis and Management of Bronchiolitis. Diagnosis and management of bronchiolitis. *Pediatrics.* 2006;118: 1774–1793

Fernandes RM, Bialy LM, Vandermeer B, et al. Glucocorticoids for acute viral bronchiolitis in infants and young children. *Cochrane Database Syst Rev.* 2010;(10):CD004878

Gadomski AM, Brower M. Bronchodilators for bronchiolitis. *Cochrane Database Syst Rev.* 2010;(12):CD001266

Zorc JJ, Hall CB. Bronchiolitis: recent evidence of diagnosis and management. *Pediatrics.* 2010;125:342–349

Community-Acquired Pneumonia

Introduction

By definition, a community-acquired pneumonia (CAP) occurs in a previously healthy child, caused by an infection of the pulmonary parenchyma that has been acquired outside of the hospital. CAP can be complicated by a pleural effusion, abscess, or necrosis, in which case the term *complicated pneumonia* is used. Although the etiology of CAP varies by age, hospitalized children are more likely to have bacterial infections. Nonetheless, viral infections (respiratory syncytial virus in particular, as well as influenza, parainfluenza, adenovirus) still play a significant role and are the most common causes of pneumonia in hospitalized infants and toddlers with CAP.

Though the universal use of the conjugate vaccine against *Streptococcus pneumoniae* has decreased the incidence of overall infections caused by this pathogen, it remains the most common cause of bacterial CAP in hospitalized children. The most frequently isolated serotypes (19A, 1) are likely to change over time, as a result of the substitution of the 13-valent vaccine for the 7-valent one.

Pathogens responsible for "atypical pneumonias," such as *Mycoplasma pneumoniae* and *Chlamydophila pneumoniae,* can be found in patients as young as 2 years, although they are more significant in children older than 5 years. Other bacteria, such as non-typable *Haemophilus influenzae* or *Moraxella catarrhalis*, are far less common.

While the overall incidence of children hospitalized for CAP has decreased since the introduction of pneumococcal conjugate vaccine-7, the incidence of local complications, such as empyema, has been steadily increasing. Most pleural fluid cultures in complicated pneumonias are culture-negative, but more extensive molecular testing, such as polymerase chain reaction (PCR), reveals *S pneumoniae* as the most common and *Staphylococcus aureus* as the second most frequent cause of complicated disease. In particular, methicillin-resistant *S aureus* (MRSA) is now a frequent and increasing cause of complicated CAP. Although group A streptococcus (*Streptococcus pyogenes*) is an uncommon pathogen of pediatric CAP, it is an important cause of severe necrotizing pneumonia.

Some rare causes of CAP include *Chlamydia trachomatis* (afebrile infants 1–4 months of age), *Coccidiodes immitis* or San Joaquin Valley fever (desert South West and California), and *Histoplasma capsulatum* or spelunker's lung (central United States, Ohio River valley, lower Mississippi River).

Clinical Presentation

History

There is usually a history of a preceding upper respiratory infection, which is then followed by fever, cough, and dyspnea. A patient younger than 5 years can present with nonspecific symptoms, such as vomiting, headache, and abdominal pain. A history of dyspnea and chest pain may be elicited in a patient with complicated disease. Overall, fever is the most consistent symptom and can often be the sole complaint, as in a so-called occult pneumonia.

Physical Examination

A patient with CAP can have a range of physical findings, from just fever with or without tachypnea to significant respiratory distress and cyanosis. Tachypnea is the most sensitive sign in children. Findings such as retractions, use of accessory muscles, nasal flaring, and grunting occur with more severe pneumonias. Auscultatory findings include localized decreased breath sounds and localized fine end-inspiratory rales. A patient who presents with wheezing is at low risk for having a radiographically confirmed bacterial pneumonia (especially pneumococcal). This is particularly true if the patient is afebrile. In addition, the patient may have signs of dehydration.

Laboratory

Leukocytosis (white blood cell count >15,000/mm^3) with a left shift is slightly more common with a pneumococcal infection than in an atypical or viral CAP; however, a normal count can be falsely reassuring. In the post-pneumococcal vaccination era, a leukocytosis 20,000/mm^3 or greater in a febrile child is associated with an "occult" pneumonia (pneumonia with radiographic evidence but no clinical signs or symptoms) in up to 9% of cases.

The yield of a blood culture is so low that it typically does not influence the clinical management. Obtain a blood culture only in a case of severe or complicated disease. When available, perform testing for atypical pathogens in a patient with a higher pretest probability of having an atypical pathogen (>5 years of age, diffuse infiltrates on chest radiograph). Cold agglutinin titers or PCR for pathogens such as *M pneumoniae* are rapid tests, which can help guide therapy.

Radiology

Virtually every patient hospitalized with CAP will have had a chest radiograph performed. An alveolar or lobar infiltrate is most commonly secondary to a bacterial infection. Diffuse or interstitial infiltrates suggest an atypical pathogen or a virus. However, since the radiographic findings often overlap, they have poor specificity for any specific particular pathogen. In addition, a normal chest radiograph does not rule out a CAP. While a repeat chest radiograph is usually not necessary, obtain one if there is no improvement after 24 to 48 hours of adequate treatment; a worsening clinical course; or a complication, such as an effusion or empyema is suspected.

Parapneumonic effusions are most commonly caused by bacteria, although viruses or atypical bacteria are sometimes implicated. Absence of "layering" in a decubitus chest radiograph is an indication of possible septations or empyema. If a complicated effusion or empyema is suspected, obtain a chest ultrasound, which is more sensitive than computed tomography scan to evaluate the presence of septations and the nature of the pleural fluid. If pleural fluid is obtained, send for Gram stain, culture, pH, lactate dehydrogenase, protein, and glucose. The most clinically useful finding in the pleural fluid is a pH less than 7.2, which is associated with failure of medical management alone. In addition, a low glucose (<40 mg/dL) and a low pH (<7.2) are consistent with a probable empyema.

Differential Diagnosis

The presentation of pneumonia can overlap with other childhood illnesses (Table 93-1). A combination of the most common symptoms, tachypnea, fever, and cough, can be seen in pulmonary diseases such as bronchiolitis, as well as non-pulmonary conditions, such as congestive heart failure (CHF), or metabolic disease, such as diabetic ketoacidosis. A pulmonary effusion can also occur in CHF and many other extrapulmonary illnesses, such as pancreatitis, and neoplastic illnesses, such as lymphomas.

Table 93-1. Differential Diagnosis of Community-Acquired Pneumonia

Diagnosis	Clinical Features
Aspiration pneumonia	Chronically ill, special needs, or technology-dependent patient
Bronchiolitis	<1–2 years of age Wheezing with or without coarse rales
Foreign body aspiration	May have a history of a choking episode Recurrent pneumonia in same site Localized hyperluceny on chest x-ray
Pertussis	Coughing paroxysms (many coughs without breathing) Whoop (>3–6 months of age) Lymphocytosis
Tuberculosis	(+) Risk factors Ghon complex on chest x-ray Purified protein derivative (+)

Treatment

The increasing resistance of pneumococcus to penicillin has not been shown to affect clinical outcomes. Most treatment failures are secondary to the development of complications, such as empyema, noncompliance, and other factors not related to antibiotic susceptibility. As a result, β-lactams remain first-line treatment for suspected bacterial infections. Start treatment with oral amoxicillin (90 mg/kg/day divided every 8 hours, 2 g/day maximum) or intravenous (IV) ampicillin (200 mg/kg/day divided every 6 hours, 6 g/day maximum). Alternatives include a third-generation cephalosporin, such as IV ceftriaxone (50–100 mg/kg/day divided every 12–24 hours, 4 g/day maximum) or cefotaxime (150 mg/kg/day divided every 8 hours, 8 g/day maximum). Add IV clindamycin (40 mg/kg/day divided every 6–8 hours, 4.8 g/day maximum) or vancomycin (45 mg/kg/day divided every 8 hours, 4 g/day maximum) if the patient has severe or complicated disease in an area with a significant prevalence of MRSA. When potential penicillin allergy is a concern, give either a closely monitored trial of a cephalosporin or clindamycin (as above).

The use of antibiotics for atypical infections is controversial, as there are no randomized, controlled trials in children with pneumonia. Modest improvement in outcomes has been noted in adult studies. If rapid testing for an atypical pathogen is positive, or there is a high suspicion of an atypical infection and rapid testing is not available, add azithromycin (10 mg/kg in a single dose followed by 5 mg/kg daily on days 2–5, 500 mg/dose maximum). However, do not use a macrolide as monotherapy for CAP, as up to 40% of community-acquired *S pneumoniae* are resistant. While fluoroquinolones, such as oral or IV levofloxacin (10 mg/kg dose every 12 hours, 500 mg/day maximum), have activity against *S pneumoniae* and atypical pathogens, reserve them for teenagers or a patient with known severe allergies to other first- or second-line agents.

Medically treat an uncomplicated parapneumonic effusion that occupies less than 40% of the hemithorax. Medical management can also be attempted in a larger, uncomplicated parapneumonic effusion, provided the patient is not in significant respiratory distress. Features of a parapneumonic effusion that are likely to fail medical management and require drainage include involvement of more than 40% of the hemithorax, the fluid is loculated, or the initial fluid analysis reveals an empyema (pH <7.2). There are many choices for draining a large or complicated parapneumonic effusion, ranging from simple chest tube insertion to open thoracotomy. Early decortication with video-assisted thoracoscopic surgery (VATS) decreases length of stay, the need for pain medication, and overall costs. However, chest tube insertion with instillation of fibrynolitics may be equal to VATS in terms of length of stay and superior in terms of cost. Base the choice of therapy (VATS or chest tube and fibrynolitics) on local expertise and availability.

The length of therapy for CAP caused by typical bacteria is 10 days. Initiate the transition from IV to oral therapy as soon as there is clinical improvement. There is no established duration of therapy for a patient with complicated disease. One useful strategy is to extend the duration of antibiotics until 7 to 10 days after the resolution of fever.

Indications for Consultation

- **Infectious diseases:** Unexpected pathogen identified or nonresponsive to the appropriate initial antibiotic regimen
- **Otolaryngology:** Suspected foreign body aspiration
- **Pulmonary:** Recurrent pneumonias or other pulmonary pathology, such as cystic fibrosis, is suspected
- **Surgery:** Drainage may be necessary (large effusion, loculations, empyema)

Disposition

- **Intensive care unit transfer:** Severe respiratory distress or signs of sepsis
- **Discharge criteria:** No oxygen requirement, defervescing or no fever, tolerating maintenance oral fluids, and adequate follow-up assured

Follow-up

- **Primary care:** 2 to 3 days

Pearls and Pitfalls

- Initiation of antibiotic therapy does not mandate completing a full course if subsequent clinical or laboratory evidence suggests a viral infection.
- The initial chest radiograph can be negative if the patient has moderate to severe dehydration.
- Most infants hospitalized with CAP have a viral process and will not benefit from antibiotics.
- A patient with a complicated pneumonia can have persistent fever despite adequate treatment.
- Wheezing is not consistent with a classic pneumococcal bacterial pneumonia.

Coding

ICD-9

• Bacterial pneumonia unspecified	**482.9**
• Empyema	**510.9**
• Pleural effusion unspecified	**511.9**
• Pneumococcal pneumonia	**481**
• Pneumonia, organism unspecified	**486**
• Viral pneumonia unspecified	**480.9**

Bibliography

Bradley JS, Byington CL, Shah SS, et al. Executive summary: the management of community-acquired pneumonia in infants and children older than 3 months of age: clinical practice guidelines by the pediatric infectious diseases society and the infectious diseases society of America. *Clin Infect Dis.* 2011;53:617–630

Don M, Canciani M, Korppi M. Community-acquired pneumonia in children: what's old? What's new? *Acta Paediatr.* 2010;99:1602–1608

Kabra SK, Lodha R, Pandey RM. Antibiotics for community-acquired pneumonia in children. *Cochrane Database Syst Rev.* 201017;(3):CD004874

Mulholland S, Gavranich JB, Chang AB. Antibiotics for community-acquired lower respiratory tract infections secondary to *Mycoplasma pneumoniae* in children. *Cochrane Database Syst Rev.* 2010;(7):CD004875

Ranganathan SC, Sonnappa S. Pneumonia and other respiratory infections. *Pediatr Clin North Am.* 2009;56:135–156

Ruuskanen O, Lahti E, Jennings LC, Murdoch DR. Viral pneumonia. *Lancet.* 2011;377: 1264–1275

Complications of Cystic Fibrosis

Introduction

Cystic fibrosis (CF) is a systemic disease affecting multiple organ systems, especially the respiratory and gastrointestinal tracts and the exocrine glands. Comprehensive care is usually delivered at CF centers, but a patient with a complication may present to any hospital. The most common pulmonary complications are pulmonary exacerbations, pulmonary hemorrhage/hemoptysis, and pneumothorax. The most urgent gastrointestinal concern is distal ileal obstruction syndrome (DIOS), an acute intestinal obstruction. CF-related diabetes (CFRD) is now a frequent complication, as a result of improved survival. If possible, always coordinate the management of a patient with CF with the staff of the CF center where the child receives chronic care.

Clinical Presentation

The presentation of CF complications is summarized in Table 94-1.

History

A patient with a respiratory complication will most often complain of worsening distress, especially shortness of breath and increased respiratory rate. A pulmonary exacerbation will typically present with increased cough and secretions, and possibly bleeding. A pneumothorax causes the acute onset of

Table 94-1. Presentation of Cystic Fibrosis Complications

Complications	Clinical Findings
Distal ileal obstruction syndrome	Abdominal pain and distension Emesis No fever
Diabetes	Unexplained poor weight gain/growth Polydipsia/polyuria Elevated glucose, glycosuria but no ketoacidosis
Pneumothorax	Acute onset of chest pain and shortness of breath Ipsilateral decreased or absent breath sounds Positive chest x-ray
Pulmonary exacerbation	± Fever Increased cough, congestion, dyspnea, and tachypnea Increased diffuse/localized rhonchi and/or rales
Pulmonary hemorrhage	Pallor Shortness of breath Coughing/expectoration of bright red blood

chest pain and difficulty breathing, without an increase in secretions. A patient with hemoptysis/pulmonary hemorrhage will report coughing up frank blood with or without increased cough and worsening respiratory distress. Fever may occur with a pulmonary exacerbation, but is not usually present with pneumothorax or hemoptysis. Ask about previous history of exacerbations, as well as current medications and pulmonary toilet regimen.

A patient with DIOS will complain of some combination of a distended abdomen, abdominal pain, emesis and, rarely, blood in the emesis or per rectum. The presentation of CFRD will be more insidious, with fatigue, poor energy, and possibly polydipsia and polyuria.

Physical Examination

Perform a complete physical examination, focusing on the vital signs, pulmonary findings, and abdominal examination.

Laboratory

If a pulmonary complication is suspected, obtain a chest x-ray. This will differentiate a pneumothorax from other lung processes. With a pulmonary exacerbation, the radiograph may also demonstrate worsening infiltrates or bronchiectasis in comparison to previous films, if available. Also, obtain a complete blood cell count to quantify the degree of any blood loss and check for leukocytosis consistent with an acute infection, and consider coagulation studies (activated partial thromboplastin time, international normalized ratio, fibrinogen).

If a DIOS is suspected, obtain a plain film of the abdomen, which usually has the diagnostic finding of distended, fluid-filled loops of bowel proximal to the level of obstruction. Alternatively, obtain a Gastrografin enema, which will confirm the diagnosis and will be therapeutic. Also obtain a comprehensive metabolic panel to identify any electrolyte imbalances.

The evaluation of suspected CFRD includes a comprehensive metabolic panel and a urinalysis. Typically, the blood sugar will be high, especially post-prandially, but without an associated acidosis or ketosis. For a definitive diagnosis, arrange an oral glucose tolerance test.

Treatment

Always attempt to contact the primary CF provider for specific care recommendations until the patient can be transported to a CF facility.

Pulmonary Exacerbation

The mainstays of treatment are systemic antibiotics and vigorous airway clearance (every 4–6 hours) using the best tolerated method, such as high-frequency chest compression vest or Flutter valve. Bronchodilators via metered-dose inhaler may also be of benefit and are most useful when given prior to airway clearance. In contrast, steroids and ipratropium have not been shown to be therapeutic in this situation. Inhaled antibiotics are most effective for chronic use, but may be helpful during an acute exacerbation in a patient with a *Pseudomonas aeruginosa* airway infection. For mild to moderate exacerbations, order oral antibiotics directed against pathogens with which the patient is known to be infected. Reserve intravenous (IV) antibiotics for a severe exacerbation, manifested by increased cough or sputum production, decreased exercise tolerance, increased fatigue, and absenteeism from daily activities, especially if a prior regimen of oral antibiotics has not been effective.

Accredited CF care centers routinely obtain airway cultures at every visit, so information regarding the patient's airway flora will most likely be available. Typical organisms are *Haemophilus influenzae*, *Staphylococcus aureus* (methicillin-susceptible *S aureus* or methicillin-resistant *S aureus*), and *Pseudomonas aeruginosa*, but other gram-negative rods may be present as well. While it is best to focus therapy on organisms known to be present in the patient's airway, if that information is not known use a regimen that is effective against *P aeruginosa* and *S aureus,* such as tobramycin (10 mg/kg every 24 hours, adjust the dose based on serum levels) *and* an anti-pseudomonal semisynthetic penicillin (pipercillin/tazobactam, 400 mg of piperacillin component/kg/day divided every 6 hours, 16 g of piperacillin component/day maximum).

Pulmonary Hemorrhage/Hemoptysis

Observation and supportive care are generally sufficient until the bleeding stops. Make the patient NPO and give IV fluid resuscitation with 20 mL/kg boluses of normal saline as needed. Transfuse 20 mL/kg or up to 2 units of packed red blood cells if the hemoglobin is below 7 g/dL or it drops by 2 g/dL or more over 8 hours. Bronchoscopy may be necessary when the bleeding is severe, and embolization may be indicated either acutely or after the hemorrhage has stopped. Consultation with, and possible transport to, a CF provider is required if embolization of the offending vessel is being considered.

Pneumothorax

If a pneumothorax measuring greater than 2 cm between the lung and chest wall is documented on a chest x-ray, consult a surgeon for chest tube placement. Since the recurrence rate is high, pleurodysis may be the preferred procedure, after consultation with a CF specialist.

DIOS

Make the patient NPO, give IV fluid resuscitation (if needed), and place a nasogastric tube (NGT) if needed. Treat with polyethylene glycol orally (Miralax; 1–1.5 g/kg every day, 100 g/day maximum) if the obstruction is mild. Otherwise give oral or continuous NGT (Golytely; 20–30 mL/kg/hour until clear, 1 L/hour maximum) if the vomiting is not severe. Alternatively, a therapeutic Gastrografin enema may be necessary. However, consult a surgeon if the obstruction persists or there is concern about a perforation (rigid abdomen, guarding, rebound tenderness, increased abdominal pain).

Diabetes

Consult an endocrinologist for dietary and insulin management guidance. Order a standard insulin bolus regimen and a high-calorie, high-fat diet.

Indications for Consultation

- **Endocrinology:** New-onset CFRD
- **Primary CF provider:** All patients
- **Surgery:** Chest tube placement or control of pulmonary hemorrhage needed; bowel obstruction

Disposition

- **Intensive care unit transfer:** Impending respiratory failure, shock, tension pneumothorax
- **Transfer to CF center:** Serious CF-related complication
- **Discharge criteria**
  - Bowel obstruction: Obstruction resolved, electrolyte imbalances corrected, and patient tolerating oral maintenance fluids
  - CFRD: Blood sugar below 200 mg/dL, glucosuria resolved, insulin regimen understood by patient, follow-up with CF-provider or endocrinologist arranged
  - Pneumothorax: Affected lung re-expanded, without any re-accumulation after chest tube removed

— Pulmonary exacerbation: Afebrile for 48 hours with significant clinical and objective improvement in pulmonary function (to near baseline)
— Pulmonary hemorrhage/hemoptysis: Bleeding stopped, hemoglobin is stable

Follow-up

- **Pulmonologist or CF center:** 2 to 3 days

Pearls and Pitfalls

- Have a high suspicion for complications although they are relatively rare.
- Diabetes has an insidious onset, but few patients will present with diabetic ketoacidosis.

Coding

ICD-9

• CF with gastrointestinal manifestations	**277.03**
• CF with pulmonary exacerbation	**277.02**
• CFRD, controlled, without complications	**249.00**
• Cystic fibrosis with other manifestations	**277.09**
• Hemoptysis	**786.30**

Bibliography

American Academy of Pediatrics. Cystic fibrosis. In: Light M, ed. *Pediatric Pulmonology*. Elk Grove Village, IL: American Academy of Pediatrics; 2001:717–744

Dicken BJ, Ziegler MM. Surgical management of pulmonary and gastrointestinal complications in children with cystic fibrosis. *Curr Opin Pediatr.* 2006;18:321–329

Kirkby S, Novak K, McCoy K. Update on antibiotics for infection control in cystic fibrosis. *Expert Rev Anti Infect Ther.* 2009;7:967–980

Mogayzel PJ Jr, Flume PA. Update in cystic fibrosis 2010. *Am J Respir Crit Care Med.* 2011;183:1620–1624

O'Riordan SM, Robinson PD, Donaghue KC, Moran A. Management of cystic fibrosis-related diabetes. *Pediatr Diabetes.* 2008;9(4 pt 1):338–344

Ventilation and Intubation

Introduction

Pediatric patients may require ventilatory support to manage respiratory failure (page 613) or cardiac failure (page 19), or to provide airway protection. A patient with chronic respiratory failure is a particular challenge, often requiring adjustments to the home regimen during times of relatively minor illnesses.

Respiratory insufficiency requiring support occurs because of pathology in at least 1 of the 4 following areas:

- Loss of central nervous system (CNS) drive: vascular event, narcotic effects
- Peripheral nerve or muscle deficiency: muscular dystrophy, botulism, Guillan-Barré syndrome (GBS), myasthenia gravis
- Increased upper airway resistance: croup, tonsil hypertrophy, tracheitis, palatal insufficiency, laryngotracheomalacia
- Alveolar pathology: pneumonia, asthma, pneumothorax, chronic lung disease, cystic fibrosis

The indications for assistance with ventilation include

- Fixed or dynamic airway obstruction in the context of acute respiratory compromise: craniofacial anomaly, hypotonia with palatal insufficiency
- CNS compromise with inability to maintain airway safety (aspiration risk): traumatic brain injury, posterior fossa tumor
- High risk for progressive airway compromise: caustic airway injury, facial or chest burns, signs of smoke inhalation, upper airway swelling, mass causing upper airway obstruction
- Worsening neuromuscular weakness: GBS, spinal muscular atrophy
- Failure to adequately oxygenate or ventilate despite the use of standard oxygenation and positioning strategies: severe parenchymal lung disease

Clinical Presentation

History

For a patient with a tracheostomy or on home ventilation, note the home settings and typical response to illness. Such a patient may be particularly vulnerable to illnesses, yet often does not demonstrate typical signs and symptoms of acute respiratory failure (page 613).

Physical Examination

Determine whether the difficulty is secondary to a problem with the central respiratory drive versus a peripheral neuropathy or muscular weakness. Look for apnea or an irregular breathing rate and the loss of protective reflexes (CNS), and assess the effectiveness of chest wall movements and peak expiratory or inspiratory flow rates (neuromuscular). Focus on elements that may affect the success of ventilation, such as neurodevelopmental state (tolerance of various support methods), narrow nasal passages, scoliosis, spasticity, and significant skin impairments (severe eczema, burns, recent craniofacial surgery). Assess the airway from mouth to chest.

- Nose/mouth: Look for nasal flaring (sign of respiratory distress) and auscultate over the nares to determine if there is nasal obstruction and to detect upper airway sounds, which may be transmitted to the lungs. If a jaw thrust reduces the airway obstruction, the pathology is at the level of the hypopharynx.
- Neck: Visually assess the trachea for deviation and listen for stridor or voice changes, which indicate pathology at the laryngeal level. Auscultate over the larynx to help differentiate stridor in the upper airway from bronchospasm in the lungs.
- Chest: Visually asses the chest wall motion for asymmetry, paradoxical movement, and retractions. Auscultate both lung fields for rales (alveolar disease), rhonchi (larger airway disease), and/or wheezing (alveolar and small airway disease).

Laboratory

Blood gas, oximetry, and capnography are the most common tools used to monitor ventilation status and determine advanced airway needs. Obtain a complete blood cell count, serum chemistries, and a venous or capillary blood gas (VBG or CBG, respectively) for a patient with either acute or chronic respiratory failure or worsening respiratory distress.

An elevated hemoglobin concentration suggests chronic hypoxemia. In contrast, interpretation of the oxygen saturation in an anemic patient can be falsely reassuring, as the limited amount of hemoglobin will be entirely saturated, while the total oxygen-carrying capacity of the blood is low. Increased serum lactate is an indicator of significant tissue hypoxia, while an increased bicarbonate suggests chronic hypercapnia. Low concentrations of potassium, calcium, or phosphate can impair muscle function.

The average pH of venous plasma is 7.37, while the oxygen tension of venous blood varies dramatically depending on the sample site and is not generally useful in the assessment of respiratory failure. The carbon dioxide tension averages 46 mm Hg. Elevation of venous carbon dioxide tension greater than 50 mm Hg and reduction in venous pH indicate retention of carbon dioxide consistent with inadequate ventilation. A trend of increasing carbon dioxide tensions over time implies respiratory fatigue and impending respiratory failure.

To assess the severity of hypoxia, calculate the alveolar to arterial gradient by obtaining an arterial blood gas on stable (preferably 100%) FiO_2 for at least 15 minutes (Box 95-1).

Capnography measures carbon dioxide concentration of the expired gas. End-tidal carbon dioxide ($EtCO_2$) correlates with $PaCO_2$ (usually within 5 mm Hg) in a closed respiratory system. However, in an open respiratory system (eg, mask or cannula), the correlation is less reliable, often greater than 5 mm Hg. Consider correlating $EtCO_2$ with a VBG/CBG when $EtCO_2$ monitoring is initiated. If measured consistently, $EtCO_2$ is useful for trending carbon dioxide retention.

Radiology

Indications for a chest radiograph include an acute change in the respiratory status, failure to improve with interventions, asymmetrical auscultatory findings (possibly indicative of a bronchial foreign body), and a concern about an alternate etiology of the clinical presentation, as well as a patient who requires additional airway or ventilatory intervention. Possible findings include upper airway narrowing or deviation, lobar collapse, air leak, asymmetrical diaphragms, effusions, cardiomegaly, and pulmonary edema.

Treatment

General Treatment

If the respiratory drive is adequate, provide oxygen and open the upper airway with an oral or nasal airway. Also maintain adequate perfusion, resolve acidosis, stabilize electrolytes and glucose, maximize nutrition, and minimize energy use.

Box 95-1. Calculation of the Alveolar to Arterial Gradient[a]

A-a O_2 Gradient =

$[(FiO_2) \times (\text{Atmospheric Pressure} - H_2O\ \text{Pressure}) - (PaCO_2/0.8)] - PaO_2$ from ABG.

Abbreviations: A-a, alveolar-arterial; ABG, arterial blood gas; FiO_2, fraction of inspired oxygen; H_2O, water; $PaCO_2$, partial pressure of carbon dioxide, arterial; PaO_2, partial pressure of oxygen, arterial.

[a]Normal gradient estimate = (Age/4) + 4

Normal gradient: 20–65 mm Hg on 100% O_2 (5–20 mm Hg on room air)

Ventilatory Support and Airway Protection

Tailor the treatment modality to the patient's underlying pathology. If the patient has inadequate central respiratory drive, cautiously deliver appropriate sedation, and discontinue any offending respiratory depressant medications or toxins, if possible (Table 95-1). Apnea mandates positive-pressure ventilation with bag-mask ventilation via a sealed mask/oral airway/ambu bag laryngeal mask airway (LMA), or endotracheal tube (ETT) for initial stabilization.

Peripheral nerve or muscle deficiency produces low tidal volumes, which is improved with continuous positive airway pressure (CPAP) or bi-level positive airway pressure (BiPAP). Manage increased upper airway resistance with insertion of an oropharyngeal airway, nasopharyngeal airway, LMA, or ETT.

Since lung pathology causes abnormalities of both perfusion and ventilation, provide adequate oxygen delivered via high-flow nasal cannula, CPAP, BiPAP, LMA, or ETT. Airway and ventilation management are summarized in Table 95-2.

Intubation

Insertion of an LMA is simple but does not protect the lungs from gastric aspiration. However, insertion of an ETT requires muscle paralysis and laryngoscopy, as nontraumatic intubation is difficult during spontaneous breathing. Muscle relaxants are required but induce apnea. The rapid

Table 95-1. Airway Sizes

LMA			ETT Size = [16 + age (years)]/4	
Size	**Weight (kg)**	**Insufflation Volume (mL)**	**Weight (kg)**	**Size**
1	<5	<4	<1	2.5
1.5	5–10	<7	1–2	3
2	10–20	<10	2–4	3.5
2.5	20–30	<14	ETT Depth = 10 + (age in years) (cm marking at the lip, up to 20 cm) or 3 × [EET size (non-neonates)]	
3	30–50	<20		
4	50–70	<30	**Weight (kg)**	**Depth (cm)**
5	70–100	<40	1	7
Laryngoscope Blade (always use straight)			2	8
Age (years)	**Size**		3	9
0–1	0–1		4	10
1–2	1 or 1.5 (Wis-hippel)			
>2	2			

Abbreviations: EET, endotracheal tube; LMA, laryngeal mask airway.

Table 95-2. Airway Management and Ventilation[a]

	Oral (OA) Nasal Airway (NPA)	HFNC	Nasal or Mask CPAP
Delivers	Normal air flow Facilitates BVM ventilation	Airway stenting ↑ O_2 delivery with blender	As with HFNC ↑ FRC Distending pressure recruits closed alveoli
Patient type (selected examples)	Hypotonic cerebral palsy	Hypoxic on standard NC at 2 LPM flow (<1 year) or 4 LPM flow (>1 year) Bronchiolitis	Bronchiolitis Upper airway obstruction Muscle weakness Post-extubation
Basic procedure	*OA* Determine size by placing opening by corner of mouth, with tip no further than corner of the jaw. Suction mouth. Place OA into mouth pointing to palate, until halfway in, then turn 180 degrees. OA will be facing tip down toward trachea. Do not secure in place. *NPA* Measure from nostril to tragus of ear. Can use ETT cut to size. Lubricate the NPA. Suction nares to ensure patency. Guide NPA through nare to predetermined length Secure the NPA. Assess by suctioning through NPA.	Use heated, humidified system. Use largest size prongs/bubble possible. Start: <1 y: 2 LPM; >1 y: 4 LPM flow Titrate flow to respiratory score improvement: ↑ 1 LPM every 15 min Max flow <1 year: <10 kg = 4 LPM; >10 kg = 6 LPM Max flow >1 year: <20 kg = 6 LPM; >20 kg = 8 LPM Use blender to titrate FiO_2 to maintain appropriate oxygen saturation; max ~50%; if >50% FiO_2 needed, consider NCPAP. Wean FiO_2 until ~40%, then ↓ flow by 1–2 LPM every 2–4 hours as tolerates until at: <1 year and <10 kg: 2 LPM; <1 year and >10 kg: 4 LPM; >1 year any size: 6 LPM. Then wean FiO_2 to ~30%. Consider convert to regular cannula (100% FiO_2 from wall) when at <2 LPM flow for <1 year and <3 LPM flow for >1 year.	Choose correct nasal prong or mask size. Nasal prongs are typically not tolerated by a patient > toddler age. Use humidified system. Start at pressure of 4 cm H_2O. Start FiO_2 at 30% and titrate to maintain appropriate oxygen saturation. Titrate flow to ↑ pressure 1–2 cm H_2O every 20–30 min to max 7–8 cm H_2O (<1 y) or 10 cm H_2O (>1 y). NCPAP: Secure bonnet over patient's head to assure tight seal. Mask CPAP: secure with ties. Weaning: Wean FiO_2 to ~ 30%–35%, then titrate flow to ↓ pressure by 1–2 cm H_2O every 2–hours as tolerated until at starting pressure. Then consider change to HFNC. Note: Once adequately ventilated, some patients may need continued pressure (CPAP) but little to no assistance with oxygenation (RA).

Table 95-2. Airway Management and Ventilation[a], continued

	Oral (OA) Nasal Airway (NPA)	HFNC	Nasal or Mask CPAP
Monitoring	Standard	Standard	Standard Advanced recommended
Limitations	No oxygen delivery	Max flow 4 L (<1 y, <10 kg) or 8 L (>1 y, >20 kg). At max flow and 100% FiO_2, will provide a maximum FiO_2 = 40% at the glottis due to entrainment of room air.	Patient tolerance (may require sedation) Tight seal needed to ensure pressure provided Skilled respiratory therapist needed
Common contraindications	*OA* Conscious patient will not tolerate *NPA* Coagulopathy Nasal deformity/infection Basilar skull fracture	Apnea Severe GERD CLD patient with respiratory acidosis	As with HFNC
Common complications	*OA* Gagging *NPA* Nasal erosion Bleeding	Nasal erosion Epistaxis Nasal congestion (reduced by humidification of oxygen)	As with HFNC Pneumothorax Aspiration Skin breakdown over nasal bridge
	BiPAP	**LMA**	**ETT Airway**
Delivers	Control over inspiratory (IPAP) and expiratory (EPAP) pressure delivery and rate Can synch with patient respirations	Ventilator use for control of pressures Tracheal suctioning possible Less sympathetic stimulation compared to ETT	As with LMA but greater pressures tolerated Longer-term ventilation possible Better airway protection

Table 95-2. Airway Management and Ventilation[a], continued

	BiPAP	LMA	ETT Airway
Patient type (selected examples)	Neuromuscular disease Exacerbation of chronic lung disease Postop respiratory failure	Emergent short-term ventilation needed and ETT intubation not possible Head and neck vascular malformations Unconscious patient	Severe tracheal injury Severe head injury ARDS
Basic procedure	Fit proper sized mask and headstrap on patient. Set IPAP to obtain visible chest excursion. Set FiO_2 to 50%. Set rate (see below). ↑ EPAP until oxygen saturations are >90%.	Deflate cuff and lubricate the mask. Introduce into the pharynx and advance until resistance felt as tube enters the hypopharynx. Inflate cuff (distal opening of tube is just above glottis). Attach breathing circuit. To remove: suction airway, deflate cuff, withdraw LMA.	PALS basics (position, BVM, etc) Pre-oxygenate 3–5 min Give RSI medications Cricoid pressure Insert ETT. Verify ETT placement (auscultate lungs, stomach). Assess outcome: clinical (VS, color, aeration), blood gas, $EtCO_2$ (capnography, colorimetry best).
Ventilator settings	*BiPAP (4 modes)* Set IPAP or EPAP at 4–20 cm H_2O and rate at 4–30 breaths per minute Spontaneous (rate controlled by patient) Spontaneous/timed (timed back-up rate, in case the patient's own rate drops below a specified level) Timed (rate controlled completely by machine) CPAP *LMA/ETT* Rate: approximate for age Volume limited: Tidal volume 8–10 mL/kg; I:E ratio start at 1:3; use a longer expiratory time for obstructive disease Pressure limited: PEEP start at 3 cm H_2O and increase as indicated; set PIP at pressure required to move chest wall (assessed by using best hand bagging pressures) Air leak: ≤25 cm H_2O For cuffed tube, deflate cuff, then check leak		

Table 95-2. Airway Management and Ventilation[a], continued

	BiPAP	LMA	ETT Airway
Monitoring	Advanced	Advanced	Advanced
Limitations	Patient tolerance Skilled respiratory therapist needed Often PICU setting	Requires sedation medications Less airway protection compared to ETT Skilled ventilator management needed PICU setting	Requires RSI or similar medications (neuromuscular blockade, sedation) As with LMA
Common contraindications	Absent gag/cough reflex ARDS Inability to maintain life-sustaining ventilation in event of BiPAP failure	Hiatal hernia Severe GERD Laryngeal burns Asthma Decreased pulmonary compliance	(All are relative) Asthma Foreign body Laryngeal burns
Common complications	Pneumothorax Aspiration Gastric distention Facial pressure sores	Pharyngeal/laryngeal mucosal or nerve injury Aspiration	Esophageal placement VILI VAP

Abbreviations: ARDS, acute respiratory distress syndrome; BiPAP, bi-level positive airway pressure; BVM, bag-valve-mask; CLD, chronic lung disease; CPAP, continuous positive airway pressure; $EtCO_2$, end-tidal carbon dioxide; EPAP, expiratory positive airway pressure; ETT, endotracheal tube; FIO_2, fraction of inspired oxygen; FRC, functional residual capacity; GERD, gastroesophageal reflux disease; H_2O, water; HFNC, high-flow nasal cannula; IPAP, inspiratory positive airway pressure; LMA, laryngeal mask airway; LPM, liter per minute; NC, nasal cannula; NCPAP, nasal continuous positive airway pressure; NPA, nasopharyngeal airway; OA, oral airway; PALS, Pediatric Advanced Life Support; PEEP, positive end-expiratory pressure; PICU, pediatric intensive care unit; PIP, peak inspiratory pressure; RA, room air; RSI, rapid sequence intubation; VAP, ventilatory acquired pneumonia; VILI, ventilator-induced lung injury; VS, vital signs.

[a]For all of these interventions, use the American Heart Association Pediatric Advanced Life Support and local standards for patient placement, respiratory therapy and other staff support, and monitoring.

"Standard monitoring" is defined as oxygen saturation and cardiorespiratory monitoring.

"Advanced monitoring" is defined as capnography, venous or arterial blood gas analyses, with or without invasive central line or arterial line access.

sequence intubation (RSI) method reduces the chance for aspiration of gastric contents. Firm backward, upward, and rightward pressure (BURP) on the patient's thyroid cartilage can improve the glottic view if there is difficulty during laryngoscopy. Typically, the assistant performing the Sellick maneuver can assist, resulting in a combined Sellick-BURP maneuver.

Key medications are fast-acting intravenous (IV) muscle relaxants, such as succinylcholine, rocuronium, or vecuronium.

- Succinylcholine: Dose—1 to 2 mg/kg, onset of action 40 seconds, duration 6 to 8 minutes. Do not use in burn, trauma, rhabdomyolysis, spinal cord injuries, or muscular dystrophy patients. Hyperkalemia can occur even days later in patients with muscle disease, and there is a US Food and Drug Administration black box warning for undiagnosed skeletal muscle myopathy.
- Rocuronium: Dose—1 mg/kg, onset of action one minute, duration 30 minutes.
- Vecuronium (non-depolarizing neuromuscular blocker): Dose—0.2 mg/kg IV, onset 1 minute, duration 45 minutes.

Mechanical Ventilation

- Intermittent mandatory ventilation (IMV) delivers a preset number of mechanical breaths per minute.
- Synchronized IMV synchronizes mechanical breaths with the patient's inspiratory efforts.
- Assist control assists a patient's own spontaneous breaths and has a backup rate for safety.
- Pressure support ventilation opens a valve allowing airflow at a preset positive pressure when a patient inspires. This mode of mechanical ventilation augments all spontaneous patient breaths with positive pressure.

Basic Strategies

- To increase PaO_2: Increase positive end-expiratory pressure (PEEP), mean airway pressure, inspiratory time, or FiO_2.
- To decrease $PaCO_2$: Increase peak inspiratory pressure (PIP), rate, or tidal volume. An increased PEEP will increase $PaCO_2$.

Mechanical Ventilation Weaning Strategies

- Reduce respiratory load by relieving bronchospasm, removing secretions, reducing pulmonary edema, and treating any pulmonary infections.
- Increase muscle power (strength and endurance) by reducing hyperinflation, optimizing nutrition, and sprint weaning.
- Improve central drive by avoiding hypochloremic alkalosis and reducing CNS depressant medications.

Predictors of Successful Extubation

- Normal $PaCO_2$
- PIP less than 14 to 16 cm H_2O
- PEEP less than 2 to 3 cm H_2O (infant) or less than 5 cm H_2O (child)
- IMV less than 2 to 4 breaths per minute
- FiO_2 below 40% with PaO_2 above 70.

Respiratory Adjuncts

Heliox, a low-density combination helium-oxygen mixture, improves ventilation by making turbulent flow more laminar through narrowed airways. Its use in nonintubated patients with upper airway (croup) or certain lower airway (bronchiolitis) diseases has been associated with improved oxygenation, as well as decreased respiratory rate and retractions. Common mixtures are (helium/oxygen) 80/20, 70/30, and 6=0/40. A helium concentration less than 60% is of no benefit. Therefore, the clinical limitation to heliox use is the inability to maintain adequate oxygenation if high FiO_2 is required because of parenchymal disease.

Disposition

- **Intensive care unit**
  - FiO_2 greater than 50% necessary to maintain an oxygen saturation 92% or greater
  - Respiratory distress accompanied by progressive fatigue
  - pH less than 7.2 and/or a normal $PaCO_2$ cannot be maintained
  - Need for advanced monitoring, heliox, BiPAP, or intubation
  - Apnea or irregular respirations
- **Transfer to a tertiary center**
  - Depends on the on-site resources, including staffing, monitoring, and availability of pediatric critical care expertise

Pearls and Pitfalls

- Initially, recognition of respiratory distress is more important than determining the cause. Discuss the signs and symptoms of, and preparation for the response to, impending respiratory failure with all staff members.
- Tachypnea is the first sign of respiratory distress, but bradypnea is an ominous sign of impending respiratory arrest.
- Altered mental status may indicate presence of hypoxia and or hypercarbia.

- Bradycardia is the ultimate sign of catastrophic respiratory compromise.
- Prevent bradycardia during intubation with atropine premedication.
- Prevent aspiration during intubation with cricoid pressure and RSI.
- Proper positioning and early extubation will reduce the risk of ventilator-associated pneumonia.

Coding

CPT

A patient with acute respiratory failure meets the criteria for *CPT* coding as critical care.

- ETT, emergency: **31500.** Use this code for an emergency or crisis situation and not for elective intubation. Note that time spent on the procedure must be subtracted from the time billed for critical care services.
- Critical care, first hour (include ventilator management): **99291**
- Ventilator assist and management, initiation of pressure or volume preset ventilators for assisted or controlled breathing
  — First day: **94656**
  — Subsequent days: **94657**

Bibliography

Aly H. Ventilation without tracheal intubation. *Pediatrics.* 2009;124:786–789

Chen L, Hsiao AL. Randomized trial of endotracheal tube versus laryngeal mask airway in simulated prehospital pediatric arrest. *Pediatrics.* 2008;122:e294–e297

Deis JN, Abramo TJ, Crawley L. Noninvasive respiratory support. *Pediatr Emerg Care.* 2008;24:331–338

Kissoon N, Rimensberger PC, Bohn D. Ventilation strategies and adjunctive therapy in severe lung disease. *Pediatr Clin North Am.* 2008;55:709–733

Sankar MJ, Sankar J, Agarwal R, Paul VK, Deorari AK. Protocol for administering continuous positive airway pressure in neonates. *Indian J Pediatr.* 2008;75:471–478

Trachsel D, McCrindle BW, Nakagawa S, Bohn D. Oxygenation index predicts outcome in children with acute hypoxemic respiratory failure. *Am J Respir Crit Care Med.* 2005;172:206–211

Sedation and Analgesia

CHAPTER 96

Pain Management

Introduction

The International Association for the Study of Pain defines pain as an unpleasant sensory and emotional experience arising from actual or potential tissue damage. Historically, pediatric pain is under-recognized and undertreated. Traditional barriers to providing good pain control to children include a lack of knowledge of pain treatment and a fear of adverse effects, such as respiratory depression or addiction.

Pain Assessment

The best way to assess pediatric pain is by asking the patient, if possible. Use the parents as an alternative if the child is unable to communicate. Elevations in the pulse and blood pressure may suggest that a nonverbal child is in pain, while the absence of altered vital signs does not preclude the child being in pain, especially if the pain is chronic. Another option is to provide the patient with pain medication and then reassess. However, there are many reasons why children might deny feeling pain. These include that they were told to be brave, are concerned about medication side effects or taste, are worried that pain means they are getting sicker, do not understand that pain can be treated, are worried that pain will prevent discharge home, are attempting to protect their parents, or fear injection site pain associated with intramuscular (IM) or subcutaneous (SC) pain control.

In a neonate or infant, or a nonverbal or neurodevelopmentally disabled patient, assessing pain can present a challenge. For a child with neurodevelopmental disabilities who cannot adequately indicate the need for pain medications, special training is often required to interpret the degree of discomfort. As an aid, there are many pain scales available that combine both physiological and behavioral parameters, such as the Neonatal Infant Pain Scale and the Face, Legs, Activity, Cry, Consolability scale (Table 96-1).

Children 3 to 8 years of age are able to articulate that they have pain and may be able to localize it. They might use different words to express pain, such as "hurt" or "ouch," although they are less capable of describing the quality or intensity of the pain. In this age group, use a child pain scale that includes color or faces scales (Figure 96-1). Assess a patient older than 8 years (or cognitively >8) with the standard visual pain scale that is used for adults (Figure 96-2).

Table 96-1. FLACC Scale[a]			
Categories	**Scoring**		
	0	1	2
Face	No particular expression or smile	Occasional grimaces or frown, withdrawn, disinterested	Frequent to constant frown, clenched jaw, quivering chin
Legs	Normal position or relaxed	Uneasy, restless, tense	Kicking or legs drawn up
Activity	Lying quietly Normal position Moves easily	Squirming Shifting back and forth Tense	Arched, rigid, or jerking
Cry	No cry (awake or asleep)	Moans or whimpers, occasional complaint	Crying steadily Screams or sobs Frequent complaints
Consolability	Content Relaxed	Reassured by occasional touching, hugging, or "talking to" Distractible	Difficult to console or comfort

Abbreviation: FLACC, Face, Legs, Activity, Cry, Consolability.

[a]From Merkel S, Voepel-Lewis T, Shayevitz J, Malviya S. The FLACC: A behavioral scale for scoring postoperative pain in young children. *Pediatr Nurs.* 1997;23:293–297. ©The Regent of the University of Michigan. Printed with permission.

Figure 96-1. Faces Pain Scale[a]

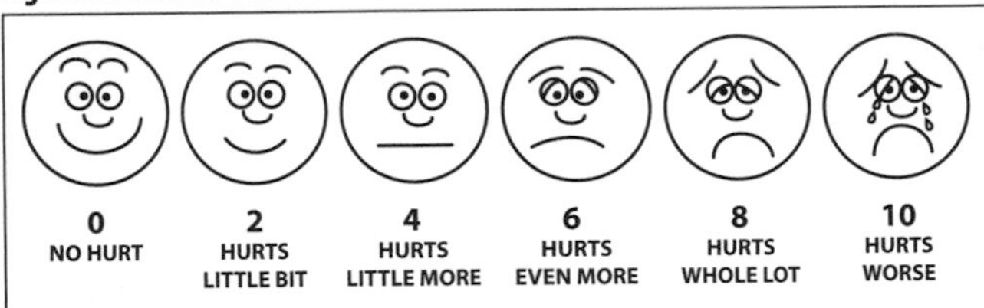

[a]From Wong DL, Wilson D. *Wong's Essentials of Pediatric Nursing*. 8th ed St Louis, MO: Mosby; 2008, with permission from Elsevier.

Figure 96-2. Visual Analogue Pain Scale

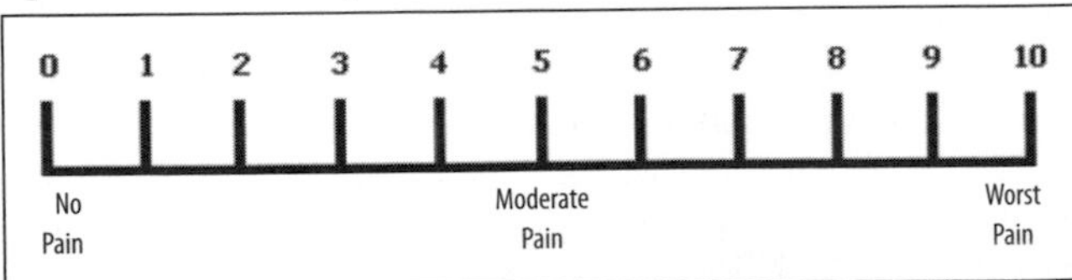

Treatment

There are a number of basic principles in pediatric pain management.

- Pediatric pain practices are not evidence-based, as most medications are used off-label, relying on extrapolation of adult study data.
- Complementary modalities, such as relaxation and breathing exercises, hypnosis, guided imagery, Reiki, biofeedback, massage, acupuncture/acupressure, or distraction (eg, art, pet, play, or music therapy), can greatly reduce the need for pharmacologic management of pain in a child.
- Treat anxiety, sadness, and fear as components of suffering that increase the child's perception of pain.
- Try to use the most painless route (oral [PO]) of administration (try to avoid IM and rectal medications).
- For an infant, start at a low dose, but titrate up quickly as needed.
- Reassess the patient frequently for continuing pain and the efficacy of treatment.
- Less medication is required to prevent pain than to eliminate it. Therefore, initially use as much as necessary to achieve pain control and then dose as frequently as needed to maintain adequate analgesia.
- A patient with advanced cancer or sickle cell pain often requires far higher doses of analgesics and adjuncts to achieve adequate pain control.
- Attempt to achieve control of long-term pain with scheduled or long-acting medications, and provide immediate-release medications for incidental or "breakthrough" pain episodes.

Medications

Acetaminophen

Acetaminophen is a mild analgesic and antipyretic that is available in PO, rectal, and intravenous (IV) (same dose as PO) forms. The onset of action occurs in 30 minutes. It is primarily metabolized in the liver and may therefore be contraindicated in hepatic failure. Also, because of a risk of chronic liver toxicity, limit the duration of around-the-clock therapy to 3 days.

Neonates 10 days or older, infants, children younger than 12 years: 15 mg/kg/dose every 4 hours. Do not exceed 75 mg/kg/day or 4,000 mg/day. A rectal loading dose up to 40 mg/kg loading can be given, followed by the standard rectal dosing. Children 12 years and older: 325 to 650 mg every 4 to 6 hours or 1,000 mg 2 to 3 times a day. Do not exceed 4,000 mg/day.

Nonsteroidal Anti-Inflammatory Drugs (NSAIDS)

NSAIDS have analgesic, anti-inflammatory, and antipyretic effects. Side effects include gastritis, nephropathy, and bleeding from platelet anti-aggregation.

Ibuprofen

The dose of ibuprofen is 10 mg/kg/dose every 6 hours (child) or 400 to 600 mg every 6 hours up to 800 mg every 8 hours (adolescent). The onset of action occurs in 30 to 45 minutes.

Ketorolac

Ketorolac is available in both PO and IV forms. The IV dose is 0.5 mg/kg every 6 hours (30 mg/dose maximum) and is particularly useful as a parenteral agent when trying to avoid opioids. The onset of action is 10 minutes. Ketorolac shares the same side-effect profile as the other NSAIDS in terms of bleeding risk and potential impact on renal function. During the course of treatment, monitor renal function and provide gastrointestinal protection (famotidine 0.6–0.8 g/kg/day IV divided every 8–12 hours, 40 mg/day maximum or ranitidine PO 2–4 mg/kg divided every 12 hours, 300 mg/day maximum). Do not use ketorolac for more than 5 days due to an increased risk of side effects.

Opioids

Opioids are available in multiple forms, including IV and PO. They are most effective when given around-the-clock (ie, on a schedule) for chronic or persistent pain, with additional when necessary (PRN) doses (every 3–4 hours for short-acting opioids) for incidental or breakthrough pain. If more than 4 to 6 PRN doses are required, increase the daily maintenance dose by 50%. If there are side effects, such as severe nausea or sleepiness, decrease the maintenance dose by 25%. Tapering is usually necessary if opioids are administered for more than 1 week.

When attempting to rapidly achieve pain control with opioids, it is helpful to do a rapid IV titration using morphine, hydromorphone or, occasionally, fentanyl. This process may take several hours and requires close attention to the patient's response to each dose. To treat pain in a patient who is already receiving opioids, increase the dose by 25% to 50% for mild to moderate pain and 50% to 100% for severe pain. Although this approach requires additional physician and nurse presence, the pain relief can be much more effectively achieved by a direct, hands-on approach.

Anticipate and treat opioid side effects. Manage nausea with ondansetron (0.05–0.1 mg/kg IV or PO every 6 hours PRN, 4 mg/dose maximum) or metoclopramide (0.1–0.2 mg/kg every 6–8 hours IV/PO, 10 mg/dose maximum). Treat pruritus with either diphenhydramine (5 mg/kg/day divided every 6 hours, 300 mg/day maximum) or hydroxyzine (2 mg/kg/day divided every 8 hours; 50 mg/day maximum <6 years, 100 mg/day maximum >6 years, 600 mg/day maximum for adults). Start a bowel regimen if multiple doses or prolonged use are anticipated.

Morphine

Morphine can be administered orally (immediate or sustained-release), sublingually, subcutaneously, intravenously, and rectally. It is indicated for moderate to severe pain. Use with caution in a patient with renal failure.

The IV morphine dose is 0.05 to 0.2 mg/kg every 2 to 4 hours and the PO dose for immediate-release morphine is 0.2 to 0.5 mg/kg/dose (adult dose 10–30 mg) every 4 to 6 hours and for controlled-release morphine 0.3 to 0.6 mg/kg every 12 hours (adult dose 15–30 mg every 8–12 hours). In an opioid-naïve child, begin at the lower dose and titrate up as needed. The maximum IV/SC/IM dose is 15 mg with close monitoring for respiratory depression. The onset is within 5 to 10 minutes with analgesia that lasts 2 to 4 hours. Therefore, with close monitoring, additional IV doses can be safely given every 30 minutes to achieve rapid pain control. The PO dose is 3 times the IV dose every 4 to 6 hours. The onset of action is typically 30 to 45 minutes later than with an enteral dose, so it is more difficult to titrate the effectiveness of PO dosing. However, if the patient has chronic pain management requirements, convert to a long-acting, PO opioid once the daily requirement has been established (either IV or PO).

One of the most common side effects is pruritus at the injection site. This is not an *allergic reaction* and therefore not a contraindication to continuing the drug. Treat with diphenhydramine or hydroxyzine (dosing as above). Hives that develop at a site remote from the injection site could be a sign of allergy and should be treated accordingly.

Morphine Patient-Controlled Analgesia (PCA)

A PCA is a programmable pump that allows the patient to control IV analgesia by choosing when to deliver a dose of opioid for quick relief as well as titration to pain needs. The lockout interval for the bolus dose is related to the onset and peak action of the opioid. The patient must be mature enough to understand how and when to push the demand button for boluses, which can be confirmed by having the child play a video game. It is generally considered fundamental to PCA use that the patient, and not the parent, control the PCA, ensuring the inherent safety built into the pump. However, some institutions' pain policies permit the parents, nurses, or other care providers to administer the demand dose with constant bedside monitoring of respirations and pulse oximetry. When parents are authorized to give the demand doses (eg, a young or disabled child), careful training is required to avoid excessive dosing.

When administered by himself or herself, the patient will not request further boluses if sedated and sleeping, and therefore cannot self-overdose. A PCA is especially useful when analgesia is required for vasoocclusive crises in a patient with sickle cell disease, postoperative pain, and cancer pain, and when goals of care have transitioned to primarily palliative.

Begin a morphine PCA regimen with a loading dose of 0.03 to 0.1 mg/kg (use the lower dose for an opioid-naïve patient and a higher one for a patient with prior opioid exposure). Then immediately start the PCA at a basal (continuous) rate of typically 0.01 to 0.03 mg/kg/hour (opioid naïve vs opioid-accommodated, respectively). Order a demand dose of 0.01 to 0.03 mg/kg with a lockout period of 6 to 10 minutes. Therefore, for a 25-kg patient, the continuous rate is 0.5 to 0.8 mg/hour with 0.25-mg PCA demand doses (up to 10 in 1 hour, if still in pain). Note that the PCA dose refers to the patient-controlled dose and has many synonyms, including intermittent dose, interval dose, interval bolus, and demand dose. Increase the basal rate by 10% to 20% if the patient requires more than 3 boluses per hour, and decrease it by the same amount if more than 3 boluses per hour are requested.

Close monitoring by trained pediatric personnel, and not the parents, is required for any patient undergoing the initiation of PCA or IV opioid treatment. A patient with advanced cancer or sickle cell pain may require significantly higher doses of PCA opioid than the typical opioid-naïve patient. Consult with a pain specialist or the palliative care service when more complex pain management is needed.

Oxycodone

Oxycodone is available in PO form and is indicated for mild to moderate pain, either alone or with acetaminophen. The dose is 0.05 to 0.15 mg/kg every 4 to 6 hours (5 mg maximum).

Fentanyl

Fentanyl can be administered IV or with a buccal tab, lozenge, intranasally, or a transdermal patch. It is indicated for severe pain, but reserve the transdermal patch for an opioid-tolerant patient and pain of anticipated long duration. Fentanyl by IV, intranasally, and buccal route has rapid onset with a relatively brief duration of action, so if a longer period of analgesia is necessary, use a continuous infusion or transdermal preparation. The dose is 1 mcg/kg every 30 to 60 minutes and 1.5 mcg/kg for intranasal dosing. Side effects of rapid administration in some patients are glottic and chest wall rigidity. Therefore, follow a careful monitoring protocol and have resuscitation equipment available when giving by infusion. Non-allergic facial pruritus can occur as with morphine (see above), but histamine release is far less common than with morphine or hydromorphone. Due to its high lipophilicity, fentanyl tends to accumulate in fatty tissues, leading to a prolonged elimination in patients on long-term treatment. Discontinuation of fentanyl following as few as 3 days' use has been associated with abstinence syndrome, necessitating close observation and consideration to weaning for patients on long-term treatment.

Hydromorphone

Hydromorphone is 5 to 7 times more potent than IV morphine. It is available in PO or IV form. The IV dose is 0.015 mg/kg/dose every 4 to 6 hours (1.2 mg maximum). It may also be used by PCA in place of morphine or in a regimen of planned opioid rotation. Consultation with a pain or palliative care service is helpful in planning a rotation of opioids.

Methadone

Methadone is available in PO and IV forms, and may be given subcutaneously as well. The IV and PO dose is 0.7 mg/kg/day divided every 4 to 6 hours with an adult maximum of 2.5 to 10 mg every 3 to 4 hours. The PO elixir is 60% to 90% bioavailable and therefore highly effective. It has a very long half-life with a slow peak and long steady state, so it is optimal for patients requiring chronic analgesia. It accumulates slowly with high partitioning to the fatty tissues, so that it can take 5 to 7 days to reach a steady state. Thus the dose of methadone that produces good analgesia acutely may lead to excess sedation within 3 to 5 days of chronic usage.

Opioid Conversion

By convention, all opioids can be related back to morphine "equianalgesic" equivalency. This approach allows the interconversion of opioids by close approximation of their equivalent activity. Several points must be noted. First, IV to PO conversion is not the same for all opioids due to first-pass elimination of the more hydrophilic compounds (eg, morphine, hydromorphone, and oxycodone), whereas the lipophilic compounds (eg, methadone and fentanyl) tend not to demonstrate the same degree of first-pass effect. Secondly, the onset of action is much slower via a PO route, making it more difficult to titrate to the patient's needs with increased risk for over- or undertreatment. Lastly, methadone equivalency is an inexact science and must be considered a "sliding scale" depending on how high a dose of other opioid the patient had been receiving prior to conversion to methadone. Thus a pharmacy, pain service, or palliative care consultation can assist with this task.

Opioid Tolerance

Opioid tolerance is the development of the need to increase the dose of the medication to achieve the same sedative or analgesic effect. Cross-tolerance among all opioids occurs, but not on a 1:1 basis. Therefore, in conversion to another opioid, it is best to administer a percentage of the equianalgesic dose

(80% for a short-acting medication) and then titrate up. Teach the family and the patient care staff that there is no upper limit of dosing in a non-naïve patient. Every child is different, and dosage must be individualized. However, in order to minimize tolerance, rotate narcotics or, in severe cases, use adjuncts such as a ketamine infusion, which enhances the response to opioids. In such complex pain management situations, consult with a pain specialist or the palliative care service.

Weaning

The goal of weaning is to prevent withdrawal symptoms (abstinence syndrome), which can occur within 24 hours of abrupt cessation of the medication, or immediately if the patient is given naloxone. The symptoms peak within 72 hours of cessation and include cramping, vomiting, diarrhea, tachycardia, hypertension, diaphoresis, restlessness, insomnia, movement disorders, and seizures.

Begin the weaning process when the patient is receiving 0.25 mg/kg/hour or less of morphine (basal + bolus). The initial step is to convert from continuous IV to around-the-clock bolus treatment. Continue the bolus treatments for 48 hours prior to weaning the dose by no more than 20% per day. Discontinue IV analgesia only when the patient is tolerating a PO regimen. Criteria for transitioning to PO analgesia are normal gastrointestinal function (tolerating PO and passing gas) and pain typically quantified as 6 or lower on a scale of 10. Begin PO analgesia when the morphine equivalent is 10 to 20 mcg/kg/hour.

When transitioning from PCA to PO medication, give a dose of the PO analgesic first, then discontinue the basal infusion 30 to 60 minutes later. Concurrently, reduce the IV bolus dose by 25% to 50%. Then discontinue the PCA if the patient has not required a bolus dose in more than 6 hours. If the patient requires 1 to 3 bolus doses over a 6-hour period and is in persistent pain following evaluation, increase the PO analgesic dose by 25% to 50%. Increase by 50% to 100% if 3 to 6 boluses are required over a 6-hour period, or add a PO adjuvant, such as acetaminophen. However, always assess if there are other, psychological motivations why the patient continues to push the button.

In some institutions the preference may be to convert the patient to PO methadone to permit continued weaning following discharge. It generally takes several days to achieve complete conversion after the parenteral opioids have been weaned to an acceptably low level, as described above. The availability of methadone for outpatient use may limit this approach in some communities.

Naloxone

Naloxone, an opioid antagonist, is indicated when a patient receiving narcotics is unresponsive to physical stimulation, has shallow respirations (<8 breaths/minute [bpm] and at risk for intubation), and pinpoint pupils. If the patient is hypoxic or hypoventilating, or there is hemodynamic compromise, discontinue the opioid and provide face-mask oxygen. For life-threatening opiate overdose, the initial dose of naloxone is 0.01 mg/kg, which can be repeated every 2 to 3 minutes until a response is seen. An alternative is 2 mcg/kg IV every 30 seconds until the patient responds. Administering higher doses may precipitate acute abstinence syndrome in patients on longstanding opioids with adverse physical and psychological consequences. Cardiac decompensation may also occur when fully reversing opiates acutely. Administer the naloxone slowly, and monitor closely for a response. Discontinue the naloxone as soon as the patient responds, but continue to monitor because the effective duration of action of naloxone is 20 to 30 minutes, which is frequently shorter than the opiate, necessitating additional doses of naloxone. The patient will then require nonopioid pain relief. However, once the patient is easily arousable with a respiratory rate greater than 9 bpm, restart the opioid at half the previous dose.

A continuous low-dose naloxone infusion may be useful in patients receiving PCA morphine. It reduces systemic side effects and may reduce the speed of tolerance development.

Special Considerations in Opioid Dosing

Infant: Morphine clearance is delayed in the first 1 to 2 months of life. Prescribe a starting dose that is one-third to one-half that used for an older child. In addition, an infant is more sensitive to the respiratory depressant effects of opioids, so close monitoring is needed. Additionally, children with central nervous system (CNS) disease (eg, perinatal asphyxia, metabolic disease affecting the CNS) may be more sensitive to the depressant effects of opioids and may require lower doses.

Child 2 to 6 years of age: Since there is an increased liver mass compared with adults, more frequent dosing is needed.

Epidural and Regional Anesthesia

Regional anesthesia is becoming routine and the standard of care in many pediatric institutions. In particular, epidural anesthesia with opiates and bupivicaine can provide both postoperative pain management as well as pain control for complex pain conditions. Regional blocks for both limb pain and intercostal blocks for pain associated with rib fractures, chest tubes, and chest wall pain are easily performed at the bedside with ultrasound guidance by pediatric pain specialists. Such approaches reduce the need for systemic medications and avoid many of the adverse effects of systemic agents, including more rapid weaning of analgesia when no longer required. Consultation with the pediatric pain service or anesthesiology is necessary for these modalities.

Specific Analgesia Recommendations

Postoperative Pain

Initially manage postoperative pain with around-the-clock analgesics, then wean as tolerated to PRN dosing. If the patient underwent abdominal surgery or cannot tolerate PO, IV morphine every 3 to 4 hours or via PCA is very useful with appropriate monitoring.

Sickle Cell Pain

Manage vasoocclusive crisis pain aggressively, and ask the patient what has worked well in the past. Depending on the patient's age and the severity of the patient's pain and disease, it may be best start with morphine PCA. If the patient is too young to use a PCA, order around-the-clock IV morphine. For any age patient, ketorolac may also be necessary (after confirmation of normal serum creatinine). See Sickle Cell Disease, page 661. Be aware of the potential need to use higher doses of opioids than required in other pain syndromes.

Orthopaedic Pain

The proper management of orthopaedic pain permits earlier mobilization, which can lead to decreased morbidity and shortened hospital stay. Around-the-clock opioids, such as IV morphine or PO Percocet, provide optimal analgesia, which can then be weaned accordingly. Ensure that adequate analgesia is given prior to mobilization or physical therapy.

Pearls and Pitfalls

- When managing pediatric pain, do it "by the child, by the mouth, and by the clock." That is, individualize an analgesia regimen for the specific patient that is given around-the-clock (every 3–6 hours) and is ideally administered orally (painless administration).
- Do not undertreat pain due to fear of adverse effects. Consult with a pain specialist when the pain severity requires you to practice outside your comfort zone.

Coding

ICD-9

- Acute pain due to trauma **338.11**
- Acute postoperative pain (other than post-thoracotomy) **338.18**
- Arthralgia, unspecified **719.40**
- Chronic pain due to trauma **338.21**
- Chronic postoperative pain (other than post-thoracotomy) **338.28**
- Long-term (current) use of NSAIDs **V58.64**
- Long-term (current) use of opiate analgesic **V58.69**
- Neoplasm-related pain (acute or chronic) **338.3**
- Other acute pain **338.19**
- Other chronic pain **338.29**
- Pain in limb **729.5**
- Sickle cell—hemoglobin C disease with vasoocclusive pain **282.64**
- Sickle cell—thalassemia with vasoocclusive pain **282.42**
- Sickle cell disease with vasoocclusive pain **282.62**

Bibliography

Ali S, Drendel AL, Kircher J, Beno S. Pain management of musculoskeletal injuries in children: current state and future directions. *Pediatr Emerg Care.* 2010;26:518–524

Anand KJ, Willson DF, Berger J, et al. Tolerance and withdrawal from prolonged opioid use in critically ill children. *Pediatrics.* 2010;125:e1208–e1225

Ellison AM, Shaw K. Management of vasoocclusive pain events in sickle cell disease. *Pediatr Emerg Care.* 2007;23:832–838

George JA, Lin EE, Hanna MN, et al. The effect of intravenous opioid patient-controlled analgesia with and without background infusion on respiratory depression: a meta-analysis. *J Opioid Manag.* 2010;6:47–54

Klick JC, Hauer J. Pediatric palliative care. *Curr Probl Pediatr Adolesc Health Care.* 2010;40:120–151

Kraemer FW, Rose JB. Pharmacologic management of acute pediatric pain. *Anesthesiol Clin.* 2009;27:241–268

Zernikow B, Michel E, Craig F, Anderson BJ. Pediatric palliative care: use of opioids for the management of pain. *Paediatr Drugs.* 2009;11:129–151

CHAPTER 97

Sedation

Introduction

The goal of pediatric sedation is to allow diagnostic and therapeutic procedures to be performed as safely, comfortably, and efficiently as possible. Consider each situation on an individual basis to determine the appropriate level of sedation needed and to address the individual patient's needs regarding control of pain, anxiety, memory, and motion during the procedure. Also consider using non-pharmacologic techniques, such as working in conjunction with a child life specialist.

Definitions

The level of drug-induced sedation is divided into 4 different states.

Minimal Sedation/Anxiolysis

The patient can respond normally to verbal commands. Although cognitive function and coordination may be impaired, ventilatory and cardiovascular functions are usually maintained.

Moderate Sedation

The patient can respond purposefully to verbal commands, either alone or accompanied by light to moderate tactile stimulation. No interventions are required to maintain a patent airway, and spontaneous ventilation is adequate. Cardiovascular function is usually maintained.

Deep Sedation

The patient cannot be easily aroused, but responds purposefully to repeated verbal or painful stimulation. The ability to maintain ventilatory function may be impaired. The patient may require assistance in maintaining a patent airway, spontaneous ventilation may be inadequate, and protective airway reflexes may be compromised. Cardiovascular function is usually maintained.

General Anesthesia

The patient cannot be aroused, even by painful stimulation. Independent ventilatory function is often impaired. The patient will often require assistance in maintaining a patent airway, and positive-pressure ventilation may be needed because of depressed spontaneous ventilation or depression of neuromuscular function. Cardiovascular function may be impaired.

Training

Each institution will have a specific training and certification program to ensure the competence of medical providers in safe sedation techniques. The program should function in conjunction with the institution's department of anesthesiology and clearly delineate hospitalist roles and limitations. Specific guidelines should include the medications that may be used, American Society of Anesthesiologists (ASA) classes that may be sedated, and the timing and location of hospitalist-run sedations. The training program must also ensure that the hospitalist is comfortable with contraindications, common side effects and complications, and basic rescue mechanisms, including airway management.

Each patient's responses to different medications can vary, so be prepared to manage deeper levels of sedation than what was intended. For example, even though moderate sedation is intended, be qualified and prepared to manage a patient who is deeply sedated. Become familiar with a small number of agents in order to simplify sedation plans and maximize safety and efficiency. For example, ketamine is useful for painful procedures, while dexmedetomidine or pentobarbital is a reasonable option for imaging procedures requiring a motionless state.

Institutional needs and resources will dictate what levels of training are available for hospitalists, and a tiered system may be appropriate in some cases. For example, a first tier of hospitalists may be approved to sedate ASA I–II patients in the emergency unit where multiple resources are in place, while a second tier may be approved to sedate ASA I–III patients in specified specialty units during daytime hours when anesthesia is available for backup, and a third tier may be approved to use a wider variety of agents or sedate after-hours.

Pre-Sedation Evaluation

Perform a screening evaluation prior to the induction of sedation. Include a focused history, guided by the mnemonic AMPLE (Box 97-1). On physical examination, pay particular attention to airway, respiratory, and cardiovascular status. Screen the patient for a personal or family history of complications from sedation; a history of snoring, wheezing, or stridor; recent illnesses; obesity; and anatomical abnormalities (small jaw, short neck, large tongue) that may make airway obstruction more likely and rescue procedures more difficult. Evaluate the patient's ASA physical status (Table 97-1) and arrange an anesthesia consultation prior to sedation if the ASA class is III, IV, or V.

Pre-Sedation Fasting

It is generally believed that fasting decreases the likelihood of aspiration. Therefore, follow the ASA recommendations for NPO times (Table 97-2) for all elective procedural sedations. For emergent sedations, carefully balance the risks of sedation with the benefits of completing the procedure quickly. In an emergent case, when the fasting interval is insufficient, use the lightest effective sedation.

Pre-Sedation Preparation

In order to guarantee patient safety, ensure the presence of a medical provider with advanced resuscitation skills at all times during the sedation. This person may also perform the procedure during moderate sedations, provided there is an assistant present who can closely monitor the patient and record vital sign data. During deep sedations, the sedation provider may offer brief,

Box 97-1. AMPLE Mnemonic for Patient History

A: Allergies to medications, food, or latex

M: Medications used regularly or recently

P: Past medical and surgical history, including history of sedations

L: Last liquid and solid intake

E: Events leading to current illness, injury, or need for procedure

Table 97-1. American Society of Anesthesiologists (ASA) Physical Status Classification

ASA Class	Disease State
I	No organic, physiological, biochemical, or psychiatric disturbance
II	Mild to moderate systemic disturbance
III	Severe systemic disturbance
IV	Severe systemic disturbance that is life-threatening
V	Moribund patient with little chance of survival

Table 97-2. NPO Guidelines for Elective Sedations

Food or Liquid	Hours
Clear liquids[a]	2
Breast milk	4
Infant formula	6
All other food and liquid	6

[a]Clear liquids include water, clear soda, clear tea, and clear fruit juice with no pulp.

interruptible assistance to a separate proceduralist if it does not interfere with the ability to closely monitor the patient at all times.

Before beginning sedation, confirm that all potentially needed rescue equipment and medications are easily accessible. Keep a crash cart nearby, with precalculated doses of common rescue medications, as well as airway rescue equipment, such as laryngoscopes with appropriately sized blades, endotracheal tubes, stylettes, and laryngeal mask airways. Have an anesthesia or continuous positive airway pressure bag readily available and connected to an oxygen source with an appropriately sized face mask attached. Connect a large-bore suction catheter to wall suction in case of emesis.

Sedation and Recovery Monitoring

During minimal and moderate sedations and recovery, continuously monitor the patient's heart rate and pulse oximetry. Also monitor end-tidal carbon dioxide ($EtCO_2$) when the sedation practitioner is at a distance and cannot directly observe the patient (eg, magnetic resonance imaging). Re-assess the blood pressure and respiratory rate every 5 minutes once a stable level of sedation has been achieved, and obtain intravenous (IV) access for moderate or deeper sedation.

For deep sedation and recovery, monitor as above, always with IV access. Monitor $EtCO_2$ during the sedation and recovery period if feasible, since ventilatory function is often compromised before oxygenation. Perform deep sedation only in an area that is familiar to the provider giving the sedation and properly supplied with all necessary equipment. Do not perform deep sedation in a routine inpatient bed.

In addition to the above-mentioned monitoring, directly observe the patient during sedation and pay particular attention to the level of consciousness, color, airway patency, ventilatory effort and adequacy, and perfusion. Continue to monitor the patient after sedation, and ensure that the institutional recovery criteria are met before the patient is discharged or returned to the inpatient floor. Follow the specific hospital's protocols for appropriate documentation of patient monitoring data during both sedation and recovery, specifically noting in the medical record all vital signs and patient information mentioned above.

Billing and Coding

Billing anesthesia codes vary across the United States, sometimes on a state-by-state or local basis. This becomes an important factor in determining the level of funding available for pediatric hospital sedation programs. The Centers for Medicare & Medicaid Services requires that sedation services be overseen by a hospital's anesthesiology division or department, necessitating a close working relationship between anesthesia and others providing moderate and deep sedation. Anesthesia codes can be used appropriately by non-anesthesiologists when the level of care provided meets the standard of those codes, with reimbursement being most successful when both teams within an institution agree on the appropriate use of these codes. In contrast, it can be difficult to get reimbursed when there is disagreement about these codes among various hospital departments.

Bibliography

American Academy of Pediatrics; American Academy of Pediatric Dentistry, Coté CJ, Wilson S; Work Group on Sedation. Guidelines for monitoring and management of pediatric patients during and after sedation for diagnostic and therapeutic procedures: an update. *Pediatrics.* 2006;118:2587–2602

American Society of Anesthesiologists Task Force on Preoperative Fasting. Practice guidelines for preoperative fasting and the use of pharmacologic agents to reduce the risk of pulmonary aspiration: application to healthy patients undergoing elective procedures. *Anesthesiology.* 1999;90:896–905

American Society of Anesthesiologists Task Force on Sedation and Analgesia by Non-Anesthesiologists. Practice guidelines for sedation and analgesia by non-anesthesiologists. *Anesthesiology.* 2002;96:1004–1017

Joint Commission. *Hospital Accreditation Standards.* Oakbrook Terrace, IL: Joint Commission on Accreditation of Healthcare Organizations; 2009:276-8, 306–307, 316–318

Surgery

Acute Abdomen

Introduction

Acute abdomen, also known as "surgical abdomen," presents with the acute onset of abdominal pain, peritoneal signs, and evidence of obstruction. Since a true "acute abdomen" is a surgical emergency, it is imperative to make this diagnosis early. However, this can be a difficult task, given the wide range of etiologies and the variation in presentations, especially among young children.

While appendicitis is the most common surgical cause, the patient's age is a major determinant of the diagnoses to consider (Box 98-1). The most common causes for infants include intussusception and incarcerated inguinal hernia.

Clinical Presentation

History

The symptoms associated with acute abdomen typically evolve over hours. The description of the pain, along with the associated signs and symptoms, helps to differentiate among potential surgical and medical causes. For example, recent sick contacts with a similar illness would make infectious conditions, such as acute gastroenteritis (AGE), more likely.

It is important to develop the pain history. Pain location can suggest a potential cause, such as appendicitis (initially periumbilical then migrating to right lower quadrant) or biliary disease (right upper quadrant). The pain time course can also be helpful. For example, appendicitis tends to be constant and

Box 98-1. Common Causes of Abdominal Pain[a]

Infant	Toddler/Child	Adolescent	
AGE	AGE	AGE	Appendicitis
Constipation	Appendicitis	Constipation	Dysmenorrhea
Hirschsprung	Constipation	Ectopic pregnancy	IBD/IBS
Intussusception	HSP	Mittelschmerz	Ovarian torsion
Incarcerated hernia	Non-accidental trauma	Pancreatitis	PID
Non-accidental trauma	Pneumonia	Pneumonia	Trauma
UTI	Trauma	UTI	
Volvulus	UTI		

Abbreviations: AGE, acute gastroenteritis; HSP, Henoch-Schönlein purpura; IBD, irritable bowel disease; IBS, irritable bowel syndrome; PID, pelvic inflammatory disease; UTI, urinary tract infection.

[a]This table is a guide to the most common causes and is not a comprehensive list.

made worse with movement. The pain of intussusception, nephrolithiasis, and intermittent volvulus is episodic or colicky.

Classic appendicitis features, such as abdominal pain, anorexia, nausea, and vomiting, are less common in a younger child and may be variably present in a patient with a retrocecal appendicitis. The fewer of these classic symptoms that are present, the less likely the patient has appendicitis.

Physical Examination

Abdominal pain can be focal or generalized, and it is typically made worse with movement. The patient may refuse to walk or walk hunched over, splinting from the pain. Bowel sounds may be present or diminished. Typically, there are peritoneal signs, such as rebound tenderness or pain when the bed is bumped. Later, with appendiceal rupture, there can be signs of generalized peritonitis, including abdominal distension and rigidity. Similarly, bloody stool is a late finding of ischemia and necrosis that can occur in conditions such as intussusception and volvulus.

A patient with appendicitis tends to find a position of comfort and lie still. In contrast, episodes of intense pain with associated movements in an attempt to find a comfortable position suggest other etiologies, such as nephrolithiasis or ischemia (ovarian torsion, intussusception, volvulus, incarcerated hernia).

A patient with a retrocecal appendicitis may not have rebound tenderness, as the pain can be limited by the overlying distended cecum, which protects the appendix. To determine if there is retroperitoneal inflammation, look for the psoas and obturator signs. The psoas sign is elicited via passive hip hyperextension, while assessing for the obturator sign involves passive internal rotation of the hip while the hip is flexed.

Laboratory

There is no universal standard for the laboratory evaluation of a possible acute surgical abdomen. The diagnosis remains a clinical one, although the young child often has an atypical presentation, making this difficult. Some laboratory testing is often required to eliminate important categories, such as pregnancy or a urinary tract infection (UTI).

In general, if a surgical abdomen is possible, obtain blood for a complete blood cell count (CBC), C-reactive protein (CRP) and /or erythrocyte sedimentation rate, electrolytes, liver function tests, and amylase and lipase, as well as urine for urinalysis and urine culture. A pregnancy test is a priority for any female who is postmenarchal or Tanner 2.

The absence of a leukocytosis and left-shift do not conclusively rule out appendicitis, but make it much less likely, especially when coupled with a low index of suspicion based on history and physical examination. Initial laboratory findings can sometimes be misleading. For example, an inflamed appendix or abscess in contact with bladder can cause pyuria and/or hematuria.

Radiology

The appropriate radiology studies depend on local preference and overall clinical suspicion. For example, some institutions successfully use ultrasound to screen for appendicitis, while others cite poor sensitivity (a negative ultrasound is not helpful) or lack of availability as reasons for its limited use. Ultrasound is the preferred imaging modality for gynecological diagnoses, especially for a possible ovarian torsion.

Classic appendicitis is a clinical diagnosis that can be made solely by physical examination, without the use of imaging. If the physical examination is not diagnostic, obtain an ultrasound if local expertise is present. However, when the clinical picture is unclear and an ultrasound is not available, a computed tomography scan may be indicated. Local preference dictates the choice of contrast (intravenous [IV], oral [PO], and/or rectal). The use of IV contrast can increase the likelihood of reliable results, without the delays and difficulties associated with the oral or rectal routes.

With the exception of a chest x-ray, when there are notable respiratory symptoms, plain films are not very helpful. Although an abdominal x-ray is often performed to look for obstruction, free air, or other gross abnormalities, up to half of plain x-rays can be normal in appendicitis, while less than 10% have a diagnostic appendicolith. Prone and supine films to look for air distribution throughout the large colon can be helpful when considering intussusception, as a lack of air suggests the diagnosis. See Table 98-2 for radiologic testing suggestions based on clinical suspicion.

Table 98-2. Radiologic Tests Based on Clinical Suspicion

Suspected Diagnosis	Radiologic Study
Appendicitis	Ultrasound (preferred) or CT with IV contrast
Constipation	Left lateral decubitus and supine x-ray or KUB
Ileus	Left lateral decubitus and supine x-ray or KUB
Intussusception	Ultrasound (diagnostic only) Air (or contrast) enema (diagnostic and therapeutic)
Malrotation Volvulus	Emergent UGI or CT with IV contrast
Ovarian torsion	Ultrasound with Doppler
Pneumonia	PA and lateral chest x-ray
Renal stone	CT without contrast

Abbreviations: CT, computed tomography; KUB, kidney, ureter, bladder; IV, intravenous; PA, posteroanterior; UGI, upper gastrointestinal.

Differential Diagnosis

Nonsurgical conditions, such as AGE, severe constipation, strep throat, and lower lobe pneumonia, can all cause severe abdominal pain and mimic an acute abdomen.

The likelihood of appendicitis increases with each additional abnormal laboratory result: mildly elevated high white blood cell count (WBC), high neutrophil % (left shift), and elevated CRP. However, a normal WBC and CRP do not rule out appendicitis. Furthermore, many other serious entities, such as volvulus and intussusception, can have a normal laboratory evaluation. The differential diagnosis of an acute abdomen is summarized in Table 98-3.

There are associations of symptoms and history that are consistent with certain diagnostic considerations. Bilious emesis suggests intestinal obstruction, ileus, or volvulus, emergencies that require prompt surgical consultation. Bloody stool is most commonly associated with bacterial gastroenteritis, but can be a late finding of intussusception or other bowel ischemia. Consider ovarian torsion, mittelschmerz, imperforate hymen, pelvic inflammatory disease, and pregnancy in a postmenarchal female. Prior abdominal surgery raises the concern for adhesions and bowel obstruction. Food intake typically decreases the pain in ulcer disease and gastritis, but worsens the discomfort in pancreatitis and biliary disease.

Treatment

When the presentation is consistent with an acute abdomen, make the patient NPO, request surgical consultation, and start antibiotics with piperacillin/tazobactam (350 mg/kg/day divided every 6 hours, 12 g/day maximum) *or* meropenem (20 mg/kg IV every 8 hours, 6 g/day maximum) *or* cefoxitin (30 mg/kg every 6 hours, 12 g/day maximum) *or* cefotetan (30 mg/kg every 12 hours, 6 g/day maximum).

If the patient is nontoxic with a presentation inconsistent with an acute abdomen, follow serial abdominal examinations every 2 hours and repeat the laboratory studies (CBC every 6–12 hours) as dictated by the degree of clinical suspicion. It is often prudent to make the patient NPO and defer starting antibiotics until the diagnosis is more certain. For example, a patient with isolated nonbilious emesis, anorexia, generalized abdominal pain, fever, and elevated WBC could have AGE, appendicitis, or a UTI. In such a case, it is useful to observe for changes in the symptoms (such as the onset of diarrhea), physical examination, fever curve, CRP, and possibly abdominal x-rays, depending on the level of concern.

Table 98-3. Differential Diagnosis of an Acute Abdomen

Diagnosis	Clinical Features
Acute gastroenteritis	Fever, nausea, vomiting, and diarrhea Pain may be relieved by vomiting Sick contacts
Appendicitis	Anorexia and fever (most patients) Patient remains still for comfort Pain precedes the vomiting (nonbilious) Pain migration periumbilical ⟶ right lower quadrant
Constipation	History of large, infrequent, painful stools Afebrile Pain does not migrate Hard stool in ampulla
Intussusception	Episodic pain with drawing up of legs or lethargy Afebrile Bloody stool or frank blood (late finding)
Irritable bowel disease Malignancy (uncommon)	Weight loss Recurrent episodes of abdominal pain Bloody stools
Nephrolithiasis	Episodic severe pain radiates to flank or groin Afebrile Hematuria
Ovarian torsion	Episodic and unilateral lower quadrant pain Afebrile Associated nausea and vomiting
Pancreatitis	Epigastric pain, which may radiate to the back Pain relieved by leaning forward Elevated amylase/lipase
Pelvic inflammatory disease	Sexually active female Vaginal discharge Cervical motion tenderness
Pneumonia	Fever, tachypnea, cough, chest pain Auscultation: rales or decreased breath sounds
Small bowel obstruction	Anorexia, bilious vomiting Crampy periumbilical pain without migration Peritoneal signs Air-fluid levels on abdominal x-rays
Urinary tract infection	Dysuria, urgency, frequency May have costovertebral angle tenderness Pyuria, bacteriuria
Volvulus	Episodic pain Afebrile Bilious emesis

About one-quarter of patients with appendicitis experience a ruptured appendix before presentation, and this typically occurs within 72 hours of the start of the symptoms. There is controversy over the best management of a patient with a ruptured appendix. After consultation with surgery, one approach is to treat with parenteral antibiotics until there is clinical improvement (afebrile >24 hours, patient tolerating maintenance oral intake, and the inflammatory markers have decreased), then transition to an oral regimen. Specific drug regimens vary by institution, but one approach is to add metronidazole (7.5 mg/kg IV every 6 hours, 4 g/day maximum) to one of the antibiotics detailed above. At discharge, change to amoxicillin/clavulanate (90 mg/kg/day of amoxicillin divided twice a day, 4 g/day maximum) with or without metronidazole (PO dose same as IV dose above). An interval appendectomy may be scheduled after about 6 weeks per surgical preference, especially if there was a fecolith.

There is no reason to withhold analgesia. Although pain medication can change some aspects of examination, this has not been associated with misdiagnosis of surgical candidates, and may actually facilitate a more thorough examination. Give morphine (0.05–0.2 mg/kg IV every 2–4 hours, 15 mg/dose maximum) as needed for pain.

Ondansetron (0.05–0.1 mg/kg IV every 6 hours as needed, 4 mg/dose maximum) may help control nausea and vomiting, although it may not be useful in an acute surgical abdomen.

Indications for Consultation

- **Gynecology or pediatric surgery:** Possible ovarian torsion
- **Surgery (immediate):** Rebound tenderness, abdominal rigidity, bilious emesis, or the presence of other findings of an acute abdomen

Disposition

- **Intensive care unit transfer:** Shock, toxic appearance
- **Discharge criteria:** Definitive diagnosis, treatment, and recovery have occurred, tolerating adequate oral intake and medications, if needed

Follow-up

- **Primary care:** 1 to 3 days
- **Surgery (if patient had a procedure or one is to be scheduled):** 1 to 2 weeks

Pearls and Pitfalls

- Laboratory tests and x-rays alone cannot be used to rule out the diagnosis of an acute abdomen.
- A patient younger than 5 years often does not have the classic presentation of appendicitis.
- Do not withhold pain medication.
- Not all cases of an acute abdomen require immediate surgery. A perforated appendix may be treated medically with or without an interval appendectomy.
- Be circumspect making a diagnosis of gastroenteritis when nausea and vomiting are not accompanied by diarrhea.

Coding

ICD-9

- Abdominal pain, unspecified site **789.00**
- Abdominal pain, right lower quadrant **789.03**
- Acute appendicitis without peritonitis **540.9**
- Acute appendicitis with peritonitis **540.1**
- Bilious emesis (vomiting) **787.04**
- Gastroenteritis, infectious **009.0**
- Intestinal obstruction, unspecified **560.9**
- Intussusception **560.0**
- Peritonitis, unspecified **567.9**
- Volvulus **560.2**
- Vomiting (alone) **787.03**
- Vomiting (persistent) **536.2**

Bibliography

Bundy DG, Byerley JS, Liles EA, et al. Does this child have appendicitis? *JAMA.* 2007;298:438–451

Kwan KY, Nager AL. Diagnosing pediatric appendicitis: usefulness of laboratory markers. *Am J Emerg Med.* 2010;28:1009–1015

Sharwood LN, Babl FE. The efficacy and effect of opioid analgesia in undifferentiated abdominal pain in children: a review of four studies. *Paediatr Anaesth.* 2009;19:445–451

Tseng YC, Lee MS, Chang YJ, Wu HP. Acute abdomen in pediatric patients admitted to the pediatric emergency department. *Pediatr Neonatol.* 2008;49:126–134

Williams RF, Blakely ML, Fischer PE, et al. Diagnosing ruptured appendicitis preoperatively in pediatric patients. *J Am Coll Surg.* 2009;208:819–825

Pyloric Stenosis

Introduction

Pyloric stenosis is the most common cause of upper gastrointestinal obstruction in infancy, with an incidence of 2 to 4 per 1,000 live births. Males are 4 to 6 times more likely to be affected, with 30% of patients being first-born males. The advent of surgical intervention over the last century has markedly improved the prognosis for these patients. With prompt evaluation and diagnosis, pyloromyotomy can prevent complications such as significant metabolic derangements, failure to thrive (FTT), shock, and death.

Clinical Presentation

History

The infant typically presents at 1 to 12 weeks of life with progressively forceful, nonbilious emesis following feeds. The vomiting may be described as projectile or fountain-like, and is almost always non-bloody. Rarely, if the symptoms have been present for a considerable amount of time, gastritis or esophageal tears can develop, leading to heme-positive vomitus.

Depending on the amount of time the symptoms have been present, the patient may have a range of constitutional symptoms, from vigorous and ravenous (especially immediately after vomiting) with adequate weight gain, to listless and emaciated with profound FTT. Other complaints may include irritability, colic, and constipation. Ask about the infant's oral intake, urine output, stooling, level of activity, and weight gain pattern.

Physical Examination

If the process has been ongoing for several weeks, the patient may appear dehydrated with significant weight loss or inadequate gain. Focus on assessing the degree of dehydration, looking for tachycardia, tachypnea, sunken anterior fontanelle, dry mucous membranes, poor skin turgor, and delayed capillary refill.

The classic finding is a palpable "olive," which is the hypertrophied pylorus, in the epigastric region or right upper quadrant. To appreciate the mass, place the patient supine with the hips flexed. Examine from the left and attempt to "slip" a hand under the edge of the right rectus muscle. Do not confuse the midline xiphoid process with an olive. While the presence of the olive is pathognomonic, it is difficult to palpate, so that its absence does not exclude the diagnosis. Another unique finding is a visible abdominal peristaltic wave seen while the infant is sucking.

Differential Diagnosis

Pyloric stenosis causes unopposed vomiting, that is, there is no diarrhea. A number of conditions, ranging from mild (gastroesophageal reflux) to life-threatening (acute adrenal insufficiency) can present with unopposed vomiting (Table 99-1).

Other causes of metabolic alkalosis in an infant include Bartter syndrome, diuretic use, cystic fibrosis, exogenous alkali, and a chloride-deficient diet.

Table 99-1. Differential Diagnosis of Pyloric Stenosis

Diagnosis	Clinical Features
Antral web	Similar presentation
Congenital adrenal hyperplasia Adrenal insufficiency/crisis	Clitoromegaly or hyperpigmented scrotum Hyperkalemia, hyponatremia No alkalosis
Gastroenteritis	May have fever Diarrhea Not ravenous after vomiting
Gastroesophageal reflux	Lower volume vomitus Nonprojectile emesis May be positional
Inborn error of metabolism	Anion gap acidosis Seizures possible Hyperammonemia
Increased intracranial pressure	Bulging fontanelle Sunsetting eyes Cranial nerve VI palsy
Overfeeding	Good/robust weight gain Nonprojectile emesis Normal electrolytes
Renal failure	Elevated blood urea nitrogen/creatinine Acidosis
Sepsis	Fever, lethargy Acidosis Elevated or low white blood cell count
Volvulus	Bilious spit-up or nonprojectile vomiting No alkalosis

Laboratory

Obtain serum electrolytes, as an infant with pyloric stenosis characteristically develops a hypochloremic, hypokalemic, metabolic alkalosis. The sodium is usually close to normal and the patient may have an elevated blood urea nitrogen and creatinine, consistent with a prerenal azotemia from dehydration.

Radiology

Abdominal ultrasonography (AUS) has replaced contrast studies as the modality of choice for diagnosing pyloric stenosis. However, if AUS is unavailable, classic findings on an upper gastrointestinal (UGI) contrast study are the "string sign" (pyloric channel filled with thin stream of barium) or "shoulder sign" (extrinsic compression of the stomach by a hypertrophied pylorus) in the presence of significant stenosis.

The pyloric ultrasound will provide measurements of both the canal length and thickness. Pyloric stenosis is confirmed if the width on a cross-sectional image is greater than 3 mm, while 2 to 3 mm is equivocal and less than 2 mm is negative. However, pyloric stenosis is a progressive process, so that a negative or equivocal pyloric ultrasound may be seen during the early stages of disease. If symptoms persist, arrange a repeat study in 1 week.

Treatment

Preoperative

Consult a surgeon to arrange a pyloromyotomy. However, this is not an emergency procedure, so the priority is correcting dehydration and any electrolyte abnormalities. Generally, the anesthesiologist will defer surgery until the bicarbonate level is below 28 mEq/L and the chloride is above 100 mEq/L.

Treat significant dehydration (≥10 %) with a normal saline (NS) bolus (or boluses) to restore intravascular volume. If renal function is normal and the patient remains alkalotic, give D5 ½ NS with 2 mEq KCl/100 mL at 150% of the maintenance rate until urine output is adequate. This will help correct the alkalosis, which is "chloride-responsive." Once the patient's hydration status and electrolytes have normalized, switch to a maintenance intravenous solution and rate. It is not necessary to make the patient NPO until the appropriate time has arrived for preoperative fasting.

Operative

Depending on individual preference, a laparoscopic or traditional open pyloromyotomy will be performed.

Postoperative

There is a range of approaches to the reinstitution of feeding. Most surgeons start within 4 to 8 hours after an open or laparoscopic procedure. Also, many surgeons are now recommending *ad libitum* feeds without stepwise volume acceleration.

Regurgitation following surgery occurs in most patients. This may be secondary to anesthesia, gastritis, and irritation from the long-standing obstruction; residual inflammation following the pyloromyotomy, or an incomplete repair. If the infant continues to vomit for more than 5 days following surgery, repeat the AUS, then obtain a UGI if the stomach does not empty properly. Consult the surgeon if fever with abdominal distension occurs within the first 24 hours, as this may be caused by an unsuspected perforation.

Acetaminophen usually suffices for postoperative analgesia.

Disposition

- **Interinstitutional transfer:** Pediatric surgeon not available
- **Discharge criteria:** Adequate oral intake without vomiting

Follow-up

- **Primary care:** 1 week
- **Surgeon:** 1 to 2 weeks

Pearls and Pitfalls

- Always consider pyloric stenosis in a young infant with unopposed vomiting.
- Pyloric stenosis is not an emergency. Correct any electrolyte abnormalities before surgery.

Coding

ICD-9

• Alkalosis	**276.3**
• Hypertrophic pyloric stenosis	**750.5**

Bibliography

Aspelund G, Langer JC. Current management of hypertrophic pyloric stenosis. *Semin Pediatr Surg.* 2007;16:27–33

Hernanz-Schulman M. Pyloric stenosis: role of imaging. *Pediatr Radiol.* 2009;39(suppl 2):S134–S139

Keckler SJ, Ostlie DJ, Holcomb GW III, Peter SD. The progressive development of pyloric stenosis: a role for repeat ultrasound. *Eur J Pediatr Surg.* 2008;18:168–170

Maheshwari P, Abograra A, Shamam O. Sonographic evaluation of gastrointestinal obstruction in infants: a pictoral essay. *J Pediatr Surg.* 2009;44:2037–2042

Panteli C. New insights into the pathogenesis of infantile pyloric stenosis. *Pediatr Surg Int.* 2009;25:1043–1052

Sola JE, Neville HL. Laparoscopic vs open pyloromyotomy: a systematic review and meta-analysis. *J Pediatr Surg.* 2009;44:1631–1637

Index

A

Index

B

C

D

Index

E

F

Index

G

H

Index

I

Index

Index

J

K

L

M

N

O

P

Index

Q

R

T

U

V

W

Y

Z